Intelligent Systems Reference Library

Volume 204

The aim of this series is to publish a Reference Library, including novel advances and developments in all aspects of Intelligent Systems in an easily accessible and well structured form. The series includes reference works, handbooks, compendia, textbooks, well-structured monographs, dictionaries, and encyclopedias. It contains well integrated knowledge and current information in the field of Intelligent Systems. The series covers the theory, applications, and design methods of Intelligent Systems. Virtually all disciplines such as engineering, computer science, avionics, business, e-commerce, environment, healthcare, physics and life science are included. The list of topics spans all the areas of modern intelligent systems such as: Ambient intelligence, Computational intelligence, Social intelligence, Computational neuroscience, Artificial life, Virtual society, Cognitive systems, DNA and immunity-based systems, e-Learning and teaching, Human-centred computing and Machine ethics, Intelligent control, Intelligent data analysis, Knowledge-based paradigms, Knowledge management, Intelligent agents, Intelligent decision making, Intelligent network security, Interactive entertainment, Learning paradigms, Recommender systems, Robotics and Mechatronics including human-machine teaming, Self-organizing and adaptive systems, Soft computing including Neural systems, Fuzzy systems, Evolutionary computing and the Fusion of these paradigms, Perception and Vision, Web intelligence and Multimedia.

Indexed by SCOPUS, DBLP, zbMATH, SCImago.

All books published in the series are submitted for consideration in Web of Science.

More information about this series at http://www.springer.com/series/8578

Janmenjoy Nayak · Margarita N. Favorskaya ·
Seema Jain · Bighnaraj Naik · Manohar Mishra
Editors

Advanced Machine Learning Approaches in Cancer Prognosis

Challenges and Applications

Springer

Editors
Janmenjoy Nayak
Department of Computer Science and Engineering
Aditya Institute of Technology and Management
Srikakulam, Andhra Pradesh, India

Margarita N. Favorskaya
Department of Informatics and Computer Techniques
Reshetnev Siberian State University of Science and Technology
Krasnoyarsk, Russia

Seema Jain
Elizabeth Grove Surgery
Elizabeth Grove, SA, Australia

Bighnaraj Naik
Department of Computer Application
Veer Surendra Sai University of Technology
Odisha, India

Manohar Mishra
Department of Electrical and Electronics Engineering
ITER, Siksha 'O' Anusandhan (Deemed to be University)
Bhubaneswar, Odisha, India

ISSN 1868-4394 ISSN 1868-4408 (electronic)
Intelligent Systems Reference Library
ISBN 978-3-030-71974-6 ISBN 978-3-030-71975-3 (eBook)
https://doi.org/10.1007/978-3-030-71975-3

This Springer imprint is published by the registered company Springer Nature Switzerland AG
The registered company address is: Gewerbestrasse 11, 6330 Cham, Switzerland

Foreword

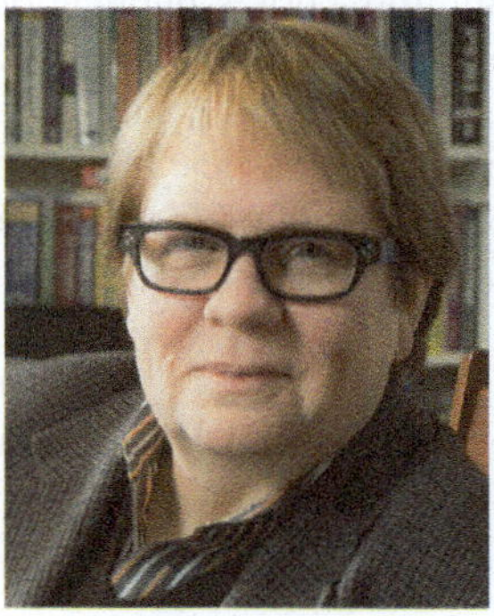

Cancer causes untold grief and exacts a heavy societal toll. Prevention is one tool in the arsenal to fight cancer. Diagnostics and prognostication are two tools of equal importance. Approximately half of all cancers are preventable with adequate knowledge of risk factors, and accurate diagnosis and survival prediction are essential for planning adequate care, strategizing treatments, and enhancing the quality of patients' lives by avoiding the discomfort and harm of inappropriate therapies.

Cancer prognosis depends on a mass of information: the age, gender, genetic makeup, and general health of the patient, the location, grade, size of tumors, as well as numerous expert appraisals of clinical, histological, and imaging (fMRI, PET, and micro-CT) data. All this information must be collected, examined, and consolidated by the attending physician to form an accurate clinical picture. The task of integrating so much information to make a reasonable prognosis is daunting and is becoming increasingly more challenging as new genomic, proteomic, and imaging technologies are being developed. This is where machine learning comes into play, as machine learning and computer image analysis offer the potential of overcoming some of the challenges posed by the massive new stores of data and the promise this treasure trove of information holds out for predictive, personalized medicine.

Historically, the focus of machine learning in cancer research has been on diagnostics. But in the last decade, especially, there has been a notable rise in research concerned with cancer prediction and prognosis. Most of this research has revolved around predicting cancer mortality, survivability, and recurrence, but researchers are also interested in risk factors predictive of cancer. In both research areas, machine learning methods are improving the accuracy of these kinds of predictions over other more traditional approaches.

This book's chapters present the very best in machine learning and image processing as applied to cancer prediction and prognosis. Topics run the gamut of research in this field: cancer data analysis using machine learning approaches, with a focus on imagery and real medical applications, prediction of cancer susceptibility on the cellular level as well as predictive drug designs for treating cancer, and the application of deep learning, especially Convolutional Neural Networks, in the detection and prediction of cancer outcomes as well as in the isolation of new gene expressions in cervical cancer.

Due to the accelerating progress in machine learning and its employment in cancer prognosis in all its complexity, this book's publication is not only timely but also much needed. This volume contains 16 peer-reviewed chapters reporting state of the art in cancer research as it relates to AI and image processing, covering many important topics in contemporary prognostics. In my opinion, this book is a valuable resource for graduate students, engineers, and researchers interested in understanding and investigating this important field of study.

Prof. Dr. Sheryl Berlin Brahnam
Department of Information Technology
and Cybersecurity
Missouri State University
National City, MO, USA

Preface

Presently, 'cancer' is a buzzword amid more than a thousand diseases. Even though cancer comprises various categories of diseases, they are all just because of abnormal growth of cells in the body. According to the World Health Organization (WHO), cancer became the second major reason behind severe deaths globally. More than 9.6 million people all over the world have died in the year 2018 due to cancer. The early detection of this abnormal growth may help doctors to save the lives of the patients. Delayed detection may increase mortality and morbidity. The most common types of cancers are Lung, Breast, Colorectal, Prostate, Skin, and Stomach cancers. Various oncologists as well as researchers consent to the truth that cancer deaths can be condensed if cases are identified and treated early. Cancer is expected to react to efficient treatment whenever identified prematurely and can result in a superior prospect of surviving, low morbidity, and low-cost treatment. Unfortunately, most of the cancer-affected patients are identified in the final phases of the syndrome. Moreover, the increased growth in the tumor size makes such dreadful disease more critical with no choice for prevention of the metastasis. Since the last decade, the efficiency of cancer management has enhanced pointedly, but, even with the surplus of novel procedures, logically acceptable beneficial results for all afflicted persons are intangible due to uncertainties in analytical accuracy. Therefore, patient-specific management/treatment could be chosen if a correct prognosis could be made. Truly, advances in prediction accuracy could significantly support physicians in formulating patient medications and reducing both physical and psychological stress caused by the diseases. Essential clinical interpretations can be combined with the application of the conventional TNM staging approach (based on the size of the tumor (T), the spread of cancer into nearby lymph nodes (N), and the spread of cancer to other body parts (M, for metastasis)) in empirical tests, but inaccurate predictions of prognoses continue to pose a bottleneck for clinicians. Enhancement in prediction accuracy owing to the use of artificial intelligence (AI) technology remains a serious challenge for medical scientists. Nowadays, the artificial intelligence (AI)-based computer-assisted diagnosis method has shown the main impact in resolving this issue. The AI application for the betterment of health care is rolling with every passing day.

Generally, identifying the cancer diseases in the early stage of their growth is quite difficult for the consultant. Furthermore, an exact forecast of cancer prognosis with higher confidence is also extremely tough. So, acquiring improved prognostic paradigms using multi-variant data and high-resolution analytic tools in clinical cancer research is essential. Automatic medical diagnosis is one of the major issues in the healthcare system. Computer-aided diagnosis schemes have been developed to identify diseases by inspecting the internal human organs through different medical image modalities. In the last decade, several types of research have included AI methods, for example, machine learning (ML) and deep learning (DL) as a decision support tool in their models for predicting cancer based on historical data. Artificial intelligence is generally used to handle and analyze multi-feature data from manifold patient inspection data to forecast cancer prognosis in addition to the survival time and the illness progress of patients more precisely. Although medicinal statistics are usually applied for cancer prognostics, uses of computational intelligence for similar jobs tend to be less familiar. Currently, researchers and oncologists have revealed strong attention in utilizing advancements in the area of machine learning (ML) to progress diagnosis, supervision, as well as improved healing alternatives of numerous illnesses, especially cancer. There is a growing concern in the ML applications in the field of healthcare to advance disease diagnosis and to widen efficient therapies. Most of the critical cancer symptoms based data are produced at the time of cancer treatment and specifically, when a patient comes under proper diagnosis. There is a particular concern in the ML applications to augment oncologic precautions.

The book will dive glare on the causes for the rising difficulty as well as a profusion of data in the treatments and symptom analysis on various cancer disease using advanced Machine Learning approaches. Additionally, the book will assist to concentrate on further research confronts and instructions for the researchers and practitioners as well. Also, a unique emphasis will be focused on assortments of valuable advanced mechanical equipment, devices, and potential directions for resolving difficult issues.

In this book, we present deep fundamental research contributions from a methodological/application viewpoint in understanding the application of advance machine learning techniques in solving cancer diagnosis system. The book contains volumes of information about advanced ML approaches that include connectionist systems, spanning the areas of neural networks (NN), evolutionary computation, fuzzy logic (FL), genetic algorithms (GA), self-organizing systems, and hybrid intelligent models in solving the cancer diseases. This Volume comprises 3 Parts and 16 chapters and is organized as follows:

Part I: Cancer Data Analysis with Machine Learning Approaches

Chapter 1 provides a brief overview of current and future trends in the application of machine learning methods for data mining in oncology.

In Chap. 2, Pati et al. specifically focus on such techniques that have been implemented and adapted for cancer data analysis. The chapter goes into quite an in-depth review of each of the proposed architectures which have been very precisely screened by authors and also do quite a lot to develop a specific sense of each one of these taxonomies by putting each of them under scanning through various evaluation metrics. Furthermore, the chapter issues several future scopes and recommendations from the perspective of the authors to ignite the thought of the ones interested in pushing this field into a further sub-stratum.

Chapter 3 includes the method for multispectral image visualization. The method proposed by Obukhova et al. supposes the synthesis of an image based on an image obtained in white light and based on a fluorescent image in the NIR channel. A feature of the method is the presentation of fluorescence data in the form of a special level map that takes into account the properties of human vision. Metric CIEDE2000 is used for visualization quality estimation. Special attention is put to preprocessing and enhancement image, obtained in white light. Methods of medical multispectral image analysis for cancer change differential diagnosis based on traditional machine learning technologies, deep learning technologies, as well as the combined approach based on both technologies are shown. The combined approach allows to effectively use the advantages of deep learning technology in conditions of limited volume of verified database for training. All the proposed methods and algorithms are illustrated by implementation in real medical applications.

Chapter 4 examines the implementation of the deep neural network for lung cancer diagnosis. Initially, the importance of deep learning among other learning methods in Artificial Neural Networks has been outlined by Maria et al. Further, deep learning for medical imaging will be focused on lung cancer detection. The usage of 3D neural networks and thermal imaging for lung cancer diagnosis will be highlighted simultaneously. 3D networks are an emerging trend due to the evolution of high-resolution images. Currently, the efficiency of 2D networks is the maximum compared to the evolving 3D networks. Hence, the chapter will implement 3D networks with more efficiency proposing ideas for higher definition networks. Additionally, the chapter will also examine the usage of the thermal imaging technique to identify short-breaths using nostril movement that is captured using thermal imaging cameras. The purpose of using short-breaths will be the ease of usage and compatibility for the high definition networks. The prediction can lead to the earliest diagnosis possible when the concerned person identifies unusual breathing habits. The prediction can also propose other tests to be done if required. The creation of networks for both will be discussed in detail as the emerging trend in deep learning. The evaluation of the networks will be conducted leaving room for future scope.

Chapter 5 presents an extensive survey done in the past on the thyroid disease prediction using data mining techniques. An extensive study on the various attributes used in thyroid prediction has been conducted by Yasir. This chapter studies various data mining techniques like Naïve Bayes, Decision Trees, etc. for thyroid prediction. Among these various feature selection algorithms, serological tests and pathological observations of the thyroid disease were also surveyed. Forty-two machine learning algorithms have been compared to find the top five best classifiers to predict whether a given patient is suffering from hypothyroidism, hyperthyroidism, or is absolutely normal. The data source has been taken from KEEL containing 7200 instances with 22 attributes. The results of various machine learning algorithms have been compared in order to find the most appropriate model for classifying whether a given patient is suffering from thyroid disease or not. The best classifier found as bagging gives an overall accuracy of 99.70 %. Another experiment to identify and remove outliers has also been conducted. With outliers' removal, 42 machine learning algorithms have been compared with the previous results. A slight improvement has been observed in the results, and this time the best classifier found achieved an accuracy of 99.95 % with the logic and analysis of data (LAD) tree.

In Chap. 6, Kamran et al. have proposed a scheme that classifies a mammographic image into normal, benign, and malignant ones. In the proposed scheme, input images are compared with a large collection of databases with the replacement of sigmoid activation function. Probabilistic neural network is used to describe nonlinear statement limits which further leads to Bayes optimal and also all the functions which bear the same properties as well. Any input data or algorithm can be pointed with the four layer neural network. Standard PNN consists of an input layer of N nodes, a pattern layer of m nodes, a summation layer of k nodes, and a pseudo layer of L nodes, which is used for decision-making which is also known as decision layer for producing output.

Part II: Prediction of Cancer Susceptibility

Chapter 7 resolves the problem of fewer data and gets the most relevant information from the available dataset. In this research, Joydev et al. implement an oversampling method on the original data while preserving the basic nature of the dataset which is followed by the clustering of the data using K-Medoid clustering, Girvan-Newman clustering, and Mahalanobis distance-based clustering for multivariate data. Once the same set of samples are predicted using clustering, the data is extrapolated based on the clusters formed using a statistical approach. To reduce complex processing and remove the irrelevant features with the intent of cleaning the dataset, a correlation-based approach for feature selection is applied and then Principal Component Analysis (PCA) is applied for dimensionality reduction.The final set of features thus obtained is then fed into an Artificial Neural Network for the classification of Colon Cancer. The result of the experiment shows that the methodology proposed has better accuracy than the available approaches which proves the effectiveness of the proposed method.

In Chap. 8, Amiya and Apurba present an automatic technique for the classification of brain magnetic resonance imaging (MRI) as abnormal, in the presence of a brain tumor or as normal in the absence of a tumor and then detect the regions of abnormal tumor cells. The exact cancerous cells from these images are then extracted. The proposed method is divided into two steps. First, a set of statistical features are generated, and then the most important features are selected using the Rough-Kernelized

Fuzzy C-Means (RKFCM) algorithm. The important features are used for accurately identifying brain MRI images containing abnormal cells. Further, a Support Vector Machine (SVM) is used to classify the images into two groups, namely, tumor-affected and tumor-free. In the second step, the tumor-affected regions in brain tumor images are detected and then segmented out from the scanned image using a rough set-based KFCM algorithm. It is followed by the use of thresholding and morphological operations to extract the exact brain tumor-affected region in the images. The proposed method is tested on different benchmark datasets such as Harvard, BRATS2013, and real-patient MRI brain images from M. R. Bangur Hospital for validation. It is observed that the proposed method performs better than existing methods in terms of accuracy, specificity, and sensitivity.

Chapter 9 illustrates the role of computational advances in the segmentation of overlapping cells. Further, a computational model based on the Voronoi-based hybrid active contour method is proposed by Adhikary et al. for segmenting the overlapping oral epithelial cells. Though the present study reports a segmentation algorithm for the isolated, slightly touching and overlapping cells, there is still some scope for the improvement of the segmenting accuracy for the high overlapping cells. The future work will address the following: (i) evaluate the segmentation algorithm more accurately, (ii) evaluate feature extraction and suitable feature selection for gaining high rate of classification, (iii) make a suitable automated algorithm for an early oral cancer diagnosis, and (iv) validate the result in medical diagnosis by taking the help of medical practitioners for developing an automated system for an early cancer diagnosis.

In Chap. 10, Sharma and Bhatia focus on the importance and latest advances of in silico modeling for the design of new and potent anti-cancer drugs. Though in silico methods have transformed the growth and design of small molecule anti-cancer drugs, but acquired resistance and intra-tumor heterogeneity, there are still challenges for which solutions need to be sought. Also, there is a shift from the 'One Ligand-One Target' approach to the 'Multi Target Drug Ligands' (MTDL)' approach for drug design for treating cancer.

In Chap. 11, Krishnan et al. implemented specific image processing methodologies to aid the appropriate diagnosis of lung cancer and provide a sterile environment for interacting with the medical data in operation theaters during treatment. Computer Tomography (CT) gives a good resolution axial slice image of the lung. The tumor's raw CT data analysis is quite impossible as the tumor's pixel characteristics would be approximately matching its neighboring pixels. Thus, a basic preprocessing algorithm is required to differentiate the target from the background. It is processed with level set segmentation to extract the tumor from the sequentially acquired multiple slices. The segmented output of each slice provides the geometric feature of the tumor. As the tumor size and shape in segmented portions are irregular, it seems appropriate to reconstruct a three-dimensional representation of 2D images for tumors' qualitative information. The volume reconstruction using the ray casting method has been applied to render the volume of tumors from a segmented stack of 2D slices. Then touch-less, computer-aided, gesture-based control of the medical images was attained using Kinect sensor, which is the best tool for human-computer interaction to maintain a sterile environment. The paper elaborates on the gestures, which is employed to interact with the medical images such as selection, drag, and swipe gestures. The selection gesture is used to open and close individual medical images. The drag gesture is used to view the patient data along with the slice image. The swipe gesture is used to view various medical datasets like 2D slices and tumor irregularity in segmented slices.

Part III: Advanced Machine Learning Paradigms for Cancer Diagnosis

In Chap. 12, a multilayer hierarchical convolutional feature integration in deep transfer learned CNN has been proposed by Mohamed et al. to achieve optimized classification. In Deep CNN, the last layer learns significant features that are highly invariant but their spatial resolutions are too stiff to exactly confine the target. In contrast, features from earlier layers offer more exact localization and hold more fine-grained spatial subtleties for exact confinement but are less invariant. This observation recommends that reasoning with multiple layers of CNN features for breast cancer detection from mammogram images is of great importance. In this chapter, the features extracted from the earlier layer and the last layer of deep CNN are integrated to train and improvise the classification accuracy of breast cancer detection in the mammogram image. The results show that the consistent improvement in accuracy is obtained by using mammogram augmentation and different weight learning factors across different layers.

Chapter 13 aims to identify the alterations of genes involved in cervical cancer. Using tools of computational genomics, Lalitha et al. have prepared a gene expression table by sorting the information from a dataset on cervical cancer as from NCBI-GEO and the Series Matrix and Platform files. The Gene expression table was then uploaded on Network Analyst for protein-protein interaction and Gene expression analysis. In N/A, genes are mapped for transcription factor, and protein-protein interactions of different pathways are identified from molecular interaction databases (KEGG, Reactome, GO_BP, and GO_MF). The pathway is studied in GeneMANIA and gene cards. Two genes CDC6 and CDKN2A are identified and are studied for alterations in cervical cancer. In cervical squamous cell carcinoma, CDC6 is amplified by 0.4%, and no mutation and deletion of genes is found. CDKN2A gene showed mutation by 1.99% and deep deleted by 0.4% but no amplification was found. In the study, the analysis is done on 607 cases in which, in cervical adenocarcinoma CDC6 gene is amplified by 2.17% with deep deleted by 2.17% gene and no mutation is found in CDKN2A whereas no amplification, deep deletion, and mutation are seen. Further, the finding would help the researchers to conduct future studies on CDC6 and CDKN2A genes for better treatments.

Chapter 14 applies some deep learning models to study the classification for the detection of clinically significant prostate cancer from the large-scale cancer image data for each patient. In this chapter, Mandal et al. have investigated the effect of deep learning architectures like Vgg16, Efficient Net, Dense Net121, and ResNext50 in the large-scale cancer image data classification setting. The main contribution of the chapter is to focus the high-level accuracy because these deep learning algorithms have the capability for transfer learning with image instant segmentation. The score of Quadratic Weighted Kappa (QWK) signifies the EfficientNet as the best net for the classification of the cancer data among other DL nets. As per the result of confusion matrix based on precision, recall, f1-score, and support, ResNeXt50 net shows the best accuracy results in comparison to other models.

Chapter 15 proposes a 16-layer deep convolutional neural network for classifying skin lesions. The network proposed by Pramanik and Chakraborty consists of 9 convolutional layers, 4 maxpool layers, and 3 fully connected layers. The validation of the proposed architecture is done on the dermatoscopic images of the Kaggle dataset archive without augmentation. The proposed work offers an accuracy value of 87.58% which is much better than the existing works on the Kaggle dataset without augmentation.

In Chap. 16, a novel 13-layer deep Convolutional Neural Network architecture to classify two types of brain tumor from MRI scans, namely Meningioma and Glioma, has been proposed by Das et al. The proposed system after performing 10-fold cross-validation gives an average validation accuracy of 100%. It is the highest attainable accuracy among existing works performed on axial MRIs, and on the same dataset.

We would like to thank all the contributors and the reviewers for their contributions and dedicated efforts for the successful completion of this book. We want to specially thank the editorial team of Springer for their valuable technical support and superior efforts. We hope that the work reported in this volume will motivate further research and development efforts in the cancer prognosis and its allied domain.

Srikakulam, India — Janmenjoy Nayak
Krasnoyarsk, Russia — Margarita N. Favorskaya
Elizabeth Grove, Australia — Seema Jain
Odisha, India — Bighnaraj Naik
Bhubaneswar, India — Manohar Mishra

Contents

About the Editors

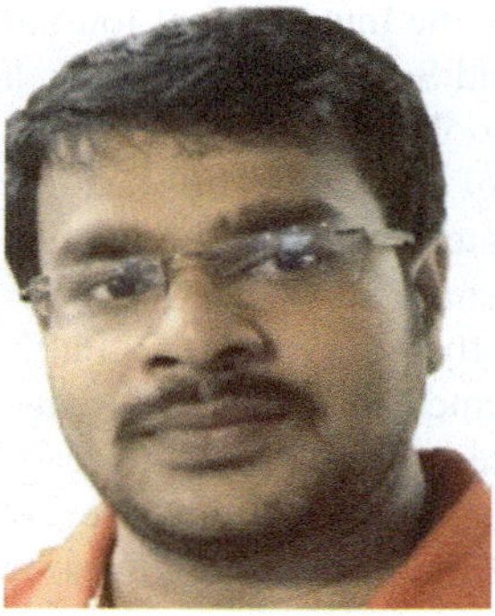

Janmenjoy Nayak is working as an Associate Professor, in the Department of CSE, Aditya Institute of Technology and Management (AITAM), (An Autonomous Institution) Tekkali, K. Kotturu, AP-532201, India. Being a two-time Gold Medallist in Computer Science in his career, he has been awarded with INSPIRE Research Fellowship from Department of Science and Technology, Government of India (both as JRF and SRF levels) and Best researcher award from Jawaharlal Nehru University of Technology, Kakinada, Andhra Pradesh, for the AY: 2018–19. He has edited 14 books and 9 Special Issues on the applications of Computational Intelligence, Soft Computing, Data Analytics, and Pattern Recognition, published by Springer and Inderscience International publications. He has published more than 140 referred articles in various book chapters, conferences, and International reputed peer-reviewed journals of Elsevier, Inderscience, Springer, IEEE, etc. He has a total of more than 11+ years of experience in both teaching and research. He is the Senior member of IEEE and a life member of some of the reputed societies like CSI India, Orissa Information Technology Society (OITS), Orissa Mathematical Society (OMS), IAENG (Hongkong), etc. He has successfully conducted and is associated with International repute series conferences such as ICCIDM, HIS, ARIAM, CIPR, and SCDA. His area of interest includes data mining, nature-inspired algorithms, and soft computing.

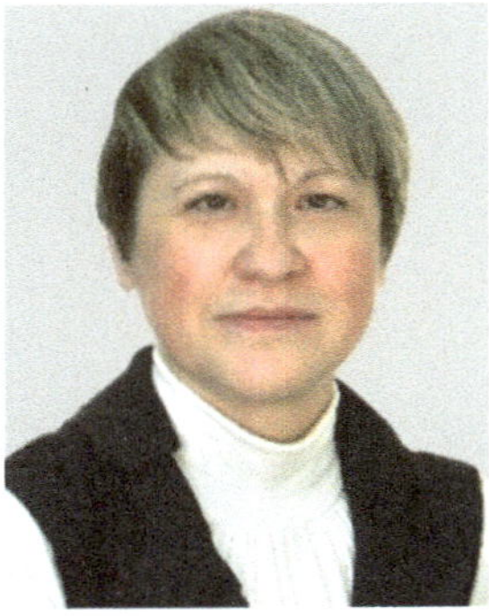

Margarita N. Favorskaya is a Professor and Head of Department of Informatics and Computer Techniques at Reshetnev Siberian State University of Science and Technology, Russian Federation. Professor Favorskaya is a member of KES organization since 2010, and the IPC member and the Chair of invited sessions of over 30 international conferences. She serves as a reviewer in international journals (Neurocomputing, Knowledge Engineering and Soft Data Paradigms, Pattern Recognition Letters, and Engineering Applications of Artificial Intelligence), an associate editor of Intelligent Decision Technologies Journal, International Journal of Knowledge-based and Intelligent Engineering Systems, International Journal of Reasoning-based Intelligent Systems, a Honorary Editor of the International Journal of Knowledge Engineering and Soft Data Paradigms, a Reviewer, Guest Editor, and Book Editor (Springer). She is the author or the co-author of 200 publications and 20 educational manuals in computer science. She co-edited seven books for Springer recently. She supervised nine Ph.D. candidates and is presently supervising four Ph.D. students. Her main research interests are digital image and video processing, remote sensing, pattern recognition, fractal image processing, artificial intelligence, intelligent computing, and information technologies.

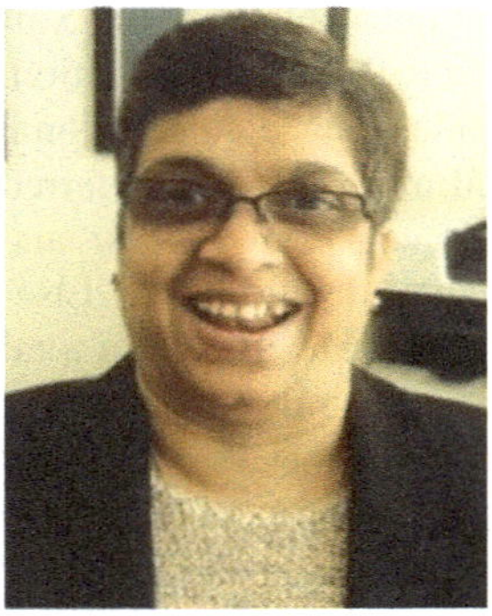

Seema Jain obtained her General Practitioner (GP) training from Flinders University of South Australia. She completed her Diploma in Child Health from the Women'sand Children' Hospital, Adelaide, South Australia. Dr. Jain has worked in numerous hospitals, including the Lyell McEwin, Modbury, Queen Elizabeth, and Women's and Children's Hospital. She also worked in Queensland for a few years. Dr. Jain is now an Integrated GP. This means she not only has the usual qualifications of a medical doctor, as well as many years' experience, but is also further qualified in one or more complementary medicine modalities, holistic approach, nutrition and environmental medicine, herbal medicine, naturopathy, and meditation. She specializes in fields such as Antenatal care, Mental Health care, Aged care, Women's health, Children's health, Diabetes, Asthma, Nutrition Vaccinations, Skin check, and so on. Dr. Jain serves various professional and social organizations in various capacities such as the Board Director of

Sonder, Committee Member of the Clinical Council of Adelaide PHN, Committee Member of the Premier Council of Suicide Prevention, Committee Member of Multifaith Association of South Australia, and so on.

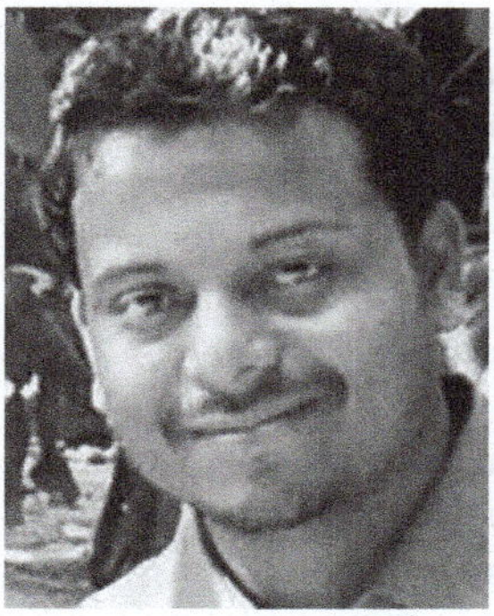

Bighnaraj Naik is an Assistant Professor in the Department of Computer Application, Veer Surendra Sai University of Technology (Formerly UCE Burla), Odisha, India. He has published more than 130 research articles in various reputed peer-reviewed International Journals, Conferences, and Book Chapters. He has edited twelve books from various international publishers such as Elsevier, Springer, and IGI Global. At present, he has more than 12 years of teaching experience in the field of Computer Science and Information Technology. He is a member of IEEE and his area of interest includes Data Science, Data Mining, Machine Learning, Deep Learning, Computational Intelligence, and its applications in Science and Engineering. He has been serving as Guest Editor of various journal special issues in Information Fusion (Elsevier), Neural Computing and Applications (Springer), Evolutionary Intelligence (Springer), International Journal of Computational Intelligence Studies (Inderscience), International Journal of Swarm Intelligence (Inderscience), etc. He is an active reviewer of various reputed journals from reputed publishers including IEEE Transactions, Elsevier, Springer, Inderscience, etc. Currently, he is undertaking a major research project in the capacity of Principal Investigator, which is funded by Science and Engineering Research Board (SERB), Department of Science and Technology (DST), Government of India.

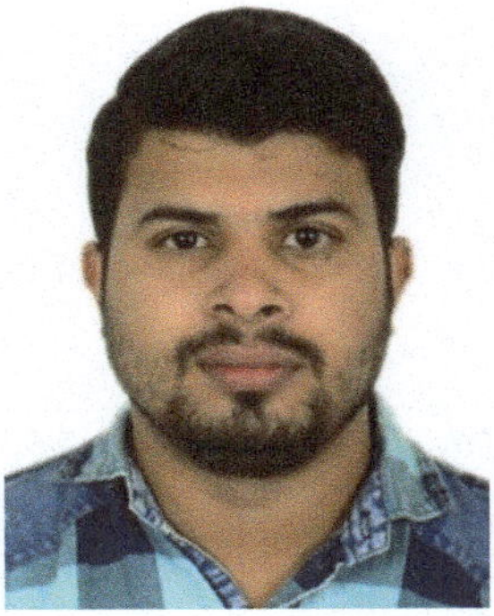

Manohar Mishra is an Associate Professor in the Department of Electronics & Electrical Engineering Department, under the Faculty of Engineering & Technology, Siksha 'O' Anusandhan University, Bhubaneswar. He received his Ph.D. in Electrical Engineering, M.Tech. in Power Electronics and Drives, and B.Tech. in Electrical Engineering in 2017, 2012, and 2008, respectively. He has published more than 40 research papers in various reputed peer-reviewed International Journals, Conferences, and Book Chapters. He has served as a reviewer for various reputed Journal publishers such as Springer, IEEE, Elsevier, and Inderscience. At present, he has more than 10 years of teaching experience in the field of Electrical Engineering. He is a Senior Member of IEEE. He is currently guiding four Ph.D. and Master scholars. His area of interest includes power system analysis, power system protection, signal processing, power quality, distribution generation system, and micro-grid. He has served as Convener and Volume Editor of International Conference on Innovation in Electrical Power Engineering, Communication and Computing Technology (IEPCCT-2019), and International Conference on Green Technology for Smart City and Society (GTSCS-2020). Currently, he is serving as Guest editor in different journals such as International Journal of Power Electronics (Inderscience Publisher), International Journal of Innovative Computing and Application (Inderscience Publisher), Neural Computing and Application (Springer).

Part I
Cancer Data Analysis with Machine Learning Approaches

Chapter 1
Advances in Machine Learning Approaches in Cancer Prognosis

Margarita N. Favorskaya

Abstract Machine Learning (ML) methods have numerous promising applications in medicine, including cancer risk assessment, lesion detection using biomarkers and image segmentation, prediction of disease grading, staging, prognosis and therapy response and so on. The ML methods have the potential to improve analysis of various medical data, such as multidimensional numerical, visual and text data, compared to conventional statistical analysis. A brief overview presented in this chapter discusses the trends in predicting some types of cancer, including the application of Deep Learning (DL) methods.

Keywords Machine learning · Deep learning · Cancer prognosis · Risk · Prediction · Precision oncology

1.1 Introduction

Large amount of cancer data collected over the past decades is enabling the creation and testing of accurate ML models that can effectively predict future cancer outcomes. The deployment of ML approaches can enhance the accuracy of cancer perceptivity, recurrence and survival prediction, achieving good results in risk assessment and lesion detection. The employed ML methods provide the basis for the utilization of innovation procedures for early cancer diagnosis and prognosis in clinical practice, for example, such as gene expression profiling.

In medical applications, the ML methods generalize the concept of inference based on the learning process in multidimensional space for a given set of biological samples. The learning process is aimed at detecting of unidentified dependencies in a given dataset with the ability to predict the output results. As well-known, there are two major common categories of learning, supervised and unsupervised [1]. Supervised learning is based on the labeled data and expert assistance, while

M. N. Favorskaya (✉)
Reshetnev Siberian State University of Science and Technology, Institute of Informatics and Telecommunications, 31, Krasnoyarsky Rabochy ave, Krasnoyarsk 660037, Russian Federation
e-mail: favorskaya@sibsau.ru

J. Nayak et al. (eds.), *Advanced Machine Learning Approaches in Cancer Prognosis*, Intelligent Systems Reference Library 204,
https://doi.org/10.1007/978-3-030-71975-3_1

unsupervised learning uses the unlabeled input data trying to find hidden structures under some hypothesis. Some modifications have been developed among supervised learning methods. Reinforcement learning generalizes the labeled input data when the actions of positive and/or adverse reinforcement affect a system as a feedback loop in a vigorous environment. Transfer learning applies the previously labeled data for a new but related task. In transfer learning, there exist three issues to resolve [2]: "What to transfer", "How to transfer" and "When to transfer". "What to transfer" concentrates on how much of the proficiency it is projected to influence across domains. The transfer learning procedures consist of four phases. They are instance, representation of feature, relational knowledge and parameter transfer. "How to transfer" concentrates on establishing the model in order to attain the transfer of knowledge. "When to transfer" concentrates on the situations where transfer learning may be utilized or may not be utilized. Transfer learning has been enforced in distinct fields of medical scinece, including cancer prognosis, due to the limited datasets [3]. However, supervised learning is most widely used in medicine, since classification tasks prevail over clustering tasks solved by unsupervised learning [1].

Typically, the ML methods include three steps, such as preprocessing, learning and post-processing. Preprocessing contains data cleaning and data modification (normalization, discretization, feature extraction and feature selection). Learning step means the model construction involving the selection of ML algorithms (or use of ML algorithm assemble) and class imbalance handling. Post-processing includes getting results, models' comparison, reliability estimation and knowledge extraction. The DL methods extract and select features automatically, providing better results than expert estimates.

Of course, all ML methods and DL methods (as a part of ML methods) have limitations and drawbacks, but compared to conventional statistical approaches, they guarantee the generalizability of the results obtained. This makes them promising for many medical applications, when data mining is an integral part.

The remaining portion of the chapter is systematized as follows. A brief overview of ML impact on data mining in oncology, with the aim of addressing the key predictive challenges, such as cancer susceptibility, cancer recurrence and cancer survival has been presented in Sects. 1.1 and 1.2. Essentially, all predictions are likelihood estimates, but we need them to be highly accurate. All predictive problems mentioned above deal with the durable temporal aspect and in this sense intersect with the problems of personalized medicine. Conclusions are drawn in Sect. 1.3.

1.2 Key Predictive Challenges

Aspects of prediction in medicine are different. Predicting disease susceptibility, called risk assessment, is a largely studied field, when lesion detection and segmentation are among the most essential application of ML in medical imaging [4]. In addition, ML methods facilitate accurate and fast assessment to determine the stage for selecting the most appropriate therapeutic approach. Predicting cancer recurrence assesses the likelihood of cancer redeveloping after complete or partial remission. Predicting cancer outcomes generally represents the cases of life duration, survivability, development and sensitivity towards treatment [5].

1.2.1 Machine Learning Methods for Cancer Susceptibility

Carcinoma is strenuous to determine at initial period or can easily replace after therapy because of its uncertain symptoms and the indistinctive control signs obtained with non-invasive scanning devices. This means that it is very hard to accurately determine the prognosis of ailment with a high degree of certainty.

Various predicting models using biomarkers are widely distributed in this sphere. Moreover, investigations in finding new cancer epigenetic and genetic biomarkers based on the ML methods, in particular, continue [6].

For predicting pancreatic cancer, a robust diagnostic model utilizing miRNA biomarkers is presented in [7]. The early detection of PDAC (Pancreatic Ductal AdenoCarcinoma), which is known as one of the deadliest cancerous disease in the world remains challenging. The objective of this study was to establish a PDAC diagnostic model using an amalgamation of bioinformatics and ML approaches. The authors selected the most essential features in the dataset in two ways: using Particle Swarm Optimization (PSO) and Artificial Neural Network (ANN) and applying Neighborhood Component Analysis (NCA). Dataset used for the experimentation consist of 671 selected miRNA expression profiles from serum samples of PDAC patients and healthy controls. These samples are downloaded from four GEO profiles i.e., GSE113486, GSE59856, GSE85589, and GSE106817. The problem was that the features representing gene expression had 28 dimensions. Feature selection was encoded in a binary format, and PSO found a binary code that reduces the classification error through the PSO iterations. Then, the selected features as microRNA signatures entered on the inputs of ANN with two hidden layers, while the output layer contained the classifying estimates of pancreatic cancer. The second way was implemented using a non-parametric method (NCA) in order to maximize the prediction efficiency of regression and classification. As a result, a combination of PSO and ANN (with about 42 epochs) selected 14 miRNAs signatures, while the NCA approach selected only 8 miRNA signatures, but with more than 1000 iterations. The Kaplan Meier plotter was utilized to perform the survival analysis of three top-ranked miRNA signatures. The results indicate that Kaplan Meier obtained P-values of 0.001, 0.001 and 0.009, respectively, and hazard ratios of 2.27, 2.27 and 0.59, respectively between the groups of high and low expressions.

In [8], the Tissue-Of-Origin (TOO) carcinoma of unknown primary was predicted by using the gene expression profiles. The commonly utilized medical image tools such as Computed tomography and positron emission tomography for predicting primary tumor lesions, provide the accuracies 20%–27% and 24%–40%, respectively. For the prediction of primary tumor, the authors suggested a systematic method based on the somatic mutation profiles from ICGC database. Feature selection and final classification are accomplished using a random forest (RF) algorithm. The evaluation indicator utilized for the feature importance is the decrease of the Gini impurity. Accuracy and F1 scores were calculated utilizing a RF that uses distinct gene sets. By using a set of 600 genes, the optimal results were attained with an accuracy of 88.22% and F1 score of 88.86% respectively.

Shao et al. [9] proposed a Multi-task Multi-modal feature selection approach for the joint identification and Prognosis of cancer (M2DP). The authors show that the identification and prophecy of cancer can be enhanced by the integrative investigation of histopathological images and genomic data. Image features, eigengene features, diagnosis information and survival information aggregated to select multi-modal features. The proposed method was evaluated by considering three cancer datasets from the Cancer Genome Atlas project.

Visual data can be facilitated by medical imaging such as MRI (Magnetic Resonance Imaging) and CT (Computed Tomography), which require the application of computer vision methods to process and extract visual features from medical images. Additionally, mammogram, ultrasound, histological and thermography images can be processed. This is a large branch of investigations because visual modalities play a significant role in clinical analysis.

By using multimodalities of the medical radiographs, review [10] provides the comparison of ML and DL methods on the determination of breast cancer in order to provide the categorization of breast cancer (i.e., having tumors, non-tumors, and dense masses) in distinct medical radiographs.

To distinguish between confirmed patients with prostate cancer and prostate benign patients, Wang et al. [11] compared DL model based on DCNN and non-DL with SIFT (Scale-Invariant Feature Transform) image feature and BoW (Bag-Of-Words). It was observed that DCNN performed superior for differentiating patients into two groups when compared with the other approaches. These outcomes demonstrated that the DL methods can be further extended to image modalities of other organs such as MRI, CT and PET (Positron Emission Tomography) scans.

By considering 3D multiparametric MRI data facilitated by the PROSTATEx challenge, a novel DL architecture known as XmasNet that is dependent on Convolutional Neural Networks (CNNs) has been developed by Xu et al. [12] for the classification of prostate cancer lesions. The results displayed that the developed model attains the AUC value of 0.84 in the PROSTATEx challenge.

A non-invasive stage classification system of melanoma skin cancer based on CNN has been proposed by Patil and Bellary [13]. The proposed approach makes use of al loss function as Similarity Measure for Text Processing (SMTP). The original data were dermoscopic images, which were subjected to edge and texture analysis. Two classification systems were introduced: one describing stage 1 and 2 type of melanoma and another defining stage 1, 2 and 3 type of melanoma.

1.2.2 Machine Learning Methods for Cancer Recurrence

It has been observed that a little literature work has been performed on the cancer recurrence [14–16]. There are more results regarding the cancer survival prediction.

For the determination of recurrence of breast carcinoma, Macías-García et al. [17] designed an approach to outline the methylation of DNA by considering the benefits of AutoEncoders (AEs). By considering the values of CpG sites of patients with and without recurrence, new features are generated by the AEs. The most heavily weighted genes in the autoencoded features developed by the AEs are all related to the literature on breast cancer. These features are categorized into five types such as confirmed-recurrence biomarkers, probable-recurrence biomarkers, obesity-related biomarkers, chemotherapeutic inhibitors and probable pesticide exposure indicators. The AEs can be useful to predict genes responsible not only for breast cancer recurrence, but also other similar ailments.

For interpreting the predictive models in cancer diagnosis, the Shapley Additive Explanations (SHAP) [19] method was adapted by Reyes et al. [18]. The proposed methodology included three main steps: ranking of weighted features, high accurate classification model based on heuristic assumptions and using the induced classifier for explaining predictions and behavior at individual and global levels respectively. The proposed methodology incorporated the expert knowledge and, at the same time, explored high-order interfeature relationships. Such approach helps to explain the results of SVM classifiers in predicting breast cancer and metastatic melanoma.

Koikea et al. [20] suggested ML-based classification of histological images of the lungs to predict recurrence of disease. They utilized an approach of color-based segmentation through clustering of K-means and recursive intensity-dependent registration.

1.2.3 Machine Learning Methods for Cancer Outcomes

Currently, the investigation on clinical cancer is focused on determining the correct outcome in response to the therapy. However, it is very strenuous to implement the more precise treatment customized for a patient, even using statistical and/or ML methods.

Faraggi and Simon [21] were the first, who utilized the ANN model to determine the prostate cancer survival by considering four clinical input parameters. However, survival data are usually high dimensional data, and the conventional ANN architecture is not suitable for this problem despite various simplifications of the input data.

Recently, a novel ANN framework known as Cox-nnet (a neural network extension of the Cox regression model) based on much richer biological information for the determination of patient prognoses both at the pathway and gene levels has been developed by Ching et al. [22]. Using dropout regularization, the authors compared three Cox-nnet architectures i.e., with no hidden layer known as standard Cox-PH model, single hidden layer having 143 nodes and two hidden layers having 143 nodes in both layers. It was observed from the evaluation that the Cox-nnet model consisting of one hidden layer performed slightly better when compared with other architectures. Cox-nnet model attained the same or better prediction accuracy in comparison with other methods such as Cox-proportional hazards regression, CoxBoost and RFs survival. For a detail overview of the Deep learning (DL) application in the prediction of carcinoma prognosis, see [23].

A weighted fuzzy decision trees (DT) has been suggested by Khan et al. [24] for determining survival analysis of patients suffering with breast carcinoma. The suggested model consists of decision tree rules, functions of fuzzy membership and inference techniques. The originality of the approach was in cooperation between DT and fuzzy theory that allowed to achieve a balance in decision making. Further, the authors discussed about the advantages of wFDTs for personalized predictive medicine.

An extensive study of the molecular characteristics, enhanced diagnosis, treatment and prevention of breast cancer has been provided by DL approaches and multi-dimensional data. Sun et al. [25] proposed a multimodal DNN that utilizes multidimensional data for the prognosis and determination of breast carcinoma. The results of the extensive analysis displayed that the developed approach surpassed other prediction models that utilizes one-dimensional data. Moreover, sometimes new deep neural network architectures such as a survival RNN (Recurrent Neural Network) has been developed to determine the survival rate of patients suffering from gastric cancer. Further, it is noticed that the outcomes are closely corresponded with the actual survival arte of gastric cancer inmates [26]. In [27], it was shown how a multistage transfer learning can be used for intermediate-stage fine-tuning by considering data from identical auxiliary domains. Some deep learning networks achieve performance close to human experts, as in the case of using a pre-trained CNN known as OverFeat for automatic classification of pulmonary perifissural nodules [28].

To predict the disease recurrence and patient survival in Non-Small Cell Lung Cancer (NSCLC) patients having brain metastases after underwent radiosurgery, an appropriate prognostic index was selected by Gao et al. [29]. Using ordinary statistical methods, further they analyzed six prognostic factors, such as age, control of primary tumor, total number of lesions, extracranial metastasis, volume of maximum lesion and score of KPS. In addition, four prognostic indices such as analysis of recursive partitioning, basic score for brain metastases, assessment of graded prognostic assessment and score index for radiosurgery were compared to determine the disease recurrence.

The ML methods provide more accurate results for devising of personalized care and patient counselling but cannot explain them. One of the ways to overcome this inconsistency is to combine conventional practical techniques with ML methods. Such approach was applied in [30]. The performance of nomogram with ML models represented by logistic regression, SVM (Support Vector Machine), decision jungle, boosted DT (Decision Tree), NB (Naïve Bayes) and decision forest were compared to determine the overall survival in tongue cancer. Among the available ML approaches, the boosted DT obtained better performance in comparison to other algorithms. Moreover, an accuracy of 88.7% was obtained by boosted decision tree while an accuracy of 60.4% was attained by the nomogram because the ML algorithms considered patient age, T stage, radiation treatment and the surgical intervention. Therefore, the ML methods provide more customized and trustworthy prophecy information of tongue cancer when compared to the nomogram. To increase the standard of explanation provided by nomogram, an integration of a nomogram and ML known as NomoML predictive model has been proposed.

Doppalapudi et al. [31] compared the performance of survival period prediction for lung cancer across three architectures—ANN, CNN and RNN—verses traditional ML approaches containing stacking ensemble, linear regression (LR), RFs and gradient boosting approaches. Data has been considered from the lung carcinoma section of SEER (Surveillance, Epidemiology, and End Results) cancer registry. The authors show that the DL models significantly outperformed in terms of classification and regression approaches when compares with the traditional ML baseline models.

1.3 Conclusions

ML methods demonstrate great assistance in many fields of oncology, enhanced screening strategies and personalized therapies. This trend leads to develop more accurate oncology models that makes use of non-intrusive and less-costly data mining approaches. The ML and DL software tools are generally open source tools and available freely for the purpose of investigation. However, medical data are often complex and require the development of well-known ML methods, especially in dynamic and long-term aspect. In addition, one of the major challenges for ML application is small medical datasets and large variability of medical personal indicators, which makes it difficult to learn ML models without overfitting and underfitting.

Currently, to train junior medical practitioners in diagnostic determination and the process of decision taking, ML approaches are utilized. However, the low ability to interpret the obtained data, both numerical and visual, brings the practice of extensive use of ML approaches in clinical practice. More precise models, such as boosted trees, RF and ANN are generally not transparent models, whereas LR, NB, KNN (K-Nearest Neighbor) and single DT are more intelligible models, that usually produces significantly worse outcomes. It is reasonable to expect that the challenges in the trade-off between accuracy and ability to explain of the results will be solved in the foreseeable future.

References

1. Choy, G., Khalilzadeh, O., Michalski, M., Do, S., Samir, A.E., Pianykh, O.S., Geis, J.R., Pandharipande, P.V., Brink, J.A., Dreyer, K.J.: Current applications and future impact of machine learning in radiology. Radiology **288**, 318–328 (2018)
2. Lu, J., Behbood, V., Hao, P., Zuo, H., Xue, S., Zhang, G.: Transfer learning using computational intelligence: a survey. Knowl. Based Syst. **80**, 14–23 (2015)
3. Wang, G., Zhang, G., Choi, K.-S., Lam, K.-M., Lu, J.: Output based transfer learning with least squares support vector machine and its application in bladder cancer prognosis. Neurocomputing **387**, 279–292 (2020)
4. Cuocolo, R., Caruso, M., Perillo, T., Ugga, L., Petretta, M.: Machine learning in oncology: a clinical appraisal. Cancer Lett. **481**, 55–62 (2020)
5. Kourou, K., Exarchos, T.P., Exarchos, K.P., Karamouzis, M.V., Fotiadis, D.I.: Machine learning applications in cancer prognosis and prediction. Computation. and Structural Biotechnology J. **13**, 8–17 (2015)
6. Liu, S., Wu, J., Xia, Q., Liu, H., Li, W., Xia, X., Wang, J.: Finding new cancer epigenetic and genetic biomarkers from cell-free DNA by combining SALP-seq and machine learning. Computational and Structural Biotechnology J. **18**, 1891–1903 (2020)
7. Savareh, B.A., Aghdaie, H.A., Behmanesh, A., Bashiri, A., Sadeghi, A., Zali, M., Shams, R.: A machine learning approach identified a diagnostic model for pancreatic cancer through using circulating microRNA signatures. Pancreatology **20**, 1195–1204 (2020)
8. He, B., Dai, C., Lang, J., Bing, P., Tian, G., Wang, B., Yang, J.: A Machine learning framework to trace tumor tissue-of-origin of 13 types of cancer based on DNA somatic mutation. BBA—Molecular Basis Disease **1866**, 165916.1–165916.7 (2020)
9. Shao, W., Wang, T., Sun, L., Dong, T., Han, Z., Huang, Z., Zhang, J., Zhang, D., Huang, K.: Multi-task multi-modal learning for joint diagnosis and prognosis of human cancers. Med. Image Anal. **65**, 101795.1–101795.10 (2020)
10. Houssein, E.H., et al.: Deep and machine learning techniques for medical imaging-based breast cancer: a comprehensive review. Exp. Syst. Appl. 114161 (2020)
11. Wang, X., Yang, W., Weinreb, J., Han, J., Li, Q., Kong, X., Yan, Y., Ke, Z., Luo, B., Liu, T., Wang, L.: Searching for prostate cancer by fully automated magnetic resonance imaging classification: deep learning versus non-deep learning. Sci. Rep. **7**, 15415 (2017)
12. Xu, Y., Hosny, A., Zeleznik, R., Parmar, C., Coroller, T., Franco, I., Mak, R.H., Aerts, H.: Deep learning predicts lung cancer treatment response from serial medical imaging. Clin. Cancer Res. **25**, 3266–3275 (2019)
13. Patil, R., Bellary, S.: Machine learning approach in melanoma cancer stage detection. J. King Saud Univ. Comput. Inform. Sci. (2020). https://doi.org/10.1016/j.jksuci.2020.09.002
14. Abreu, P.H., Santos, M.S., Abreu, M.H., Andrade, B., Silva, D.C.: Predicting breast cancer recurrence using machine learning techniques: a systematic review. ACM Comput. Surv. **49**, 52.1–52.40 (2016)
15. Colleoni, M., Sun, Z., Price, K.N., Karlsson, P., Forbes, J.F., Thürlimann, B., Gianni, L., Castiglione, M., Gelber, R.D., Coates, A.S., Goldhirsch, A.: Annual Hazard rates of recurrence for breast cancer during 24 years of follow-up: results from the international breast cancer study group trials I to V. J. Clin. Oncol. **34**, 927–935 (2016)
16. Wang, C., Cicek, M.S., Charbonneau, B., Kalli, K.R., Armasu, S.M., Larson, M.C., Konecny, G.E., Winterhoff, B., Fan, J.-B., Bibikova, M., Chien, J., Shridhar, V., Block, M.S., Hartmann, L.C., Visscher, D.W., Cunningham, J.M., Knutson, K.L., Fridley, B.L., Goode, E.L.: Tumor Hypomethylation at 6p21.3 associates with longer time to recurrence of high-grade serous epithelial Ovarian cancer. Cancer Res. **74**, 3084–3091 (2014)
17. Macías-García, L., Martínez-Ballesteros, M., Luna-Romera, J.M., García-Heredia, J.M., García-Gutierrez, J., Riquelme-Santos, J.C.: Machine learning models and gene-weight significance. Artif. Intell. Med. **110**, 101976.1–101976.16 (2020)

18. Reyes, O., Perez, E., Luque, R.M., Castano, J., Ventura, S.: A supervised machine learning-based methodology for analyzing dysregulation in splicing machinery: an application in cancer diagnosis. Artif. Intell. Med. **108**, 101950.1–101950.13 (2020)
19. Lundberg, S.M., Lee, S.-I.: A unified approach to interpreting model predictions. In: Advances in Neural Information Processing Systems 30: 31st Annual Conference on Neural Information Processing Systems (NIPS 2017), Long Beach, CA, USA, pp. 4765–4774 (2017)
20. Koikea, Y., Aokage, K., Ikeda, K., Nakai, T., Tane, K., Miyoshi, T., Sugano, M., Kojima, M., Fujii, S., Kuwata, T., Ochiai, A., Tanaka, T., Suzuki, K., Tsuboi, M., Ishii, G.: Machine learning-based histological classification that predicts recurrence of peripheral lung squamous cell carcinoma. Lung Cancer **147**, 252–258 (2020)
21. Faraggi, D., Simon, R.: A neural network model for survival data. Stat. Med. **14**(1), 73–82 (1995)
22. Ching, T., Zhu, X., Garmire, L.X.: Cox-nnet: an artificial neural network method for prognosis prediction of high-throughput omics data. PLoS Comput. Biol. **14**, (2018)
23. Zhu, W., Xie, L., Han, J., Guo, X.: The application of deep learning in cancer prognosis prediction. Cancers **12**, 603.1–603.19 (2020)
24. Khan, U., Shin, H., Choi, J.P., Kim, M.: wFDT—Weighted fuzzy decision trees for prognosis of breast cancer survivability. In: Roddick, J.F., Li, J., Christen, P., Kennedy, P.J. (eds.) Proceedings of the 7th Australasian Data Mining Conference, Australian Computer Society, Glenelg, South Australia, pp. 141–152 (2008)
25. Sun, D., Wang, M., Li, A.: A multimodal deep neural network for human breast cancer prognosis prediction by integrating multi-dimensional data. IEEE ACM Trans. Comput. Biol. Bioinform. **16**(3), 841–850 (2018)
26. Oh, S.E., Choi, M.-G., Seo, S.W.: ASO author reflections: use of the survival recurrent network for prediction of overall survival in patients with gastric cancer. Ann. Surg. Oncol. **25**, 1153–1159 (2018)
27. Samala, R.K., Chan, H.-P., Hadjiiski, L., Helvie, M.A., Richter, C.D., Cha, K.H.: Breast cancer diagnosis in digital breast tomosynthesis: effects of training sample size on multi-stage transfer learning using deep neural nets. IEEE Trans. Med. Imaging **38**, 686–696 (2019)
28. Ciompi, F., de Hoop, B., van Riel, S.J., Chung, K., Scholten, E.T., Oudkerk, M., de Jong, P.A., Prokop, M., van Ginneken, B.: Automatic classification of pulmonary perifissural nodules in computed tomography using an ensemble of 2D views and a convolutional neural network out-of-the-box. Med. Image Anal. **26**, 195–202 (2015)
29. Gao, H.X., Huang, S.G., Du, J.F., Zhang, X.C., Jiang, N., Kang, W.X., Mao, J., Zhao, Q.: Comparison of prognostic indices in NSCLC patients with brain metastases after radiosurgery. Int. J. Biol. Sci. **14**, 2065–2072 (2018)
30. Alabi, R.O., Makitie, A.A., Pirinen, M., Elmusrati, M., Leivo, I., Almangush, A.: Comparison of nomogram with machine learning techniques for prediction of overall survival in patients with tongue cancer. Int. J. Med. Inform. **145**, 104313.1–104313.9 (2021)
31. Doppalapudi, S., Qiu, R.G., Badr, Y.: Lung cancer survival period prediction and understanding: deep learning approaches. Int. J. Med. Inform. 104371 (2020)

Chapter 2
Data Analysis on Cancer Disease Using Machine Learning Techniques

Soumen K. Pati, Arijit Ghosh, Ayan Banerjee, Indrani Roy, Preetam Ghosh, and Chiraag Kakar

Abstract Coherent and systematic analysis for finding complex patterns in structured and unstructured cancer data has seen quite a rich and diverse implementation of distinct techniques in the recent past. The delicate and life-threatening aspect of Cancer has led to the huge need as well as the attraction of everyone to propose optimized techniques to garner a commendable result for the prediction of cancer subtypes. As a result, several Data Analysis techniques have led a revolution to provide the best outcomes, among which several have shown mammoth results. In this chapter, the focus is put directly on such techniques that have been implemented and adapted for cancer data analysis. The chapter goes into quite an in-depth review of each of the proposed architectures which have been very precisely screened by us and also do quite a lot to develop a concrete sense of each one of these taxonomies by putting each of them under scanning through various evaluation metrics. Furthermore, the chapter issues several future scopes and recommendations from the perspective of the authors to ignite the thought of the ones interested in pushing this field into further sub-stratum.

Keywords Data analysis · Pattern recognition · Optimized technique · Cancer data · Bioinformatics

---

S. K. Pati (✉)
Department of Bioinformatics, Maulana Abul Kalam Azad University of Technology, Nadia, West Bengal, India

A. Ghosh · I. Roy
Department of Electronics and Communication Engineering, Calcutta Institute of Engineering and Management, Kolkata, West Bengal, India

A. Banerjee · P. Ghosh · C. Kakar
Department of Computer Science and Engineering, Jalpaiguri Government Engineering College, Jalpaiguri, West Bengal, India
e-mail: ab2141@cse.jgec.ac.in

C. Kakar
e-mail: ck2222@cse.jgec.ac.in

J. Nayak et al. (eds.), *Advanced Machine Learning Approaches in Cancer Prognosis*, Intelligent Systems Reference Library 204,
https://doi.org/10.1007/978-3-030-71975-3_2

2.1 Introduction

In 2020, cancer has spread its wrath among a staggering 29% of the total population of the entire world (2.2 Billion people) with 6 million people having already lost their battles and a further 18 million still fighting it in the square rings (Cancer Statistics, 2020 [1]). But with the upsurge of the novel CoVID-19 virus and its subsequent rise in the number of cases, the focus has entirely shifted to suppress the pandemic and has thereby retracted all the focus from the research of the deadly cancer disease, making it more fatal than ever. But the negligence would result in the disease being more lethal, and as such need a rushed prompt to have a dedicated discussion along with dealing with the deadly pandemic. With the evolving computational techniques (Artificial Intelligence, Machine Learning, Deep Learning, Pattern Recognition etc.), the past decade has seen numerous potential approaches being presented with very diverse ideas as such it bears a lot of missing links among them. Hence, the focus of this chapter is to present a static roadmap to get a grasp of these techniques in a precise and compact manner.

2.1.1 Overview of the Cancer Disease

Cancer disease is an irregular development of cells derivative with mutated oncogene from a particular abnormal cell [2]. Usually, the affected cells lose their standard control mechanisms and mutate rapidly, attack adjacent tissues, migrate to obscure body parts, and facilitate the development of blood circulation vessels to derive nutrients. Malignant cells from the host tissue can spread all over the body due to metastasis. These malignant tissues can be separated according to the blood and making of blood tissues (leukemia and lymphoma) and tumors which can be further classified as sarcomas or carcinomas. Leukemia [3] and Lymphoma [4] are the cancers of blood and blood-creating cells and tissues of the resistant system. The production of standard blood cells crowds out by the Leukemia in bone marrow. The lymphoma cancer cells inflate nodes of lymph, thereby accumulating big clumps in the regions of the chest, groin, armpit, or abdomen. Carcinomas [5] are cancer cells that are lined in the lungs, skin, digestive tract, and other internal organs. Some examples of the carcinomas are the cancer of the different internal organs and skin. Naturally, carcinoma cancers occur regularly in old people. The Sarcomas [6] are cancer of mesodermal cells. The mesodermal cells generally instigate the formation of blood vessels, muscles, bones, and connective tissues. Sarcomas can be classified as osteosarcoma (type of bone cancer) and leiomyosarcoma (generally found in the wall of digestive tissues). The young generation is much more vulnerable than the elderly by the effects of Sarcoma cancer cells.

2.1.2 *Overview of the Cancer Data*

All the publicly available datasets can be broadly classified into several categories:

A. Structured dataset—Structured data are always available in the form of microarray dataset [7] or gene expression data where the rows represent the genes (g_1, g_2,………,g_n) related to the disease and the columns represent the samples (s_1, s_2,……,s_n) from where the genes are collected.

B. Unstructured data—The unstructured data is again classified into the two categories.

   (a) Image Dataset [8]—Consisting of various types of tumor images for analysis.
   (b) Sequence dataset [9]—Consisting of DNA sequence information with their nitrogen bonding (adenine (A), cytosine (C), guanine (G), and thymine (T)—ATGC) which can be used to analyse how cell DNA changes their nitrogen bonding from normal to cancer cells.

C. Statistical dataset [10]—It has been made publicly available to obtain the tumor characteristics (e.g. primary tumor site, year of diagnosis, behaviour, histology, stage at diagnosis etc.) with the demographic knowledge (e.g. age, sex, race, etc.) for public awareness.

Till date, International Collaboration on Cancer Reporting (ICCR) categorized all the cancer databases in the following anatomical sites. Figure 2.1 provides an overview of these types of cancer databases.

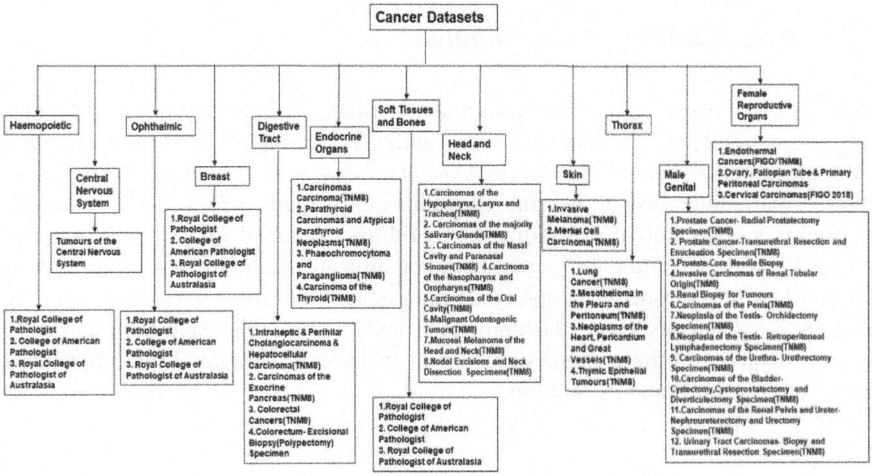

Fig. 2.1 Overview of cancer databases

2.1.3 *Objective and Proposed Outcomes*

In the past few decades, several researchers made their notable contribution to obtain novel data analyzation techniques, so that a lot of information is obtained from the available dataset to build a protective wall against the cancer disease. But now this research field is going to be saturated and with the evolving deep learning techniques, it is in the way of obscurity. Nowadays, it is badly needed to obtain a detailed review of the existing data analysis techniques, so that future generations can get an essence of how the computational techniques help the world to obtain a preliminary defence against the disease. Though, there are some good surveys that already exist, they are mainly focused on classification and mostly bounded with a single source of data (e.g. structured or unstructured). This chapter provides robustness over the existing ones and tries to cover all possible aspects. The chapter is mainly divided into three broad classes: (1) **Supervised,** (2) **Semi-Supervised** and (3) **Unsupervised**. These classes are further subcategorizes until they reach unit level. Section 2.2 shows a detailed description of existing analysis techniques with the authors obtaining a notable contribution in the corresponding fields. Not only that, this chapter provides a quality checking of all the algorithms based on the well-defined validation techniques (e.g. error rate, classification accuracy, specificity, sensitivity, Precision, F1-score, Area Under the Curve (AUC), Receiver Operating Characteristics (ROC), Cohen's kappa, etc.) for a detailed comparison to obtain the problems faced in times of implementation. Besides that, this chapter provides some valuable insights on these algorithms for the betterment of the existing ones and also provides all possible future aspects that guide the researchers to jump into a new era.

2.1.4 *Organization of the Chapter*

This chapter is structured into the subsequent sections. Section 2.2 provides a detailed description of all possible data analysis techniques. Section 2.3 provides the possible Challenges and issues of the Cancer Data Analysis work. Section 2.4 obtains all possible parameters to validate the algorithms explained in Sect. 2.2. Section 2.5 highlights a comparative study of the algorithms discussed in Sect. 2.2 in accordance to number of publications, number of citation and a country-wise contribution. Section 2.6 throws some lights upon the future aspects that come out from this survey. Section 2.7 discusses about the findings from the comprehensive review. Lastly, Sect. 2.8 concludes the chapter summary of the overall study and the information conserved for the future generation.

2.2 Review Report

Data analysis [11] is a method of examining, cleaning, transforming and exhibiting dataset with the objective of learning usefulness of information, informing summaries and supporting decision-making. It has several sides and methods, surrounding diverse procedures to be used in various medical domains. In the recent medical world, analysis of data shows a vital role in making decisions more scientific thereby helping medical operations more effectively. This chapter throws a light on possible data analysis applications to treat the cancer disease in the following subsections.

2.2.1 Supervised Learning

Supervised Learning adheres to optimize the required algorithms based on the presence of the desired output. The algorithm learns to map from the given labels as if being supervised in each of its steps to proceed in the optimum direction. Supervised Learning has been here for decades and is typically the conventional method used by researchers for not only cancer data but also in several other applications, such as Image Recognition, Natural Language Processing, Sentiment Analysis, etc. This section of the chapter is focused on the ever-present, simple and rudimentary learning algorithms as shown in Fig. 2.2. The section also tabularizes the best possible methodologies adopted as per the view of the authors and segregates the advantages and disadvantages of each one of them. Since, a significant amount of time and focus has been given in each of these Supervised Learning algorithms for Cancer Data Analysis, only a handful of these major techniques could be handpicked and described as such it will "supervise" the learners on to the right path.

2.2.1.1 Logistic Regression

Logistic Regression utilizes the statistical probability to determine the occurrence of an event or a class ($y = 1$ or cancer) given a cancer dataset of $\{g_1, g_2, g_3 \dots g_n \in \text{G}\}$. It does so with the help of logit or sigmoid function given in Eq. (2.1).

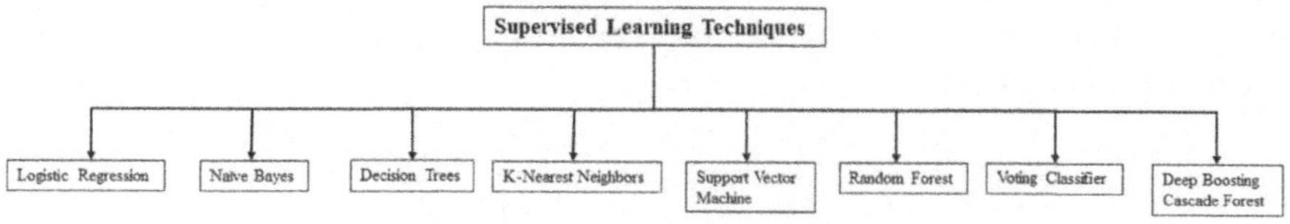

Fig. 2.2 Flowchart of supervised learning algorithms used for cancer data analysis

$$P(y = 1|G) = h = \frac{1}{1 + \exp(-(\beta_0 + \sum_{i=0}^{n} \beta i.gi))} \tag{2.1}$$

where, $\boldsymbol{\beta}_0$ is the intercept and $\boldsymbol{\beta}_i$ is a n * 1 vector of learnable coefficients of the features.

The logistic regression algorithm predicts the probability of occurrence of class 1 by minimizing the loss function given by Eq. (2.2).

$$\iota(\beta 0, \beta 1, \ldots\ldots \beta n) = -\sum_{j=1}^{m} (y_j * \ln(h_j) + (1 - (y_j) * \ln(1 - h_j)) \tag{2.2}$$

The simplistic nature of the Logistic Regression has over the years led to many concerning disadvantages, one such is over fitting of the model due to the higher dimension of the dataset. One such technique to fight the problem of over fitting was stated in [12] where a more robust approach of penalizing the coefficients was undertaken. The process follows the simple algorithm but adds a regularizing term to the cost function to reduce the potency of the coefficients thereby preventing the model to over fit, given in Eq. (2.3).

$$\xi(\beta_0, \beta_1, \ldots \beta_n) = \iota(\beta_0, \beta_1, \ldots \beta_n) + \lambda * \sum_{i=1}^{n-1} \sum_{j>i} \left(\frac{(\beta_i - \beta_j)^2}{1 - v_{ij}} + \frac{(\beta_i + \beta_j)^2}{1 + v_{ij}} \right) \tag{2.3}$$

where, *ij* is the correlation between the *i*th and *j*th genes and is the regularization parameter.

2.2.1.2 Naive Bayes

Naive Bayes follows suit to prediction by separating out the positive and negative classes of a given cancer dataset with a feature set of $\{g_1, g_2, g_3 \ldots g_n \in \mathrm{G}\}$ and thereby finding the probabilities of each class (*i* or cancer and *j* or non-cancer) given each of the features $\mathrm{P}(g_k|C_i)$ and $\mathrm{P}(g_k|C_j)$. Once, all the probabilities are initiated, new predictions are given by first calculating the $\mathrm{P}(C_i|\mathrm{G})$ and $\mathrm{P}(C_j|\mathrm{G})$ given in Eqs. (2.4) and (2.5) and thereby predicting the class *i* or class *j* based on the higher probability of either $\mathrm{P}(C_i|\mathrm{G})$ or $\mathrm{P}(C_j|\mathrm{G})$.

$$\mathrm{P}(C_i|\mathrm{G}) = \mathrm{P}(C_{\mathrm{prior(i)}}) \prod_{k=1}^{n} \mathrm{P}(g_k|C_i) \tag{2.4}$$

$$P(C_j|G) = P(C_{\text{prior(j)}}) \prod_{k=1}^{n} P(g_k|C_j) \tag{2.5}$$

where, $P(C_{\text{prior}(i)})$ and $P(C_{\text{prior}(j)})$ are the prior probabilities of class i and class respectively, which are considered by simply considering that the new sample is a class *i* or *j* irrespective of checking it. It faces a dilemma when faced with a gene whose probability is 0 for a given class *i* or *j* as it strikes down the probability to 0 without considering any other thing. This is corrected via the Laplacian Correction, which suggests adding a value of 1 to each of the features of the dataset as followed by [13].

2.2.1.3 Decision Tree

Based on a cancer dataset given by $\{g_1, g_2, g_3 \ldots g_n \in G\}$, the decision tree approach follows a questionnaire type evaluation as it goes node to node asking questions of alternatives if another child node is to be added to it or not, based on the increment of Information Gain or the decrement of Entropy thereby providing a non-linear induction of dividing between the classes. It goes on to be classified by first initializing the "root" or top-most node which has the highest weighted average Information Gain or lowest weighted average Entropy with the targeted output. One such entropy validation technique, known as Gini Impurity, is given in the Eq. (2.6).

$$\varepsilon(t_i) = 1 - p^2(i|t) \tag{2.6}$$

where, $p^2(i|t)$ is the square of the probability of that node in that level of the branch. The evaluation of the correct node is decided based on the sum of the weighted average of the entropies also known as the total Gini Impurity generated by the question or addition of a node and is given by the Eq. (2.7).

$$g(t_i) = \sum_{i=1}^{c} p(i|t) * \varepsilon(t_i) \tag{2.7}$$

where, *c* is the class number of of the dataset and $p(i|t)$ is the weighted average of that node. The feature which generates a question with the lowest $g(t_i)$ is selected as the node at that level. The algorithm stops if at the leaf node adding any other question of remaining features doesn't bring out lower entropy or if no other feature is remaining, thereby causing the node to be fixed at the previously generated value. Decision Trees can be oriented in a lot of ways, one such way is described in [14] which follows a Classification and Regression Technique (CART) based decision tree which selects the decision nodes after checking the entropy of all the other nodes. Even though Decision Trees are quite handy and are computationally less expensive, they suffer a lot from overfitting, which does more harm than good and is thereby referred only when the order of the dataset is smaller.

2.2.1.4 K-Nearest Neighbors

This algorithm classifies the new data of a given cancer dataset $\{g_1, g_2, g_3 \ldots g_n \in G\}$ by looking at the distance annotated cells (nearest neighbors) given in Eq. (2.8).

$$d(q, p) = \sqrt{\sum_{i=1}^{n}(h - gi)^2} \tag{2.8}$$

where, h is the new cell and g is the dataset. (h–g) is the distance between the new cell from the nearest cells. K-Nearest Neighbor's (KNN) main focus is to find a small set from the training set with full of informative genes to get a better classification accuracy. Its utility has been provisioned in many such gene selection tasks from the cancer expression data and has been quite clearly described in [15] among many others.

2.2.1.5 Support Vector Machine

The main goal of this algorithm is to obtain a hyperplane in N dimensional space, that helps in classifying between the different classes of the given cancer dataset $\{g_1, g_2, g_3 \ldots g_n \in G\}$. The algorithm achieves a far superior classification accuracy by posing a larger margin between the nearest points and the separating plane. It achieves so by deriving "landmarks" and thereby computing similarity functions or kernels to push the data into higher dimensionality functions leaving the entire dataset for classification. The most potent aspect of this algorithm lies in the selection of these kernels, which can be of various types, namely linear, Radial Basis Function (RBF), polynomial, etc. all assigned to replicate the task of pushing the feature set into higher dimensions. A lot of work has been focused attributing to the usage of Support Vector Machine (SVM) in unstructured Magnetic resonance imaging (MRI) image classification dataset proposed in [16] and also in structured Breast Cancer Dataset proposed in [17], with SVM achieving fruitful results irrespective of the orientation of the data.

2.2.1.6 Random Forest

This algorithm prepares a different subset from the original cancer dataset of $\{g_1, g_2, g_3 \ldots g_n \in G\}$ by randomly selecting a number of features by a method called Bootstrapping and prepares different Decision Tree algorithms based on the features. When a dataset is fed to the algorithm, the classification is done via a voting classifier (discussed in Sect. 2.2.1.7) which predicts the class of the sample. The Random Forest algorithm has been quite a pioneering algorithm as it can enforce its classification even with a lot of noise. A number of proposed methodologies [18] have been adopted which utilizes the CART based decision tree algorithms for splitting different models.

2.2.1.7 Voting Classifier

A voting classifier is one of the most unique classifying tools of Supervised Learning. It takes into account the prediction out of several models and filters out the result class C, based on the maximum votes or predictions received from the models which feed in the data from a cancer dataset given by $\{g_1, g_2, g_3 \ldots g_n \in G\}$. This unique technique derives through two possible ideologies—with one being based on the number of votes fed to it by the models (known as Hard Voting Classifier) or via the probabilities (known as Soft Voting Classifier). This type of algorithm is an important supplementary method for the ensemble techniques. Some unique methodologies [19, 20] have been proposed, which have shown the door for the implementation of various ensemble techniques.

2.2.1.8 Deep Boosting Cascade Forest

This algorithm follows a relatively similar footstep as that of a Deep Neural Network, but to ease out the progresses of forward and backward propagation, utilizes an ensemble of ensembles techniques based on Random and Completely Random Forest algorithms. Given a feature set of $\{g_1, g_2, g_3 \ldots g_n \in G\}$ of a cancer dataset, L layers each with Q Random Forests in each layer trained to glorify the best possible path for a decision point as displayed in Fig. 2.3. Since each of the layers consists of Q Random Forests, each layer pushes out a probability for the respective output classes of the dataset and are stored in a feature vector. To select the best possible path of Decision Trees contributing to the Random Forests, the top K height levels of each of the Random Forest are selected and their standard deviations are derived which are weighted with the class probabilities. The class probabilities along with the initial input features are concatenated and fed to the next layers of the Deep Boosting Cascade Forest.

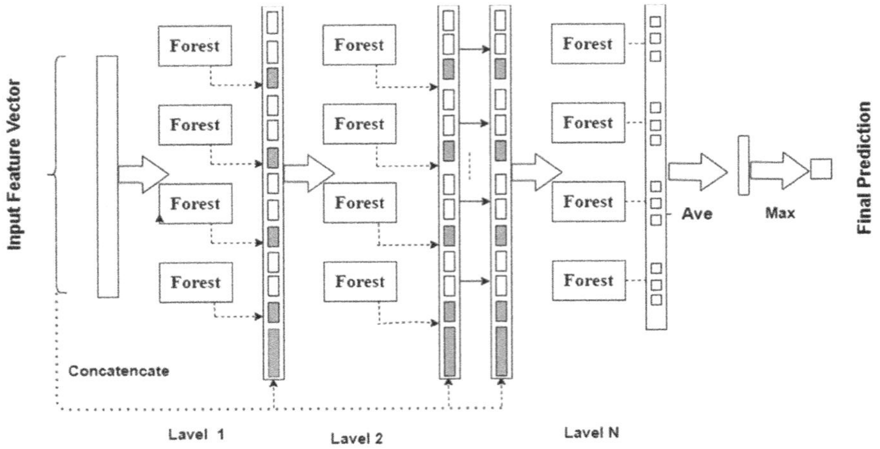

Fig. 2.3 Illustration of a typical deep boosting cascade forest [10]

Deep Boosting Cascade Forest provides quite an exceptional accuracy and that too with an excellent time complexity due to its simplistic nature. This new algorithm has been proven to be a great methodology for cancer data analysis in [21]. The following Table 2.1 provides the comparative analysis of the studies carried on caner using different supervised learning techniques along with pros and cons

2.2.2 *Semi-supervised Learning*

This is a machine learning technique that trains the combination of a slight amount of labelled data with a massive amount of unlabelled dataset. Let **G** be an identical independently distributed set whose examples $g_1, g_2,\ldots,g_n$ are labelled and $i_1, i_2,\ldots,i_n$ are unlabelled are going to be processed with semi-supervised learning. To outshine the classification performance through inductive learning it provides a correct mapping from $g_i \longrightarrow s_i$. Figure 2.4a shows the Venn diagram representation and Fig. 2.4b shows a small example for a proper understanding of semi-supervised learning.

2.2.2.1 Literature Details of Semi-supervised Cancer Data Analysis

In 1970, Semi-Supervised (transductive or inductive) learning was formally introduced by Vapnik et al. [29]. Till then numerous researchers obtained a notable contribution in this field with new methodologies that evolved this technology into a supreme level. But, all the existing methodologies can be broadly classified into several categories. Figure 2.5 provides an overview of this classification.

Table 2.1 Literature review of supervised learning

Approach	Author and References	Objective	Method	Dataset	Pros	Cons
Logistic regression	Algamal and Lee [12]	Classification of cancer microarray data	The method follows a Correlation Based Penalized Logistic Regression(CBPLR), where the coefficients of the Logistic Regression are penalized for higher values such that it prevents overfitting. The classification is similar to that of a conventional Logistic Regression and gives out a probability for the occurrence of class 1	Colon (6000 genes), Prostrate (5966), DLBCL (7129) datasets	1. Time Complexity is very low 2. The penalized approach prevent overfitting 3. Selected a very minimal 10, 16 and 17 genes from the Colon, Prostrate and DLBCL dataset respectively	1. The CBPLR directly depends on the Correlation between the genes, which might make the calculation very sensitive since microarray data has a lot of genes and there might be outliers leading to bad formulations 2. If the correlation factor between two genes is equal to 1, then the methodology of CBPLR doesn't fetch a convex function

(continued)

Table 2.1 (continued)

Approach	Author and References	Objective	Method	Dataset	Pros	Cons
	Park et al. [22]	To predict the response of anti-drugs on the predicted features	The method follows a Wilcoxon Rank Sum Test (WRST) for gene ranking of the and a penalty based L1 Logistic Regression algorithm optimizes the classification by lowering the potency of the low ranked genes found by the WRST	Sanger dataset	The methodology attributes to best feature selection as well as classification resulting in a filtered output	The methodology mainly focuses on the statistical standpoint and classifies almost ignoring the biological point of view. Further studies based on both the biological and statistical standpoints need to be presented

(continued)

Table 2.1 (continued)

Approach	Author and References	Objective	Method	Dataset	Pros	Cons
Naive Bayes	Rashmi et al. [13]	To categorizes tumors as malignant and benign	The method follows the conventional Naive Bayes algorithm where each of the features of the Breast Cancer dataset are taken as independent sets of features and are used for prediction based on the Bayes theorem	Breast cancer dataset	The method is quite a simple one, and provides a good result if the dataset features are independent of one another	For cancer dataset, since the feature set are not microarrays the Naive Bayes algorithm performs without any hiccups, but for microarray analysis the consideration of independency of the genes might lead to sensitive calculation and the process needs to be reconsidered

(continued)

Table 2.1 (continued)

Approach	Author and References	Objective	Method	Dataset	Pros	Cons
Decision tree	Mohammadzadeh et al. [14]	To predict the mortality rate of the people suffering from gastric cancer and also to extract the most important features leading to the mortality	The methodology implemented decision trees based on CART architecture and progressed by first dividing the patients into two distinct groups of dead or alive. 80% of the total dataset was utilized for training purposes and node formation was done without any stopping rules thereby producing maximum depths. To remove unwanted branches the pruning process was utilized which trimmed down the extra splits	Own dataset consisting of 216 gastric cancer patients	The methodology is quite simple and effective and can be easily structured with medical data	Decision Tree based methodology is quite unstable and a smaller change can make volatile changes to the classification. A Random Forest is much more reliable in such a scenario

(continued)

Table 2.1 (continued)

Approach	Author and References	Objective	Method	Dataset	Pros	Cons
	Carmona-Bayonas et al. [23]	To classify patients suffering from cancer or pulmonary embolism as higher risk of complications within the 15 days time period	The method follows an exhaustive Chi-square automatic interaction detection or CHAID based algorithm for the Decision Trees where Chi-Square test is utilized to split the nodes, until no significant statistical differences were observed. The chosen significance statistical value was set at 0.05, which acts as the driving criteria for splitting	Observational cancer-associated pulmonary embolism registry who suffered consecutive cases and had received care at several (14) Spanish hospitals between the years of 2004–2015	Time complexity is quite lower and decision trees provide quite a simpler approach to solving such a necessary problem	1. The decision tree models are sometimes unstable and sensible to bad evaluation and a better approach of random forest could be adopted for better confidence 2. The dataset utilized has higher intrinsic constraint and a work on a better dataset would have set the tone of better confidence

(continued)

Table 2.1 (continued)

Approach	Author and References	Objective	Method	Dataset	Pros	Cons
K-Nearest neighbors	Kar et al. [15]	To precisely classify cancer subgroups of microarray data based on Particle Swarm Optimization and KNN	The method utilizes a particle swarm optimization algorithm for the gene selection of cancer subgroup categorization microarray dataset and follows it up with k-fold cross-validation of the KNN algorithm. The hyperparameter K of the KNN is enforced in-between range 3–20 and the accuracy is evaluated based on the validation average	SRBCT (2308 genes), ALL_AML (7129), MLL (12,582) datasets	1. The methodology shows a simpler method to find out the precise classification of the cancer subgroups 2. The method forks out a whopping 6,3 and 4 genes from SRBCT, ALL_AML and MLL dataset respectively, and that too without dipping the accuracy percentage	1. Even though the methodology lands in great results it somehow falls short since several methods like Partial Least Square Variant Importance in Projection (PLSVI) and Partial Least Square Independent Variable Explanation Gain (PLSIEG) have resulted in better accuracy 2. The model overfits the data for an average of 3% in the ALL_AML data

(continued)

Table 2.1 (continued)

Approach	Author and References	Objective	Method	Dataset	Pros	Cons
	Ayyad et al. [24]	To derive a much accurate and robust classification based on a simpler weighted KNN	The methodology utilizes a modified K-nearest neighbor method to push out the classification results where it segregates classes regarding the highest weighted sum of the points lying within the radius of the new data point from the class centers	Colon Tumor (2000 genes), Leukemia (7129), Lung Cancer (12,533), Lymphoma-DLBCL (4026), Ovarian Cancer (15,154), Prostate Cancer (12,600)	1. Efficiently increases the computational time 2. It doesn't require dimensionality reduction for the prediction of microarray data	The proposed methodology wasn't validated on biological interphase and evaluations were drawn from a statistical standpoint
Support vector machine	Islam et al. [17]	To detect breast cancer utilizing a supervised machine learning algorithm namely SVM	A simple support vector machine approach was utilized which classified the data by pushing them into a higher (n−1) dimensional space and thereby separating them based on a separable hyperplane	Wisconsin breast cancer dataset	1. The proposed approach is quite simple and time-efficient 2. The approach gets a 98% accuracy, which is worthwhile based on the simplistic nature of the model	The SVM methodology even though its simple and fetches a great accuracy in this data, for a much larger dataset it crumbles. A better approach like that of a Random Forest is far superior when it comes to larger datasets

(continued)

Table 2.1 (continued)

Approach	Author and References	Objective	Method	Dataset	Pros	Cons
	Alquran et al. [25]	To detect Melanoma, risky Skin Cancer diseases using image processing and classifying based on the SVM algorithm	The methodology utilizes image processing, and extracts features using PCA, thereafter feeding a support vector machine for classification of cancer as benign or malignant, The SVM architecture follows a radial basis similarity function or a kernel, which instigate the classification by creating a separating hyperplane	In-house database of images collected from several Melanoma websites	1. Time complexity is very low 2. Accuracy achieved is above 92% which is great for a simple model	Even though the approach is very simple, its main stream accuracy falls quite below par and for a bigger dataset it is not suitable. Moreover, the entire process could be far better optimized by utilizing a convolutional neural network

(continued)

Table 2.1 (continued)

Approach	Author and References	Objective	Method	Dataset	Pros	Cons
Random Forest	Geetha et al. [18]	To detect cervical cancer, the most common malignant disease among the women, which gets intensified by the presence of certain features	The feature dependencies are extracted via a combination of principal component analysis or PCA and recursive feature elimination along with Synthetic Minority Oversampling Technique (SMOTE) [26] which then feeds forward to a CART based Random Forest, which classifies the classes of cancer based on its highest voted architecture	Cervical cancer dataset	The proposed methodology achieved an average of above 94% in all the tests namely cytology test, Biopsy test, Hinselmann test, Schiller test, thereby preserving the efficiency of the model	1. SMOTE is highly inefficient when used in higher dimensional data and an extension of it is highly necessary to evaluate for other bigger datasets 2. Evaluation metrics utilized were highly ambiguous from a biological perspective and a better and more biologically proven metric is necessary to better realize the performance

(continued)

Table 2.1 (continued)

Approach	Author and References	Objective	Method	Dataset	Pros	Cons
	Alquraishi et al. [27]	To detect the recurrence among patients suffering from breast cancer	A Random Forest classifier was utilized as the proposed methodology which was fed after the balancing of the dataset through SMOTE	Wisconsin prognostic breast cancer dataset	1. The methodology outperforms even a much fancier Deep Neural Network in its accuracy 2. Simpler and bears a lower time complexity	Even though the proposed methodology performed well with respect to a Deep Neural Network, the SMOTE architecture used is quite volatile when used with a heavier and higher dimensional dataset and presents an overall threat of volatility in performance
	Dai et al. [28]	To analyze the breast cancer diagnosis by utilizing a machine learning algorithm	A CART based random forest architecture was utilized whose trees were split up based on the Gini Impurity criterion, which set up for the voting of the classifier	Wisconsin breast cancer dataset	1. The repeated orientation of the architecture prevents overfitting 2. Accumulates a staggering 99.3% ROC accuracy	The precision achieved for the methodology was ~93%, which for a cancer like disease prediction is quite below par
Voting classifier	Kumar et al. [19]	To compare the efficiency of normal Machine Learning algorithms and the voting based algorithm on the breast cancer data	The method involves classifying based on the combination of the votes fed from three models namely Naive Bayes, SVM and J48	Obtained datasets from the University of Wisconsin Hospital, Madison	Combining the three architectures resulted in a far superior result when compared with the potency of their individual accuracy	There is a high possibility of overfitting and the methodology didn't provide a concrete way to prevent it

(continued)

Table 2.1 (continued)

Approach	Author and References	Objective	Method	Dataset	Pros	Cons
Deep boosting cascade forest	Guo et al. [21]	To classify cancer subtypes by utilizing an alternative of Deep Neural Network process	The architecture follows a multilayered Random Forest based approach which pushes out a classification by selecting out the top K level features of the decision trees contributing to the random forests	Microarray dataset: adenocarcinoma, colon and brain RNA-sequence dataset	1. The methodology solved any underfitting issues present while solving a smaller cancer dataset 2. The proposed methodology outperformed any other conventional architecture in classifying the microarray and sequence data	Even though methodology is quite precise the architecture suffers from a huge time complexity since it has to keep on making a huge number of Random Forests which itself has several decision trees linked to them

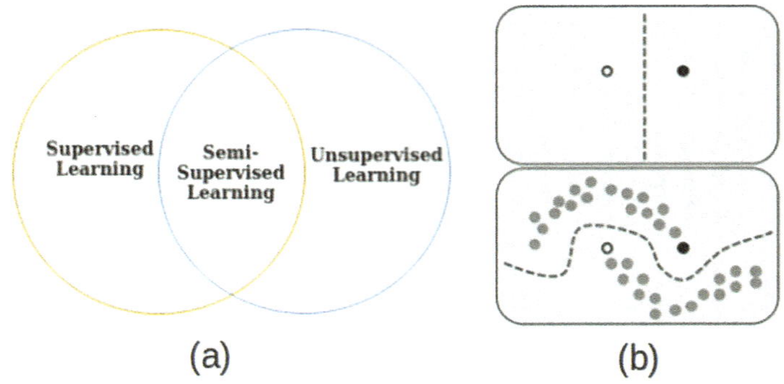

Fig. 2.4 **a** Venn diagram of sem-supervised learning. **b** The decision boundary formed from the knowledge of labelled data (white and black circles) for unlabelled data (grey circles)

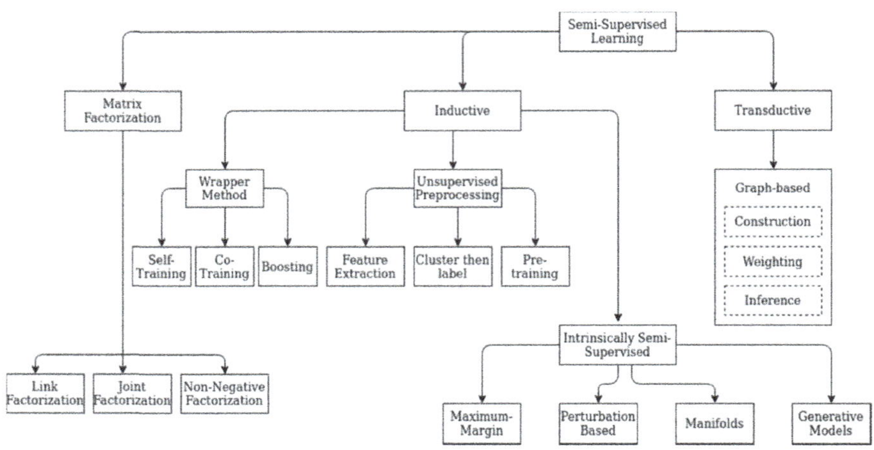

Fig. 2.5 Overview of semi-supervised learning

In the following subsections, a detailed review of each and every subgroup has been obtained at the molecular level.

2.2.2.2 Inductive Learning

It makes a decision tree from the known cancer cases to automate the knowledge acquisition process which can predict the properties of the given dataset [30]. The working principle of this algorithm is as follows:

Let, G = (g_1, g_2,……,g_n; s_i) is a cancer dataset where, $g_i \in D_j$; D_j is the domain of the attribute A_j and s_i is the class of i. The algorithm is structured as follows:

Algorithm 2.1; Inductive Learning

Begin

1. root node = G,
2. for given G do:
   a. $\forall_j \in A_j$ do:
      i. find g_i to decompose into two subsets.
      ii. compute entropy and decomposition.
      iii. decompose for the largest entropy value.
   b. $\forall_j \in A_j$ compute entropy to decompose G in i.
   c. find the attribute A^* for largest entropy value after decomposition to divide G into mutually exclusive subset G_i, i = 1,2,.....k<n. //the total number of subset(k) less than total number of points(n)
   d. label A^* as the root and G_i as it leaves.
3. for x=1 to k do:
   a. if ($G_i \in$ i) do:
      i. $G = G_i$.
      ii. repeat 2.
   b. else:
      i. Stop.

End.

The advantages and disadvantages are listed in Table 2.2.

To overcome the above shortcomings this algorithm is further improved. In the way of improvement, Inductive Learning is subdivided into three major categories. These are as follows:

Wrapper Methods: To identify the optimal feature set of gene expression data with the combination of model hypothesis and search space classifier [31]. This algorithm begins with a population (the entire microarray data) and ends with the feature subset evaluated through the learning strategy by optimizing the fitness function. Figure 2.6 obtain the flowchart of the wrapper method.

These methods provide some notable contribution in the data analytics fields namely, Genetic Algorithm (GA) [32], Artificial Bee Colony (ABC) [33], Particle Swarm Optimization (PSO) [35], Ant Colony Optimization (ACO) [34], Bat Algorithm (BA) [36], Black Hole Algorithm (BHA) [37], Grasshopper Optimization Algorithm (GOA) [38], Firefly Algorithm (FA) [39], Harmony Search Algorithm (HSA) [40], etc. But when it comes to analyzing the cancer disease high computational costs have to be paid along with a higher risk of overfitting. But it provides

Table 2.2 Advantages and disadvantages of inductive learning

Advantages	(i) Taken care of marginal values (ii) Time Complexity $O(n\log_2 n)$ (n is the data-points number)
Disadvantages	(i) Overfits the training dataset (ii) Sensitive to noise (iii) Error directly affects the entropy value

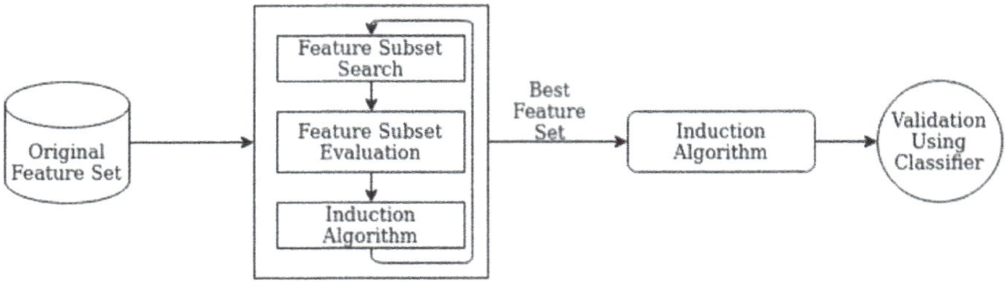

Fig. 2.6 Flow diagram of wrapper method

better performance than the filter and induction algorithm by generating an optimal feature set by reducing the noise sensitivity.

Self-training: Self-training is an exceptional semi-supervised methodology to diminish the shortcoming of labelled data classification through iterative learning. For cancer data analytics this algorithm works on differential evolution with density peaks of the dataset. It uses the structure of the dataset space to find the density peaks and train a classifier with this knowledge. Later it optimizes the positioning of newly labelled data points through differential evolution. Here, the density peaks for a cancer dataset can be calculated using Eq. (2.9), and the differential evolution is calculated using Eq. (2.10). Figure 2.7 shows the flow diagram of the self-training algorithm for cancer data analysis and Table 2.3 provides some notable contribution to this algorithm.

$$\rho_i = \sum_j \Phi(d_{ij} - d_c), \Phi(\mathrm{t}) = 1, \forall \mathrm{t} < 0 \tag{2.9}$$

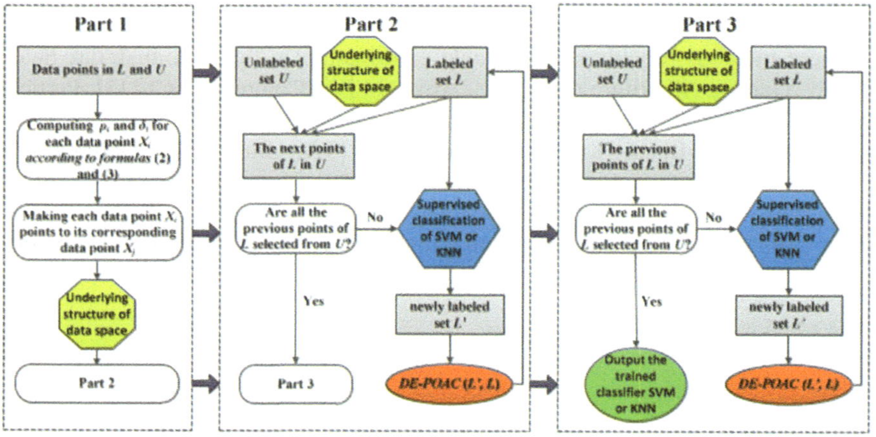

Fig. 2.7 Flow diagram of self-training algorithm [41]

Table 2.3 Literature review for self-training

Author and References	Objective	Dataset	Validation model	Pros	Cons
Xia et al. [42]	To accurate identification and classification of cancer data with Low-Rank Representation (LRR) in self-training subspace	GCM (218 tumor samples, 14 classes, 16,030 gene expression data) MBD (76 samples, 4 classes, 54,675 gene expression data)	Recall, false positive rate, matthews correlation coefficient	1. LRR helps to find the intrinsic structure of cancer data and its subtypes 2. To discriminate the key genes sparse matrix encoding has been used with better time complexity	1. Unannotated data problems exist 2. Lots of memory space has been wasted as in the sparse matrix most of the entry contains a null value
Wang et al. [43]	To train high-quality pseudo-labeled samples of cancer datasets for improvement of classification accuracy	Generate own dataset of (300 samples, 600,000 genes, 2 classes benign)	AUC, sensitivity, specificity, ROC	1. This learning algorithm has ~94% accuracy 2. Reduce the noise of the sample	1. imbalance data problem 2. Cost-sensitive issues
Azmi et al. [44]	Segment suspicious lesions of breast Functional Magnetic Resonance Imaging (FMRI)	PIDER Breast MRI dataset	Volume overlap ratio, specificity, sensitivity, precision, accuracy	1. High performance in image segmentation 2. Remove the cost of labeling	1. FMRI provides lots of information along with the suspicious lesions Ignorance of this information may produce a weak analytical model

(continued)

Table 2.3 (continued)

Author and References	Objective	Dataset	Validation model	Pros	Cons
Ting et al. [45]	Classification of breast cancer data with self regulated multilayer perceptron	MIAS dataset (56 benign cases, 39 malignant cases and 75 normal cases)	Accuracy, specificity, sensitivity and AUC	A quick solution to assist the doctors for early stage detection breast cancer	Neural Network is not the efficient solution for all cases as here AUC is very low 0.0227
Zhou et al. [46]	Provide a balanced data distribution for cancer pre-diagnosis by reducing the chance of oversampling and undersampling	GSE1456, GSE2034, GSE22210, GSE103479	Recall, precision, specificity, F1-score, G-mean	Reduce noise of imbalanced samples, redundant features to find suitable subsets for improving classification accuracy	Latest updated paper in this field. No such cons in it
Advantages	i. Simplest form of semi-supervised learning method for cancer data analysis ii. Produce Optimal subset of the cancer data iii. Reduce noise and redundant data				
Disadvantages	i. Mistakes can also reinforce themselves				

where, ρ_i is the density index, d_{ij} = distance between i and j, d_c = cutoff distance

$$U_i = X_i + K \cdot (X_{r1}, \mathrm{L} - X_i) + F_i \cdot (X_{r2}, \mathrm{L} - X_{r3}, \mathrm{L}) \quad (2.10)$$

where, F_i is the scaling factor, K ∈ [0, 1] a random number, X_{r1}, X_{r2}, X_{r3} are the data points of the labeled set L.

Though there exist several approaches to cancer data analysis with self-training, the survey of the previous five years (since 2016) is listed in Table 2.3.

Co-training: This semi-supervised learning algorithm takes two conditionally independent views of data as inputs. In the first steps, it trains two separate classifiers for two different views (labelled data) and later merges both the knowledge for further predictions over unlabelled data. The Algorithm 2.2 obtains the applications of co-training in cancer data analysis and Table 2.4 obtains some notable contribution in this field and Table 2.5 displays its advantages and disadvantges.

Table 2.4 Literature review for co-training

Author and References	Objective	Dataset	Validation model	Pros	Cons
Xia et al. [47]	A unified framework for biomedical image processing with multi view co-training	NIH pancreas segmentation dataset	DSC score	Estimate the uncertainty to survive from the stage	Work with fixed and predefined views has to consider the randomness
Yavuz and Eyupoglu [48]	Co-training with effective blood analysis features for breast cancer diagnosis	Breast Cancer Coimbra Dataset (BCCD) (9 features, 116 subjects)	Mean accuracy rate	Detect the disease in the inception phase Reduce the noise to prevent overfitting	Expensive computational cost for PCA + median filtering
Huang et al. [49]	Construct unified multi-cancer segmentation network with co-training	LiTS, KiTS, Pancreas, MOBA	DSC score HD score	Superior performance, better utilization, less inference computational cost	The most advanced work with detail description till date

Table 2.5 Advantages and disadvantages of co-training

Advantages	1. Each classifier's high confidant data points are IID samples to the other classifier
Disadvantages	2. Only works when one classifier correctly labels a data that the other classifier misclassified

Algorithm 2.2: Co-Training
Input: The labelled cancer dataset CL and unlabelled cancer dataset CU.
Output: Prediction model obtained from each view points $v_1, v_2, \ldots\ldots v_n$.
Begin

1. while(True):
   a. Sample batch $b_{cl} = (x_{cl}, y_{cl}) \in$ CL and $b_{cl} = (x_{cl}, y_{cl}) \in$ CL
   b. Compute multi view inputs $T_i(x_{cl}), T_i(x_{cu})\ \forall\ i \in \{1,2,\ldots\ldots,N\}$
   c. for j in all views:
      i. obtain predictions of each view and perform inverse rotation permutation.
      ii. $p_j(x_{cl}) = T_j^{-1} \oplus f_j \oplus T_j(x_{cl})$
      iii. $p_j(x_{cu}) = T_j^{-1} \oplus f_j \oplus T_j(x_{cu})$
   d. for j in all views:
      i. Compute label for b_{cu}.
      ii. $y_j = \prod_{j=1}^{n} p_j(x_{cu})$
   e. $l_{sup} = {}^{1}/_{b_{cl}} * \sum_{(x_{cl}, y_{cl}) \epsilon b_{cl}} \sum_{i=1}^{n} p_i(x_{cl})$
   f. $l_{cot} = {}^{1}/_{b_{cu}} * \sum_{(x_{cu}, y_{cu}) \epsilon b_{cu}} \sum_{i=1}^{n} p_i(x_{cu})$
   g. $l = l_{sup} + \lambda_{cot} l_{cot}$
   h. Optimize loss function land perform back propagation until best fit of parameters.

End.

Boosting: It is a meta semi-supervised learning method that wraps with the supervised algorithm discussed in Sect. 2.1 to increase the performance of the unlabelled dataset [50]. The objective function of this algorithm is obtained in Eq. (2.11). Figure 2.8 obtain the working principle of this algorithm and Table 2.6 obtain a literature review of boosting over the past five years and its advantages and disadvantages are listed in Table 2.7.

$$F_u(y_u, \mathrm{S}) = \sum_{ij=1}^{n_u} S^{un}\left(y_i^u - y_j^u \mathrm{uj}\right) \tag{2.11}$$

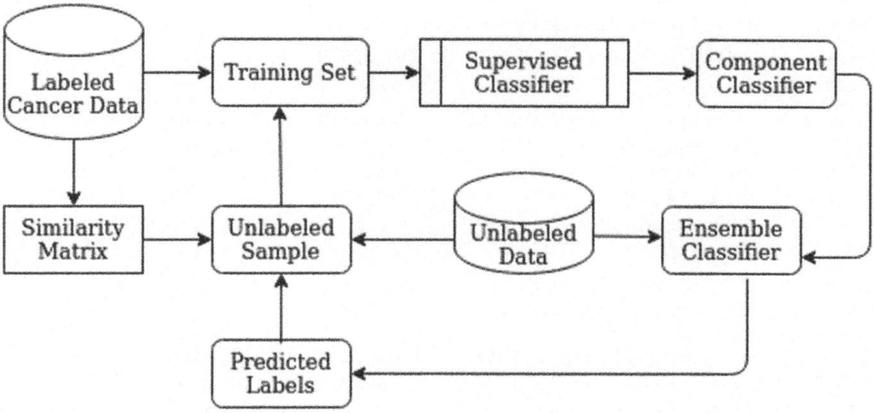

Fig. 2.8 Overview of boosting algorithm

Unsupervised Preprocessing: It is the most argumentative topic of semi-supervised learning. Some researchers treated it in unsupervised learning some treated it in semi-supervised learning. This topic is further classified into three sub-topic (a) Feature Extraction (b) Cluster then label and c) pre-training. As this chapter performs a detailed review in the later section (Sect. 2.2.3) it is decided to produce a brief literature review in this section. Tosado et al. [54] proposed a novel methodology for discriminative groupings Oropharyngeal Head and Neck Cancer Patients to progress the output predictions. Shi et al. [55] performs semi-supervised convolutional neural networks with noisy labels for historical analysis of image for cancer classification. In pre-training, Kim et al. [56] proposed a novel methodology to improve survival analysis with shared genomic information using a pan cancer database. Last but not the least, in Hsu et al. [57], breast cancer was predicted using generative adversarial networks for strong with limited size of data. It is the most advanced and effective methodology till date.

Intrinsically Semi-supervised: It is the latest subclass of the inductive learning where the unlabelled data are directly incorporated into an objective function to optimize by the learning paradigm [58, 59]. The objective function of intrinsic learning is obtained in Eq. (2.12). The main disadvantages of these sections are: Continuity assumption, Cluster assumption, Manifold assumption. In the further subclasses (e.g. Maximum-margin, perturbation, manifolds, generative models) these problems are removed simultaneously.

$$min_{w,b}\{C * \sum_{i=1}^{n} max\{1 - y_i\left(w^T x + b\right)\}^2 + (1 - C) * ||w||_1\} \tag{2.12}$$

Table 2.6 Literature review of boosting algorithm

Author and References	Objective	Dataset	Validation model	Pros	Cons
Qi et al. [51]	Adaptive functions with light driven transformable optical agents for surgery outcomes	DTE-TPECM	Sensitivity, specificity, f1-score, Cohen's kappa	Fluorescence and acoustic photo imaging	One of the most complex methodology It is impossible to implement in a normal laboratory
Kwak et al. [52]	Prostate cancer detection with morphological characteristics from multiview boosting	TMA1, TMA2, TMA3, TMA4, TMA5	AUC, confidence interval (CI)	Accomplished incorporating information from various resolutions Excessive potential for developing digital pathology	Lack of robustness Experiments perform on very less data
Koyasu et al. [53]	Radiomics approach to figure out Estimated glomerular filtration rate (EGFR) mutation of lung cancer by gradient tree boosting	(32 squamous cell carcinomas and 156 adenocarcinomas) (38 mutant and 100 wild-type samples)	AUC, ten-fold cross validation	Useful for classifying EGFR mutation grade and histological subtypes in lung cancer	Very low accuracy Bayesian optimization is not a good optimization algorithm

Table 2.7 Advantages and disadvantages of boosting

Advantages	1. Performance improvement with multitude unlabeled data 2. Effective calculation and iterative boosting algorithm 3. Exploiting manifold and cluster assumption with classification
Disadvantages	1. Time and computation are expensive 2. Hard to implement in real time platforms 3. Complexity of the classification increases

where, w = weight vector, b = base value, C = constant normalizer. This algorithm doesn't rely on any supervised base learners, it is an extension of existing supervised learners by including the unlabelled samples.

Maximum Margin: In cancer data analysis, the gene microarray data is given as (x_1, y_1), (x_2, y_2).... (x_n, y_n) ∈ Rm × {C_1,..., C_l}. Where, x_i and y_i are the m-dimensional vector and class marker, respectively. The supreme margin goals after transformation to maximize the distances between classes using Eq. (2.13).

$$J = 1/2 * \sum_{i=1}^{l} \sum_{j=1}^{l} p_i * p_j * d(c_i, c_j) \tag{2.13}$$

In the past few decades, several researchers obtained a notable contribution in cancer data analysis, using this algorithm. Table 2.8 provides a brief literature review on it and Table 2.9 provides its advantages and disadvantages.

Perturbation Method: To overcome the disadvantages of the maximum-margin method perturbation is proposed in 2016 [63]. This methodology combines knowledge of semi-supervised learning with the convolutional neural network to obtain its

Table 2.8 Literature review on maximum margin

Author and References	Objective	Dataset	Validation model	Pros	Cons
Cui et al. [60]	Gene selection on microarray data with sparse maximum margin discriminant analysis	Colon, Acute Leukemia, Breast, Glioma, Prostate	Accuracy, AUC, sensitivity, specificity	Obtain a proper decision boundary between each and every class	Prone to overfitting, high variance
Niijima and Kuhara [61]	Recursive gene selection with maximum margin	Colon, Prostate, Leukemia, Medulloblastoma, Breast cancer, MLL, SRBCT, CNS, NCI60	Standard and average error rates	Less sensitive to noise normally extends to multi-class problems No parameter tuning	A little high error rate (close to 13%)
Holmes et al. [62]	Evaluate the success rate of metastatic castration-resistant prostate cancer with CT–guided bone biopsies	mCRPC dataset	Success rate, HU index	Easy to implement Implemented in real-time scenario	Very low accuracy (~69%)

Table 2.9 Advantages and disadvantages of maximum margin

Advantages	(i) Efficiently taken care of the non-linear datasets (ii) Provide stability
Disadvantages	(i) Feeding the data into the objective function needs lots of preprocessing (ii) Required a long training time

objective function (Eq. 2.14). Figure 2.9 gives a brief overview of the structure of perturbation and its advantages and disadvantages are displayed in Table 2.10. As it is a new technique it is not rigorously applied in cancer data analysis till now but this algorithm has the potential to prove its efficiency in near future.

$$l_u^{TS} = \sum_{i=1}^{N} \sum_{j=1}^{n-1} \sum_{k=j+1}^{n} \left|\left| f^j\left(T^j(x_i)\right) - f^k\left(T^k(x_i)\right)\right|\right|^2 \tag{2.14}$$

where, l_u^{TS} = loss function of the neural networks, f^j = cost function, T^j and T^k are the transpose with rank j and k respectively.

Manifolds: This is a method of a finite sample analysis using unlabelled data to quantify the potential gain. It computes the Helinger distance and size-constrained spectral

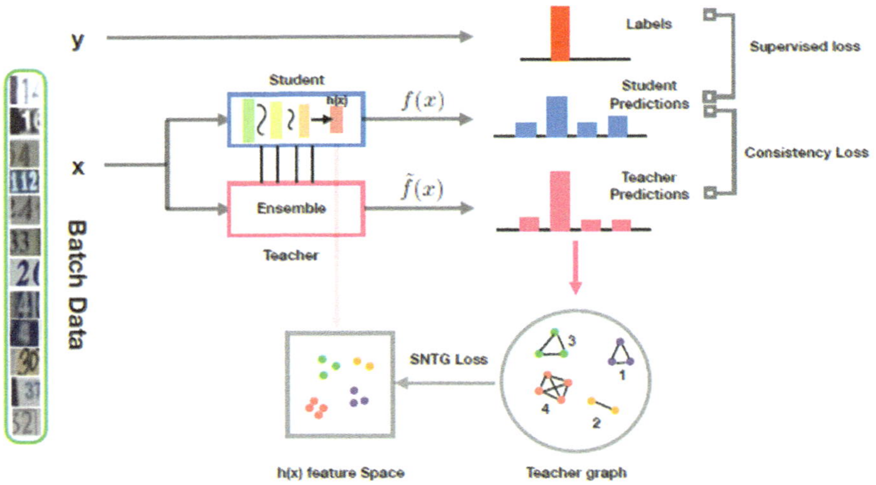

Fig. 2.9 Overview of the perturbation methods [64]

Table 2.10 Advantages and disadvantages of perturbation method

Advantages	(i) Regularization capabilities (ii) Work as classifier as well as clusterer
Disadvantages	(i) Difficulty to choose proper kernel size

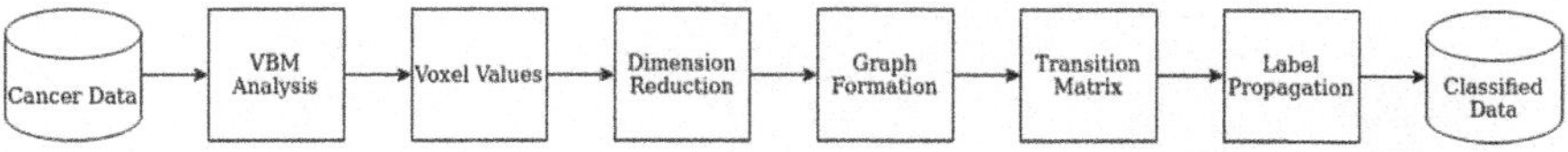

Fig. 2.10 Application of manifolds in cancer data analysis

Table 2.11 Literature review of manifolds

Author and References	Objective	Dataset	Validation model	Pros	Cons
Cruz-Barbosa and Vellido [65]	Human brain tumor analysis with partly labeled MRS data by manifold learning	SV1-H	Accuracy, sensitivity, specificity	High accuracy Perform better than SVM and Laplacian method	Should be compared with other validation accuracy, sometimes high accuracy tends to overfitting
Feng [66]	Differentiation based optimization to classify the microarray data	SRBCT, DLBCL and brain tumor	Accuracy, precision, recall	Effective method with high accuracy	Demonstrates with very less amount of data

Table 2.12 Advantages and disadvantages of manifold

Advantages	(i) Provides reliability in terms of cross validation (ii) Lucid mathematical framework
Disadvantages	(i) Optimization is difficult due to bad local optima

clustering to extend the benefits of semi-supervised learning. Figure 2.10 shows the application of manifolds in cancer data analysis and Table 2.11 and Table 2.12 obtains the literature review and advantages and disadvantages of this methodology.

Generative Models: Here, the joint probability has been used for the curriculum learning. It first estimates the likelihoods for the unlabelled data then tuning the parameters for the best fit. Later it calculated log likelihood jointly with labelled and unlabelled data and lastly it balanced the output of the objective function to obtain the final result. Figure 2.11 obtained an overview of the generative models and Table 2.13 provides a brief literature review about this methodology.

With these generative models, the inductive learning section has been concluded. The next section provides a detailed overview of transductive learning.

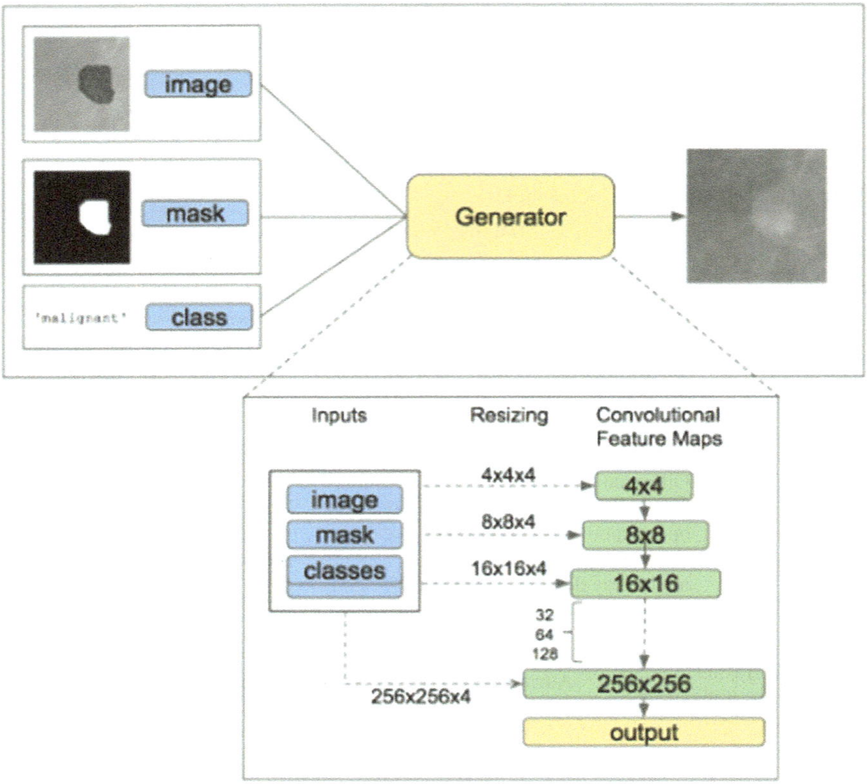

Fig. 2.11 Overview of the generative models [68]

2.2.2.3 Transductive Learning

It provides all possible sets of predictions for the unlabelled dataset. Basically, it defines a graph for all data points (labelled and unlabelled) with pairwise similarity encoding for all data points corresponding to their weighted edges. An optimized objective function is written in Eq. (2.15).

$$f(x) = \lambda * (y_i' - y_i)^2 + \sum_{i=1}^{n} \sum_{j=1}^{n} W_{ij} * (y_i' - y_i)^2 \tag{2.15}$$

where, W_{ij} = weighted edges, λ = normalization factor, y_i' = predicted label, y_i = actual label. As this transductive learning is a graph based approach, it can be further sub-categorised into three subclasses.

Table 2.13 Literature review of generative models

Author and References	Objective	Dataset	Validation model	Pros	Cons
Ding et al. [67]	Interpretable reduction of dimension of a cell transcriptome dataset with deep generative models	CyTOF, GPLVM	Accuracy, sensitivity, specificity	A detailed evaluation from all the perspectives	Too complex to implement
Chang et al. [68]	Analysis of pediatric wbMRIs using generative models	90 de-identified patients	FID, DFD, FPR	Opens a new era of cancer research	High false positive rate (~30%)
Wu et al. [69]	Perform data augmentation for mammogram classification	DDSM	AUC	Able to generate realistic lesions Improve classification performance	Need more validation parameters to evaluate

(i) Construction model, (ii) Weighted model, and (iii) Inference model. Table 2.14 provides a brief literature review of each of these techniques. Table 2.15 describes its advantages and disadvantages.

The transductive learning section has been concluded here. In the next section a new semi-supervised learning approach has been surveyed.

2.2.2.4 Matrix Factorization

It is the last section in the review of semi-supervised learning where a class of collaborative filter algorithms first implemented for a recommender system. In cancer data analysis, it decomposed the gene interaction matrix into the product of two lower dimensionality matrices for molecular level analysis. Algorithm 2.3 gives a brief overview of the sparse non-negative matrix factorization [76]. Along with that, Fig. 2.12 provides a brief overview of the joint non-negative matrix factorization and Table 2.16 provides a literature review of this ultimate class of semi-supervised learning.

Table 2.14 Literature survey of the transductive learning

Methods	Author and References	Objective	Dataset	Validation model	Pros	Cons
Construction model	Khan et al. [70]	Apply transductive learning to find the influence of prostate tumor with image based prognostics employing	3390 images of 226 patients	CI, sensitivity, specificity, criterion	beneficial in ensuring robust results High accuracy	Theoretical model, experiments not conducted with human subjects
	Khan [71]	Predicting advanced prostate cancer with prostatectomy sample for early indications through transductive semi-supervised survival analysis	262 patients, 8 clinical features, 37 PSAR 342 patients, 43 PSAR	CI, sensitivity, specificity, criterion	Rapidly integrating different information domains	Not evaluating supplementary existence analysis algorithms Have to discover other performance standards
Weighted model	Li et al. [72]	Gene expression profile based cancer classification with transductive local fisher discriminant analysis	GCM, acute leukemia	Sensitivity, specificity	Provides a combination of the discriminative criterion in supervised learning High performance	Very simple mathematical model. It can be implemented in real-life scenario

(continued)

Table 2.14 (continued)

Methods	Author and References	Objective	Dataset	Validation model	Pros	Cons
	Zemmal et al. [73]	CAD based automated classification of Mammographic abnormalities	DDSM	Sensitivity, Specificity, Accuracy	For unlabelled data it provides better accuracy	Lack of analysis how they overcome the problem
Inference model	Khan [74]	Combining biometric measurements of prostate samples through interval kernels	Prostatectomy data, prostate biopsy data	CI, sensitivity, specificity, criterion	Provides better guidance in treatment decision making	Does not perform experiments on any human subjects
	Khan and Kulikowski [75]	Expecting progressive prostate cancer endpoints from primary warnings via transductive semi-supervised regression	43 sample PSAR and 12 samples CF	CI, sensitivity, specificity, criterion	For prostate cancer this model provides higher performance accuracy	This model is not generic and also suffers from detailed analysis

Table 2.15 Advantages and disadvantages of transductive learning

Advantages	(i) Best mathematical framework (ii) Provides high accuracy if the graphs fit at the first attempt (iii) works for both directed and undirected graphs
Disadvantages	(i) Feature sets might not be able to split (ii) Performance will be decreased if the graph does not fit in the first attempt (iii) Less stable: vulnerable to graph structure and edge weights

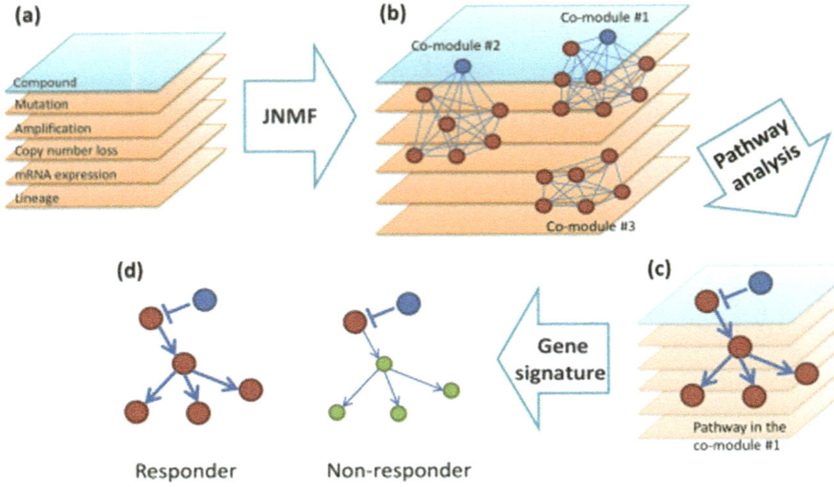

Fig. 2.12 Joint non-negative matrix factorization in cancer data analysis [80]

Algorithm 2.3 Sparse Non-Negative Matrix Factorization

Begin:

1. Initialize W and H two random matrices having (N x K) and (K x M) dimension, respectively.
2. Reset the column of W to make a unique normalization.
3. Repeat until touch the maximum number of allowable repetitions.
   a. Solve $W_{(ia+1)} = W_{ia}(AH^T)_{ia}/(WHH^T)_{ia}$
   b. Reset the column of H for a unit normalization.
   c. . Solve for each j
   $$min_{H_1} = \{0.5 * ||A_j - WH_j||^2\} + 0.5 * \lambda||H_j||^2$$

End

After matrix factorization the gene expression data has been coagulated into several modules then a pathway analysis has been performed to get the molecular structure. After that, gene signature provides a detailed analysis which module responds to a particular drug field. Table 2.16 provides the rest of the survey.

Table 2.16 Literature survey

Methods	Author and References	Objective	Dataset	Validation model	Pros	Cons
NMF	Wang et al. [77]	Non-negative matrix factorization model with Huber loss and sparse graph regularization for cancer data analysis	TCGA	Accuracy, Macro-R, Macro-P, Macro-F	Differentially expressed genes can be selected Enhance robustness Preserve data geometry	Detailed analysis of sparsity based approach has been needed
	Gao et al. [78]	Gene co-expression network analysis with integrated graph regularized NMF	TCGA	CHOL, PAAD	Node relationships are improved due to construction of the network Superior data fusion and reconstruction	Clinical validation and analysis are very much required
jNMF	Zhang and Zhang [79]	Joint non-negative matrix factorization for integrative cancer data analysis	Colon, Leukaemia, DLBCL, TCGA	AUC, time	High competitive performance with attractive computational speed	Needs to improve on statistical analysis
	Deng et al. [80]	Multi-constrained joint non-negative matrix factorization with application to imaging genomic study of lung metastasis in soft tissue sarcomas	FDG-PET with DNA Methylation	AUC	It can exactly find modules connected to lung diseases or sarcoma Mine more complex biological mechanisms	No prior cons at all

Along with that, Link matrix factorization is a new concept in this field but till now it is not applied to any cancer data analysis. That's why it will be discussed in the future scope of this chapter. This section tries to cover a detailed analysis of the existing semi-supervised approach applied on cancer databases. In the subsequent section a detailed review of the unsupervised learning has been provided.

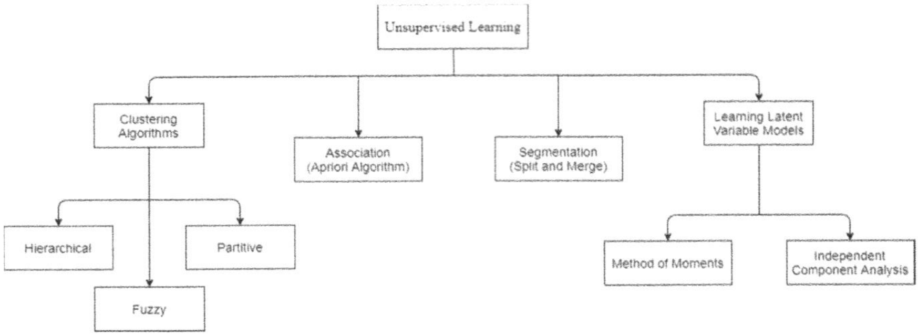

Fig. 2.13 Broad classification of unsupervised learning methods

2.2.3 *Unsupervised Learning*

Unsupervised Learning is another branch of Machine Learning which is utilized to identify patterns in data with no pre-existing information about the labels and with very little human intervention. Unlike supervised learning where human-labelled data is necessary, unsupervised learning uses unlabelled data and provides an insight on the probable classes present in the dataset which is then used to broadly classify the data. The main benefit of unsupervised learning lies in the fact that it does not require any human-labelled data which saves a lot of manual effort that is otherwise used to individually label every data point in a particular dataset. The broad classification of unsupervised learning methods has been depicted in Fig. 2.13.

2.2.3.1 Split and Merge Algorithm

The split and merge is an image segmentation algorithm that recursively splits an image into four quadrants regarding some homogeneity principles and then merges the quadrants back together. The homogeneity criterion is responsible for determining if a given quadrant needs to be split any further. The homogeneity criterion can be defined as per the requirement of the work to be done and the features of images to be processed. For cancer data analysis this algorithm is mainly used as a filtering step to get the region of interest from the images of tumours.This process has been successfully used to help detect breast cancer from mammogram images as shown in [87, 88].

2.2.3.2 Various Types of K-means Methodology

K-means is a partition grouping approach in which each group or cluster is related with a centroid and every data point is assigned to the group with the closest centroid. It segments n samples into precisely k various groups in which each item has a place with the closest mean based on the Eq. (2.16). The best number of k clusters prompting the best partition (separation) isn't previously known and must be initialized.

$$J = \sum_{j=1}^{k} \sum_{i=1}^{n} d(x) \tag{2.16}$$

where the objective function is referred to as J, the cluster number is initialized by k, the sample number is n and $d(x)$ is the distance function. Some variants to deal with the limitations of traditional k-means like centroid initialization, accuracy, outliers etc. are mentioned below along with their use for cancer data analysis.

K-means++ guarantees a more intelligent introduction of the centroids and improves the nature of the clustering though it is computationally more costly than the traditional K-means. Thus, the run-time for convergence to optimal is definitely decreased for K-means++.

Spherical K-means, uses cosine uniqueness and standardizes all the vectors. Spherical K-means is equivalent to anticipating our perceptions to the unit circle and afterward using any suitable distance measure [98].

Mini-Batch K-means is an adjusted variant of k-means that makes updates to the centroids of clusters utilizing scaled down clusters of samples as opposed to the whole dataset, which can make it quicker for huge datasets, and maybe more robust to statistical noise.

Rough K-means is used in [94] where a novel algorithm for image segmentation of leukaemia is explained whichmerges the powers of a soft rough set and rough k-means clustering algorithm. As determination of the cluster numbers is a problematic work in segmentation. The hybrid histogram-based soft covering rough k-means (HSCRKM) algorithm overcomes this limitation, and is presented to accurately segment the image of the nucleus of leukaemia.

EK means (Kernel K means): Although, the Kernel k-means is an extension of the original k-means algorithm recognizes nonlinearly distinct clusters to overcome the initialization issue of clustering and because of its steady nature and search technique, it situates itself close to optimal solutions dodging helpless neighbourhood minima. However Number of cluster centres should be predefined and the algorithm is quite complex in nature with large computational complexity. In [95], the EK-means clustering algorithm is utilized for segmentation of the pre-processed CT images followed by dimension reduction using Gray Level Co-occurrence matrix or GLCM which increases the accuracy of classification of Back Propagation Neural Network up to 90.87%. In [96], the goal to cluster lung cancer from non-involved (blood) samples using chromosome-wide spatial Copy Number Variation (CNV)s is achieved by utilizing kernel k means.

Quantum K-means: clustering unlike classical K-Means, that takes O(LNpK) time, this new approach takes only O(LNK) time after L iterations with N data points of dimension p. This algorithm, thus, subsequently, performs in a way that is better than conventional algorithms when dimension p of data is enormous [97].

H-k-means: A hybrid k-mean and k-medoid algorithm which is efficient to deal with datasets containing noise and outliers [98]. At first cluster centres are recognized by utilizing the procedure of k-mean algorithm in the main emphasis. Cluster-means are recalculated after transitory expulsion of the most distant cluster from each respective cluster's centre and a reference point (medoid) is picked as a new group mean for each bunch which is closest to the recalculated mean. Same cycle is followed for ensuing iterations until the calculation joins.

2.2.3.3 Self-organizing Map

Self-organizing Map (SOM) is a type of neural network (artificial) utilized for representation and examination of high-dimensional datasets. SOM encourages introduction of high dimensional datasets into lower dimensional ones, typically 1-D, 2-D and 3-D. A SOM is shaped from a matrix of nodes or units to which the dataset is introduced. Each node is linked with the input and there is no association among them. SOM is a topology saving strategy and keeps the local relations in its mapping presentation. In [102] SOM is applied to pre-processed data to create patient cohort clusters and then DBSCAN divides the clusters into 9 cohorts based on survivability time. Finally, these 9 cohorts are fed to the Multilayer Perceptron (MLP) model for overall survival prediction.

2.2.3.4 Density-Based Spatial Clustering of Applications with Noise (DBSCAN)

It is a clustering method regarding density based that recognizes particular clusters in the dataset, in view of the possibility that a cluster in the dataset is a continuous area of high point thickness, isolated from other such clusters by contiguous areas of depressed point thickness. The algorithm does not work admirably when managing clusters of differing densities. While it is extraordinary at isolating high thickness clusters from low thickness clusters, it battles with clusters of comparative thickness and dataset with high dimensionality. In [104] 268 collected breath samples were pre-processed and dimensionally reduced before DBSCAN clustering was performed to improve e-nose model's performance for detection of lung cancer.

2.2.3.5 Model Based Clustering

It is a probabilistic based approach that gives a principled alternative over heuristic approaches to overcome the issue of selecting 'good clusters'. [101] utilizes a Bayesian Hidden Markov model (HMM) with Gaussian Mixture (GM) method to model the DNA duplicate number alteration over the genome. In [100], Bayesian Hidden Markov Model & GM Clustering technique is utilized to model the DNA with a scalable approach and performs well as compared to the existing approaches.

Here Table 2.17 is listed for the overall literature review on Unsupervised Learning methods for cancer data analysis.

2.3 Challenges and Issues in Data Analysis of Cancer Disease

Over the years, even though meticulous learning approaches have been induced and have resonated and enriched the field of Cancer Data Analysis, most of the work has been improvised based on old techniques, which are novelized with minor improvements. Moreover, most of the work has focused on the statistical perspective, even though a precise care on Biological inference was needed, which was absent, but was of utter importance due to the Biological output the work adheres to. The supervised based learning techniques on cancer data ushers a somewhat slow increase in newer ideas due to the higher amount of saturation it has achieved over the years, thereby curving old techniques with minor alterations. The unsupervised techniques even though catching a higher popularity still resembles somewhat the decade long techniques when dealing with cancer data. Moreover, the introduction of Deep Learning has thwarted the entire Machine Learning based approaches on cancer data analysis, since it has somewhat been synonymous to low accuracy, which is very critical in medical field.

2.4 Comparative Study Through Validation Parameters

All the methodologies discussed in Sect. 2.2, with respect to the cancer data analysis are validated in the context of several parameters. Among them, error rate, classification accuracy, specificity, sensitivity, Precision, F1-score, AUC, ROC, Cohen's kappa, are frequently used to validate the models. Figure 2.14 shows a detailed comparison of supervised, semi-supervised, and unsupervised learning regarding these validation parameters.

From Fig. 2.14, it can be clearly concluded that Semi-Supervised Learning provides slightly enhanced validation performance than its counterparts in the case of cancer data analysis.

Table 2.17 Literature review for unsupervised learning methods

Approach	Author and References	Objective	Method	Dataset	Pros	Cons
Hierarchical clustering [83]	Nidheesh et al. [82]	To identify potential new subtypes of cancer from genomic dataset	The method used is based on Ward's framework for hierarchical clustering algorithm and it uses the average value of the Silhouette index as the objective function to get the optimal cluster numbers	NCBI GEO [89] Data from consensus clustering [90] RNA-Seq Pan-Cancer gene expression dataset [91]	1. The estimated cluster numbers closer to the ground truth 2. The quality of the clusters are also better 3. The results produced are stable as it takes a deterministic approach	1. In case of clusters with greater inter-cluster distances this method tends to go for a lower number of clusters
	Xie et al. [84]	To identify the differential genes that can be used to check if a person is affected with colon cancer	Three step optimal gene process, using Fisher function, Chameleon algorithm and Information index for classification to obtain the subset	Colon cancer dataset (2000 genes, 62 samples 40 cancerous and 22 normal)	This method selects a very low number of genes which is 1/400 th of the original dataset and yet manages to get a respectable classification accuracy of around 85%	Some other methods manage to get a bit more accuracy (around 89%) by selecting just a few more genes

(continued)

Table 2.17 (continued)

Approach	Author and References	Objective	Method	Dataset	Pros	Cons
	Sharma et al. [81]	To implement a divisive hierarchical clustering algorithm with lower computational complexity and equivalent accuracy to its Hierarchical Agglomerative Clustering counterparts	A novel divisive hierarchical algorithm is implemented (named DRAGON) which removes clusters from a set based on a likelihood function	AML (25 AML, 47 ALL, 7129 genes), MLL (24 ALL, 20 MLL, 28 AML, 12582 genes) Mutation dataset (416 + 90 samples, 1636 genes)	Even with divisive hierarchical clustering it has a time complexity of O (n^2c) compared to O (2^nc) complexity of most other such algorithms	The clustering accuracy is reasonably good for some datasets but it fails for other datasets
	Weghorn and Sunyaev [85]	Determining the coding point mutation using a hierarchical framework to find cancer driver genes and highly mutated genes	The expected distribution of per gene synonymous mutation is calculated which is then compared to the observed distribution to get the count of expected synonymous mutations in the genome-wide distribution	17 cancer types with 4476 patients from tumour portal dataset	Good classification accuracy across a number of different datasets and can detect a considerable amount of negative selection signals for some of the datasets	There is room for further improvement for detection of negative selection signals in tumors which play an equivalent role as positive selection but are considerably harder to detect
K means [93]	Clayman et al. [92]	To assess the extent to which the 978 landmark genes of L1000 dataset improves clustering results w.r.t random set of non landmark genes	PCA K-means	L1000 dataset (129 157 samples, 22 678 total genes, 978 landmark genes, & 1300 non-landmark genes)	Study successfully assessed how selected landmark genes improves clustering performance & can be more predictive	Non linear or independent correlations are ignored in PCA so there is loss of information

(continued)

Table 2.17 (continued)

Approach	Author and References	Objective	Method	Dataset	Pros	Cons
	Inbarani and Azar [94]	To accurately segment the image of leukemia nucleus using HSCRKM clustering	HSCRKM clustering	ALL-IDB dataset (368 images—175 benign & 193 malignant were occupied for analysis of experiment)	A suitable hybrid method for accurate segmentation of leukemia nucleus images with an overall estimation accuracy of 82%	The method is not suitable in terms of computation cost for multiple color images
	Sangamithraa et al. [95]	To show that EK means clustering is a better segmentation method for CT images	CT images are pre-processed using median filter & wiener filter followed by segmentation using EK-mean clustering	CT images	Effectively addresses the problem of Lung Tumour Segmentation Has an accuracy of 90.87%	With the computational complexity of O (n^2), the method is not suitable for very large datasets
	Haq and Bonny [97]	To detect the cancer type utilizing the mRNA-seq dataset by applying Quantum K-Means clustering	Quantum K means	Normal 'gene expression cancer RNA-Seq' data from UCI database	Gives evidence of the idea of ease of use of the Quantum Algorithms in clinical and medical care applications that can provide high accuracy in future	The methodology dooms to a larger inaccuracy through the probabilistic dependencies and a far robust approach is necessary for better accuracy

(continued)

Table 2.17 (continued)

Approach	Author and References	Objective	Method	Dataset	Pros	Cons
DBSCAN	Li et al. [104]	To design an e-nose system regarding ten gas sensors and two humidity sensors for detection of lung cancers	Preprocessing & dimensional reduction was followed by DBSCAN & AP to detect high density samples & estimate clusters from them. For classification SVM was used	268 breath samples were taken (153 from healthy samples including 10 healthy smokers and 115 from lung cancer patients)	1. It is a very new method with a promising performance 2. Gets accuracy above 85%	1.The lab setup is complex and expensive 2. The system performance though good in experimental conditions should be validated against a larger cohort
Apriori	Akshaya et al. [86]	To find an effective set of rules for analysing association item sets which can help predict cancer	Rules were derived by association rule mining which were further filtered and grouped by using an interest measure named Confidence	GBSG2 (Breast cancer dataset) BIOPSY (Tumour dataset) WPBC (Prognostic Breast Cancer dataset)	1. High accuracy across all the datasets used 2. False alarm rate is much lower as compared to other methods	More datasets could have been used to prove its robustness across multiple sets of data
Split & merge	Jothilakshmi and Raaza [87]	To increase the diagnostic accuracy in the image processing field by finding the region of interest by using image segmentation and thus reduce mis-classification	Following data collection and pre-processing the region of interest were identified by the split and merge segmentation algorithm which were then utilized for dimension reduction and classification	Mini-MIAS (50 images) UC Irvine machine learning repository (569 images)	Has appreciable prediction accuracy of 94%	The accuracy can be further improved by fine tuning the parameters for segmentation and feature selection

(continued)

Table 2.17 (continued)

Approach	Author and References	Objective	Method	Dataset	Pros	Cons
	Kaur and Sharma [88]	To classify cancer cells from normal cells in Mammograms using segmentation to analyze features and Bayesian classifier for classification	The images are scanned using morphological scanning and then split and merge segmentation is used to extract the features which are finally fed into the Bayesian classifier for classification	MIRE breast cancer image dataset	Quick and easy to understand implementation of the algorithms. Faster than other weight based classification approaches	Evaluation results are not properly presented and no quantitative values are available for depicting accuracy of the approach
Fuzzy based	Rundo et al. [99]	To propose a fully automated prostate segmentation method on Multispectral MRI anatomical data	Fuzzy C means	Prostate cancer patient dataset comprising 7 patients	1. A novel approach that performs clustering on co-registered T1W & T2W MR image series 2. FCM on MRI anatomical dataset enhanced the attained prostate ROI considerably	Experiment performed on a smaller cohort (7 patients)

(continued)

Table 2.17 (continued)

Approach	Author and References	Objective	Method	Dataset	Pros	Cons
Model based [101]	Bulut et al. [100]	To identify the genetic disorder (copy number change) and the model of disease diagnosis	Bayesian hidden Markov model & GM clustering method is utilized to model the DNA	Array-based comparative genomic hybridization (CGH) dataset from sample PA.C.Dan.G	1. A scalable approach to deal with infection of tumor in tissue specimens and normalization errors 2. Model performs well as compared to existing approaches	This method has high computational complexity
	Kasa et al. [103]	To perform patient subtyping using High Dimensional Gaussian mixture Copula model method	Copula based Gaussian mixture model	Gene expression datasets used: Leukemia, Colon-cancer, Prostate cancer, Breast cancer, khan500 & NC160, lusc-Methyl & lusc-rnaseq Clinical dataset used: SCADI	1. Outperforms the state-of-art model based clustering techniques 2. Robust in dealing with outliers 3. LASSO penalized BIC prevents component calculation errors	Even though the efficiency is great, the detection of the cancer subtypes is based on statistical abstract and the paper doesn't showcase any biological evaluation
SOM	Shukla et al. [102]	To develop a model to understand breast cancer survivability in occurence of missing value, get insights of factors connected with survival of patients and to group patients with similar characteristics	A divide and conquer approach is applied to the pre-processed dataset. SOM is utilized to produce patient cohort groups which are fed into the MLP for final classification	SEER program dataset	The SOM method is more efficient than ad hoc methods in capturing similarities of the linear combination of features and handling missing data points	The use of 2D SOM causes an important compression of the dataset and there is a risk of information loss

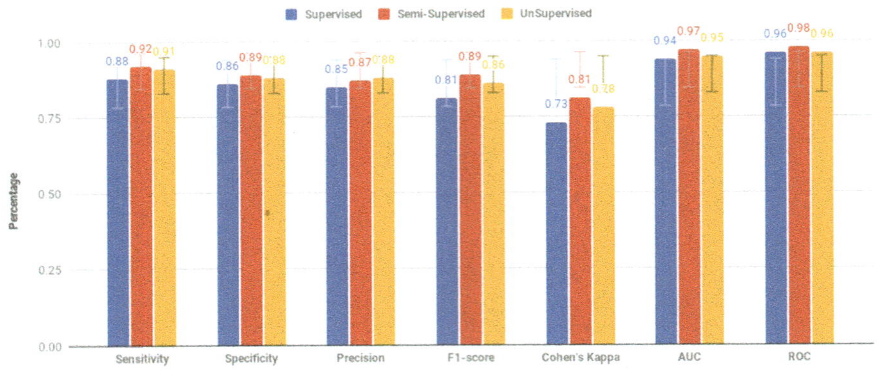

Fig. 2.14 Comparison of the supervised, semi-supervised and unsupervised learning regarding validation parameters

2.5 Comparative Study of Data Analysis in Cancer Disease

In Sect. 2.3, a precise analysis of all the existing cancer data analysis methodologies has been obtained in terms of validation parameters. But in review, besides the validation comparison, an overall performance evaluation needs to be obtained with appropriate statistical analysis. This section compares all the data analysis models related to cancer data analysis based on time analysis, implementation details, input data, computational complexities, Real-time implementation, Reliability. Table 2.18 shows a comparative study of these above-mentioned approaches and Figs. 2.15, 2.16 and 2.17 obtained a statistical comparison based on research publications, their

Table 2.18 Comparison of data analysis techniques

Characteristics	Supervised	Semi-supervised	Unsupervised
Input data	Known and labelled cancer dataset	Both labelled as well as unlabelled cancer dataset	Only unlabelled cancer data
Computational complexity	Very Complex due to stricts rules	Less complex than supervised but more than unsupervised	Less complex as no such strict rules
Problem-faced during the implementation	As all the rules are previously defined the dataset has to be modified according to the rules	As it has to tackle both labelled and unlabelled data so its implementation became very complex	No prior problem faced during the implementation
Reliability	Accurate and reliable	Accurate and reliable	Moderate accurate and reliable
Time analysis	Moderate pace	Very high	Very fast

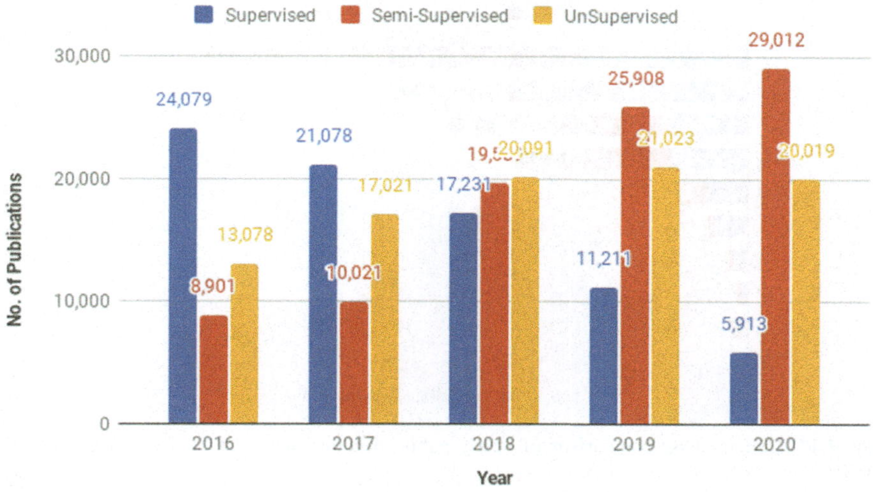

Fig. 2.15 Number of publications on cancer data analysis in the last five years

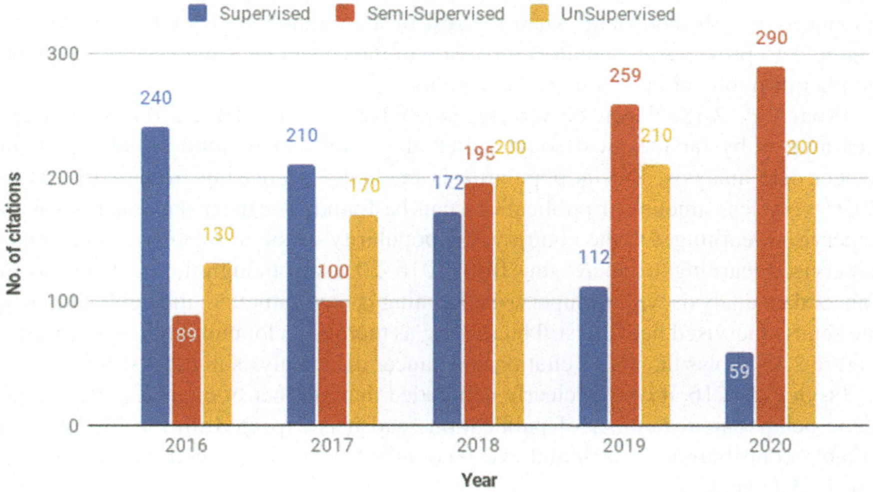

Fig. 2.16 The number of citations on cancer data analysis in the last five years

citations, and country-wise contribution for a better understanding of how the data analysis trend has been changed in the past five years.

From Table 2.11 it can be concluded that supervised learning is easy to implement but a huge problem is faced in the data preprocessing phase that's why it takes much more time than unsupervised learning but it always provides highly accurate results. Besides that, unsupervised learning is a highly responsive algorithm that returns a quick output without any label but compromises its accuracy. Lastly,

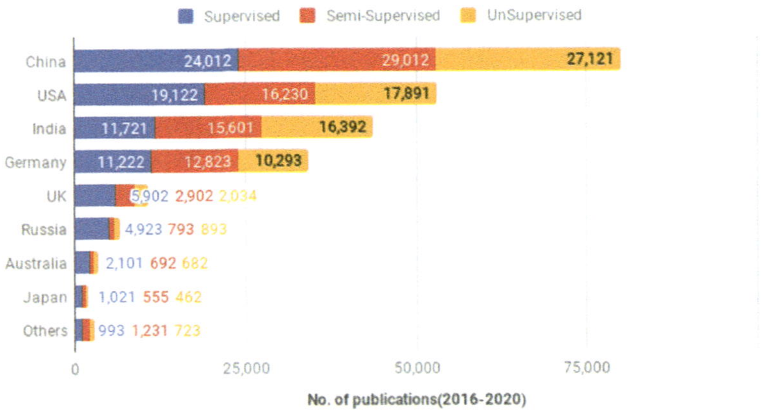

Fig. 2.17 Country-wise comparison of yearly publication on cancer data analysis from 2016 to 2020

Semi-Supervised Learning is a very slow-moving approach but it provides very accurate results and also tackles both labeled and unlabeled cancer data that's why it's popularity is still increasing when the rest of the methodologies take a back seat. Figure 2.15 provides an overall comparison of the cancer data analysis based on the number of publications in the past five years.

From Fig. 2.15, it can be clearly concluded that, in 2016, 2017 Supervised Learning is by far the most sought after algorithm and is quite broadly used in cancer data analysis. But its popularity is gradually decreasing from 2018 and in 2020, very less amount of publications can be found on cancer data analysis with supervised learning. On the contrary, the popularity of the unsupervised and semi-supervised learning are increasing from 2016–20. Even though the publications in cancer data analysis with unsupervised learning is now saturated, the publications in the semi-supervised field are still increasing as there are a lot more things to explore. Figure 2.16 shows the no. of citations on cancer data analysis in the last five years.

From Fig. 2.16, it can be clearly concluded that number of citations follows the same behaviour as number of publications and it is expected. In the Fig. 2.17, a notable contribution of each and every country has been obtained with respect to cancer data analysis.

From the Fig. 2.17, it can be concluded that China made a notable contribution to cancer data analysis and published more than 75,000 research articles in the past five years. India comes in 3rd in this list with 42,000 + publications made in the last five years. Since 2016, this field has got close to 2 lakhs publication, as such it is now going to be saturated and will reach its highest level of accuracy with the provided information. So, in the near future, some new techniques had to be developed to emphasize the information gain.

2.6 Future Scope

Currently, Deep Learning and Artificial Intelligence have reached immense popularity which has suppressed other data analysis techniques. But after this extensive review, this chapter finds some fields which are still unexplored. These are as follows:

(i) **Deep Boosting Cascade Algorithm**: It is a deep neural network with ensemble technique to ease out the forward and back propagation. In the literature review of supervised learning, Deep Boosting Cascade with Random Forest has been explored. In place of Random Forest, researchers can try other classifiers (i.e. Decision tree, Voting Classifier etc.) to obtain a detailed analysis and comparative study with cancer data thereby fueling its potential to a much higher reach.

(ii) **Link Matrix Factorization**: It belongs to the class of semi-supervised learning where each dataset has been subdivided into the lower rank matrix until it reaches the molecular level analysis. Already this chapter explored the potential of joint matrix factorization and non-negative matrix factorization. But still the researchers do not apply link matrix factorization on cancer data. It was first proposed by the Menon et al. [105]. The objective function of this methodology is depicted in Eq. (2.17) and Fig. 2.18 show a case study which can also be applied in cancer data analysis.

$$min_{U,A,V,\omega,b}\frac{1}{|O|}\sum_{i=1}^{n}\sum_{j\varepsilon O_j^+ k\varepsilon O_j^+} l\left(L\left(u_i^T \Lambda\left(u_j - u_k\right)\right) + b_i + b_j + x_i^T V x_j + w^T z_{ij}\right)$$
$$+ \frac{\lambda_u}{2}||U||_F^2 + \frac{\lambda_\Lambda}{2}||\Lambda||_F^2 + \frac{\lambda_V}{2}||V||_F^2 + \frac{\lambda_W}{2}||W||_F^2 \quad (2.17)$$

With this discussion, this chapter concludes the future scope as the rest of the data analytics techniques have already been explored. For further information gain, the researchers have to shift in the domain of deep learning.

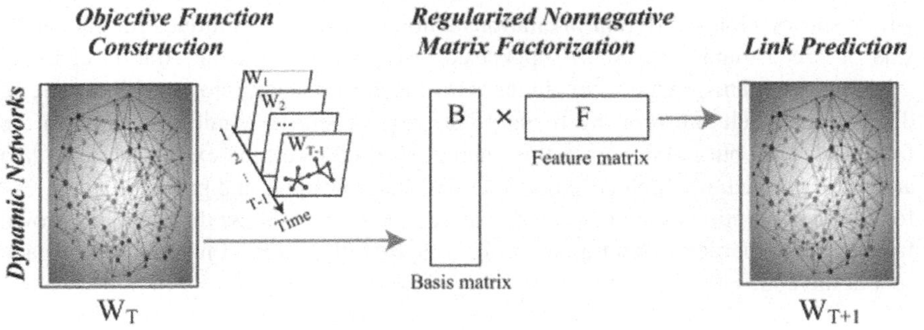

Fig. 2.18 A case study of the link matrix factorization [106]

2.7 Discussion

The comprehensive review in Sect. 2.2 majorly implies that the supervised learning techniques are being saturated with lesser amount of work on cancer data analysis being dedicated to it, thereby acknowledging the shifting trend from supervised learning field. The chapter also puts forward the fact that even though the utility of unsupervised learning is reckoned in recent years the techniques utilized for cancer data analysis are still concentrated on the decade long improvised algorithms with very few advancements. The recent thrive can be dedicated with Semi-Supervised Learning with newer and novel techniques popping out in the limelight of the cancer data analysis, thereby enforcing new researchers to a new pathway.

2.8 Conclusion

This chapter explores all possible evaluation that exists in the field of cancer data analysis. It starts with the analysis of cancer disease where it finds out the types of cancer disease with its characteristics. Later, it explores all the types of databases available in the open source repository. Once the database has been explored, it is obtained a detailed review of various types of data analysis techniques applied on the cancer dataset with their advantages and disadvantages. The chapter also includes a brief implication to the issues and challenges faced when studying about the predominant Cancer Data Analysis techniques adding in another layer for new researchers to follow. In the later section, a detailed comparison of all these approaches has been developed along with a statistical backdrop. The chapter puts forward the fact that Supervised Learning algorithms are having a downward trend in recent years with Semi-Supervised techniques gaining the larger popularity as years go on. Moreover, the data analysis of cancer data is being taken as a serious concept by researchers all over the world as well as India with India ranking third for total publications based among the countries with Supervised Learning possessing the lowest publications among the three techniques. Furthermore, the chapter also proves the point of an increasing popularity of Semi-supervise based techniques through Fig. 2.16, which shows a huge different in citations among the three techniques for data analysis of cancer data, with Semi-supervised technique leading the citation chart by a log margin. This chapter concludes with the future scope along with a concise discussion which can turn the focus of the researchers to regain this topic in the front seat. Last but not the least, this chapter showcases all the existing cancer data analysis approaches which have taken a back seat nowadays and provides a pathway for future generations such that it helps them to understand how this field has grown from scratch, thereby extending its limits, touching the saturation and taking a back seat at the end.

References

1. Siegel, R.L., Miller, K.D., Jemal, A.: Cancer statistics, 2020. CA Cancer J. Clin. **70**(1), 7–30 (2020). https://doi.org/10.3322/caac.21590. Epub 2020 Jan 8 PMID: 31912902
2. Carr, L.K.: Microwave radiometry: its importance to the detection of cancer. In: IEEE Transactions on Microwave Theory and Techniques, vol. 37, no. 12, pp. 1862–1869, December 1989. https://doi.org/10.1109/22.44095
3. Foran, J.D., Comaniciu, D., Meer, P., Goodell, A.L.: Computer-assisted discrimination among malignant lymphomas and leukemia using immunophenotyping, intelligent image repositories, and telemicroscopy. IEEE Trans. Inf Technol. Biomed. **4**(4), 265–273 (2000). https://doi.org/10.1109/4233.897058
4. Sertel, O., Lozanski, G., Shana'ah, A., Gurcan, N.M.: IEEE Trans Biomed Eng. Author manuscript; available in PMC 2011 May 16. Published in final edited form as: IEEE Trans Biomed Eng. October 2010; **57**(10): 2613–2616. Accessed 28 June 2010. https://doi.org/10.1109/tbme.2010.2055058. PMCID: PMC3095036
5. Stenman, S.E., Bychkov, D., Kucukel, H., Linder, N., Haglund, C., Arola, J., Johan, L.: Antibody supervised training of a deep learning based algorithm for leukocyte segmentation in papillary thyroid carcinoma. IEEE J. Biomed. Health Inform. (2020)
6. Hermessi, H., Mourali, O., Zagrouba, E.: Deep feature learning for soft tissue sarcoma classification in MR images via transfer learning. Expert Syst. Appl. **120**, 116–127 (2019). https://doi.org/10.1016/j.eswa.2018.11.025
7. Jiang, D., Tang, C., Zhang, A.: Cluster analysis for gene expression data: a survey. IEEE Trans. Knowl. Data Eng. **16**(11), 1370–1386 (2004)
8. Veta, M., Pluim, J.P., Van Diest, P.J., Viergever, M.A.: Breast cancer histopathology image analysis: a review. IEEE Trans. Biomed. Eng. **61**(5), 1400–1411 (2014)
9. Albrecht, J.C., Kotani, A., Lin, J.S., Soper, S.A., Barron, A.E.: Simultaneous detection of 19 K-ras mutations by free-solution conjugate electrophoresis of ligase detection reaction products on glass microchips. Electrophoresis **34**(4), 590–597 (2013)
10. Centers for Disease Control and Prevention: National Program of Cancer Registries and Surveillance, Epidemiology, and End Results SEER Stat Database: NPCR and SEER Incidence—USCS 2001–2014 Public Use Research Database, Released August 2017, based on the November 2016 submission (2017)
11. Ni, L., Zhou, L., Zhou, M., Zhao, J. and Wang, D.W.: Combination of western medicine and Chinese traditional patent medicine in treating a family case of COVID-19 in Wuhan. Front Med. 1–5 (2020)
12. Algamal, Z.Y., Lee, M.H.: Regularized logistic regression with adjusted adaptive elastic net for gene selection in high dimensional cancer classification. Comput. Biol. Med. **67**, 136–145 (2015)
13. Rashmi, G.D., Lekha, A., Bawane, N.: December. Analysis of efficiency of classification and prediction algorithms (Naïve Bayes) for Breast Cancer dataset. In: 2015 International Conference on Emerging Research in Electronics, Computer Science and Technology (ICERECT), pp. 108–113. IEEE (2015)
14. Mohammadzadeh, F., Noorkojuri, H., Pourhoseingholi, M.A., Saadat, S., Baghestani, A.R.: Predicting the probability of mortality of gastric cancer patients using decision tree. Irish J. Med. Sci. (1971–), **184**(2), 277–284 (2015)
15. Kar, S., Sharma, K.D., Maitra, M.: Gene selection from microarray gene expression data for classification of cancer subgroups employing PSO and adaptive K-nearest neighborhood technique. Expert Syst. Appl. **42**(1), 612–627 (2015)
16. Nandpuru, H.B., Salankar, S.S., Bora, V.R.: MRI brain cancer classification using support vector machine. In: 2014 IEEE Students' Conference on Electrical, Electronics and Computer Science, pp. 1–6, March 2014. IEEE (2014)
17. Islam, M.M., Iqbal, H., Haque, M.R., Hasan, M.K.: Prediction of breast cancer using support vector machine and K-Nearest neighbors. In: 2017 IEEE Region 10 Humanitarian Technology Conference (R10-HTC), pp. 226–229, December 2017. IEEE (2017)

18. Geetha, R., Sivasubramanian, S., Kaliappan, M., Vimal, S., Annamalai, S.: Cervical cancer identification with synthetic minority oversampling technique and PCA analysis using random forest classifier. J. Med. Syst. **43**(9), 286 (2019)
19. Kumar, U.K., Nikhil, M.S., Sumangali, K.: Prediction of breast cancer using voting classifier technique. In: 2017 IEEE International Conference on Smart Technologies and Management for Computing, Communication, Controls, Energy and Materials (ICSTM), pp. 108–114, August 2017. IEEE (2017)
20. Bashir, S., Qamar, U., Khan, F.H.: Heterogeneous classifiers fusion for dynamic breast cancer diagnosis using weighted vote based ensemble. Qual. Quant. **49**(5), 2061–2076 (2015)
21. Guo, Y., Liu, S., Li, Z., Shang, X.: BCDForest: a boosting cascade deep forest model towards the classification of cancer subtypes based on gene expression data. BMC Bioinform **19**(5), 118 (2018)
22. Park, H., Shiraishi, Y., Imoto, S., Miyano, S.: A novel adaptive penalized logistic regression for uncovering biomarker associated with anti-cancer drug sensitivity. IEEE/ACM Trans. Comput. Biol. Bioinf. **14**(4), 771–782 (2016)
23. Carmona-Bayonas, A., Jiménez-Fonseca, P., Font, C., Fenoy, F., Otero, R., Beato, C., Plasencia, J.M., Biosca, M., Sanchez, M., Benegas, M., Calvo-Temprano, D.: Predicting serious complications in patients with cancer and pulmonary embolism using decision tree modelling: the EPIPHANY index. Br. J. Cancer **116**(8), 994–1001 (2017)
24. Ayyad, S.M., Saleh, A.I., Labib, L.M.: Gene expression cancer classification using modified K-nearest neighbors technique. Biosystems **176**, 41–51 (2019)
25. Alquran, H., Qasmieh, I.A., Alqudah, A.M., Alhammouri, S., Alawneh, E., Abughazaleh, A., Hasayen, F.: The melanoma skin cancer detection and classification using support vector machine. In 2017 IEEE Jordan Conference on Applied Electrical Engineering and Computing Technologies (AEECT), pp. 1–5, October 2017. IEEE (2017)
26. Zhu, T., Lin, Y., Liu, Y.: Synthetic minority oversampling technique for multiclass imbalance problems. Pattern Recogn. **72**, 327–340 (2017)
27. Alquraishi, T.: Predicting breast cancer risk, recurrence and survivability candidate declaration (2020)
28. Dai, B., Chen, R.C., Zhu, S.Z., Zhang, W.W.: Using random forest algorithm for breast cancer diagnosis. In: 2018 International Symposium on Computer, Consumer and Control (IS3C) pp. 449–452, December 2018. IEEE
29. Vapnik, V.N., Chervonenkis, A.Y., Moskva, N.: Pattern Recognition Theory. Statistical Learning Problems (1974)
30. Jeng, B., Jeng, Y.M., Liang, T.P.: FILM: a fuzzy inductive learning method for automated knowledge acquisition. Decis. Support Syst. **21**(2), 61–73 (1997)
31. Moradi, P., Gholampour, M.: A hybrid particle swarm optimization for feature subset selection by integrating a novel local search strategy. Appl. Soft Comput. **43**, 117–130 (2016)
32. Reddy, G.T., Reddy, M.P.K., Lakshmanna, K., Rajput, D.S., Kaluri, R., Srivastava, G.: Hybrid genetic algorithm and a fuzzy logic classifier for heart disease diagnosis. Evol. Intel. **13**(2), 185–196 (2020)
33. Zhou, G., Moayedi, H., Bahiraei, M., Lyu, Z.: Employing artificial bee colony and particle swarm techniques for optimizing a neural network in prediction of heating and cooling loads of residential buildings. J. Clean. Prod. **254**, (2020)
34. Uthayakumar, J., Metawa, N., Shankar, K., Lakshmanaprabu, S.K.: Financial crisis prediction model using ant colony optimization. Int. J. Inf. Manag. **50**, 538–556 (2020)
35. Rajagopal, A., Joshi, G.P., Ramachandran, A., Subhalakshmi, R.T., Khari, M., Jha, S., Shankar, K., You, J.: A deep learning model based on multi-objective particle swarm optimization for scene classification in unmanned aerial vehicles. IEEE Access **8**, 135383–135393 (2020)
36. Yildizdan, G., Baykan, Ö.K.: A novel modified bat algorithm hybridizing by differential evolution algorithm. Expert Syst. Appl. **141**, (2020)
37. Qasim, O.S., Al-Thanoon, N.A., Algamal, Z.Y.: Feature selection based on chaotic binary black hole algorithm for data classification. Chemometrics and Intelligent Laboratory Systems, 204, International Journal of Mathematical, Engineering and Management Sciences, vol. 5, no. 4, pp. 697–706 (2020). https://doi.org/10.33889/IJMEMS.2020.5.4.056

38. Abualigah, L., Diabat, A.: A comprehensive survey of the grasshopper optimization algorithm: results, variants, and applications. Neural Comput Appl **32**, 15533–15556 (2020). https://doi.org/10.1007/s00521-020-04789-8
39. Zhou, J., Nekouie, A., Arslan, C.A., Pham, B.T., Hasanipanah, M.: Novel approach for forecasting the blast-induced AOp using a hybrid fuzzy system and firefly algorithm. Eng. Comput. **36**(2), 703–712 (2020)
40. Zhu, Q., Tang, X., Li, Y., Yeboah, M.O.: An improved differential-based harmony search algorithm with linear dynamic domain. Knowl.-Based Syst. **187**, (2020)
41. Wu, D., Shang, M., Wang, G., Li, L.: A self-training semi-supervised classification algorithm based on density peaks of data and differential evolution. In: 2018 IEEE 15th International Conference on Networking, Sensing and Control (ICNSC), pp. 1–6, March 2018. IEEE
42. Xia, C.Q., Han, K., Qi, Y., Zhang, Y., Yu, D.J.: A self-training subspace clustering algorithm under low-rank representation for cancer classification on gene expression data. IEEE/ACM Trans. Comput. Biol. Bioinf. **15**(4), 1315–1324 (2017)
43. Wang, Q., Xia, L.Y., Chai, H. and Zhou, Y.: Semi-supervised learning with ensemble self-training for cancer classification. In: 2018 IEEE SmartWorld, Ubiquitous Intelligence & Computing, Advanced & Trusted Computing, Scalable Computing & Communications, Cloud & Big Data Computing, Internet of People and Smart City Innovation (SmartWorld/SCALCOM/UIC/ATC/CBDCom/IOP/SCI), pp. 796–803, October 2018. IEEE
44. Azmi, R., Norozi, N., Anbiaee, R., Salehi, L., Amirzadi, A.: IMPST: a new interactive self-training approach to segmentation suspicious lesions in breast MRI. J Med Signals Sens **1**(2), 138 (2011)
45. Ting, F.F., Sim, K.S.: Self-regulated multilayer perceptron neural network for breast cancer classification. In: 2017 International Conference on Robotics, Automation and Sciences (ICORAS), pp. 1–5, November 2017. IEEE
46. Wang, Q., Zhou, Y., Zhang, W., Tang, Z., Chen, X.: Adaptive sampling using self-paced learning for imbalanced cancer data pre-diagnosis. Expert Syst. Appl. **152**, (2020)
47. Xia, Y., Yang, D., Yu, Z., Liu, F., Cai, J., Yu, L., Zhu, Z., Xu, D., Yuille, A., Roth, H.: Uncertainty-aware multi-view co-training for semi-supervised medical image segmentation and domain adaptation. Med. Image Anal. **65**, (2020)
48. Yavuz, E., Eyupoglu, C.: An effective approach for breast cancer diagnosis based on routine blood analysis features. Med. Biol. Eng. Comput. (2020)
49. Huang, R., Zheng, Y., Hu, Z., Zhang, S., Li, H.: Multi-organ segmentation via co-training weight-averaged models from few-organ datasets. In: International Conference on Medical Image Computing and Computer-Assisted Intervention, pp. 146–155, October 2020. Springer, Cham
50. Mallapragada, P.K., Jin, R., Jain, A.K., Liu, Y.: Semiboost: boosting for semi-supervised learning. IEEE Trans. Pattern Anal. Mach. Intell. **31**(11), 2000–2014 (2008)
51. Qi, J., Chen, C., Zhang, X., Hu, X., Ji, S., Kwok, R.T., Lam, J.W., Ding, D., Tang, B.Z.: Light-driven transformable optical agent with adaptive functions for boosting cancer surgery outcomes. Nat Commun **9**(1), 1–12 (2018)
52. Kwak, J.T., Hewitt, S.M.: Multiview boosting digital pathology analysis of prostate cancer. Comput. Methods Programs Biomed. **142**, 91–99 (2017). https://doi.org/10.1016/j.chempr.2019.07.015
53. Koyasu, S., Nishio, M., Isoda, H., Nakamoto, Y., Togashi, K.: Usefulness of gradient tree boosting for predicting histological subtype and EGFR mutation status of non-small cell lung cancer on 18 F FDG-PET/CT. Ann. Nucl. Med. **34**(1), 49–57 (2020)
54. Tosado, J., Zdilar, L., Elhalawani, H., Elgohari, B., Vock, D.M., Marai, G.E., Fuller, C., Mohamed, A.S., Canahuate, G.: Clustering of largely right-censored oropharyngeal head and neck cancer patients for discriminative groupings to improve outcome prediction. Sci. Rep. **10**(1), 1–14 (2020). https://doi.org/10.1038/s41598-020-60140-0PMID:32123193PMCID: PMC7051972

55. Shi, X., Su, H., Xing, F., Liang, Y., Qu, G., Yang, L.: Graph temporal ensemble based semi-supervised convolutional neural network with noisy labels for histopathology image analysis. Med. Image Anal. **60**, 101624 (2020). PMID: 31841948, https://doi.org/10.1016/j.media.2019.101624
56. Kim, S., Kim, K., Choe, J., Lee, I., Kang, J.: Improved survival analysis by learning shared genomic information from pan-cancer data. Bioinformatics **36**(Suppl 1), July 2020, i389–i398 (2020). https://doi.org/10.1093/bioinformatics/btaa462
57. Hsu, T.C., Lin, C.: Generative adversarial networks for robust breast cancer prognosis prediction with limited data size. In the 2020 42nd Annual International Conference of the IEEE Engineering in Medicine & Biology Society (EMBC), pp. 5669–5672, July 2020. IEEE Published online 2 October 2018. https://doi.org/10.3390/genes9100478pmcid: PMC6210393, PMID: 30279327
58. Gong, H., Pan, C., Yang, Q., Lu, H. and Ma, S.: A semi-supervised framework for mapping data to the intrinsic manifold. In: Tenth IEEE International Conference on Computer Vision (ICCV'05), vol. 1, pp. 98–105, October 2005. IEEE
59. Sun, S., Xie, X.: Semi supervised support vector machines with tangent space intrinsic manifold regularization. IEEE Trans. Neural Netw. Learn. Syst. **27**(9), 1827–1839 (2015)
60. Cui, Y., Zheng, C.H., Yang, J., Sha, W.: Sparse maximum margin discriminant analysis for feature extraction and gene selection on gene expression data. Comput. Biol. Med. **43**(7), 933–941 (2013). https://doi.org/10.1016/j.compbiomed.2013.04.018
61. Niijima, S., Kuhara, S.: Recursive gene selection based on maximum margin criterion: a comparison with SVM-RFE. BMC Bioinformatics **7**, 543 (2006). https://doi.org/10.1186/1471-2105-7-543
62. Holmes, M.G., Foss, E., Joseph, G., Foye, A., Beckett, B., Motamedi, D., Youngren, J., Thomas, G.V., Huang, J., Aggarwal, R., Alumkal, J.J., Beer, T.M., Small, E.J., Link, T.M.: CT–guided bone biopsies in metastatic castration-resistant prostate cancer: factors predictive of maximum tumor yield. J. Vasc. Intervent Radiol. **28**(8), 1073–1081.e1 (2017). https://doi.org/10.1016/j.jvir.2017.04.019
63. Sajjadi, M., Javanmardi, M., Tasdizen, T.: Regularization with stochastic transformations and perturbations for deep semi-supervised learning. Adv. Neural. Inf. Process. Syst. **29**, 1163–1171 (2016)
64. Luo, Y., Zhu, J., Li, M., Ren, Y., Zhang, B.: Smooth neighbors on teacher graphs for semi-supervised learning. In: 2018 IEEE/CVF Conference on Computer Vision and Pattern Recognition (CVPR), Salt Lake City, UT, USA, 2018, pp. 8896–8905. https://doi.org/10.1109/cvpr.2018.00927
65. Cruz-Barbosa, R., Vellido, A.: Semi-supervised analysis of human brain tumours from partially labeled MRS information, using manifold learning models. Int. J. Neural Syst. **21**(1), 17–29 (2011),DOI:https://doi.org/10.1142/S0129065711002614
66. Feng, H.: Gene classification using parameter-free semi-supervised manifold learning. IEEE/ACM Trans. Comput. Biol. Bioinf. **9**(3), 818–827 (2011)
67. Ding, J., Condon, A., Shah, S.P.: Interpretable dimensionality reduction of single cell transcriptome data with deep generative models. Nat Commun **9**, 2002 (2018). https://doi.org/10.1038/s41467-018-04368-5
68. Chang, A., Suriyakumar, V.M., Moturu, A., Tewattanarat, N., Doria, A., Goldenberg, A.: Using generative models for pediatric wbMRI (2020). arXiv preprint arXiv:2006.00727
69. Wu, E., Wu, K., Cox, D., Lotter, W.: Conditional infilling GANs for data augmentation in mammogram classification. In: Image Analysis for Moving Organ, Breast, and Thoracic Images, pp. 98–106. Springer, Cham (2018)
70. Khan, F.M., Kulikowski, C.A.: Impact of prostate biopsy tumor amount on imaging based prognostics employing transductive semi-supervised regression. In: 2016 38th Annual International Conference of the IEEE Engineering in Medicine and Biology Society (EMBC), pp. 5604–5607, August 2016. IEEE. https://doi.org/10.1109/embc.2016.7591997
71. Khan, F.M.: Predicting advanced prostate cancer from modeling early indications in biopsy and prostatectomy samples via transductive semi-supervised survival analysis. BioMed. Res. Int. **2018**, Article ID 2178645, 12 p. https://doi.org/10.1155/2018/2178645

72. Li, D., Wang, L., Wang, J., Xue, Z., Wong, S.T.C.: Transductive local fisher discriminant analysis for gene expression profile-based cancer classification. In: 2017 IEEE EMBS International Conference on Biomedical and Health Informatics, BHI 2017, pp. 49–52. Institute of Electrical and Electronics Engineers Inc. https://doi.org/10.1109/BHI.2017.7897202
73. Zemmal, N., Azizi, N., Sellami, M., Dey, N.: Automated classification of mammographic abnormalities using transductive semi supervised learning algorithms. In: Proceedings of the Mediterranean Conference on Information & Communication Technologies, pp. 657–662. Springer, Cham (2016)
74. Khan, F.M.: Interval kernels for combining biometric measurements from multiple prostate samples per patient in prognostic models with transductive semi-supervised support vector regression. In: 2018 40th Annual International Conference of the IEEE Engineering in Medicine and Biology Society (EMBC), pp. 3967–3970, July 2018. IEEE
75. Khan, F.M., Kulikowski, C.A.: Predicting advanced prostate cancer endpoints from early indications via transductive semi-supervised regression. In: 2016 IEEE 29th International Symposium on Computer-Based Medical Systems (CBMS), pp. 19–23, June 2016. IEEE (2016)
76. Gao, Y., Church, G.: Improving molecular cancer class discovery through sparse non-negative matrix factorization. Bioinformatics **21**(21), 3970–3975 (2005)
77. Wang, C.Y., Liu, J.X., Yu, N., Zheng, C.H.: Sparse graph regularization non-negative matrix factorization based on huber loss model for cancer data analysis. Front. Genet. **10**, 1054 (2019). https://doi.org/10.3389/fgene.2019.01054
78. Gao, Y.L., Hou, M.X., Liu, J.X., Kong, X.Z.: An integrated graph regularized non-negative matrix factorization model for gene co-expression network analysis. IEEE Access **7**, 126594–126602 (2019)
79. Zhang, L., Zhang, S.: A general joint matrix factorization framework for data integration and its systematic algorithmic exploration. IEEE Trans. Fuzzy Syst. **28**(9), 1971–1983 (2020). https://doi.org/10.1109/tfuzz.2019.2928518
80. Deng, J., Zeng, W., Kong, W., Shi, Y., Mou, X.: The study of sarcoma microenvironment heterogeneity associated with prognosis based on an immunogenomic landscape analysis. Front Bioeng Biotechnol. **8**, 1003 (2020). https://doi.org/10.3389/fbioe.2020.01003 Accessed 21 Aug 2020
81. Sharma, A., López, Y., Tsunoda, T.: Divisive hierarchical maximum likelihood clustering. BMC Bioinform **18**, 546 (2017). https://doi.org/10.1186/s12859-017-1965-5
82. Nidheesh, N., Nazeer, K.A., Ameer, P.M.: A hierarchical clustering algorithm based on silhouette index for cancer subtype discovery from genomic data. Neural Comput. Appl. **32**, 11459–11476 (2020). https://doi.org/10.1007/s00521-019-04636-5
83. Kruger, D.T., Beelen, K.J., Opdam, M., et al.: Hierarchical clustering of activated proteins in the PI3K and MAPK pathways in ER-positive, HER2-negative breast cancer with potential therapeutic consequences. Br. J. Cancer **119**, 832–839 (2018). https://doi.org/10.1038/s41416-018-0221-8
84. Xie, J., Wang, Y., Wu, Z.: Colon cancer data analysis by chameleon algorithm. Health Inf. Sci. Syst. **7**(1), 23 (2019)
85. Weghorn D, Sunyaev S (2017) Bayesian inference of negative and positive selection in human cancers. Nat Genet. **49**(12), 1785–1788. https://doi.org/10.1038/ng.3987. Accessed 6 Nov 2017. PMID: 29106416
86. Akshaya, V., Krishnamoorthy, V., Sivanantham, S.: Performance evaluation of association rule based classification in cancer diagnosis. In: 2020 Second International Conference on Inventive Research in Computing Applications (ICIRCA), pp. 14–17, 15 July 2020. IEEE (2020)
87. Jothilakshmi, G.R., Raaza, A.: Effective detection of mass abnormalities and its classification using multi-SVM classifier with digital mammogram images. In: 2017 International Conference on Computer, Communication and Signal Processing (ICCCSP), pp. 1–6, January 2017. IEEE. https://doi.org/10.1109/icccsp.2017.7944090

88. Kaur, N., Sharma, A.S.: Detection of breast cancer on mammograms using neural network approach. In: 2018 International Conference on Computing, Power and Communication Technologies (GUCON), pp. 544–547, September 2018. IEEE
89. Barrett, T., Wilhite, S.E., Ledoux, P., Evangelista, C., Kim, I.F., Tomashevsky, M., Marshall, K.A., Phillippy, K.H., Sherman, P.M., Holko, M., et al.: NCBI GEO: archive for functional genomics data sets-update. Nucleic Acids Res. **41**(D1), D991–D995 (2012). https://doi.org/10.1093/nar/gks1193
90. Monti, S., Tamayo, P., Mesirov, J., Golub, T.: Consensus clustering: a resampling-based method for class discovery and visualization of gene expression microarray data. Mach. Learn. **52**(1), 91–118 (2003). https://doi.org/10.1023/A:1023949509487
91. Lichman, M.: UCI machine learning repository (2013). http://archive.ics.uci.edu/ml
92. Clayman, C.L., Srinivasan, S.M., Sangwan, R.S.: K-means clustering and principal components analysis of microarray data of L1000 landmark genes. Procedia Comput Sci **168**, 97–104 (2020). https://doi.org/10.1016/j.procs.2020.02.265
93. Choudhary, A.: Survey on K-means and its variants. Int. J. Innov. Res. Comput. Commun. **4**(1) (2016)
94. Inbarani H.H., Azar, A.T.: Leukemia image segmentation using a hybrid histogram-based soft covering rough k-means clustering algorithm. Electronics **9**(1), 188 (2020)
95. Sangamithraa, P.B., Govindaraju, S.: Lung tumour detection and classification using EK-Mean clustering. In: 2016 International Conference on Wireless Communications, Signal Processing and Networking (WiSPNET), pp. 2201–2206, March 2016. IEEE
96. Kachouie, N.N., Shutaywi, M., Christiani, D.C.: Discriminant analysis of lung cancer using nonlinear clustering of copy numbers. Cancer Invest. **38**(2), 102–112 (2020). https://doi.org/10.1080/07357907.2020.1719501
97. Haq, A.U., Bonny, T.: Cancer transcriptome analysis with RNA-Seq using quantum K-means clustering algorithm. In: 2020 Advances in Science and Engineering Technology International Conferences (ASET) (2020). https://doi.org/10.1109/aset48392.2020.9118341
98. Rustam, Z., Fijri, A.L.: Breast cancer clustering using modified spherical K-Means. J. Phys: Conf. Ser. **1490**, (2020). https://doi.org/10.1088/1742-6596/1490/1/012028
99. Rundo, L., Militello, C., Russo, G., D'Urso, D., Valastro, L.M., Garufi, A., Mauri, G., Vitabile, S., Gilardi, M.C.: Fully automatic multispectral MR image segmentation of prostate gland based on the fuzzy c-means clustering algorithm. In: Multidisciplinary Approaches to Neural Computing, vol. 69, pp. 23–37 (2018)
100. Bulut, H., Onan, A., Korukoğlu, S. (2020). An improved ant-based algorithm based on heaps merging and fuzzy c-means for clustering cancer gene expression data. Sādhanā **45**(1). https://doi.org/10.1007/s12046-020-01399-x
101. Manogaran, G., Vijayakumar, V., Varatharajan, R., Kumar, P.M., Sundarasekar, R., Hsu, C.: Machine learning based big data processing framework for cancer diagnosis using hidden markov model and GM clustering. Wireless Pers. Commun. **102**(3), 2099–2116 (2017). https://doi.org/10.1007/s11277-017-5044-z
102. Shukla, N., Hagenbuchner, M., Win, K.T., Yang, J.: Breast cancer data analysis for survivability studies and prediction. Comput. Methods Programs Biomed. **155**, 199–208 (2018). https://doi.org/10.1016/j.cmpb.2017.12.011
103. Kasa, S.R., Bhattacharya, S., Rajan, V.: Gaussian mixture copulas for high-dimensional clustering and dependency-based subtyping. Bioinformatics **36**(2), 621–628 (2020)
104. Li, W., Jia, Z., Xie, D., Chen, K., Cui, J., Liu, H.: Recognizing lung cancer using a homemade e-nose: a comprehensive study. Comput. Biol. Med. **120**, (2020). https://doi.org/10.1016/j.compbiomed.2020.103706

105. Menon, A.K., Elkan, C.: Link prediction via matrix factorization. In: Joint European Conference on Machine Learning and Knowledge Discovery in Databases, pp. 437–452, September 2011. Springer, Berlin, Heidelberg (2011)
106. Ma, X., Sun, P., Wang, Y.: Graph regularized nonnegative matrix factorization for temporal link prediction in dynamic networks. Physica A: Stat. Mech. Appl. **496**, 121–136 (2018). https://doi.org/10.1016/j.physa.2017.12.092

Chapter 3
Learning from Multiple Modalities of Imaging Data for Cancer Detection/Diagnosis

Nataliia A. Obukhova, Alexander A. Motyko, and Alexander A. Pozdeev

Abstract Methods of automatic analysis and visualization of multispectral medical images are considered. In particular, the chapter includes method for multispectral images visualization. Proposed method supposes the synthesis of image based on an image obtained in white light and image based on a fluorescent image in the NIR channel. A feature of the method is the presentation of fluorescence data in the form of a special level map that takes into account the properties of human vision. Metric CIEDE2000 is used for estimation of visualization quality. Special attention is paid to preprocessing and enhancement image obtained in white light. Methods of medical multispectral images analysis for cancer changes differential diagnosis based on traditional machine learning technologies, deep learning technologies, as well as the combined approach based on both technologies are shown. The combined approach allows to effectively use the advantages of deep learning technology in conditions of limited volume of verified database for training. All the proposed methods and algorithms are illustrated by implementation in real medical applications.

Keywords Multispectral medical images · Laparoscopy image enhancement · Multispectral medical image visualization · Medical images enhancement · Deep learning

---

N. A. Obukhova (✉) · A. A. Motyko · A. A. Pozdeev
Saint Petersburg Electrotechnical University "LETI", ul. Professora Popova 5, St. Petersburg 197376, Russian Federation
e-mail: natalia172419@yandex.ru

A. A. Motyko
e-mail: motyko.alexandr@yandex.ru

A. A. Pozdeev
e-mail: puches4@gmail.com

J. Nayak et al. (eds.), *Advanced Machine Learning Approaches in Cancer Prognosis*, Intelligent Systems Reference Library 204,
https://doi.org/10.1007/978-3-030-71975-3_3

3.1 Introduction

During a diagnostic examination or treatment, a physician needs to quickly and accurately identification and localization of anomalies and diseases using available technical means. Rapid advances in sensor and imaging technologies, as well as diagnostic techniques are driving to the widespread use of Clinical Decision Support Systems (CDSS).

CDSS is a new generation of automatic medicine diagnostic systems. CDSS supposes the integration of the diagnostics results obtained by a physician, results obtained by means of automatic analysis and system database information. This integration provides high sensitivity and specificity of the diagnosis. The values of these characteristics exceed the results of diagnostics realized only by a physician or only by an automatic system. CDSS can be used to solve a variety of medical problems such as screening, diagnosis and treatment.

Important role in CDSS belongs to imaging and image analysis, especially in different endoscopy systems. The special type of endoscopy is laparoscopy. Laparoscopy is a surgery method in which operations on internal organs are performed through small holes. Laparoscopy is usually performed on organs inside the abdominal or pelvic cavity. The main instrument in laparoscopic surgery is the laparoscope: a telescopic tube containing a lens system and attached to a video camera. The range of surgical interventions performed by laparoscopic access is wide: from cholecystectomy and hernioplasty, to gastrectomy, pancreatoduodenal resection and operations on the colon and rectum.

The endoscope has a flexible optical path, the laparoscope has a rigid one, but both systems obtain video images. These images are base as for diagnostics as for surgery manipulation. Automatic analysis, effective enhancement and visualization are very important part in CDSS for endoscopy and laparoscopy systems.

Thus, CDSS in endoscopy and laparoscopy requires to solve tasks of image processing and analysis. There are two approaches for solving these tasks. The first approach is improving the methods of processing and analysis for images obtained in white light, as result nowadays there are a lot of new "state of the art" methods for endoscopic images enhancement and analysis. But another very important approach based on possibility to get new diagnostic information is multispectral images formation and analysis. Multispectral images make it possible to increase the efficiency CDSS and medical video systems in general.

A multispectral image is an image consists of several color planes (channels), each of which contains information obtained in a certain spectral range of wavelengths (spectral channel). Spectral channel is a continuous, relatively narrow portion of the spectral range, recorded by one of the sensors and displayed on one color plane.

According to the number of color planes can be defined next type of images: multispectral (the number of channels up to 15), hyperspectral (the number of channels up to 1000) and ultraspectral systems (the number of channels is more than 1000).

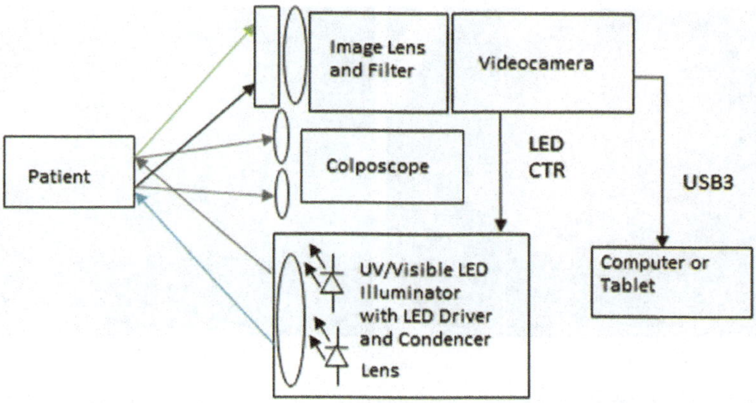

Fig. 3.1 Formation of fluorescent images in the multispectral complex

Multispectral images are widely used in video systems for various purposes. This class of images is used in systems for segmentation and tracking objects of interest, geosystems, preventive access systems, document authentication systems, and space television. This type of images is in great demand in medicine. First of all, on the base multispectral images is the fluorescent images are formed.

When forming fluorescent images, tissues (biological object) are illuminated with narrow-spectrum radiation in order to excite endogenous or exogenous fluorescent tissue biomarkers. Next, the sensor registers the image in the light formed by the reflected object, while the exciting radiation is blocked. A possible hardware solution for the formation of fluorescent images in the multispectral complex for the diagnosis of oncological changes in the cervix is shown in Fig. 3.1.

In Fig. 3.1, one can see blocking (cut-off) filter in front of complementary metal–oxide–semiconductor sensor. The cutting edge of the filter is located at a wavelength of 400 nm, because in complex the excitation radiation with a wavelength of 360 nm was used to form fluorescent images. Fluorescent images contain additional diagnostic information based on changes in concentration and restructuring of fluorophores.

Diagnostic methods are based on determining the differences in the fluorescent image between the pathological tissues and surrounding normal tissues that occurs when the surface of the tissue is irradiated by narrow-spectrum radiation. These differences, for which the term “fluorescent contrast” is used, can be of endogenous or exogenous origin.

In the first case (endogenous fluorophores), the method is called autofluorescence diagnosis. It is based on differences in the intensity and spectral changes of endogenous (autofluorescent) radiation from normal and pathological tissues. For example, in multispectral colposcopy system on the base of fluorescent images (Figs. 3.2 and 3.3) the following changes in cervical tissues: Norm, CNI (Chronic Nonspecific Inflammation), CIN I, CIN II, CIN III (Cervical Intraepithelial Neoplasia refers to

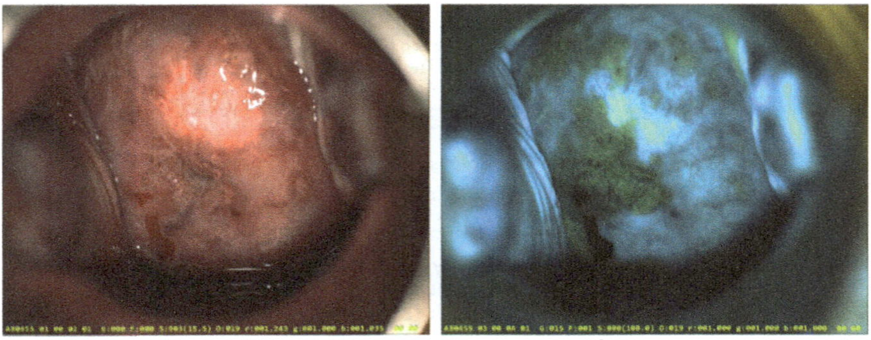

a b

Fig. 3.2 Examples of images: **a** reflection image, **b** fluorescence image attributed to NADH by exciting 360 nm

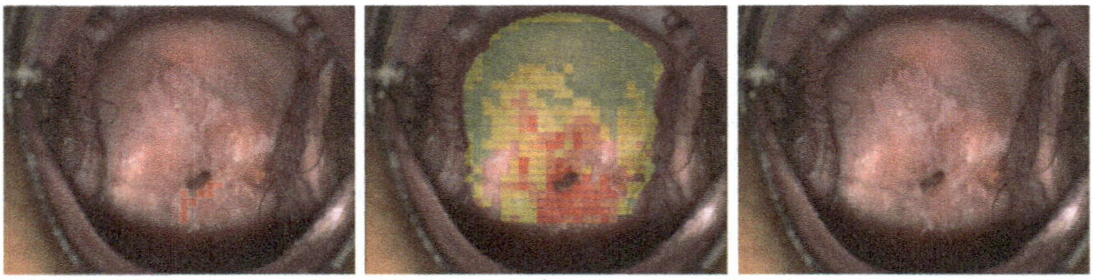

a b c

Fig. 3.3 Examples of images resulted in precancerous cervical tissues by histopathological diagnosis (Pap-HSIL, Histopathology-CIN): **a** images of cervix with acetic acid, **b** pathology map, **c** guiding site for biopsy sampling

various types of oncological changes)were determined as a result of the implemented differential diagnosis.

For differential diagnostics classification performed in fluorescent images obtained with excitation at wavelength mode 360 nm with features Cr, Cb in color space YCrCb and b in color space Lab. Classification strategy is random decision forest. For the border CIN/CNI sensitivity 87% and specificity 75% are achieved [1].

In the second case, the fluorescent contrast arises as a result of selective staining of pathological tissue with exogenous dyes or fluorescent markers. For example, these include photosensitizers used for Photo Dynamic Therapy (PDT) oncological and non-oncological diseases. As a result of selective accumulation of photosensitizers gives pathological tissue brightly fluoresce.

When conducting PDT of the cervix for the dysplasia of varying severity treatment, photosensitizers belonging to the porphyrin families (Photofrin, derivatives of 5-aminolevulenic acid (5-ALA)) and chlorins (Photolon, Photoditazin) are used. The control of photosensitizers in tissues accumulation and photo-burnout dynamics can be effectively implemented in the generated fluorescent images at 360 nm excitation radiation.

In the given examples, fluorescent images were formed by exciting ultraviolet radiation. A demanded direction today is the use of the Near Infrared Range (NIR) in the formation of fluorescent images as exciting radiation. For high fluorescence contrast between the normal and pathology, IndoCyanineGreen (ICG) as a non-targeting NIR contrast is used.

During surgery, the physician needs to see structures to avoid, such as blood vessels and nerves. Absorption and scattering of light prevent its penetration into tissues and blood, which make invisible important objects deeper than the surface. NIR has a higher penetrating power, which is used in near infrared fluorescence imaging technology [2].

Near-infrared fluorescence imaging provides a cheaper and more sensitive real-time molecular visualization method [3] and works by penetrating near infrared photons into tissue. The fluorophore in the tissue is excited by the light emitted diode or laser diode. A charge-coupled device detects fluorescence. In this way, a fluorescence image is formed to detect exogenous contact substances emitting fluorescence from 700 to 900 nm [4].

NIR fluorescent light is practically invisible to the human eye, so special imaging systems are required to provide information from the NIR channel in a form convenient for the physician. In modern imaging systems, information from the NIR channel is applied to an image obtained in white light, and a new synthesized image is formed. For this purpose, the alpha blending technology [5] is used to superimposing the NIR channel onto a color image using green.

Multispectral images in medicine are widely used not only for fluorescence diagnostics, but also for more effective visualization of vascular structures and other features of the mucous tissues that are not displayed in white light. For endoscopy one of the very effective visualization technologies is electronic chromoendoscopy.

Electronic chromoendoscopy realizes the diagnostic value of medical images increase by highlighting the features of the analyzed tissues, mucous features and vascular structures with color. Electronic chromoendoscopy can be based on optical and digital technologies. Optical electronic chromoendoscopy is implemented in hardware by forming images in narrow spectral ranges. The most famous are the technologies of the largest companies manufacturing endoscopic equipment–Olimpus and FujiFilm.

Olimpus implements Narrow Band Imaging (NBI) technology, which provides illumination of the examined tissues with blue (415 ± 15 nm) and green (540 ± 15 nm) light. Blue light in NBI mode with a wavelength of 415 ± 15 nm penetrates only the surface layers of the mucous membrane and is absorbed by the surface capillaries. The mode helps to detect tumors, since they most often contain a large number of vessels and change the capillary pattern. Green light in NBI mode with a wavelength of 540 ± 15 nm penetrates deeper and is absorbed by blood vessels located in the deeper layers of the mucous membrane. The mode allows to visualize deeper vessels and the presence of suspicious focal formations.

FujiFilm's Multilight technology includes Blue Light Imaging (BLI) and Linked Color Imaging (LCI). In the BLI mode, certain part of the spectral range in the emitted light are isolated and enhanced. One of such part is the blue-violet part with a wavelength of 410 nm, which is referred to the zone of maximum light absorption by hemoglobin. The resulting image provides a better visualization of superficial vessels and mucous features, changes in which make it possible to differentiate polyps and neoplasms. In LCI mode, the matched illumination spectrum and subsequent image processing allows for more efficient differentiation of red colors. Image processing algorithms highlight small differences between different shades of colors. Initially red areas of the image become redder, and initially white areas become whiter, retaining their original tone. An increase in color contrast leads to a more pronounced drawing of contours and facilitates the detection of pathologically altered areas.

At the same time, a demand direction is the post-processing of images obtained in white light in order to simulate visual effects obtained by optical filters—virtual chromoendoscopy. The most famous technologies of virtual chromoendoscopy are implemented by FujiFilm, Pentax and STOLZ, these are FICE, i-scan and SPICE technologies, respectively. In recent years, researchers have proposed a number of new technologies for virtual chromoendoscopy [6, 7] only on digital image processing. It has been proven that the use of images obtained in narrow spectral ranges or by virtual chromoendoscopy can significantly increase the efficiency of diagnostics.

Thus, we can see that multimodal (multispectral) images used for effective diagnostic and also for advanced visualization, as by the way of fluorescent images generation as in the way narrow-band imaging. In chapter, we would like to present our experience in multispectral images enhancement, analysis and visualization. It should be noted that each of these tasks requires special processing and analysis methods that take into account the features of multispectral images.

The main feature of NIR channel in conditions of diagnosis and therapy of different cancer diseases is the ability of special injected reagents to glow in IR spectrum (see Fig. 3.4).

The drawbacks of IR representation are high presence of noise and weak ergonomics of visualization. So, in the case of enhancement and visualization for

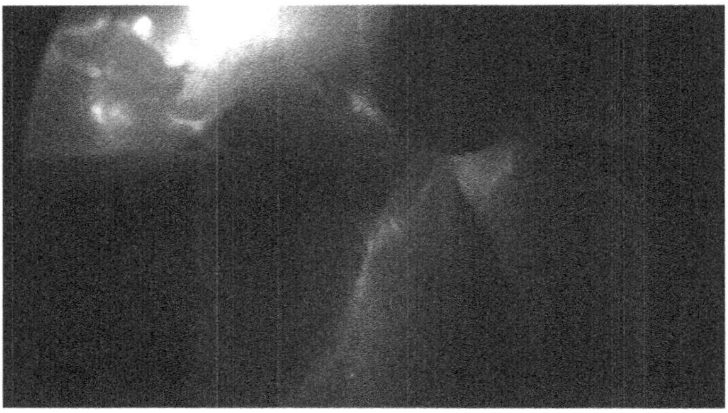

Fig. 3.4 Glowing in NIR channel

NIR images, the main task is to make effective combination in one image of information from NIR fluorescent image and information from image obtained in white light. This combination should ensure the preservation of information about fluorescence: different fluorescence levels of tissues with different pathology levels should be clearly reflected. Additionally, the synthesized image should retain the appearance of organs and tissues in white light familiar to the physician.

In the case of analysis, the fluorescence images can be used for obtaining more high specificity and sensitivity. For this aim, method must realized simultaneous analysis of different image types, such as the images obtained in white light and fluorescent images.

Accordingly, the chapter is structured as follows. Section 3.2 discusses methods of synthesizing a composite image that includes information from white light and NIR images. Section 3.3 is devoted to diagnostics based on multispectral images and features of Convolutional Neural Network (CNN) application in this case. Section 3.4 is devoted to a general explanation of the proposed methods, i.e. the tasks they solve and their areas of applicability. In conclusions (Sect. 3.4), the main results are summarized.

3.2 Development of a Method to Visualization of Multispectral Endoscopic Images

This section describes the stages of developing a method for image synthesis based on data obtained in various spectral ranges. The structure of the section is as follows. The main idea presents in Sect. 3.2.1. Methods of improving the quality of color images obtained in white light are considered in Sect. 3.2.2. Objective metrics for quality estimation for choosing an optimal processing method are described in Sect. 3.2.3. Experimental results with examples of processed images and calculated metrics are presented in Sect. 3.2.4, and finally, an algorithm for superimposing color and NIR images is proposed in Sect. 2.3.5.

3.2.1 The Main Idea

Improving the visualization of multispectral images captured by the endoscopic system requires several procedures. The physician should be well oriented in the scene which he/she is observing on the display. A habitual three-component color image obtained in white light with an RGB sensor is used for visualization as the reference. Digital processing techniques such as luminance equalization, contrast correction should be applied to improve overall visual quality. Additional information contained in the NIR channel should be added to the image while preserving important information on the main color image.

3.2.2 Methods and Algorithms for Endoscopic Images Enhancement

Contrast enhancement methods are divided into global and local. Global methods use a single brightness transform function for all image structural elements. Conversely, local methods apply individual brightness transform function for each image element. Its type is based on the analysis of the neighborhood of processed element. Contrasting endoscopic images using global methods is ineffective due to their features caused by complicated imaging conditions and the specifics of objects of interest. For example, when we use gamma correction to contrast dark areas of the image, it is necessary to decrease the slope of the transform function with increasing brightness. As a result, the contrast of dark areas of the image is increased. The shift of the image brightness to the high range will inevitably lead to a loss of contrast in the light area, which is a serious disadvantage in relation to images with uneven brightness and contrast. Due to the presence of large areas of light and dark areas, more complex methods are required to ensure brightness and contrast enhancement.

Contrast correction methods can be divided into two groups according to the data domain they are applied to:

- Methods with changing the value of the brightness of a pixel directly (pixel-domain).
- Methods with transforming into a new space (discrete cosine transform [8, 9], wavelet transform [10], curvelet transform [11], etc.) for further processing (transform-domain).

Methods of the first group have become more widespread in modern systems due to lower requirements for computational complexity and flexible configuration. According to the principle of implementation, methods of this group, in turn, can be divided into the following subgroups:

1. Histogram-based methods.
2. Retinex-like methods.
3. Local correction methods based on the use of nonlinear brightness transform curves, where the shape and type of curves used depend on the local distribution of halftones.

Among the histogram methods, the most effective and, therefore, often used is the adaptive histogram equalization with contrast limiting (CLAHE) [12]. It is important to note that all of the following brightness and contrast enhancement methods are applied to a single-channel image. To process a color image, it is required to convert the image to another color space, including the luminance channel (HSV, Lab), and process only it. The second option is to process all three channels independently, but this can affect the performance of the methods.

The Retinex method is based on nonlinear spatial/spectral transformation that provides localized contrast enhancement and color consistency [13]. The most widespread is the multiscale version of this method, known as MultiScaleRetinex (MSR) (Eq. 3.1):

$$L_{MSR}(x, y) = \sum_{n=1}^{N} w_n\left[\log L(x, y) - \log(G_n(x, y) * L(x, y))\right] \quad (3.1)$$

where $L(x, y)$ is the initial brightness of the processed pixel with coordinates (x, y), $L_{MSR}(x, y)$ is the pixel brightness after processing, * is the sign of two-dimensional convolution, $G_n(x, y)$ is the Gaussian filter mask of N different scales, $\mathbf{w}$ is a set of weights for each scale (often $\mathbf{w} = \{1/3, 1/3, 1/3\}$).

Retinex-like methods are usually applied to images with a narrow dynamic range, such as frames from traffic cameras or a runway in poor visibility conditions (rain, fog). Retinex can significantly distort the image, making it visually "flatter" or providing "cartoon effect". Such undesirable effects can mislead the physician and complicate navigation during the endoscopic examination, so the use of such methods in endoscopy is not advisable.

A simple method based on the use of the transformation function is gamma correction (Eq. 3.2):

$$L_{Gamma}(x, y) = A \cdot L(x, y)^{\gamma}, \quad (3.2)$$

where A is a coefficient, usually equal to 1, γ is the parameter that determines the degree of curvature of the transformation function. There are many options for the implementation of gamma correction, where the authors offer options for choosing the parameter γ [14–16].

Local adaptive gamma correction is more effective. Parameter γ is determined by the features of the neighborhood of the processed pixel. We have proposed an implementation option with Eq. 3.3 as transformation function:

$$L_{Gamma}(x, y) = L(x, y)^{B(0.65 + L_m(x, y))} \quad (3.3)$$

where $L_m(x, y)$ is the brightness value averaged over the neighborhood for processed pixel with coordinates (x, y), B is a parameter that determines the power of correction.

Figure 3.5 shows a variety of transformation functions for two different B. The larger the value of B, the stronger the curvature of the transformation function for a given L_m value, and the more pronounced correction effect.

Another, more efficient brightness correction method is Locally Tuned Sine Non-Linear Enhancement (LTSNE) [17]. This method includes two sequential stages. The first stage implements adaptive nonlinear brightness correction, and the second one implements adaptive nonlinear contrast correction. Let's consider the first stage in detail. A transform function that reduces the brightness of high-brightness pixels while increasing the brightness of low-brightness pixels is written by the following equation:

$$L_{LTNSE}(x, y) = \sin^2\left(L(x, y)^q * \frac{\pi}{2}\right), \quad (3.4)$$

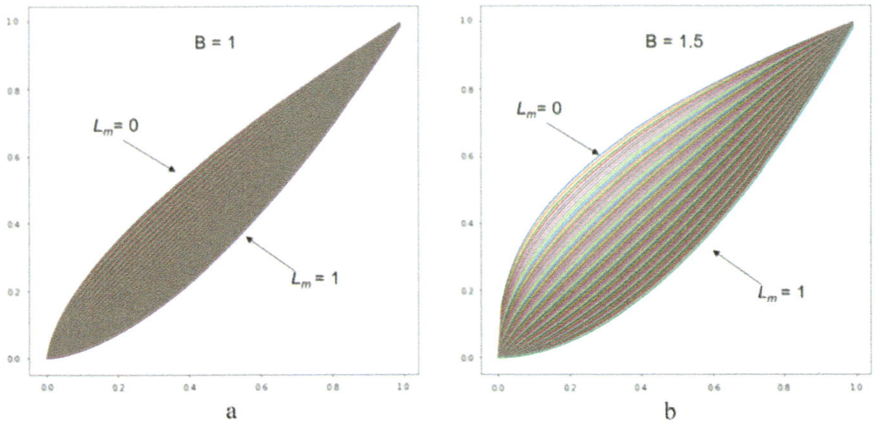

Fig. 3.5 The transformation function for the local adaptive gamma correction method for the set of $L_m(x, y)$ values in range [0, 1] with the parameter: **a** B = 1, **b** B = 1.5

$$q = \tan\left(\frac{L_m(x, y) * \pi}{c1}\right) \tag{3.5}$$

where $L(x, y) \subset [0, 1]$ is the brightness of the processed pixel with coordinates (*x*, *y*), $L_{LTNSE}(x, y)$ is the brightness of the pixel after processing, c_1 and c_2 are the method parameters that determine the curvature of the transformation function, and $L_m(x, y)$ is the brightness of the processed pixel, averaged over the neighborhoods of various scales:

$$L_m(x, y) = \sum_{n=1}^{N} w_n[G_n(x, y) * L(x, y)], \tag{3.6}$$

where * is the sign of two-dimensional convolution, $G_n(x, y)$ is the Gaussian filter mask of *N* different scales, **w** is a set of weights for each scale (often **w** = {1/3; 1/3; 1/3}).

Figure 3.6 shows a graph of the set of transformation functions (Eq. 3.4) for various values of *q* (Eq. 3.5). Unlike the nonlinear adaptive gamma correction method, the function used in the LTSNE method is more flexible and more symmetric, which has a positive effect on the processing quality.

The authors of [17] note that the noise level increases significantly in the region of extremely dark values. As we can see from Fig. 3.6, even the slightest positive brightness value increases extremely after processing if the average brightness of the neighborhood a close to zero value. To avoid this, the authors introduce an additional function for calculating *q* for low brightness levels:

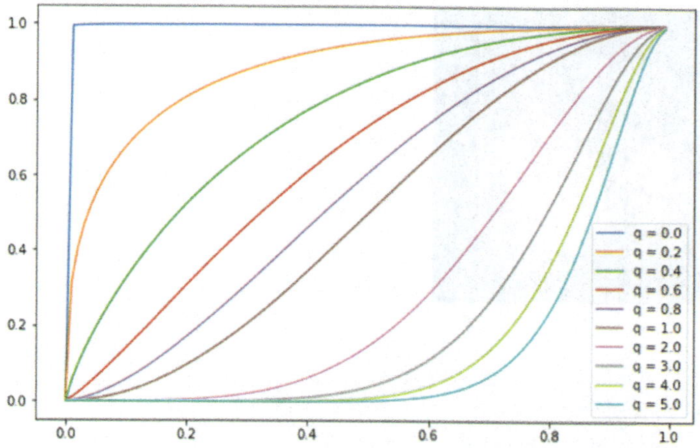

Fig. 3.6 LTSNE local adaptive transformation function for brightness correction for different q

$$q = \log(2L_m(x, y) + 2)/2 \tag{3.7}$$

Figure 3.7 represents examples of the brightness correction of initial image (Fig. 3.7a) using this method without additional function for calculating q value for low average brightness (Fig. 3.7b) and using this function (Fig. 3.7c). The values suggested by the authors were taken as the parameters of the method: $c1 = 2.25$, $c2 = 0.0085$. The figure clearly shows that the use of Eq. 3.7corrects the excessively "steep" transformation function, increasing the quality of the correction.

It should be noted that the parameters proposed by the authors are not suitable for application to endoscopic imaging. Strong overcorrection significantly changes the image, makes it dissimilar to the original, which negatively affects perception and can confuse the physician. Correction methods should be soft, provide emphasis on small details, equalize brightness and at the same time preserve the perception of the image. Strong changes are allowed as additional rendering modes that can be disabled. In this chapter, we are developing a correction procedure to improve the quality, and not as an additional mode to give the image new properties, so we chose other correction parameters. Figure 3.7d shows the result of the correction with the parameters $c1 = 2.7$, $c2 = 0.46$. Note that changing the parameters solved the problem of the extremely sharp transformation function in the region with low brightness. Therefore, Eq. 3.7 is not required for the calculation.

An important parameter of the method is the spatial scale for determining the average brightness in the neighborhood of the processed pixel. (The size of the Gaussian filter aperture $G_n(x, y)$ in Eq. 3.6). A small scale affects the appearance of halo artifacts, while a large scale weakly increases contrast. To provide a balance between halo artifacts and contrast enhancement, the method uses three different scales to capture the low, average and high frequency features of the image.

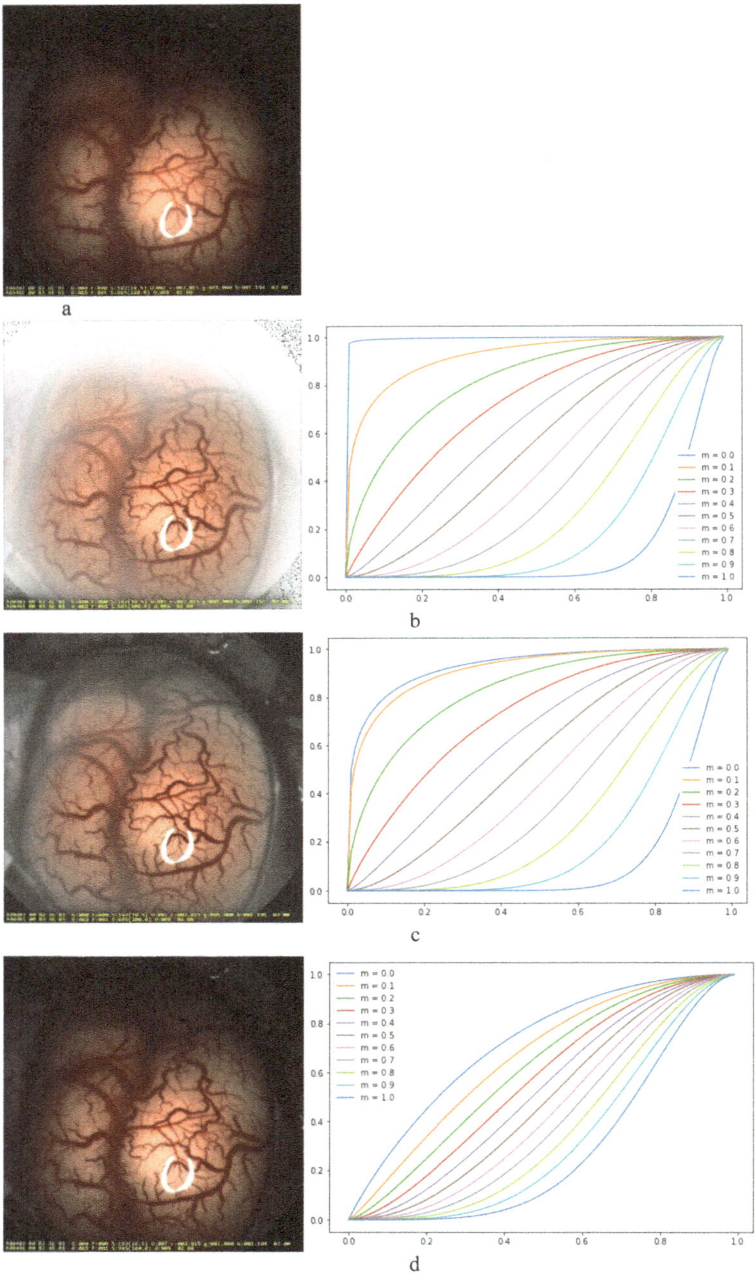

Fig. 3.7 Result of applying local adaptive LTSNE brightness correction: **a** original image, **b** image and graph without an additional function for calculating q at low brightness values, **c** image and graph with using an additional function, **d** image and graph with new correction parameters

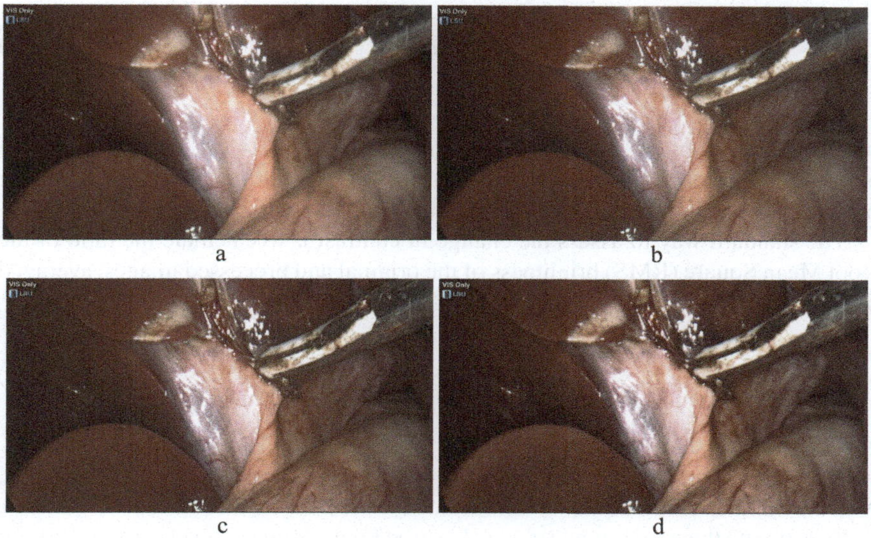

Fig. 3.8 Results of image enhancement by method LTNSE with different spatial scales: **a** initial image, **b** (7 × 7, 15 × 15, 31 × 31), **c** (31 × 31, 63 × 63, 127 × 127), **d** (197 × 197, 621 × 621, 981 × 981)

Figure 3.8 shows the correction results for three different sets of scales. In the case of (197 × 197, 621 × 621, 981 × 981), insufficient brightness equalization is observed. This is due to the fact that the original image has a resolution of 2608 × 1474, which does not greatly exceed the dimensions of the spatial dimensions of the apertures in comparison with another variants. For endoscopic images with this resolution, we have chosen option (31 × 31, 63 × 63, 127 × 127) as providing the best result.

We also want to note that to reduce the processing time, the search for the mean value of the processed pixel neighborhood can be performed using a simple averaging filter without significantly affecting the final result in comparison with applying the Gaussian filter, but the aperture size in this case remains the same important.

3.2.3 Objective Metrics for Assessing Image Quality Enhancement

Objective quality metrics used in digital image processing can be divided in two large classes. The *first class* includes metrics based on mathematical search for the difference between images: Mean Square Error (MSE), Mean Absolute Error (MAE), Signal-to-Noise Ratio (SNR), Peak Signal-to-Noise Ratio (PSNR). Finding the difference between images can be summarized by the following formula (Eq. 3.8) in the Minkowski metric:

$$D = \left(\sum_k \left(|L_k - L'_k|^\beta \right) \right)^{1/\beta} \tag{3.8}$$

where β is a constant, usually chosen in the range [1..4], L_k and L'_k are the corresponding components of the original and processed image, which are either brightness values or coefficients of discrete cosine transform or wavelet transform.

The standard way to assess the change in contrast is to calculate the ratio of the Root Mean Square (RMS) brightness of the original and processed images, averaged over image blocks:

$$\Delta C = \frac{1}{N} \sum_k \frac{\sigma_k}{\sigma'_k}, \tag{3.9}$$

where σ_k and σ'_k are the standard deviation of the original and processed image block, N is the number of blocks.

To estimate the image contrast, we also used Focus Value (FV) [18] metric, representing the ratio of the discrete-cosine transform corresponding to the energy of the constant component (DC) and the energy of the remaining components (AC) of the image.

The *second class* includes metrics, which are based on an attempt to use the physiology of the human perception system in such a way that the change in the objective quantitative assessment corresponds to the change in the person's subjective perception of the processed image in comparison with the original [19]. Currently, due to its high correlation with subjective perception of a person, the Structural Similarity Index Measure (SSIM) [20] has become widespread. A version with block-by-block averaging (Mean SSIM) [21] was used in this work.

An example of perceptual approach is the transition from the Euclidean metric to the CIEDE2000 [22] metric when calculating the difference in color coordinates. A color space is considered as uniform color space if the Euclidean distance between two colors corresponds the difference in perception by the human vision system [23]. There are color spaces designed to achieve this correspond. For example, the CIE recommended the CIE Lab as a roughly uniform color space in 1976. However, the CIE Lab cannot be considered as uniform, especially in the high saturation domain. At the moment, there are no uniform color spaces. Therefore, instead of the Euclidean metric, other metrics are additionally introduced, which provides a more accurate correspondence of the numerical values of the color difference to the human visual perception. These metrics include the following: CIE76, CIE94, CIEDE2000 and DIN99D. Today the standard is the CIEDE2000 as the most advanced and most accurate metric [24].

CIEDE2000 metric can be used not only to calculate the color difference between the initial and processed images. Using this metric, we can estimate the color contrast taking into account the peculiarities of human visual perception. In [25], the authors proposed using a metric to calculate color gradients in Sobel operator. The Sobel operator is calculated according to Eq. 3.10:

$$G = \sqrt{G_x + G_y}, \tag{3.10}$$

where G_x and G_y are the approximate values of derivatives at the point (i, j) which calculated as:

$$G_x(i, j) = \Delta E(L_{i-1,j+1}, L_{i-1,j-1}) + 2\Delta E(L_{i,j+1}, L_{i,j-1}) + \Delta E(L_{i+1,j+1}, L_{i+1,j-1}),$$
$$G_y(i, j) = \Delta E(L_{i-1,j-1}, L_{i+1,j-1}) + 2\Delta E(L_{i-1,j}, L_{i+1,j}) + \Delta E(L_{i-1,j+1}, L_{i+1,j+1}).$$

The value of ΔE in the original Sobel operator calculates as the difference between the corresponding coordinates of the grayscale image. By applying a color difference formula such as CIEDE2000, we can obtain contours that more accurately corresponds the color differences perceived by a human visual system in a color image. Examples of contour preparations calculated using the CIEDE2000 metric are shown in Fig. 3.9.

The left image shows that the contour obtained using the CIEDE2000 metric provides a lower contour intensity in the upper left area compared to the central area. This is fully consistent with the sharpness perception of a human. In the right image, the border of the transition from one color to another in the central area is better visible.

In this research, we propose a quantitative metric for assessing contrast correction based on human perception. The contrast level of a fragment of an image can be estimated by counting the number of brightness drops or by averaging the magnitude of these drops over a neighborhood. According to Rosenfield and Troy, the contrast value in the image fragment can be described by the Eq. 3.11 [26]:

$$R_k = \sum_{i=1}^{M} \sum_{j=1}^{N} \| gradL(x_j, y_i) \|, \tag{3.11}$$

where M is the number of rows, N is the number of columns in the bit matrix, grad L (x, y) is the gradient vector composed of the first partial derivatives of the image $L(x, y)$ along the x and y directions for each image point:

$$\text{grad}L(x, y) = \left(\frac{dL(x, y)}{dx}, \frac{dL(x, y)}{dy} \right)^T. \tag{3.12}$$

We used the difference in color coordinates in the corresponding direction, calculated using the CIEDE2000 metric $\Delta L_{CIEDE}(x, y)$ as an approximate value of the gradient in Eq. 3.12:

$$\text{grad}_{CIEDE} L(x, y) = \left(\frac{\Delta L_{CIEDE}(x, y)}{\Delta x}, \frac{\Delta L_{CIEDE}(x, y)}{\Delta y} \right)^T. \tag{3.13}$$

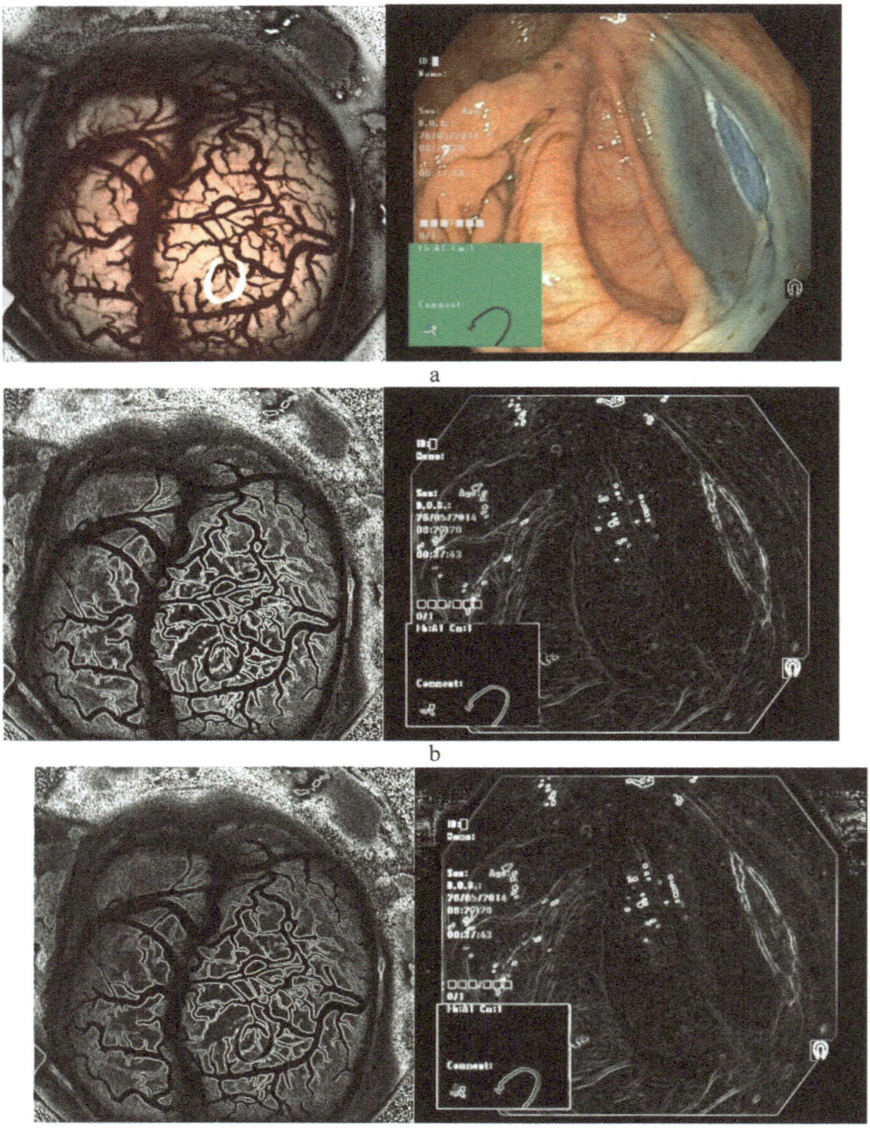

Fig. 3.9 Contours of images: **a** initial images, **b** contour native Sobel, **c** contour CIEDE Sobel

Substituting the value $grad_{CIEDE}L(x,y)$ from Eq. 3.13 into Eq. 3.9, we obtain the final equation for evaluating the contrast enhancement:

$$\Delta C_{CIEDE} = \frac{1}{N}\sum_{k}\frac{R_k}{R'_k} \tag{3.14}$$

Increasing the contrast of the image leads to an increase in the high-frequency component. In turn, the contribution to high frequencies can be either positive (emphasizing the vascular structure and other small details) or negative (increasing noise). In order to be able to evaluate the efficiency of contrast processing, it is important to have information about the noise level. A corresponding estimate of ΔSNR can be obtained using Eq. 3.9, especially for low-detail blocks, the changes in RMS of which are due to a change in the noise level. In the next section, we used this approach to assess the noise level increasing after correction.

3.2.4 Experimental Results

We have implemented the previously described algorithms and tested their effectiveness to improve the quality of laparoscopic color images. Experimental analysis, which involved subjective assessment and calculation of quantitative estimates according to the objective criteria described above, followed by the choice of the best processing approach was performed on the laparoscopic images database.

Figures 3.10 and 3.11 show the results of contrast enhancement by methods CLAHE, adaptive gamma correction and LTSNE. Method parameters are the following:

- CLAHE – clip limit = 2.0.
- Adaptive gamma correction – B = 1.2, window size = 31 × 31.
- LTSNE – c1 = 2.7, c2 = 0.46, window sizes = (31 × 31, 63 × 63, 127 × 127).

Objective assessment results are summarized in Table 3.1. The first metric ΔSNR is the estimate of the noise level, the value of which is equal to 1 corresponds to the fact that no noise increasing is observed on dark parts of the image with low detail. We want to preserve sufficient visual corresponding between the original and processed images, so the MSSIM value close to 1 is preferred. Higher values of FV, ΔC (Eq. 3.9), ΔC_{CIEDE}(Eq. 3.14) indicate stronger contrast enhancement. A significant increase in contrast leads to an increase in the noise level, therefore requires a balance between all evaluated parameters.

The adaptive gamma correction method provides best noise level, but at the same time weak contrast enhancement. The ability to flexibly change the shape of the transformation function of the LTSNE method by varying the parameters makes it possible to achieve better enhancement in comparison with the adaptive gamma

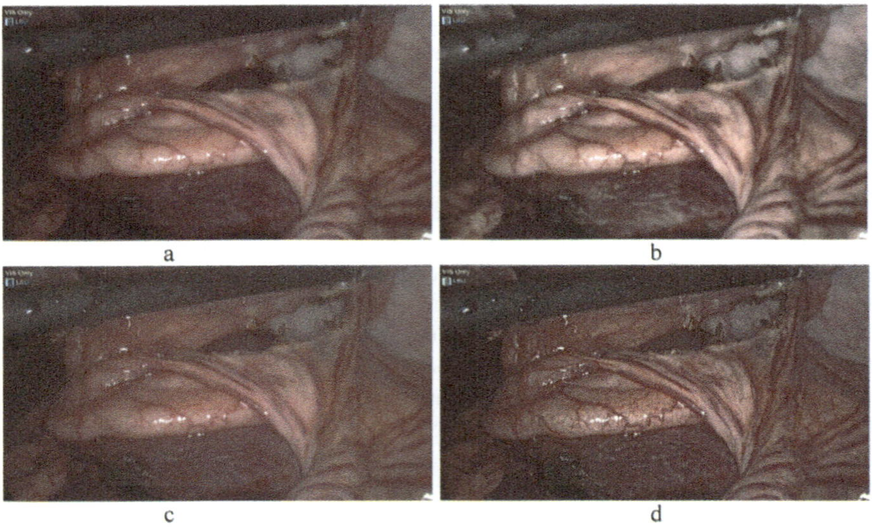

Fig. 3.10 Contrast enhancement results: **a** original image, **b** CLAHE, **c**adaptive gamma correction, **d** LTSNE

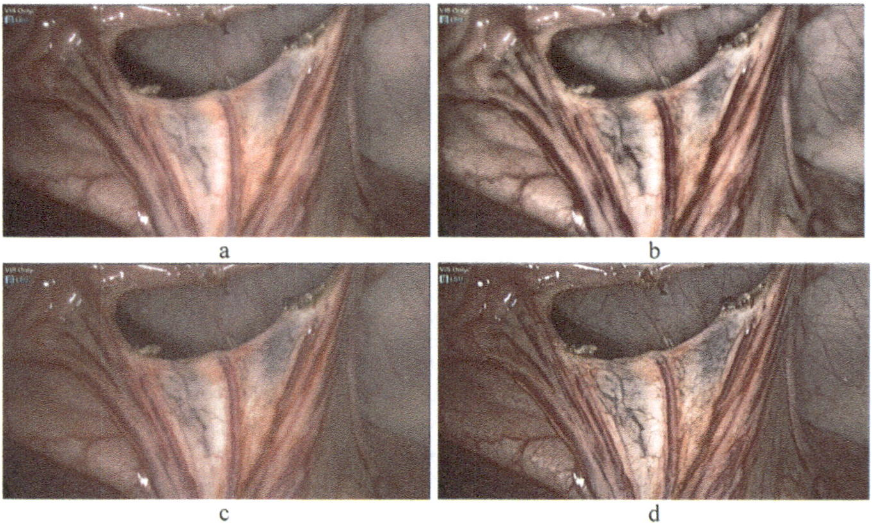

Fig. 3.11 Contrast enhancement results: **a** original image, **b** CLAHE, **c**adaptive gamma correction, **d** LTSNE

Table 3.1 Comparison of contrast enhancement methods by objective criteria

Method	ΔSNR	FV after corr	MSSIM	ΔC	ΔCCIEDE
CLAHE	1.36	0.0069	0.80	1.79	1.58
Adaptive gamma	1.15	0.0044	0.94	1.12	1.20
LTSNE	1.21	0.0062	0.95	1.43	1.31

Table 3.2 Color values for $k = 4$

Color №	1	2	3	4
sRGB values	[0, 112, 0]	[0, 147, 0]	[0, 197, 0]	[0, 253, 0]
ΔE_{00}	15.19	15.21	15.13	15.13

correction method, which is clearly seen from the results obtained. CLAHE significantly redistributes the brightness over the image, the sensation of illumination by a point light source disappears, which negatively affects the perception of the image and can disorient the physician. Despite the good contrast enhancement, the MSSIM metric is much lower compared to the other two methods.

Based on the results obtained, we propose to use LTSNE, which performs a noticeable and at the same time soft correction. The processed image is then used to combine with the NIR channel. The superimposing algorithm is described below.

3.2.5 *Superimposing Color and NIR Channels in Laparoscopic Imaging*

Let $\mathbf{O_w} = (O_{wR}, O_{wG}, O_{wB})$ and $\mathbf{O}_m = (O_{mR}, O_{mG}, O_{mB})$ be vectors of RGB pixel values with (x, y) coordinates of a color image obtained in white light respectively, and O_{nir} be the brightness of the corresponding pixel of the single-channel NIRimage. Then, the result of the synthesis of two images using alpha blending is described by following expression:

$$P = (1 - \alpha)\mathbf{O_w} + \alpha \mathbf{O_m} O_{nir} \tag{3.15}$$

where α is the transparency coefficient. In general, $\mathbf{O_m}$ image is filled with green:

$$\mathbf{O}_m = (0, 255, 0) \forall x, y. \tag{3.16}$$

Green is chosen to provide significant contrast of fluorescent areas against the reddish background of body tissues. It is important to note that before imposing a NIRchannel on a color image, it is required to perform geometric alignment of the channels, removing possible shifts or geometric distortions. Our database included

4 K video for white images and 2 K for NIR images, so a scaling procedure was also performed. An example of channel alignment is shown in Fig. 3.12. Figure 3.12a shows the original image obtained in white light, and Fig. 3.12b depicts corresponding NIRimage. Figure 3.12c shows the result of combining channels (left) according the Eqs. 3.15 and 3.16 and the mask used for this (right).

In [27], authors mention that green overlay is not robust as it relies on a predominantly reddish tissue background. When the background changes, it can lead to low contrast and incorrect visualization. The authors propose to produce the alpha blending procedure in HSV color space. Moreover, the value $\mathbf{O}_m$ is selected in such a way as to lie on the opposite side of the color tone relative to the value of the color tone of the image in white light averaged over the neighborhood O_{wHavg} :

$$\mathbf{O}_{\boldsymbol{mHSV}} = \left(\mathrm{mod}\left(O_{wHavg} + 180\,\mathrm{deg}, 360\,\mathrm{deg}\right), 255, 255\right). \tag{3.17}$$

Figure 3.12d represents the result of applying the Eq. 3.17 to align the images. Although the contrast of the highlighted area has improved, the highlight color has changed significantly, which can confuse the physician. Such a significant change in color tone should not be present in the mask image, otherwise it can be mistaken for pathology. Instead, we propose a different visualization approach based on cluster analysis and alpha blending.

Let $L^n = \{L_1, L_2, \ldots L_n\} \subset (0, 255]$ be the set of nonzero (or higher than a certain threshold τ) values of the brightness of the image pixels $\mathbf{O_{nir}}$. Let's divide the set L^n into clusters by brightness levels: $L^k = \{L_1, L_2, \ldots L_k\}$, where k is the number of clusters. Each cluster is assigned a color tone value $C^k = \{\mathbf{C_1}, \mathbf{C_2}, \ldots \mathbf{C_k}\}$. Then the value $\mathbf{O}_m \in C^k$ will be determined by the belonging of the brightness of the corresponding pixel of the NIR channel to one of the clusters: $O_{nir} \in L^k$. In the simplest case, colors C^k are selected from a set of primary and complementary colors. An example of such visualization is shown in Fig. 3.12e. The use of colors with a large tone difference makes it possible to better emphasize the color contrast, but at the same time prevents the interpretation of the objects in the image.

The second implementation assumes to use as colors C^k the set from dark green for the cluster with the lowest values brightness to light green for the cluster with the highest brightness values. Moreover, the choice of patches of green should be due to the peculiarities of the human visual system. As a criterion we chose the equality of threshold changes at different points of the sRGB color space with the introduction of an additional condition for the red and blue components:

$$\Delta E_{00}(\mathbf{C_i}, \mathbf{C_{i-1}}) \approx \Delta E_{00}(\mathbf{C_{i+1}}, \mathbf{C_i}) \approx d, \quad i \in [1, k-1]; \tag{3.18}$$

$$C_i = (0, G, 0), \quad G \in [0, 255], \tag{3.19}$$

where ΔE_{00} is the color difference between two colors, calculated using the CIEDE2000 metric (for more information about this metric, see Sect. 2.3), d is the threshold value of color difference.

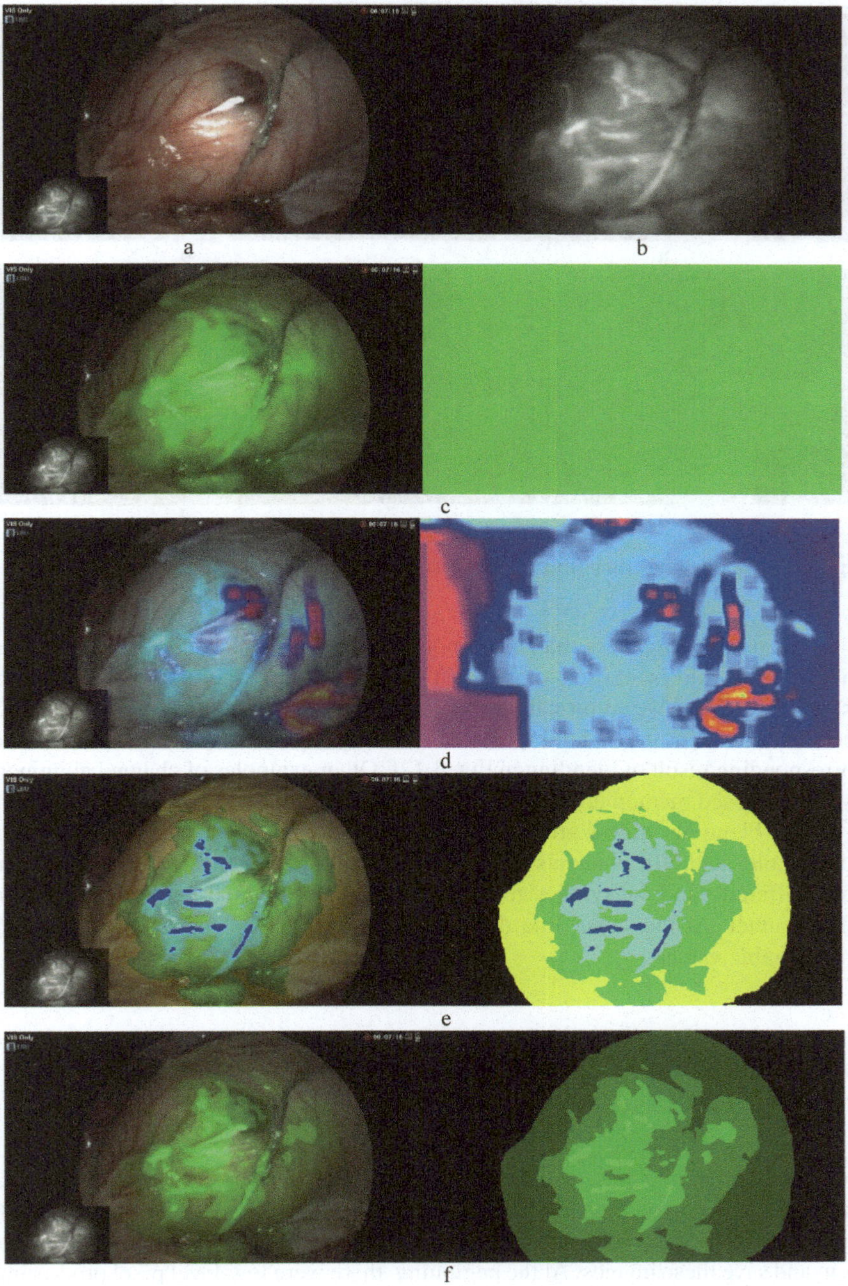

Fig. 3.12 Superimposing color and NIR channel results: **a** color image, **b** NIR image, **c** simple blending, **d** adaptive HSV blending, **e** cluster blending with custom colors, **f** cluster blending with green colors. The left picture **b–f** represents the result of blending, and the right picture represents the mask

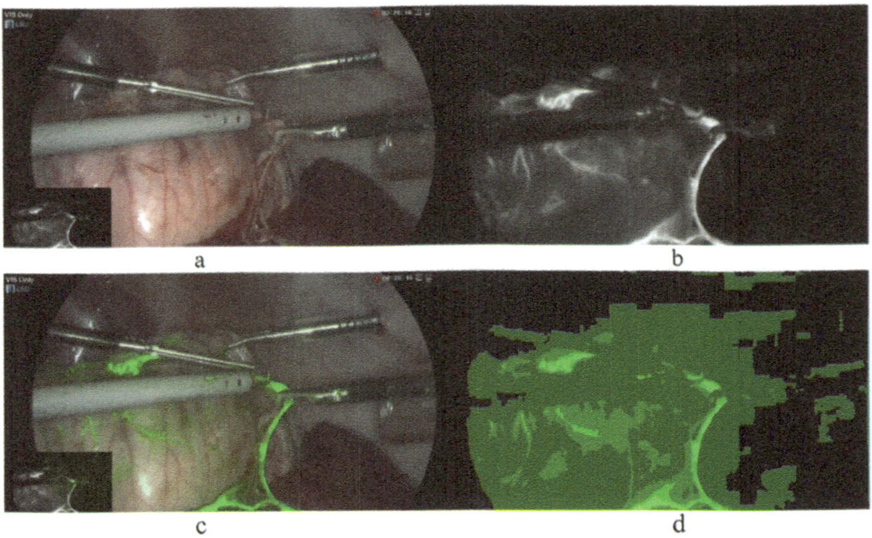

Fig. 3.13 The result superimposing: **a** color image, **b** NIR image, **c** blending result, **d** mask

Color pairs with d less than 1 are not visually distinguishable for human. The value of d should be chosen such that it covers a wide range of green colors. For example, for $k = 4$ we empirically set the value $d = 15$. The colors found taking into account criteria formalized in Eqs. 3.18 and 3.19 are presented in Table 3.2, and the corresponding result of blending in Fig. 3.12f. Other examples of channel alignment by the proposed method are shown in Fig. 3.13 and Fig. 3.14.

Alpha-blending with a green mask is the most common method for superimposing color and NIR channels. We proposed an implementation that enhances the color differences in the synthesized image depending on the brightness level of the NIR channel. At the same time this approach does not change the color tone to unacceptable values.

3.3 Anatomical Landmarks Detection for Laparoscopic Surgery Based on Deep Learning

Deep learning approaches, or, to be more specific CNN, have become a most popular and rapidly developed tools for medical images analysis. Of course, people began to solve the task of automatic analysis of medical images as soon as it became possible to form and save these images. At the beginning, there were low-level pixel processing, edge detection, watershed segmentation etc. and different mathematical modeling (fitting lines, circles and ellipses, other shape detectors) to construct compound rule-based systems that solved particular tasks. New methods of analysis were introduced

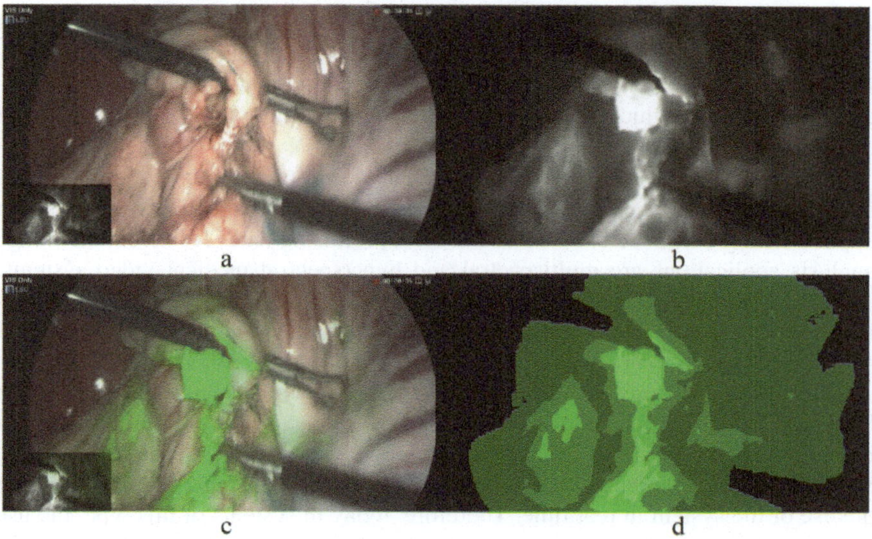

Fig. 3.14 The result superimposing: **a** color image, **b** NIR image, **c** blending result, **d** mask

as the sciences of digital image processing, computer vision and machine learning developed. But after deep learning became extremely popular in computer vision, the number of publications about attempts to use CNNs in medical systems increased tremendously [28]. In fact, every year several hundred papers are published on the application of deep learning approaches in the analysis of medical images. Largely for marketing reasons, the words "AI" or "Smart" are used in the names of medical video systems that use CNN technologies.

Nevertheless, this explosive increase in the number of studies has not yet led to an adequate level of implementations in the actual practice of creating and operating medical vide systems. There are many reasons for this, among which we can highlight the main ones:

- Well-known failures of attempts to build automatic diagnostic systems in medicine based on automatic analysis [29].
- The justifiable skepticism of the medical community that modern systems with automatic visual information analysis are capable to make diagnosis.
- There are objective difficulties in collecting a training data of sufficient volume, in ground truth forming, in covering the whole variety of cases (for example, in histology, the same diagnosis can have a lot of manifestations on the image completely different from each other and the training data will need to be collected over the years).
- Incomparable price of an error in the medical system making a diagnosis and in the recommendation system on the shop's website, a very long period of approbation and validation of the results.

Existing problems in building full featured AI video systems in medical diagnostic do not interfere with successful development of CDSS systems that extract new non-visual features from images through data analysis and somehow convert them to displayable result, which is useful for the doctor and help him to make the right diagnosis.

Although, there is also a sufficient number of serious and credible publications and there are areas, where methods of automatic medical images analysis have been applied with great success. Some of the most promising areas for automatic image analysis applications are multispectral and hyperspectral medical video systems. This is due to the fact that, on the one hand, multispectral and hyperspectral sensors have recently started to develop actively, and on the other hand, the performance of solutions for processing large amounts of video data is increasing.

Nevertheless, the processing and analysis of really hyperspectral images (with at least several tens of channels) is still at a rather early stage of development. First, it is difficult to produce a medical camera (e.g., endoscopic) with such characteristics. Second, a huge amount of data needs to be processed, which calls into question the use of the system in real time. Therefore, today in systems of this type, the use convolution neural networks are quite limited [30]. They are not deep, only up to 5–10 layers, to perform some specific task of the whole analysis process (for example, to cluster data at a certain stage), but not to solve for example detection or segmentation tasks (which require deep networks).

Many researches are devoted to the use of CNN in automatic analysis of multi-spectral RGB-NIR images [31]. This was made possible after the maturation of 4-sensor (Red, Green, Blue, near IR) line scan camera technology (Fig. 3.15) and the appearance of the corresponding datasets in large quantities.

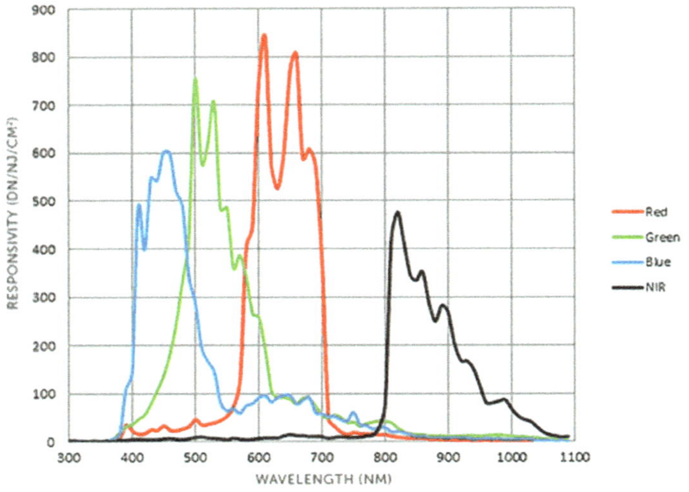

Fig. 3.15 Spectral characteristic of Piranha4 multispectral camera [32]

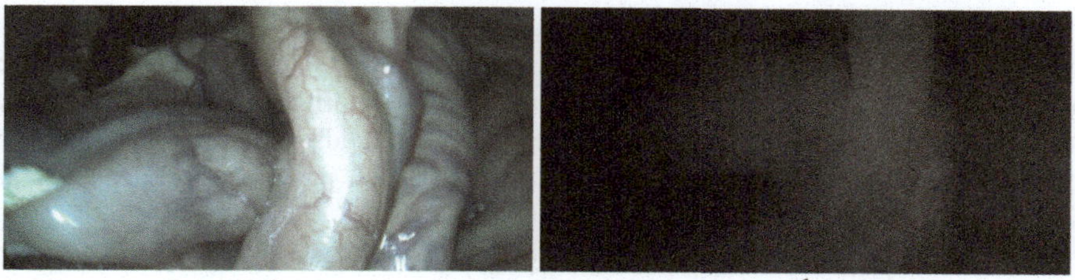

Fig. 3.16 RGB-NIR image: **a** RGB, **b** NIR image of intestine

As a rule, the following RGB-NIR image (Fig. 3.16) property is used: the RGB image has rich color features and the NIR image has sharp edge features or reveals some specific information of the tissues and organs.

It should be noted that in fact the potential of RGB-NIR cameras exactly for medical image analysis is much higher. It is a question of using fluorescent medical images. Medical video systems that use (record) fluorescence are quite well developed. One of the best-known examples is ICG endoscopy and laparoscopy [33].

ICG is wide used to visualize the location of blood vessels and define the perfusion in tissues and organs in medical diagnostics. It absorbs light around 800 nm and emits light around 830 nm. Therefore, it is possible to use narrow-band NIR illuminator and sensor to ICG exciting and registration. Although the typical use of ICG is to superimpose NIR on an RGB image to display the blood flow in tissues, organs and vessels, the information contained in the IR channel can be useful for automatic analysis. Automatic detection of anatomical landmarks (Fig. 3.17) during endoscopic or laparoscopic operations is a rather popular area of intelligent data analysis in medical video systems [34].

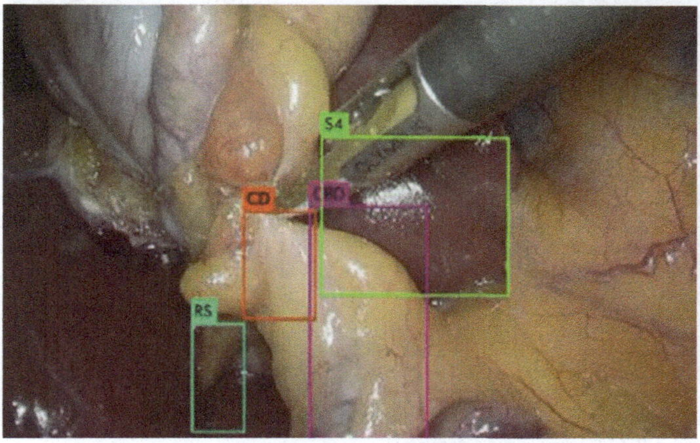

Fig. 3.17 Illustration of anatomical landmarks detection from [34]

This can be explained by the fact that in this area, despite the difficulties, it is possible to gather a minimum required amount of video data, and sometimes the annotation does not require the involvement of highly qualified doctors. In addition, the task of objects detection on images is quite well solved by modern CNNs. There is a family of architectures (like YOLO and SSD) that provide good accuracy at sufficiently high performance.

Anatomical landmarks detection is useful in training systems. It helps the doctor during the operation and can be used for automatic registration of examination stages (the task interesting today to companies engaged in insurance in the medical sphere).

Of course, when ICG endoscopy is in demand and widespread, it seems logical to train the model using not just RGB image (as it is done in conventional medical video systems with RGB images), but with additional data obtained in NIR. Still, at the moment there are no reports of successful use of NIR channel (in ICG systems) in training networks. Most likely, this can be explained by the fact that the intensity of the fluorescence itself depends on many reasons (the characteristics of the illuminator and sensor, the processes of blood flow, the nuances of the reagent injection), is dynamically changing and in general is not a reliable feature for detecting an object.

However, the information contained in the NIR channel can be very useful at the post-processing stage of neural network results. Knowing the peculiarities of a particular object of interest (some anatomical landmark) allows us to perform effective filtering and, for example, to fight against false positives as a quite often being a problem. Let us imagine that the target for object procedure is an artery. Then it will always be characterized by a strong glow in the NIR channel (Fig. 3.18). In areas, where tissues are saturated with vessels, it is also easy to highlight characteristic patterns.

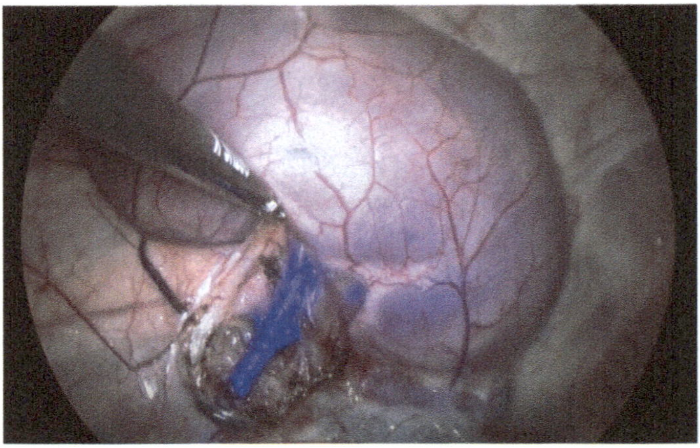

Fig. 3.18 Artery in the kidney (highlighted in purple color) viewed in fused channel (NIR applied on RGB) during ICG laparoscopic operation

As an illustration, let us consider an example of developing a procedure for detecting anatomical landmarks for the ICG laparoscopic video system. In described example, the goal was to detect an artery in a kidney.

The following main tasks should be solved while developing the procedure:

- Acquisition of training dataset.
- Questions related to the used framework for network training and deployment.
- Choice of network architecture.

The formation of a quality training dataset is a key procedure that determines the success of the task as a whole. There are basic principles that should be strictly followed:

- Despite the network's ability to generalize, the model is able to detect only what has been encountered at least once in a training sample. Each shape, relative size, angle, illumination of one object from human viewpoint are different objects from the model viewpoint.Thus,they should be covered in train dataset.
- Images in the dataset should not have a strong correlation with each other because this does not give any new information. Although, video fragments of endoscopic operations are characterized by a small changing context for long periods of time (Fig. 3.19).
- For successful detection, an anatomical landmark must be represented on at least 2000–3000 images.

A good dataset for anatomical landmarks detection should be obtained on the base of 2–3 hundred video sequences collected during the corresponding operations. Video

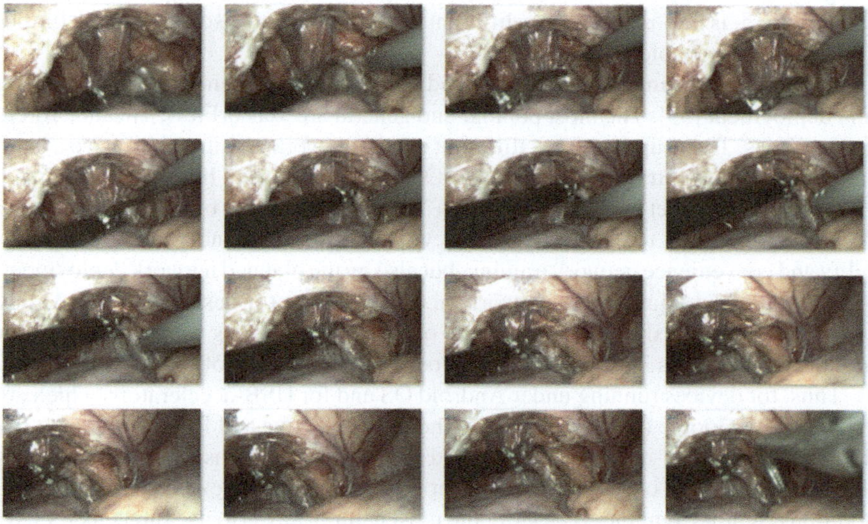

Fig. 3.19 Correlated images from endoscopic surgery

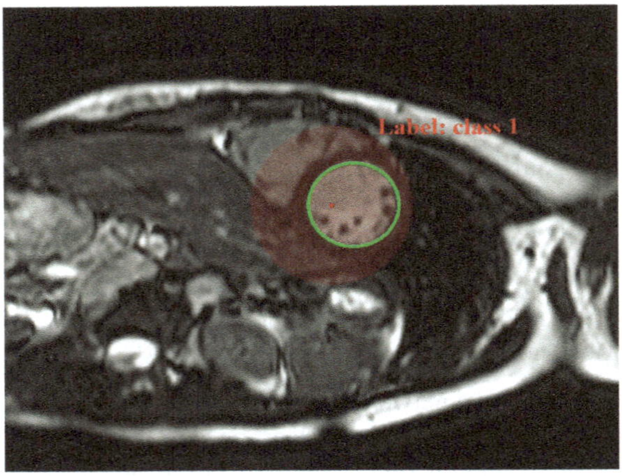

Fig. 3.20 Illustration to data annotation process in cardiac surgery video

sequences should represent the work of different doctors with different patients. It is necessary to create the variety of data. Received video sequences should be manually thoroughly cleaned from cases with poor quality shooting, excessive bleeding, erroneous recordings, etc.The images for training are extracted from the remaining videos. Then the duplicates (images with a degree of similarity that exceeds certain threshold) are removed with the help of special software.

The next important stage is data annotation (Fig. 3.20). There are methods to ensure accurate annotation, which include cross-working of several experts with the same images and calculation of their concordance. The peculiarity of medical images is that often only qualified specialists (doctors) can correctly annotate them. In this case, it is impossible to use different services like crowdsourcing. This further complicates the whole procedure.

Today there are many frameworks and extensions for neural networks training and deployment [35]. The most popular and general are TensorFlow, Theano, Torch, Caffe, Keras. They support many different neural network architectures, have a large toolkit for network training and design. Other packages may be more specialized. For example, Darknet is used to work with YOLO networks for object detection [36].

To a large extent, the choice of a framework is determined not only by the possibility and convenience network training, but also by the planned network deployment. If it is assumed not just to use network on a workstation (or desktop), but to deploy it on some embedded device, the choice of the framework (as well as the network architecture itself) is influenced by the type and specification of this device.

Thus, for devices running under Android OS and for USB-accelerators, which are produced by Google (Coral Edge TPU) the most effective and logical way is to use TensorFlow Lite for deployment [37] and therefore "big" TensorFlow for network design and training on workstation, or in cloud. For many devices based on Intel solution (Neural Compute Stick etc.), the most natural way is to use Intel OpenVINO [38] for deployment and, thus, various frameworks for training (TensorFlow, Caffe, MXNet, etc.), for which the conversion to OpenVINO format is supported. For

NVidia Jetson [39] solutions, the stack TensorRT and PyTorch is very popular. The choice of network architecture is determined based on the following questions:

- Which task should be solved by neural network?
- Which device will be used for deployment and what are the requirements to performance on inference?
- Which specification has environment for training?

First of all, specific architectures are suited best for specific tasks. For example, for segmentation task, there are SegNet, U-Net, MaskRCNN, Fast-FCN, Gated-SCNN [40]. For object detection, best scores are achieved by various YOLO, SSD, RetinaNET. There are architectures for object classification, time-series prediction and other tasks.

Each architecture depending on the number of layers and filters has a computational complexity that directly affects performance. As a rule, there is a trade-off between network accuracy and performance. As a rule, there is a trade-off between network accuracy and performance (Fig. 3.21). Therefore, if it is supposed to receive answers from the network in real time conditions, preference is given to lighter models optimized for performance. So, for example, for mobile devices MobileNet architecture is very useful.

The learning outcomes of some architectures are significantly affected by the environment used for training. So, many architectures use batch normalization, i.e. the more memory (for large batches of data) has the system, the better. Modern networks

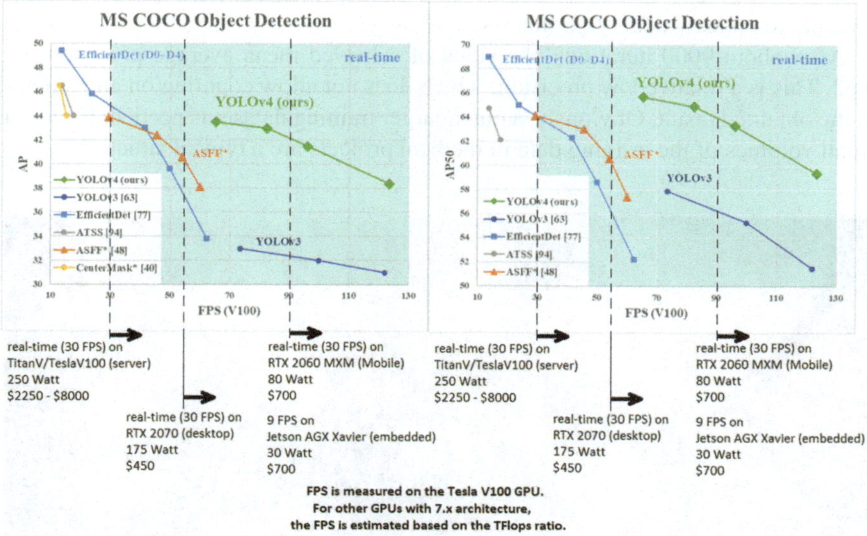

Fig. 3.21 Dependence accuracy/performance for the COCO dataset for various object detection models [40]

may have cross GPU batch normalization. In this case, one should understand that one cannot get the declared results without using several GPUs during training.

Let us summarize the above for the case in question. When designing a medical endoscopic video system, the requirement for performance is quite high. The doctor needs to see the result of the neural network prediction during the operation. Thus, at least 12–15 frames per second should be provided. If the system is designed mobile, it may be necessary to deploy the network on the appropriate device. Thus, the model should have some "mobile" or "tiny" version and should be as fast as possible.

Search of anatomical landmarks is the object detection task. So, the question is to choose architecture for object detection with good performance, mobile version and ability to be deployed on embedded devices.

According to analysis of current state-of-the-art solution one can conclude that the YOLO networks family [41] meets these requirements. The latest version "Yolo v4 tiny" can be trained using different environments. As a framework, it makes sense to use the Darknet, the native framework for Yolo. It is reported that Yolo-based models obtained with a Darknet are superior in accuracy to analogues (ported versions) trained in other frameworks. The model weights obtained with Darknet can be easily converted into TensorFlow format and then into TensorFlow Lite for deploy on some Android device, or, for example, on Raspberry Pi 4 with Coral Edge TPU on which it is possible to achieve near real-time performance.

The artery in the kidney is a very simple landmark for annotation (Fig. 3.22) and the process doesn't require high qualification of a physician. Since the frames have a high temporal correlation, it is necessary to perform undersampling of the dataset. So, for some small dataset that consists of videos from 10 surgical operations it was possible to collect about 3000 images.

After about 9000 iterations, the value of achieved mean average precision was 0.62. This is a relative low precision, which does not allow counting on any real use of the obtained result. Obviously, a much larger training dataset is needed. However, small volumes of the training data in medical projects are a typical situation.

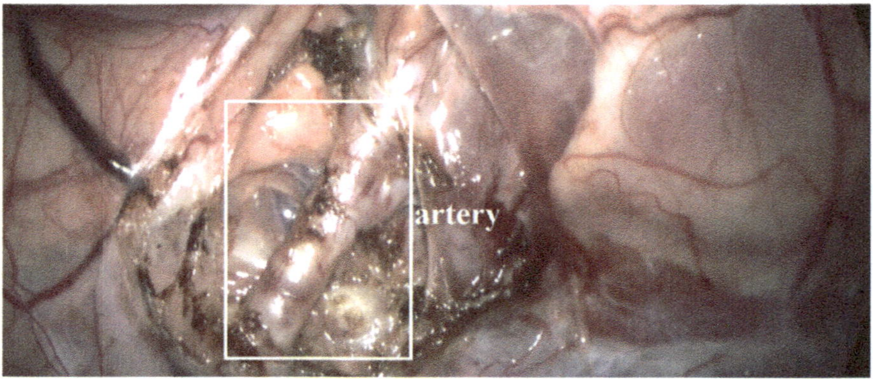

Fig. 3.22 Annotated artery on a kidney image

To perform filtering with information in the NIR channel it is useful to lower the threshold of accepted network predictions (default value is usually 0.5). The exact value depends on specific case, but make it twice lower will be a good starting point. The idea isto use a lowered threshold. In this case, the network will give outputs containing many false positives, but probably also with correct true positive (unseen with default threshold).

All false positives can be divided on two cases. The first case is misses. That is, completely erroneous rectangles containing no object at all. The second case, as a rule, is the groups of overlapping rectangles, bounding with varying precision the target object. Both cases are represented in Fig. 3.23.

Using the characteristic property of the detected object (artery)—the presence of high-intensity fluorescence in ICG endoscopy, it becomes possible to filter out a significant number of cases from the first group by analyzing the level of fluorescence in the area bounded by the rectangle received from the network.

In the second case, it is reasonable to select the rectangle that has the largest intersection over union (IoU or Jaccard index, see Fig. 3.24) with the area where fluorescence is present in Eq. 3.20:

$$IoU(A, B) = \frac{|A \cap B|}{|A \cup B|}, \tag{3.20}$$

where A is the area, bounded by predicted rectangle, $B$is the area with high level of fluorescence.

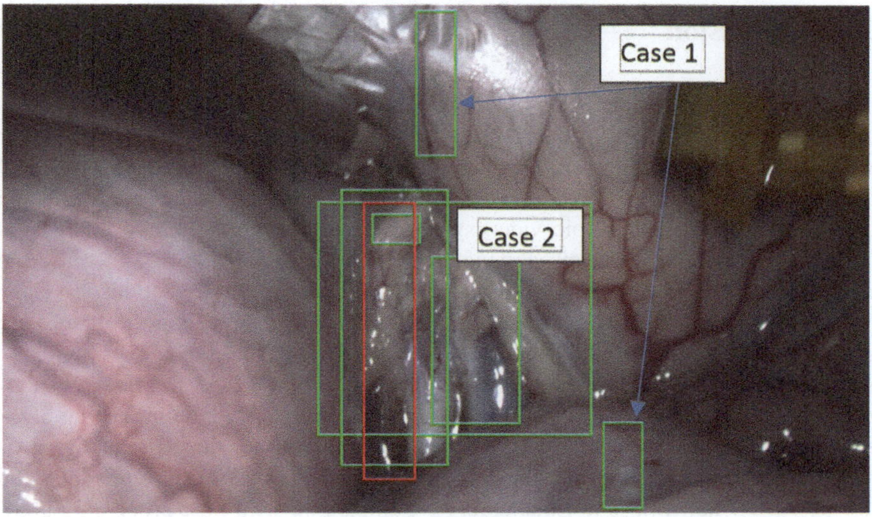

Fig. 3.23 Different cases of false positives and the ground truth rectangle (red color)

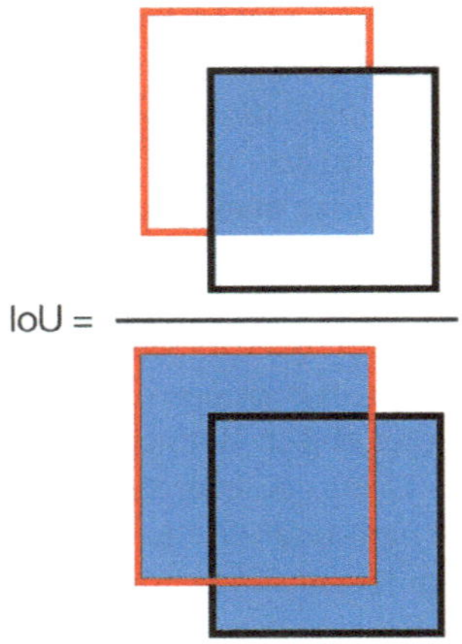

Fig. 3.24 Intersection over union (ratio of blue areas)

This relatively uncomplicated approach makes it possible to effectively increase the accuracy of the algorithm for detecting anatomical signs. The result depends on the type of anatomical landmark and the presence of its characteristic features in the NIR channel, but on average it is equivalent to an increase in the initial mAP value by 10–15%, which often allows one to speak about the practical utility of the obtained neural network model. This example clearly illustrates the benefits of multimodal medical video systems in terms of automated analysis and diagnosis.

3.4 Discussion

As part of the discussion, we would like to clarify that the described approaches are not steps of some "all-in-one" algorithm for medical data analysis. This chapter describes a set of methods for visualization and analysis of video sequences typical for endoscopy. The considered visualization and analysis approaches are applicable to a wide class of endoscopic video systems. They help to solve two main tasks of computer medical video processing: to improve visualization and increase the diagnostic value of video data for a doctor during visual analysis and also to carry out automatic analysis and, if possible, diagnostics. Thus, the enhanced images are shown to doctor, while initial images are used for network inference.

It should also be noted that for the considered approach in the field of automatic analysis, it was difficult to make a comparative analysis with existing algorithms, since the approach consists in increasing the accuracy through outputs post-processing of modern state-of-the-art CNN-based detection algorithms (actually, the use of YOLO network is not mandatory). Comparison with post-processing algorithms as a whole would not be correct, since all of them, one way or another, are tuned to a certain specificity of the initial data.

3.5 Conclusion

Multispectral images give new possibilities for CDSS development, because this type of images contain a lot of new diagnostic information associated both with fluorescence (endogenous and exogenous) and with the possibility of narrow-spectrum radiation to penetrate into deeper tissues layers. Thus, multispectral images can be used as advanced visualization for physician analysis or for automatic analysis.

For the task of multispectral images visualization, we proposed method based on combination image obtained in white light and NIR. On the first stage, image obtained in white light is processed with modified LTSNE method. This method was chosen after experimental research realizing it comparing with such methods as CLAHE, Retinex, standard LTSNE and adaptive gamma correction for endoscopic and laparoscopic images enhancement. Comparison was realized on the base of two metrics classes. The first class includes metrics based on mathematical search for the difference between images: ΔSNR, MSSIM, FV. The second class includes metrics, which are based on an attempt to use the physiology of the human perception system in such a way that the change in the objective quantitative assessment corresponds to the change in the person's subjective perception of the processed image in comparison with the original—metric CIEDE2000.

Based on the results obtained, we propose to use the modified LTSNE, which performs a noticeable and at the same time soft correction. The second stage of proposed method realizes fluorescent map (level map) creation, which was overlayed on result combine image. The main feature of this stage—fluorescent map (level map) is based on features of human vision. For the task of multispectral images analysis, we proposed method based on CNN for landmark detection for laparoscopic surgery (our landmark is artery in the kidney).

According to analysis of current state-of-the-art solutions we choose the YOLO networks family, the latest version "Yolo v4 tiny" was trained for landmark detection. Deep learning technologies are very strong and effective especially if input images have high level of variability. But deep learning technologies demands very big (extremely big) data bases for classifier training. In real condition, big data base of medical images verified by physician is hard problem. The main task of our research was to propose method that gives a possibility to obtain satisfactory result of CNN application in conditions of small data base.

To solve this task, we proposed to use the characteristic property of the detected object (artery)—the presence of high-intensity fluorescence in ICG endoscopy. It gives a possibility to filter out a significant number of error cases by analyzing the level of fluorescence in the area bounded by the rectangle received from the network. It gives to obtain an increase in the initial mAP value by 10–15%.

References

1. Obukhova, N., Motyko, A.: Image analysis in clinical decision support system. In: Favorskaya, M.N., Jain L.C. (eds.) Computer Vision in Control Systems – 4: Real Life Application.Intelligent Systems Reference Library, vol. 136, pp. 261–297. Springer, Cham (2018)
2. Chance, B.: Near-infrared images using continuous, phase-modulated, and pulsed light with quantitation of blood and Blood oxygenation. Ann. N. Y. Acad. Sci. **838**, 29–45 (1998)
3. Zhu, B., Sevick-Muraca, E.M.: A review of performance of near-infrared fluorescence imaging devices used in clinical studies. Br. J. Radiol. **88**, 20140547 (2015)
4. Gioux, S., Choi, H., Frangioni, J.: Image-guided surgery using invisible near-infrared light: fundamentals of clinical translation. Mol. Imaging **9**, 237–255 (2010)
5. Porter, T., Duff, T.: Compositing digital images. ACM Siggraph. Comput. Graph. **18**(3), 253–259 (1984)
6. Imtiaz, M.S., Mohammed, S.K., Deeba, F., Wahid, A.: Tri-scan: a three stage color enhancement tool for endoscopic images. J. Med. Syst. **41**(6), 1–16 (2017)
7. Obukhova, N.A., Motyko, A.A., Pozdeev, A.A.: Image processing algorithm for virtual chromoendoscopy (Tone Enhancement) in clinical decision support system. In: Proceedings of the Conference of Open Innovations Association FRUCT (Finnish-Russian University Cooperation in Telecommunication) and ISPIT, pp. 293–299 (2018)
8. Agaian, S., Silver, B., Panetta, K.: Transform coefficient histogram based image enhancement algorithms using contrast entropy. IEEE Trans. Image Process. **16**(3), 741–758 (2007)
9. Mukherjee, J., Mitra, S.K.: Enhancement of color images by scaling the DCT coefficients. IEEE Trans. Image Process. **17**(10), 1783–1794 (2008)
10. Fattal, R.: Edge-avoiding wavelets and their applications. ACM Trans. Graph. **28**(3), 1–10 (2009)
11. Starck, J.-L., Murtagh, F., Candès, E.J., Donoho, D.L.: Gray and color image contrast enhancement by the curvelet transform. IEEE Trans. Image Process. **12**(6), 706–717 (2003)
12. Yadav, G., Maheshwari, S., Agarwal, A.: Contrast limited adaptive histogram equalization based enhancement for real time video system. In: 2014 International Conference on Advances in Computing, Communications and Informatics (ICACCI-2014), Delhi, India, pp. 2392–2397 (2014)
13. Jobson, D.J., Rahman, Z., Woodell, G.A.: A multiscale retinex for bridging the gap between color images and the human observation of scenes. IEEE Trans. Image Process. **6**, 965–976 (1997)
14. Huang, S.-C., Cheng, F.-C., Chiu, Y.-S.: Efficient contrast enhancement with adaptive gamma correction. IEEE Trans. Image Process. **22**(3), 1032–1041 (2013)
15. Huang, L., Cao, G., Yu, L.: Efficient Contrast Enhancement with Truncated Adaptive Gamma Correction, pp. 189–194. BioMedical Engineering and Informatics, IEEE, Datong, China, IEEE International Congress on Image and Signal Process (2016)
16. Cao, G., Huang, L., Tian, H.: Contrast enhancement of brightness-distorted images by improved adaptive gamma correction. Comput. Electr. Eng. **66**, 531–544 (2017)
17. Arigela, S., Asari, V.K.: A locally tuned nonlinear technique for color image enhancement. WSEAS Transl. Signal Process. **4**(8), 514–519 (2008)
18. Shen, C. H., Chen, H.H.: Robust focus measure for low-contrast images. In: International Conference on Consumer Electronics (ICCE'06) IEEE, Las Vegas, NV, USA, pp. 69–70 (2006)
19. Winkler, S.: Vision models and quality metrics for image processing applications. Ph.D. Thesis (2000)
20. Wang, Z., Bovik, A.C., Sheikh, H.R., Simoncelli, E.P.: Image quality assessment: from error visibility to structural similarity. IEEE Trans. Image Process. **13**(4), 600–612 (2004)
21. Wang, Z., Simoncelli, E.P., Bovik, A.C.: Multiscale structural similarity for image quality assessment. In: Thirty-Seventh Asilomar Conference on Signals, Systems and Computers, IEEE, Pacific Grove, CA, USA, vol. 2, pp. 1398–1402 (2003)

22. Sharma, G., Wu, W., Dalal, E.N.: The CIEDE2000 color-difference formula: implementation notes, supplementary test data, and mathematical observations. Color Res. Appl. J. **30**(1), 21–30 (2004)
23. Acharya, T., Ray, A.K.: Image processing principles and applications. Wiley, Chichester (2005)
24. Huertas, R., Melgosa, M.: Performance of a color-difference formula based on OSA-UCS space using small–medium color differences. J. Optic. Soc. Am. A **23**, 2077–2084 (2006)
25. Li, X., Zhang, X.: A perceptual color edge detection algorithm. In: International Conference on Computer Science and Software Engineering, Wuhan, China, pp. 297–300 (2008)
26. Rosenfeld, A., Troy, E.B.: Visual Texture Analysis. Technical Report, Maryland University, College Park, Computer Science Center,USA (1970)
27. Glatz, J., Symvoulidis, P., Garcia-Allende, P.B., Ntziachristos, V.: Robust overlay schemes for the fusion of fluorescence and color channels in biological imaging. J. Biomed. Opt. **19**(4), 040501 (2014)
28. Litjens, G., Kooi, T., Bejnordi, B.E., Setio, A.A.A., Ciompi, F., Ghafoorian, M., van der Laak, J.A.W.M., van Ginneken, B., Sánchez, C.I.: A survey on deep learning in medical image analysis. Med. Image Anal. **42**, 60–88 (2017)
29. Strickland, E.: How IBM Watson overpromised and underdelivered on AI Health Care (2019). https://spectrum.ieee.org/biomedical/diagnostics/how-ibm-watson-overpromised-and-underdelivered-on-ai-health-care
30. Grigoroiu, A., Yoon, J., Bohndiek, S.E.: Deep learning applied to hyperspectral endoscopy for online spectral classification. Sci. Rep. **10**, 3947 (2020)
31. Monno, Y., Teranaka, H., Yoshizaki, K., Tanaka, M., Okutomi, M.: Single-sensor RGB-NIR imaging: high-quality system design and prototype implementation. IEEE Sensors J. **19**(2), 497–507 (2019)
32. Multispectral Imaging devices. https://www.teledynedalsa.com/en/products/imaging/cameras/piranha4-multispectral/. Accessed 7 September 2020
33. Cho, W.S., Kim, J.E., Kim, S.H., Kim, H.C., Kang, U., Lee, D.S.: Endoscopic fluorescence angiography with indocyanine green: a preclinical study in the Swine. J. Korean Neurosurg. Soc. **58**(6), 513–517 (2015)
34. Tokuyasu, T., Iwashita, Y., Matsunobu, Y., Kamiyama, T., Ishikake, M., Sakaguchi, S., Ebe, K., Tada, K., Endo, Y., Etoh, T., Nakashima, M., Inomata, M.: Development of an artificial intelligence system using deep learning to indicate anatomical landmarks during laparoscopic cholecystectomy. Surg. Endosc. (2020) (in press)
35. https://en.wikipedia.org/wiki/Comparison_of_deep-learning_software. Accessed 7 September 2020
36. Darknet: Open Source Neural Networks in C. https://pjreddie.com/darknet/. Accessed 7 September 2020
37. Tensorflow framework. https://www.tensorflow.org/lite. Accessed 7 September 2020
38. Deep Learning & Vision Tools, OpenVino. https://software.intel.com/content/www/us/en/develop/tools/openvino-toolkit.html. Accessed 7 September 2020
39. NVIDIA Jetson. https://developer.nvidia.com/embedded-computing. Accessed 7 September 2020
40. Bochkovskiy, A., Wang, C.-Y., Liao, H.-Y.M.: Yolov4: Optimal Speed and Accuracy of Object Detection. arXiv preprint arXiv:2004.10934 (2020)
41. YOLO: Real-Time Object Detection. https://pjreddie.com/darknet/yolo/. Accessed 7 September 2020

Chapter 4
Neural Network for Lung Cancer Diagnosis

T. Maria Patricia Peeris, P. Brundha, and C. Gopala Krishnan

Abstract This chapter examines the implementation of deep neural network for lung cancer diagnosis. The chapter will first outline the importance of deep learning amongst other learning methods in Artificial Neural Networks. Further, deep learning for medical imaging will be focused on lung cancer detection. The usage of 3D neural networks and thermal imaging for lung cancer diagnosis will be highlighted simultaneously. 3D networks are the emerging trend due to the evolution of high resolution images. Currently, the efficiency of 2D networks is the maximum compared to the evolving 3D networks. Hence, the chapter will implement 3D networks with more efficiency proposing ideas for higher definition networks. Additionally, the chapter will also examine the usage thermal imaging technique to identify short-breaths using nostril movement that is captured using thermal imaging cameras. The purpose of using short-breaths will be the ease of usage and compatibility of the network. The prediction can lead to earliest diagnosis possible when the concerned person identifies unusual breathing habits. The prediction can also propose other tests to be done if required. The creation of networks for both will be discussed in detail as the emerging trend in deep learning. The evaluation of the networks will be conducted leaving room for the future scope.

Keywords Neural networks · Deep learning · Lung cancer diagnosis · 3D networks · Thermal imaging · Short-breaths

---

T. M. P. Peeris · P. Brundha
Department of CSE, Francis Xavier Engineering College, Tirunelveli, India

C. G. Krishnan (✉)
GITAM School of Technology, GITAM University, Bengaluru, Karnataka, India
e-mail: gchandra@gitam.edu

J. Nayak et al. (eds.), *Advanced Machine Learning Approaches in Cancer Prognosis*,
Intelligent Systems Reference Library 204,
https://doi.org/10.1007/978-3-030-71975-3_4

4.1 The 'AI' Motto

Intelligent systems have become the recent code word that has overtaken computational concepts giving insights to a completely new technicality. Earlier, computation evolved around few lines of code that compiled the expected output when scripted into the corresponding platform. Nonetheless, intelligent systems have overcome the perception of coding revolving around making the computers behave like humans. The systems are trained with huge amount of data without the necessity of coding. The underlying terminology of making computers adapted to human-like thinking is called Artificial Intelligence i.e., 'AI'. Most industries have already redesigned their working protocol transforming their products or services to AI based kind. This catchy phrase has completely changed the future of technology to a great extent.

Taking a deeper dive into the 'AI' concept is Machine Learning also called as 'ML' which is said to be a part of artificial intelligence but not AI itself. ML is considered to be a sub-set of AI that has gained popularity in the recent years conquering numerous sectors. This is a technique that trains computers to predict the output without coding so as to make machines learn from experiences. Machine learning has eased out computation in various fields like education, medicine, business etc. The ultimate aim of machine learning is to mould computers to think and behave like a human without the usage of codes. This type of intelligence has developed new insights to computing creating a whole new concept of prediction, logic based decision making, voice recognition and classification. For instance, for a human being to predict if it will rain or not depends on the previous experiences like the humidity of the climate, temperature, windiness, colour of the cloud, etc. Hence, if any change as mentioned is identified by the individual then it is expected to rain. The same behaviour is expected out of computers as a result of learning. Nevertheless, in the case of a computer, the machine learns to predict the climate as a result of series of training phases. When the machine is given the situation wherein the changes are identified, it learns to automatically predict if it is going to rain. Thus, they begin to think and behave like humans.

Further exploring machine learning, today deep learning has gained more focus compared to the other machine learning methods due to the ability of the network to study the model in depth. As the name mentions, this technique helps the computer to unleash the hidden parameters by learning the medical images and other inputs layer by layer in deep. This model has the ability to distil complicated information from the given input data. The progressive arrangement of layers enables the model to pick up patterns on its own by implementing a step-wise accumulation of the same in order of these hidden connected layers. Besides, the model abides continuous learning where the machine learns its mistake on its own as a consequence of continuous training. The more number of samples fed into the model, the better the training process. In the training phase, the model is taught to detect anomalies in the given input by the subsequent application of an algorithm and multiple genres of raw data. This mechanism helps the model to increase the accuracy of the prediction when compared to the other training models. Furthermore, most deep learning models have been successfully yielding increased performance with an extensive learning capability.

4.2 Limitations of AI/ML

Despite the fact that AI/ML is a revolution that has gained familiarity lately and that its performance has been better than human beings over proper training, there are certain limitations.

- AI/ML have 100% accuracy: There has not been any model so far that has had 100% accuracy like us, human beings. Machines learn to predict and classify based on the input that is given to them and they do not have the ability to logically think beyond these sets of training and testing raw data. However, research and implementation of producing a 100% accurate model is under progress.
- AI/ML model can be a total disaster if taught the wrong way: The possibility of false positives may arise in case the machine does not learn properly. Suppose an unsupervised training model is considered, the machine will not be taught if the answer is right or wrong. Based on the weights designated for every node, the model will try to make corrections on its own. Hence, if the model learns the wrong interpretation, the entire might become a failure ruining the time and energy invested on the same.
- AI/ML model cannot take authoritative decisions: The trained models can only be able to predict or classify the raw data but will not be able to suggest the next step to be taken. For instance, in the case of lung cancer diagnosis, the model will be able predict if the individual has cancer or not but will not be able to suggest any treatments. Also, in the case of law and order, the model can be trained with previous experiences and case studies. However, they will not be able to analyse and pass judgements like how human beings do. The model will be able to give a general statement without mentioning to which party the statement is put forth.
- AI/ML model cannot be relied on for correctness in medical imaging: Today, most of the AI/ML model in medical fields reflect on medical imaging for prediction purposes. Also, taking the fact that there is no correct answer for machine learning, the correctness of the model may not be reliable. Every raw data processed will not be subjected to the correctness, rather the model will undergo a series of training where the machine will learn the more instances fed into the training phase to be accurate and continue learning.

4.3 Deep Learning in Medical Imaging

Deep learning is known for its complicated feature extraction from the raw input data wherein the network or the model learns on its own. This learning has confiscated a major part of the medical imaging field accounting for its feature extraction process. The features mentioned here may be the dimensionality of the pictures that the model considers as the input that can be extracted using various tools like keras. The ability of the network to recognise patterns without the parameters to be mentioned by the model developer makes it crucial for medical imaging. Pattern recognition is the fundamental of a machine learning model that acts as the baseline on which the entire model functions. Therefore, the initial model development process involves a few lines of code where the parameters and variables to determine the output are mentioned. These codes are developed mainly using python where in-built functions are present. The presence of in-built functions makes coding simpler and easier reducing the lines of code. The datasets piled for training purpose is then fed into the network one by one. As the model undergoes the training phase, it becomes more accurate gaining experience. Every image sent to the model is slowly analysed and the possible features predicted is extracted without the help of an external source to justify the selection of features.

For example: The model is initially developed to detect lung nodules in a CT scan which means dot like structures are the anomalies to be detected. A python code is developed and the network is created using the relevant functions required for the scope of the model. However, the size of the dot is not mentioned and the model learns the size consequently from the training phase with the idea that dotted structures are to be predicted, be it big or small. This implies that the model does not require the presence of both the doctor and engineer for developing the model, rather ample amount of data from medical resources and an engineer to generate and train the model would be more than enough. In clinical imaging, medical resources like CT scans, X-rays and many other image-based raw data are used to train model to detect anomalies [1]. The model ideally identifies if the texture of the image is the same all across the image. In case of any variables in the density of the texture, the model crops that particular area where the change is identified and further classifies if it is an anomaly. Thus, deeply learning is mainly preferred in medical analysis compared to the other methods.

Most of the healthcare providers contain huge quantities of data that are available both digitally and physically at data centres that can be used for research purposes. Datasets are usually divided into two for training and testing purposes. In the training phase, a different set of images are used so as to teach the model. As mentioned above, in the case of lung nodule detection, images with different sizes of lung nodules are put together. For the testing purposes a different set of images are used with a variety in nodule sizes. This way the deep learning model becomes familiar with diversified data increasing the accuracy of the prediction [2]. The process might look simplified but involves a series of layers of perceptron that contributes to the model to deep learn. Therefore, deep learning is preferred over any other learning in medical imaging.

4.4 Neural Networks for Lung Cancer Diagnosis

Lung cancer is the most dominating terminal disease that has increased the mortality rates in both men and women. There are many reasons that make for lung cancer like alcohol, tobacco, increased accumulation of harmful substances etc. Many institutions are finding ways to enrich the detection and treatment of lung cancer lately. Though lung cancer is a deadly disease, recent innovation in technology has made it possible to treat lung cancer efficiently. However, the main reason that might be behind the increased death rates is the detection of lung cancer at a much developed state. The realisation of symptoms occurs at a very later stage where treatment becomes very tedious and sometimes impossible too. In order to detect cancer numerous ways are being implemented among which a few have become very common. Lung cancer can be diagnosed using chest x-rays and scans. The more reliable way to predict lung cancer is the use of lung nodules or lumps present in the medical images. Lately, deep learning has been largely implemented in detecting lung nodule for lung cancer prediction [3]. These nodules are dot like structures that appear on the scans and x-rays which varies in size depending on the severity of the cancerous cells present. A more detailed discussion of implementing the same for early diagnosis will be given below.

Neural networks are connected layers of perceptrons that look similar to the neuron connection in a human brain. They look like the connection made between brain cells where each neuron is connected either in a single or multiple manner. A deep neural network consists of many layers that help the model enhance the accuracy, given the output required. The hidden layers consist of perceptrons that act like the neurons of the brain studying every minute detail of the input fed into the network [4]. The number of layers depends on the expectation of the model so as to make correct predictions. Here, algorithms serve as the means of teaching the network to learn the details of the input according to the model developed. Furthermore, deep learning has gained importance in the field of medical imaging which will be discussed more in detail. The classification and prediction of anomalies in medical images such as scans, x-rays etc. is easier and efficient using deep learning. They allow the model to segregate dense and less dense regions based on the texture, area under selection and many other parameters. Research has given credibility to deep learning in the field of medical imaging compared to the other types of learning methods.

A deep neural network consists of many hidden layers that enhance feature extraction. The neural network looks like as shown in Fig. 4.1.

The image is a depiction of how a neural network looks like in the form of layers. Each dotted structure is a perceptron (i.e.) neurons of the brain that are called as perceptrons in the case of neural networks. The different colours are used to show different layers that act as the hidden layers of the deep neural network which are connected to each other. These layers shown in the image depict a typical deep neural network where the input layer takes the raw data and the hidden layers extract explicit and hidden complex features. Each perceptron is assigned a weight by the network that sorts the variables manipulated by the network during the prediction process.

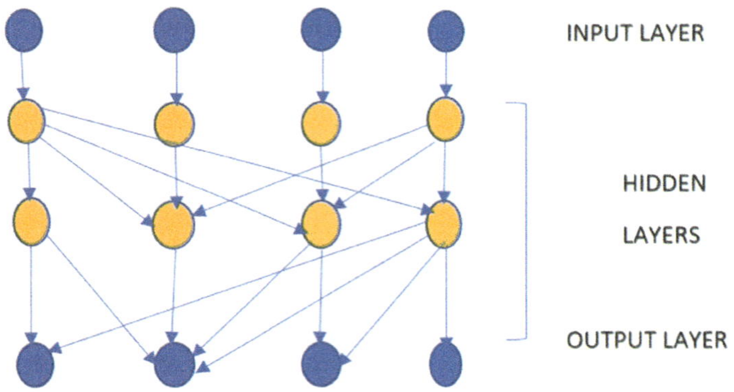

Fig. 4.1 Deep neural network with hidden layers

The output layer is the expected outcome of the model. The hidden layers connect the perceptrons with identical parameters to draw out possible characteristics of the given input image.

For an illustration: when a clinical image is given as input to the network, the image is passed to the next immediate hidden layer where the necessary features like texture of the image, width of the area of selection, etc. are segregated. The images are further sent to the next hidden layer for another set of investigation like the size of the lung nodule as mentioned above. The layers are interconnected in such a way that each perceptron carry a weight and similar weights or weights close to the previous ones are connected to the other perceptrons [5]. The picture describes the interconnection through the connected lines where multiple connections represent the similar parametric acquaintances. The number of hidden layers may vary depending on the complexity of the model. Thus, is the working of a deep neural network.

4.4.1 Convolution Neural Networks

Most deep learning models use Convolution Neural Networks (CNN) for prediction purposes as they require very few parameters for training purposes. A general CNN consists of convolution layer and pooling layers. In the case of a deep neural network, the convolution layer acts as a medium for selecting the area under investigation whilst the pooling layer acts as a connecting joint that pools or segregates similar structures [6]. Currently, 2D CNNs are implemented in most of the deep learning models and 3D CNNs are beginning to gain importance. The deep neural network that will be used in lung cancer diagnosis and the working of 2D CNNs is depicted in Fig. 4.2.

The image here is a demonstration of the working of a 2D convolution neural network for the convenience of the reader. The segregation process of the intense

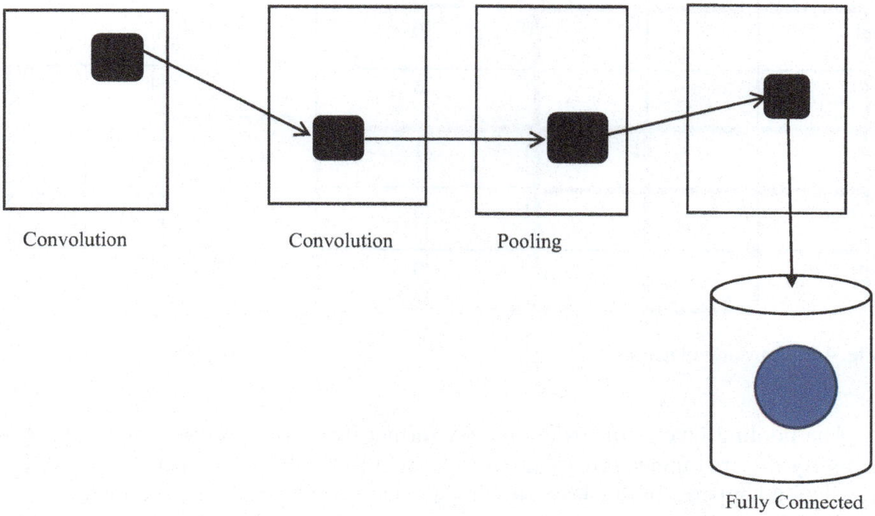

Fig. 4.2 Working of a 2D convolution neural network

textures takes place in a similar manner. The patches here represent the area under investigation based on the dimensions used for investigation in the convolution layer. The patch in the pooling layer shows the grouping of all the similar structures (lung nodules). The fully connected layer represents the entire hidden layer based on which the prediction is done [7].

In a 2D CNN, two convolution layers are used so as to isolate the two dimensional variables. What happens here is that a matrix is applied that convolutes layers with similar values are tries minimize the matrix i.e. when a picture is fed into the network, the density of the texture in both dimensions are investigated and the similar density areas are grouped together. The grouping happens individually amongst the two convolution layers with respect to dimensions. An example matrix of convolution is shown below in Fig. 4.3.

The representation showed above is an imaginary matrix of how the convolution takes place. The areas are separated based on the weight values of the perceptrons as shown in the deep neural network architecture. Based on the weights, the parametric values are convoluted and converted to a smaller matrix. The matrix conversion is not visible with the human eye but takes place within the network. The image fed into the network is split into a matrix where the texture of the image is taken into consideration. According to the dimensions, the convolution matrix assigns the values. The matrix cross is determined by the model developer based on the requirement [8]. Therefore, in the case of a 2D convolution layer, 2 matrices are convoluted. The matrix is further simplified to make it easier for pooling purposes. The thicker the texture of the image, higher is the value of the matrix if the medical image is of an infected person and vice-versa [9].

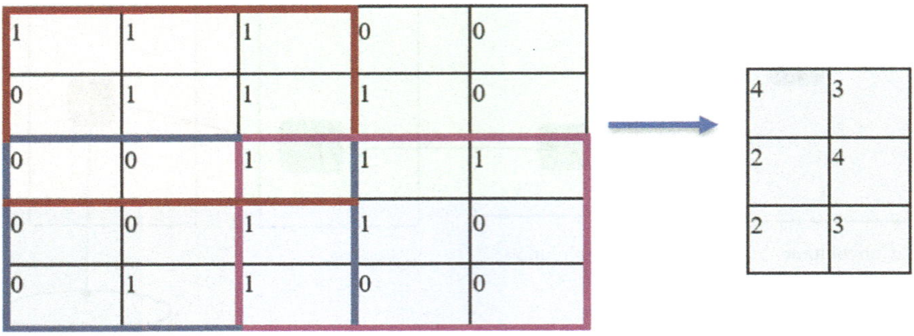

Fig. 4.3 Convolution matrix

The pooling layer reduces the matrix further down to a limited one in order to simplify the area under investigation to be sent to the fully connected layer where prediction happens. In this layer, the image is left behind and only the matrix value is taken for the next level. As machine learning is basically a mathematical model designed for respective intelligences, the entire network except for the initial layers work mathematically. An example matrix is shown below in Fig. 4.4.

The colour based representation of the matrix is to show the pooling process where isolation of similar parameters is combined into one. This simplified form of the matrix disregards the frames of the image and instead groups same valued features together. The two convolution matrices are grouped together and the simplified form of matrix is obtained. Here, the resultant matrix is a single matrix which is the average value of the convoluted matrix. The sectional area where the thickness is likely to be more is further examined for the prediction of lung cancer. Since most lung cancers are diagnosed based on the lung nodules, the model will isolate the area where the presence of lung nodules is expectantly more.

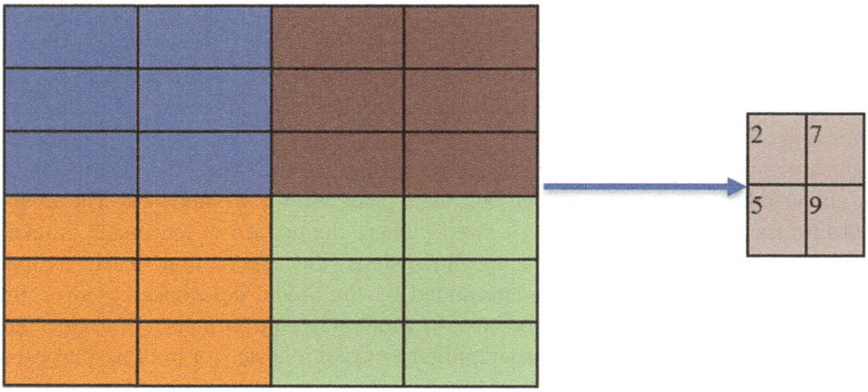

Fig. 4.4 Pooling matrix

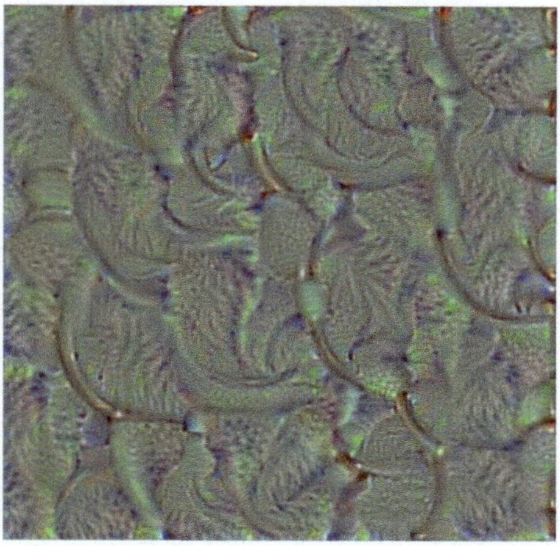

Fig. 4.5 An area of the cropped texture

The fully connected layer further considers the cropped portion of the image (Fig. 4.5) and conducts an analysis for the same.

The image is a cropped texture of the lung nodule that might be detected during the runtime of the model. The cropping is a part of the zoomed portion taken from the input image fed into the network. This zoomed portion of the image when passed through the fully connected layer, the network analysis the picture based on the algorithm with which it is trained imparting the functional parameters to be examined. The layers then inculcate variables like colour, size, etc.

Now, when the neural networks are trained, before the outcome is produced, there is an expectation of epoch generation. Epochs are nothing but the full training cycle that has been completed successfully nevertheless the correctness is void at this stage [10]. If the model is able to generate epochs, then the cycle of training phase is expected to be successful. Only if the epochs are successful the model can be subjected to training. Initial, the model is trained with a single image to test if the cycle is complete. Therefore, more the number of images, more the epochs are generated. These epochs are a part of the algorithm that is used for implementation. Most machine learning models use python for code generation as it is easier to implement and require very few lines of code due to the inbuilt functions in the language. Though many other languages like JAVA, Ruby are being used, python has made a stronghold in machine learning. The epoch generation of the neural network is depicted in Fig. 4.6.

Once the epoch is successfully completed, the model is subjected to a training phase where huge amount of data are docked in the train case folder of the running platform at the backend. As mentioned earlier, the data is either accessed online or offline depending on the subscription or membership respectively. This one epoch generation used the entire CNN model expect for the fully connected layer [11]. Fully connected layers are used for the prediction purposes. The successful outcome will further enhance the successful implementation of the predictive model. On achieving epochs, the next step is the actual prediction of the model where the ultimate goal is

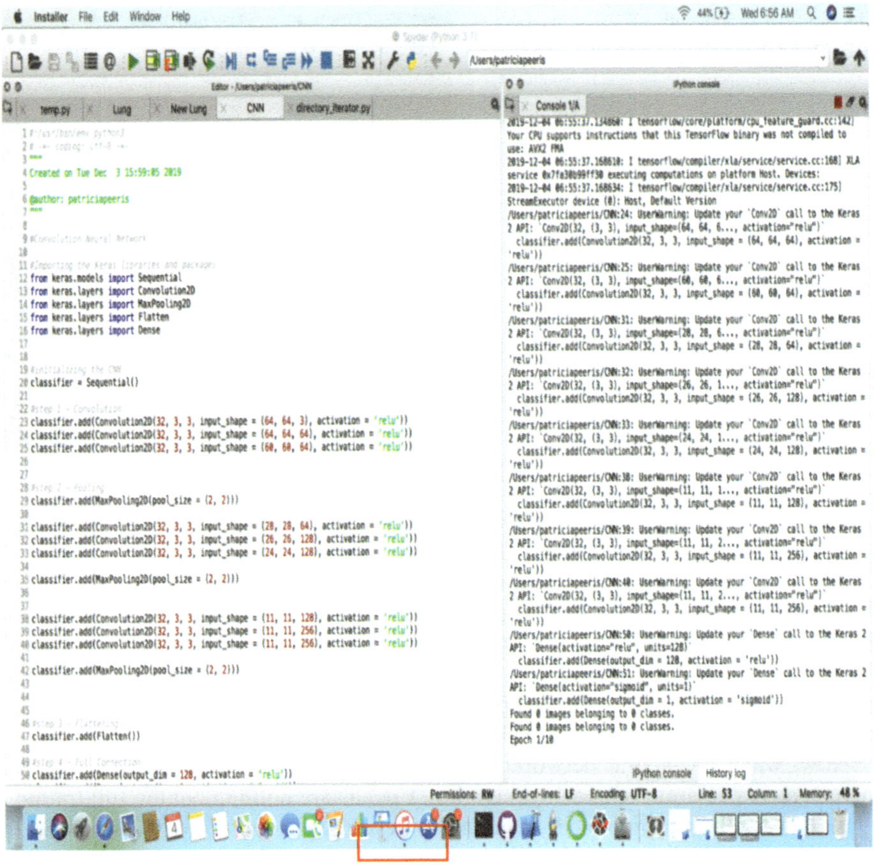

Fig. 4.6 Epoch generation of neural network

to predict cancer or not. As mentioned earlier, the initial code is then iterated to fit in the required functions that help in the parametric analysis of the lung cancer cells present in the input image [12]. The train and test functions are used to differentiate if the particular image is used for training purpose or testing purpose [13]. Mostly, CT scan images or x-rays are used for a 2D model. Once the mode is trained, test images are fed into the network and the model is tested for the lung cancer. The outcome will be 'CANCER' or 'NO CANCER'. The results will be displayed in the console of the platform and discrepancies if any will be specified in the same.

The expected outcome is as shown in Fig. 4.7.

The resultant image is the output obtained from the self-trained model that has predicted 'CANCER' for the particular individual for the corresponding image shown in the diagram.

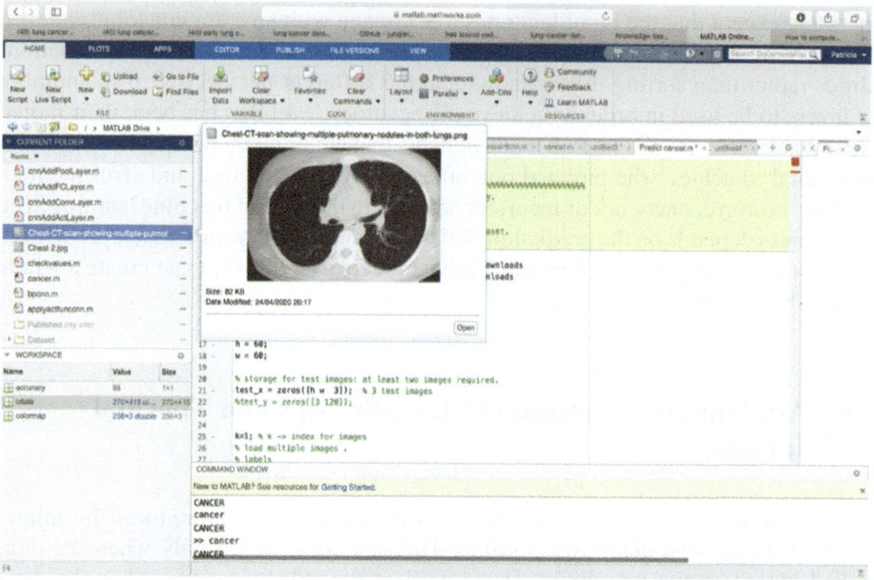

Fig. 4.7 Cancer prediction

4.5 Proposing a 3D Neural Network

The revolution of artificial intelligence has paved way for much better types of prediction such as using 3-Dimensional (3D) neural networks actualising in-depth learning of the images. The possibility of using 3D neural networks increases the variability of the medical images that can be used as the input. Photographic images like jpeg, jpg can also be used for prediction purposes. Due to technological advancements, the quality of pictures has been improvised. The existing CNN networks are more prone to lesser quality predictions as they are trained to access two dimensions only. The accuracy level although is reaching the maximum, applying 3D networks will altogether contribute to a whole new better quality of prediction.

The implementation of 3D CNN networks may be a breakthrough to gain 100% accuracy as the quality and variability of the image is high flocking even more huge quantity of data. The difference might be the number of convolution layers, pooling layers and the dimensions of the image. However, the functionality will remain the same.

Implementing 3D layers for predictive models can also pave way to experiment other 5D, 8D networks in future. The dimensions of the matrix and the number of matrix might vary. Additionally, when the convolution takes places, a better quality can be expected as the dimensions are individually examined giving rise to a better quality the area under selection making the machine more intelligent by feeding any type of images which has 3 dimensions. The architecture of the network might remain the same except that the input layer has a 3D image with an extra convolution layer. The pooling layer however will remain the same as it has only grouping functionalities rather than sorting. Every individual has different perspective of the number of layers to be used in order to achieve the accuracy level that has been their target. Neural networks are just human made puppets that are implemented by the particular individual to achieve the targeted outcome from a series of trial and error method. There is no correct network or incorrect network in the case of machine learning. The correctness depends on the prediction of the system and not the process of prediction. This concept can generate more innovative models in future that can create a whole new technical aspect.

4.6 Applying the Concept of Short-Breaths and Thermal Imaging

The mortality rates resulting as a result of lung cancer can be reduced by implementing the earliest diagnosis possible. This can be achieved only when the individual identifies an abnormality at the earliest possible stage. Short-breaths are a symptom of many illnesses amongst which is lung cancer, asthma, etc. [14, 15]. The shortness of breaths can be an easy and early identification of an abnormality in an individual. For example, if an individual averagely breaths 5 times every minute then an increase in the number of breaths will show an abnormality in the breathing pattern which means when an individual breaths more than 5 times they fall short of breath.

Short-breaths are easily identifiable when compared to the other symptoms. A person climbing the ladder before being diagnosed with cancer or any other ailments has a different breathing pattern when compared to a person who is not infected by any disease. Any individual falling short of breath will be able to feel that he is exhausted than usual or unusually. This alerts the individual to go for a check-up wherein cancer if present can be predicted. As a result, they can undergo further tests and treatments for the same. However, if there is no lung cancer predicted, then the individual may be subjected to tests related to shortness of breath resulting in the diagnosis of any other ailments if present. Hence, the patient will be able to undergo treatments for the diagnosed disease and take curative measures. Therefore, short-breaths can have a positive impact in predicting lung cancer at early stages.

Now, to make tasks easier and innovative, implementing a new concept of predicting short-breaths handily is proposed. Thermal imaging can be used for detecting short breaths that can be used to predict lung cancer. Thermal cameras are now easily available both online and offline. The advantage of using thermal imaging is that the camera can keep a track of black and white motions at the exposed area. Suppose, a person holds the camera focusing the eyes, the eye movement of the individual is recorded for the speculated interval of time. The camera will be able to predict the number of eye movements, the dimensions at which the eyes are capable of moving, the extent to which the eye balls move and many more features. Therefore, an initiative of applying thermal imaging to capture short-breaths in order to predict lung cancer is proposed which is a resultant of the earliest approach possible.

4.6.1 Components and Arrangements

This ideology requires a thermal imaging camera placed at a distance of 15 m from the individual diagonally because the focus is to be laid on the movement of the nostrils. These cameras are available on e-commerce websites like Amazon, Flipkart, etc. at an affordable price. The camera is to be placed from a lower angle at the mentioned distance so as to capture the nostrils from below. The camera is connected to the smartphone via Bluetooth and the distance between the phone and the rest of the components are immaterial as the phone is used to record the video and make a connection to the smart phone. The arrangements of components is depicted in Fig. 4.8.

When the connection is established, the thermal camera is switched on. Keeping the camera at the mentioned angle will result in capturing the diaphragm movement as well. A timer of say 10 s is kept and the breathing pattern of the individual is recorded for the stipulated time. The pattern is to be identified as short breaths or not and depending on the investigation, the individual subjected to the particular diagnosis required. This way the person is able to undergo treatment for cancer or any other similar ailments related to short-breaths at the earliest possible stage without further delay. This accounts for an early diagnostic approach of lung cancer resulting in the decrease of the mortality rates.

Having put forth the setup, it is also required to build a deep neural network that will be able to identify the breathing pattern of the recorded person. A CNN network will be ideal as it is believed to be the best deep neural network so far and will be able to derive complex patterns from the input data. Collecting datasets for the model can be a huge task but developing a consistent model can change the field of medical analysis. The pattern recognition of breathing places a major role in developing the model.

The pattern to be observed is expected to look like as shown in Fig. 4.9.

The pattern shown is a simulation of the self-worked model that has a gradient descent showing the differences in the textures using different colours. The change in the pattern will be easily identified by the neural network when the simulation is similar to that in the image. This will help the model predict of the person has short-breaths and evaluate the breathing habit for the same.

Speech recognition having changed the entire notion of artificial intelligence is a result of simulation that has boomed AI. Similarly, if video recognition with simulation is also created, then AI in medical field will gain emphasis over other existing technologies. The idea of thermal imaging and short-breaths creates space for a completely new literature in the field of machine learning. However, lately researchers are beginning to adapt to the new normal of the AI world which is

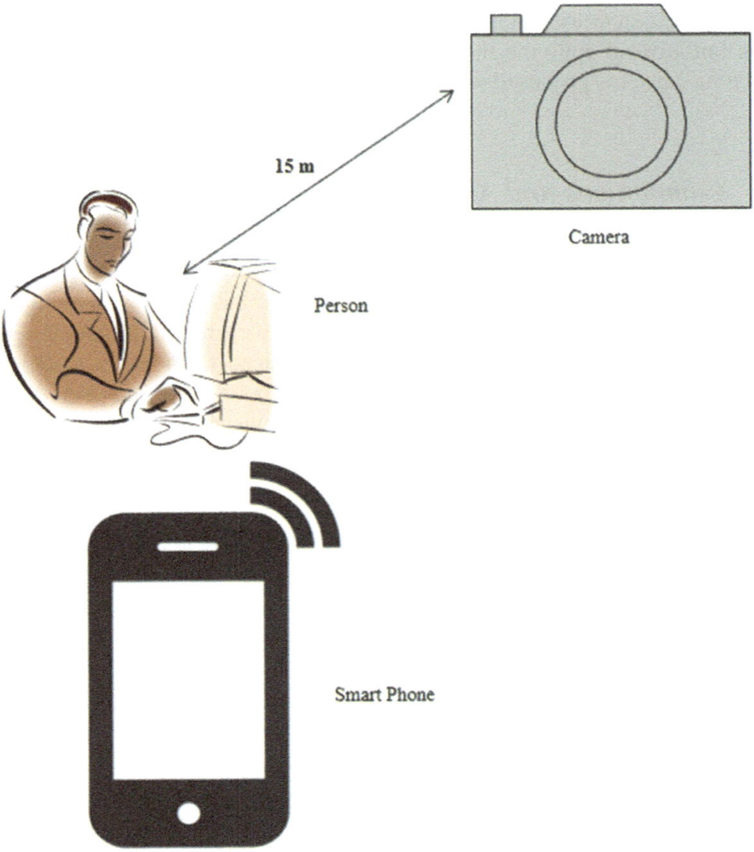

Fig. 4.8 Arrangement of components

expected to rule the globe in the upcoming years. Having said that, simulation based technologies are expected to provide more insights in the near future in overcoming human intelligence for machine intelligence.

4.7 Contemplation

The chapter has outlined the revolution of AI with the growing focus on machine learning technology especially deep learning. The growing demand and supply for intelligent systems and their perspectives are also skimmed through. Deep learning has revolutionized technical thinking and intelligent computation owing to new innovative technologies. Also, the creation and function of a deep neural network has been simplified. Based on the discussions above, this chapter leaves room for

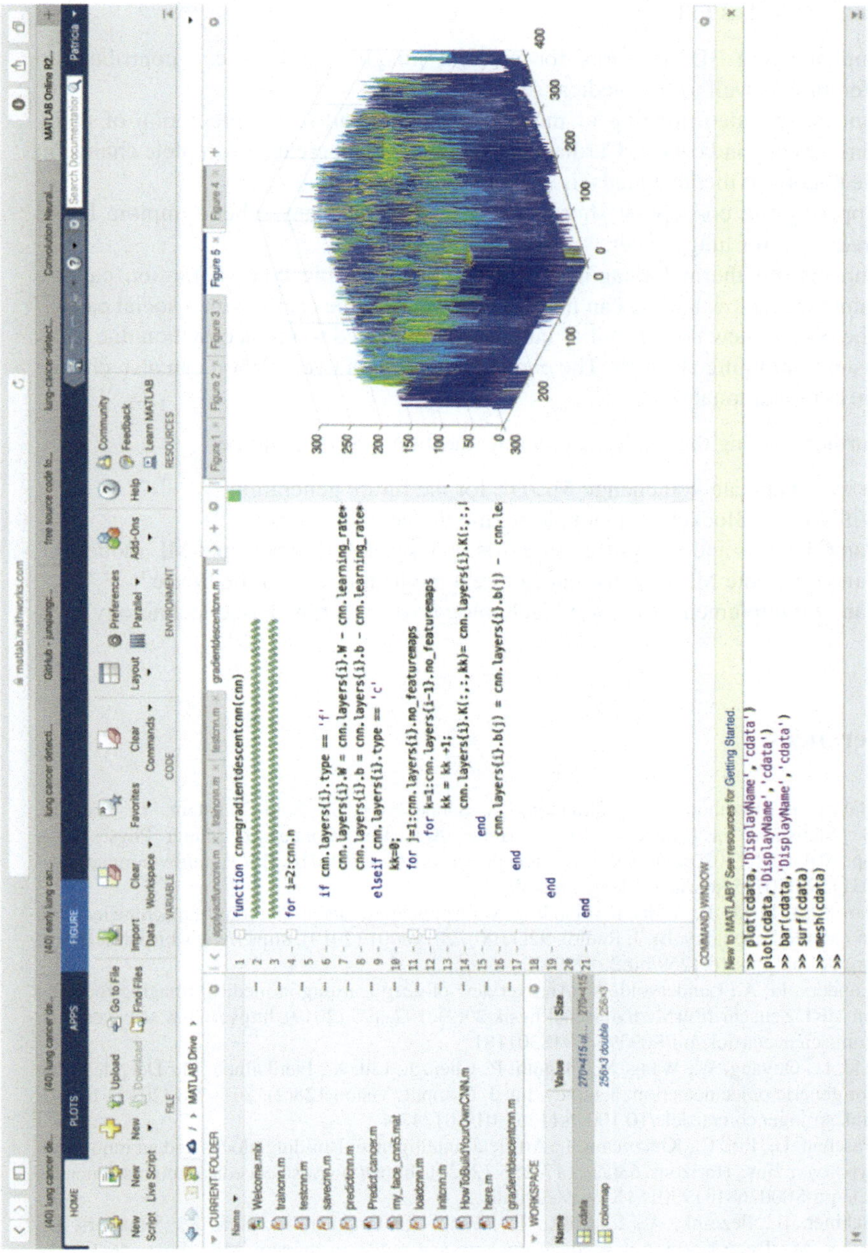

Fig. 4.9 Pattern recognition

upcoming researchers and scientists to implore 3D, 5D and 8D networks dissipating insights on cultivating a new diagnostic technology. The scope of neural networks are summarised as follows:

- Implementing 3D networks for medical imaging analysis can contribute to literature as well as the medical sector.
- Innovative video imaging of medical field can lead to the prediction of many illnesses beyond cancer. Cardiac analysis via AI can create a complete change in the history of medical analysis.
- Applying the concept of short-breaths can unveil many other symptom based prediction for lung cancer.
- Improvising thermal imaging and any other possible type of motion capture cameras at a low budget can make facilities available easily with a social cause.
- The current new comer 'Julia' language is expected to replace python due to its faster computing abilities. The exploration of Julia over Python can also change the computational time.

Further, leaving the reader with a few questions to contemplate:

- In what way can you change ML/DL for the future generation?
- Will AI and Blockchain technology rule the next 20 years?
- Can CT scans and x-rays for diagnosis be replaced by robots and ML models?
- Can you create ML models that can treat medical illness in the future?
- Can you implement chip based technology over machine based technology?

References

1. Bahri, Y., Kadmon, J., Pennington, J., Schoenholz, S., Sohl-Dickstein, J., Ganguli, S.: Statistical mechanics of deep learning. Ann. Rev. Condensed Matter Phys. **11**(1), pp. 501–528 (2020). https://www.annualreviews.org/doi/abs/10.1146/annurev-conmatphys-031119-050745?journalCode=conmatphys
2. Jarrett, D., Stride, E., Vallis, K., Gooding, M.: Applications and limitations of machine learning in radiation oncology. Br. J. Radiol. **92**(1100), 20190001 (2019). https://www.birpublications.org/doi/pdfplus/10.1259/bjr.20190001
3. Lundervold, A., Lundervold, A.: An overview of deep learning in medical imaging focusing on MRI. ZeitschriftfürMedizinischePhysik **29**(2), 102–127 (2019). https://www.sciencedirect.com/science/article/pii/S0939388918301181
4. Liu, L., Ouyang, W., Wang, X., Fieguth, P., Chen, J., Liu, X., Pietikäinen, M.: Deep learning for generic objectdetection: a survey. Int. J. Comput. Vision **128**(2), 261–318 (2019). https://link.springer.com/article/10.1007/s11263-019-01247-4
5. Paschen, U., Pitt, C., Kietzmann, J.: Artificial intelligence: Building blocks and an innovation typology. Bus. Horizons **63**(2), 147–155 (2020). https://www.sciencedirect.com/science/article/pii/S000768131930151X?via%3Dihub
6. Sahiner, B., Pezeshk, A., Hadjiiski, L., Wang, X., Drukker, K., Cha, K., Summers, R., Giger, M.: Deep learning in medical imaging and radiation therapy. Med. Phys. **46**(1), e1–e36 (2018). https://aapm.onlinelibrary.wiley.com/doi/full/10.1002/mp.13264%4010.1002/%28ISSN%292473-4209.Reviewarticles

7. Suri, J.: State-of-the-art review on deep learning in medical imaging. Front. Biosci. **24**(3), 392–426 (2019). https://www.researchgate.net/profile/Mainak_Biswas/publication/328130500_State-of-the-art_review_on_deep_learning_in_medical_imaging/links/5ee8c67f299bf1faac59c6d0/State-of-the-art-review-on-deep-learning-in-medical-imaging.pdf
8. Morocho-Cayamcela, M., Lee, H., Lim, W.: Machine learning for 5G/B5G mobile and wireless communications: potential, limitations, and future directions. IEEE Access **7**, 137184–137206 (2019). https://ieeexplore.ieee.org/stamp/stamp.jsp?arnumber=8844682
9. Mendelson, E.: Artificial intelligence in breast imaging: potentials and limitations. Am. J. Roentgenol. **212**(2), 293–299 (2019). https://www.ajronline.org/doi/full/10.2214/AJR.18.20532
10. Bradley Wendel, W.: The promise and limitations of artificial intelligence in the practice of law, 72 Okala L. Rev. 21 (2019)
11. Prasannavenkatesan, T., Menakadevi, T.: Futuristic speed prediction using auto-regression and neural networks for mobile ad hoc networks. Int. J. Commun. Syst. **32**(9), e3951 (2019)
12. Usha Ruby, A., Theerthagiri, P., Jeena Jacob, I., Vamsidhar, Y.: Binary cross entropy with deep learning technique for image classification. Int. J. Adv. Trends Comput. Sci. Eng. **9**(4), 5393–5397 (2020)
13. Theerthagiri, P., Gopala Krishnan, C., Nishan, A.H.: Prognostic analysis of hyponatremia for diseased patients using multilayer perceptron classification technique. EAI Endorsed Trans. Pervasive Health Technol. (2021). https://doi.org/10.4108/eai.17-3-2021.169032. Online First
14. Komarasamy, G., Archana, K.V.: An efficient approach for identification and classification of brain tumors using optimized deep learning techniques (2019, July 30). SSRN eLibrary, Elsevier Publication. https://ssrn.com/abstract=3428863
15. Pillai, B.G., Jecob, I.J., Madhurya, J.A., Saritha, A.K.: Predicting the possibility of cancer with supervised learning algorithms. Int. J. **8**(9) (2020)

Chapter 5
Improved Thyroid Disease Prediction Model Using Data Mining Techniques with Outlier Detection

Yasir Iqbal Mir

Abstract Thyroid disease is one of the most common diseases worldwide. Thyroid gland in human body controls the metabolic activities of human body. Any malfunctioning in thyroid gland will lead to serious health issues. Diagnosis of thyroid is an important task. There has been enormous growth in thyroid cases worldwide and it needs serious attention as soon as possible. According to the survey conducted in India on thyroid disease, approximately 42 million people suffer from thyroid disease. This paper presents an extensive survey done in the past on the thyroid disease prediction using data mining techniques. In this paper, an extensive study on the various attributes used in thyroid prediction has been conducted. This paper studies various data mining techniques like Naïve Bayes, Decision Trees etc. for thyroid prediction. Amongst these various feature selection algorithms, serological tests and pathological observations of the thyroid disease were also surveyed. The forty-two machine learning algorithms are compared to find the top five best classifiers to predict whether a given patient is suffering from hypothyroidism, hyperthyroidism or is absolute normal. The data source has been taken from KEEL which contains 7200 instances with 22 attributes. The results of various machine learning algorithms have been compared in order to find most appropriate model for classifying whether a given patient is suffering from thyroid disease or not. The best classifier found as bagging gives an overall accuracy of 99.70 percent. Another experiment is also conducted to identify and remove outliers. With outliers' removal, a comparison of forty-two machine learning algorithms with the previous results has been performed. Here, a slight improvement in results is observed and this time the best classifier found, achieved an accuracy of 99.95 percent with logic and analysis of data (LAD) tree.

Keywords Thyroid prediction model · Data mining · Classification · Machine learning model · Outlier detection · LAD tree

---

Y. I. Mir (✉)
Department of Computer Science and Engineering, Poornima University, Jaipur, Rajasthan, India

J. Nayak et al. (eds.), *Advanced Machine Learning Approaches in Cancer Prognosis*, Intelligent Systems Reference Library 204,
https://doi.org/10.1007/978-3-030-71975-3_5

5.1 Introduction

Thyroid disease is the most common endocrine disorder worldwide. In India too, it has been roughly calculated that about 42 million people suffer from thyroid disease. Thyroid [1] is a butterfly shaped gland located in the anterior of the neck. Thyroid produces two hormones which are essential for controlling the speed of metabolism. Thyroid releases two hormones Triodothyroxine (T3) and Levothyroxine (T4) into the blood stream [2], Triodothyroxine is named as T3 because it contains three atoms of iodine per molecule and T4 contains four atoms of iodine per molecule. Hormones secreted by the thyroid gland control the metabolic, cardiovascular and developmental activities of the human body. Thyroid gland uses iodine to produce vital hormones i.e., it uses one milligram of iodine per week for normal functioning. Productions of the hormones are controlled by pituitary gland and hypothalamus; both are found at the base of the brain. Any malfunctioning in the production of the thyroid hormone leads to thyroid disease and thus causes several health problems like hyperthyroidism, hypothyroidism.

At present, more than 200 million people are suffering from thyroid disease. Although, the cause of thyroid disease still remains unknown, its symptoms could be detected if the thyroid illness is discovered at an early stage. Classification is one of the important processes in data mining where a given patient's information can used to predict whether he/she is suffering from thyroid disease or not [3]. There are various classification algorithms which can be used for prediction of thyroid [4]. The results of forty-two machine learning algorithms including ensemble learning methods are compared to find out the best five classifiers. The data set has been taken from KEEL repository which includes the data taken from Garavan institute, Sydney, Australia. The reason for selecting data source from keel is that the data set available is preprocessed and hence doesn't require any pre-processing techniques. The data set comprises of 7200 instances with 22 attributes. The class variable is taken as "class" that is whether a given patient is suffering from hyperthyroidism, hypothyroidism or is absolutely normal.

In thyroid prediction, the main objectives of study are

- First, finding out the top classifiers for this work.
- Secondly, finding out the various data sets used by the previous researchers with the intent of finding the best data set for proposed prediction model.
- Thirdly, improving the accuracy of founded top classifiers.

Rest of this paper is arranged as follows. Summary of data mining and medical data mining is discussed in Sect. 5.2. In Sect. 5.3, a brief literature survey on attributes, thyroid prediction is presented. Data set description, tool used, outlining of machine learning algorithms and performance metrics are presented in Sect. 5.4. The implementation of algorithms and results achieved are discussed in Sect. 5.5. Lastly, Sects. 5.6 and 5.7 summarize conclusion and future work respectively.

5.2 Data Mining and Medical Data Mining

Data mining is all about describing the past and finding out useful information from data using data analysis. Data mining helps us in better decision making with the help of past knowledge. Many medical organizations have collected and stored large amounts of data and data mining techniques will help us in finding useful knowledge. In health care, data mining techniques are used in disease diagnosis and prognosis. Doctors can find best and effective practices to improve patient's health [5].

Predictive modeling is the process in which a model is built for predicting results. If the result is numerical, it is called as regression while as if the result is nominal, then it is referred to as classification. In clustering, similar observations are grouped together to form a cluster.

Medical data mining is the evolving area that deals with the development of various methods to explore medical data. Medical data mining finds the patterns and relationships hidden inside the data. Medical Data mining uses different computational approaches to analyze medical data for studying medical queries [6]. Data mining is also referred to as knowledge discovery in database (KDD). KDD is the process of extracting meaningful information from large collection of data by applying various methods. KDD can be used to learn new model, predict and evaluate useful information from the historical data [7].

5.3 Related Work

Extensive work has been done in the past for prediction of thyroid disease. Various classifiers like Decision Trees, Naïve Bayes, and Support Vector Machines etc. have been used for thyroid prediction. Many researchers have shown importance of data-pre-processing, feature selection and attributes used for thyroid disease prediction. In this section, an extensive survey of the various attributes and methods used in the prediction of thyroid disease is presented.

Sharpe et al. [8], has used multilayer perceptron (MLP) and linear vector quantization (LVQ) for thyroid diagnosis. MLP was trained by back propagation algorithm (BP). Both the networks were efficient during training and testing phase. Zhang et al. [9] trained forward feed neural network with resilient back propagation (RPROP). Four-fold cross validation method was used to validate results. However, dataset contained large number of missing values and hence required pre-processing. Brameier et al. [10] compared linear genetic programming and neural network. Four kinds of datasets were used. The results showed that genetic programming is able to achieve same classification. Hoshi et al. [11] showed Bayesian regularized neural network (BRNN) achieved higher accuracy than self-organizing maps. Dataset contained 215 instances. The author could use tenfold cross validation for validating results. Temurtas [12] used MLP, LVQ and probabilistic neural network (PNN) for thyroid diagnosis. The data source was UCI and PNN and showed better results than other two neural networks. Polat et al. [13] obtained classification accuracy over 81% with artificial immune recognition system (AIRS). Fuzzy weighted technique was used for data pre-processing. Saiti et al. [14] concluded that support vector machines (SVM) and PNN showed classification accuracy of 99% and 96.8% respectively. In this experiment, two kinds of thyroid data sets were used and genetic algorithm was used as a feature selection technique. Shariati et al. [15] compared adaptive neuro fuzzy interface system (ANFIS) with several artificial neural networks for thyroid and hepatitis prediction. The data was collected from hospital with 250 records for hepatitis and 221 records for thyroid. The overall accuracy achieved for thyroid disease was 96.8%. Dogantekin et al. [16] proposed wavelet SVM and generalized discriminant analysis (GDA) for thyroid diagnosis. The proposed framework incorporated three stages. In first stage, features were extracted from the dataset. The second stage incorporated classification and finally in third stage GDA_SVM was tested for classification results. Accuracy of 91.86% was achieved with 60–40 partition for training and testing. However, data set contained only 150 instances. Chen et al. [17] proposed three stage expert system (FS-PSO-SVM). In first stage, features were selected by Fischer score method, in second stage, features obtained were to SVM classifier for training, and meanwhile the parameters of the SVM were optimized using particle swarm optimization (PSO). In the last stage, thyroid prediction was done with SVM classifier. The data source was UCI with 215 clinical instances. Khanale et al. [18] used fuzzy interface system for hypothyroidism diagnosis. The dataset contained pathological observation along with T4 and TSH blood report and data was collected from Aurangabad. An accuracy of 88% was achieved for hypothyroidism. The proposed model predicts whether a patient has hypothyroidism or not.

Rani et al. [19] investigated decision trees on different kinds of medical data sets. Her studies show that CART performed well on different medical data sets. Liu et al. [20] achieved accuracy of 98.82% via tenfold cross validation analysis. Principle component analysis (PCA) algorithm extracted features and formed a new feature space on which PSO and fuzzy k nearest neighbour (FKNN) was used for thyroid diagnosis. In this work, the author developed computer aided diagnosis (CAD) system, PCA-PSO-FKNN for thyroid prediction. However the model could assist only laboratory technicians as dataset contained only clinical data rather than both clinical and non-clinical data. Jaganathan et al. [21] used Fischer score feature selection method with MLP and C4.5 for diagnosis of thyroid. The results of both the classification models were compared and MLP achieved accuracy of 93.49%. The data source was UCI with 215 instances. Margret et al. [22] predicted thyroid using decision tree splitting rules. Her work used different splitting criteria for constructing decision tress. Her dataset contained 21 attributes and accuracy of 88.34% was achieved using distance measure splitting rule. Li et al. [23], proposed principle component analysis (PCA)-extreme learning machine (ELM) CAD system for thyroid disease diagnosis. Dimension reduction was obtained using PCA, then new features were fed into ELM classifier for disease diagnosis. Results were validated with tenfold cross validation and number of hidden neurons were 46 to create training model. Classification accuracy of 97.3% was obtained with PCA-ELM.

Gharehchopogh et al. [24] achieved classification accuracy of 98.6% with MLP trained with BP. The author used trail error method for achieving highest accuracy. The data source was UCI. Kaya [25], proposed ELM model for thyroid prediction. The author compared results of ELM with other models MLP, SVM, J48 and came to conclusion that ELM performed better than other models. The classification accuracy obtained with ELM was 96.79% for 70–30% training testing partition. Rawte et al. [26] Roy proposed ontology based expert system for thyroid diagnosis. The author argued drawbacks of machine learning techniques and created knowledge base and rules for disease diagnosis.

Mayanjaya et al. [27] compared results of various classification models for thyroid disease prediction. The author came to a conclusion that MLP performed well than other methods. Prerana et al. [28] implemented predictive neural model for thyroid disease classification. Her experiments concluded that Levenberg Marquardt shown better performance in comparison with simple gradient descent algorithm. Prasad et al. [29] proposed hybrid architecture for thyroid diagnosis. The architecture consists of rough set theory (RST), string matching system (SMS) and PSO. Data source was UCI with accuracy of 93%. Razia et al. [30] compared two neural networks MLP and radial basis function (RBF). Her experiments showed that both the networks could be used for thyroid prediction. MLP and RBF achieved highest accuracy of 99% and 87% respectively. Taneja et al. [31] used association rule and simple K means clustering algorithm. The data source was taken from UCI machine learning repository with 29 attributes; however, after feature selection, 10 attributes were selected. The author buil the rules for thyroid prediction based on age and gender. Biyouki et al. [32] proposed neuro-fuzzy classification method, K-means algorithm for generating initial rules and scaled conjugate gradient (SCG) for obtaining optimum rules. Data pre-processing was dome by consulting endocrinologist and achieved accuracy of 89.09%. Ionita et al. [33] used data mining techniques for thyroid prediction. In this work, results of naïve bayes, decision tress, MLP and RBF network were compared and decision tree achieved highest accuracy of 96.91%. However, data pre-processing was not done. Bekar et al. [34] used decision trees, MLP, naïve bayes and RBF networks for thyroid prediction. The author carried out two experiments on different data sets to find optimum accuracy. The results showed that decision trees achieved highest accuracy of 96.5% on UCI data. Mirza et al. [35] came to the conclusion that data mining techniques are useful in medical applications. Data mining techniques can be used for disease diagnosis. Random forest classifier [36] are helpful in reducing over fitting, bias and variance random forest works on bagging algorithm to replace data for constructing the tree. For better prediction results, it inter mixes various decision trees together. Sundaram et al. [37] selected UCI data source and trained neural network with back propagation algorithm. Her results concluded that Elman neural network achieved greater accuracy (97.8%) than forward feed neural network. Dewangan et al. [38] used various classification techniques for thyroid disease classification. In this paper (classification and regression tree CART) CART-Info Gain and CART-Gain ratio achieved highest accuracy of 99.47% in 90–10% training testing partition. Dash et al. [39] worked on hypothyroid dataset and applied Ranker search as feature optimization method. Optimized data was fed in naïve bayes classifier for hypothyroid prediction. Naïve Bayes classifier achieved 98.38% accuracy. The experiment was carried in WEKA software which is one of the most popular graphical user interfaces (GUI) machine learning tool. Agarawal et al. [3] applied auto associative neural network (AANN) for thyroid prediction. Data source was selected as UCI. After data preprocessing, co-relation based feature selection (CFS) selected 10 attributes. Overall accuracy of 95.1% was achieved. Hameed [40] used multilayer forward feed network for thyroid diagnosis on the dataset with only 3 attributes. Data was collected from laboratory with 655 samples and this model achieved accuracy of 99.2% with 80–20 training testing partition. Pavya et al. [41] focused on feature selection algorithms to predict thyroid, the data set was taken from UCI and her studies showed that filter and wrapper based methods combined with extreme learning classifier produced maximum accuracy. Umadevi et al. [42] selected data source as UCI and applied data mining classification algorithms which are K-nearest neighbour (KNN), ANN and fuzzy ANN. After feature selection, it was found fuzzy ANN achieved highest accuracy. Venugopal et al. [43] classified data source from UCI with random forest algorithm. However, only hypothyroid disease was predicted with best accuracy of 71.62%, data preprocessing was not done for improving accuracy. Mahurkar et al. [44] applied k-means algorithm on attribute named as T3 and rest of the five attributes were fed into ANN for thyroid diagnosis. Prediction accuracy of 98.21% was achieved in results. Shrivas et al. [45] used rapid minor tool for thyroid disease classification. The author obtained highest accuracy of 97.61 by forward and backward elimination method for feature selection with ensemble model as a base classifier. Gurram et al. [46] did comparative study of SVM and logistic regression for the diagnosis of thyroid. Classification accuracy of both the networks was about 98%. Jatav et al. [47] used data mining techniques for pattern extraction and getting useful knowledge for disease prediction. The author built a model for diabetic data set and used support Vector machine (SVM) for disease classification. According to Turki et al. [48] the prediction of thyroid cancer can be best classified by using support vector machines (SVM). The researcher has used four machine learning methods but SVM yielded highest accuracy. The accuracy was calculated on the basis of area under curve (AUC) with data set partitioned into five folds for training and testing sets. Deepika et al. [49] compared various mining techniques on heart, diabetes and thyroid dataset to check which classifier shows best results. In her experiment on thyroid data set SVM classifier gave an accuracy of 98.62%. Razia et al. [50] compared various data mining algorithms on KEEL data set and she came to the conclusion that decision tress showed best results than SVM, Naive Bayes and multiple linear regression models. Yadav et al. [51] proposed two ensemble models for classification of thyroid prediction model on women. First ensemble model was built using decision tree and neural network. Second ensemble model was built on the combination of boosting and bagging. After experimentation second ensemble model showed better results than first ensemble model. Begum et al. [52] proposed Naïve Bayes, Id3, KNN and SVM for finding the correlation between T3, T4,TSH, gender and thyroid patients. Sindhya [53] used weka tool for prediction of thyroid disease. The author compared naïve bayes, J48 and random forest model to find out best classifier on the basis of accuracy and time taken to built the model. After experimentation it was concluded that J48 achied tha highest accuracy of 99%, however least period of time was taken by Naïve bayes to build the model. Chaubey et al. [54] presented intuition on how data mining techniques could be applied to UCI data set for classification of thyroid disease. The author focused of k-nearest neighbor, logic regression and decision trees for model building. Mir et al. [55] identified five machine learning techniques and built the two-tier ensemble model on these classifiers. The work was carried in weka with 99.05% accuracy on ensemble model. Mir et al. [56] proposed three novel models on primary dataset. The experimentation was carried out in weka. The author achieved the highest accuracy of 99.08% with SVM on pathological parameters of dataset.

A survey on attributes, methodology used in the diagnosis of the thyroid disease is shown as in Table 5.1. The attributes of table are further explained in Tables 5.2, 5.3, 5.4, 5.5, 5.6, 5.7 and 5.8.

A complete list of attributes (serological tests and pathological observations) used by various researchers is shown below

5.4 Methodology

This section explains about the process of selecting database, the tools and major classification algorithms used in the proposed methodology.

5.4.1 Selecting Database

The thyroid data set has been taken from KEEL (knowledge extraction based on evolutionary learning) repository available at https://sci2s.ugr.es/keel/dataset.php?cod=1072. The reason of selecting data source from KEEL is that it is pre-processed data with no missing values and hence doesn't require any sort of prepossessing. The data set contains 7200 instances with 22 attributes; the class attribute has three possible values: 1 for normal, 2 for hyperthyroidism and 3 for hypothyroidism. The KEEL data set is originally extracted from UCI (https://archive.ics.uci.edu/ml/datasets/thyroid+diseasemachine) learning repository. The description of attributes used in the data set is given in Table 5.9. The data set used contains 6 attributes with numeric values (Age, TSH, T3, TT4, T4U, FTI) and 15 attributes (Sex, On thyroxine, Query on thyroxine, On antithyroid medication, Sick, Pregnant, Thyroid surgery, I131 treatment, Query hypothyroid, Query hyperthyroid, Lithium, Goitre, Tumor, Hypopituitary, Psych having two possible values (0 for No and 1 for Yes). The class attribute can have 3 possible values (0 for normal, 1 for hyperthyroidism or 2 for hypothyroidism).

Table 5.1 Literature review

Author	Attribute table no. used/data source	Methodology	Accuracy in %age/results	Remarks	References
Sharpe et al. (1993)	No._4	MLP with BP LVQ	98.9–99.2 96.7–96.3	Only clinical data was used	[8]
Zhang et al. (1998)	No._2	ANN trained with Rprop Logistic regression	98.16 92.71	Large number of missing values, no-pre-processing done	[9]
Brameier et al. (2001)	No._2	Linear Genetic programming, MLP trained with Rprop	72.40	Comparison of GP and ANN done in this paper and concluded GP is better. No pre-processing done	[10]
Hoshi et al. (2005)	No._3	Kohonen neural network, Bayesian regularized neural network	91.40 (hyper), 83.30 (hypo), 98.70 (normal)	BRNN showed better accuracy,only 215 instances used, only clinical data used	[11]
Feyzullah Temurtas (2007)	No._3	MLNN, PNN, LVQ	93.19, 94.81, 90.50	Comparison of methods done, only 215 instances all clinical	[12]
Polat et al. (2007)	No._3	AIRS with fuzzy weighted pre-processing	85.00	Only clinical data used	[13]
Saiti et al. (2009)	No._2, No._3	PNN with GA feature selection, SVM with GA feature selection	96.80 99.02	Comparative study of both networks done. UCI dataset is having many missing values and hence require pre-processing	[14]
Saeed Shariati [57]	No._4, No._5	ANFIS	96.80	Important pathological observations were ignored	[15]
Dogantekin et al. (2010)	No._3	GDA-WSVM	91.86	Only clinical data used	[16]

(continued)

Table 5.1 (continued)

Author	Attribute table no. used/data source	Methodology	Accuracy in %age/results	Remarks	References
Chen et al. (2011)	No._3	FS-PSO-SVM	97.49	PSO downs the computing performance	[17]
Khanale et al. (2011)	No._6, No._7	Fuzzy interface system	88.00	Only 45 instances used	[18]
Lavana et al. (2011)	No._1	ID3 C4.5 CART	77.99 92.44 94.68	Decision tress could be used for thyroid prediction	[19]
Liu et al. (2012)	No._3	PCA-FSO-FKNN CAD system	98.82	Small dataset used	[20]
Jagannathan et al. (2012)	No._3	Improved F-score with MLP & C4.5	93.49 92.09	This method can be combined with other data mining techniques	[21]
Margret et al. (2012)	No._2	I.G G.I Chi square G.R D.M	68.925 73.222 77.769 84.190 88.340	Normalization based splitting rules have high accuracy, however no pre-processing done & UCI dataset is having many missing values	[22]
Li et al. (2012)	No._3	PCA-ELM CAD system	97.73	Dataset having only 215 instances	[23]
Gharehchopogh et al. (2013)	No._3	Min max normalization with MLP	98.60	Used trial and error method for increasing accuracy	[24]
Yilmaz Kaya [58]	No._3	Min max normalization with ELM	96.79	Only clinical dataset used for classification	[25]
Rawte et al. (2015)	No._6, No._7	Ontology based	94.00	Only 3 clinical values used	[26]
Mayanja et al. (2015)	No._3	RBF, LVQ MLP BPA AIRS Perceptron	95.35 93.50 96.74 69.77 93.50 91.16	Only serological attributes used	[27]

(continued)

Table 5.1 (continued)

Author	Attribute table no. used/data source	Methodology	Accuracy in %age/results	Remarks	References
Prerana et al. (2015)	No._1	BP algo	Not shown	ANN could be used for thyroid prediction	[28]
Prasad et al. (2015)	No._1	SMS, ABC, PSA,RST	99.00	Hybrid model of rough sets along with machine learning algorithms should be introduced	[29]
Razia et al. (2015)	No._3	RBF, MLP trained with BP	87.00 99.00	Only clinical dataset used	[30]
Taneja et al. (2015)	No._1	Apriori Predictive Apriori	Not shown	Old patients and females are most affected by thyroid	[31]
Biyouki et al. (2015)	No._3	Neuro-fuzzy based on k means & SCG	89.09	Only clinical dataset used	[32]
Ionita et al. (2016)	No._2	Naïve bayes Decision tree MLP RBF	91.63 96.91 95.15 96.03	Pre-processing not done, dataset contains missing values	[33]
Bekar et al. (2016)	Data collected from hospital	NB tree J48 LAD tree BFT tree LMT Random forest FT Random tree REP tree CART DS	75.00 66.25 66.25 65.00 65.00 65.00 63.75 62.50 62.50 62.50 58.75	Neither Attributes of dataset nor count of dataset mentioned Pre-processing not done	[34]
Sundaram et al. (2016)	No._2	ERNN	97.8	Pre-processing not done	[37]
Dewangan et al. (2016)	No._1	CART	99.47 99.33 99.07 99.20	Dataset is binary class, no processing done Could use k fold cross validation	[38]
Dash et al. (2016)	No._1	Ranker search naïve bayes	95.38	Feature reduction could be applied	[39]

(continued)

Table 5.1 (continued)

Author	Attribute table no. used/data source	Methodology	Accuracy in %age/results	Remarks	References
Agarawal et al. (2016)	No._1	CFS, AANN	95.10	Neither data pre-processing nor feature selection clearly mentioned	[3]
Hameed [59]	No._7 and T3 attribute	Multilayer forward feed network	99.20	Only 3 attributes used and other pathological observations ignored	[40]
Umadevi [60]	No._2	ANN KNN Fuzzy ANN	85.00 80.00 90.00	Pre-processing not done, no of attributes selected not mentioned	[42]
Venugopal et al. (2017)	No._1	Random forest	70.52	Neither Pre-processing nor attribute selection Done	[43]
Mahurkar et al (2017)	No._3	Improvised k-means	98.13	Pre-processing not done. Used only clinical data	[44]
Shrivas et al. (2017)	No._1	Random forest Naive bayes KNN Ensemble model	91.39 92.67 90.06 93.55	UCI database is having many missing and duplicate values and hence requires pre processing before experimentation	[45]
Gurram et al. (2018)	No._3	SVM, Logic regression	98.30 98.9	Only clinical data used	[46]
Deepika et al. (2018)	No._1	SVM Decision tree ANN	98.62 95.00 98.60	UCI database is having many missing and duplicate values and hence requires pre processing	[49]

(continued)

Table 5.1 (continued)

Author	Attribute table no. used/data source	Methodology	Accuracy in %age/results	Remarks	References
Razia et al. (2018)	No._2	Multiple linear regression SVM Naive bayes Decision tree	91.59 96.04 6.31 99.23	Ensemble learning methods can give better results	[50]
Yadav et al. (2019)	Rahul pathology	Ensemble 1st and 2nd method	98.80	Dataset taken from UCI repository	[51]
Begum et al. (2019)	No._1	Naïve bayes Id3 KNN SVM	Not shown	Data mining techniques are useful for detecting thyroid illness at an early stage	[52]
Chaubey et al. (2020)	No._3	Logistic regression Desision tree KNN	81.25 87.5 96.875	Various other data mining techniques could be used	[54]
Mir et al. (2020)	Sawai Man Singh Hospital, Jaipur, India	Bagging Boosting SVM Naive bayes J48	98.56 98.29 97.61 97.59 96.41	In future, more instances could be added for strong results	[55]
Mir et al. (2020)	Sawai Man Singh Hospital	Two tier ensemble classifiers	99.05	More instances could be added for strong results	[56]

5.4.2 *Tools Used*

To select the best data mining tool following important factors were took in consideration

- Data mining tool must support the machine learning algorithms
- Format of data available
- The data mining tool must support the platform
- Tools used by various researchers for building thyroid prediction model

These factors were kept in view and various data mining software's were compared; WEKA (Waikato Environment fir knowledge Analysis) is selected for the experimentation. WEKA is open source software that was developed at Waikato University. WEKA is used for data mining tasks that contains the algorithms of

Table 5.2 Attribute table no_1

Attribute number	Attribute name	Value type	Attribute description
1	Age	Integer	Age of the person
2	Sex	M, F	Gender
3	On thyroxine	f, t	Is patient taking thyroxine drug
4	Query in thyroxine	f, t	Query on thyroxine content report
5	On antithyroid medication	f, t	Is patient taking any antithyroid drug or not
6	Sick	f, t	Sick / weakness / drowsiness
7	Pregnant	f, t	Is patient pregnant of not
8	Thyroid surgery	f, t	Has done thyroid surgery or not
9	I131 treatment	f, t	Prescribed on i131 treatment
10	Query hypothyroid	f, t	Identification of hypothyroid or not
11	Query hyperthyroid	f, t	Identification of hyperthyroid or not
12	Lithium	f, t	Is patient on lithium medication
13	Goitre	f, t	Is patient have goitre
14	Tumor	f, t	Is patient having tumor or not
15	Hypopituitary	f, t	Patient is hypopituary
16	Psych	f, t	Patient has psychological symptoms
17	TSH measured	f, t	Tsh measured or not
18	TSH	Continuous	Thyroid stimulating hormone test results
19	T3 measured	f, t	T3 measured or not
20	T3	Continuous	T3 test results
21	TT4 measured	f, t	Tt4 measured or not
22	TT4	Continuous	Tt4 test results
23	T4U measured	f, t	T4u measured or not
24	T4U	Continuous	T4u test results
25	FTI measured	f, t	FTI calculated or not
26	FTI	Continuous	FTI calculated from TT4 and T4U values

(continued)

Table 5.2 (continued)

Attribute number	Attribute name	Value type	Attribute description
27	TBG measured	f, t	Thyroxine binding globulin test results
28	TBG	Continuous	Laboratory blood test
29	Referral source	WEST, STMW, SVHC, SVI, SVHD, other	Source of the data

Table 5.3 Attribute table no_2

Attribute number	Attribute name	Value type	Attribute description
1	Age	Integer	Age of the person
2	Sex	M, F	Gender
3	Sick	f, t	Sick/weakness/drowsiness
4	Thyroid surgery	f, t	Underwent thyroid surgery or not
5	Pregnant	f, t	Is patient pregnant of not
6	I131 treatment	f, t	Prescribed on i131 treatment
7	Hypothyroid indicator	f, t	Patient responses indicate likelihood of hypothyroidism
8	Hyperthyroid indicator	f, t	Patient responses indicate likelihood of hyperthyroidism
9	Lithium	f, t	Is patient on lithium medication
10	Thyroxine indicator 1	f, t	Patient on thyroxine treatment
11	Thyroxine indicator 2	f, t	Patient thyroxine treatment status unknown or unreported
12	Goitre	f, t	Is patient have goitre
13	On antithyroid medication	f, t	Is patient taking any anti thyroid drug or not
14	Tumor	f, t	Is patient having tumor or not
15	Hypopituitary	f, t	Patient is hypopituary
16	Psychology	f, t	Patient has psychological symptoms
17	TSH	Continuous	Thyroid stimulating hormone
18	T3	Continuous	T3 test results
19	TT4	Continuous	Tt4 test results
20	T4U	Continuous	T4u test results
21	FTI	Continuous	FTI calculated from TT4 and T4U values

Table 5.4 Attribute table no_3

Attribute number	Attribute name	Value type	Attribute description
1	Class attribute	1, 2 or 3	1 = normal, 2 = hyper, 3 = hypo
2	T3-resin	Continuous	T3-resin uptake test
3	Total Serum thyroxin	Continuous	Total Serum thyroxin as measured by the isotopic displacement method
4	Total serum triiodothyronine	Continuous	Total serum triiodothyronine as measured by radio immuno assay
5	Thyroid-stimulating hormone	Continuous	Measurement of amount of TSH present in blood by radio immuno assay
6	Absolute difference	Continuous	Absolute difference of TSH value after injecting 200 mg of TRH in blood

Table 5.5 Attribute table no_4

Attribute number	Attribute name	Value type	Attribute description
1	T4	Continuous	Total thyroxine
2	FT4	Continuous	Free thyroxine
3	T3	Continuous	Triiodothyroxine
4	T3U	Continuous	T3uptake test
5	TSH	Continuous	Thyrotropin
6	TBG	Continuous	Thyroxine-binding globulin

Table 5.6 Attribute table no_5

Attribute number	Attribute name	Value type	Attribute description
1	Hair fall	Yes/no	Symptom of hair fall
2	Weight gain	Yes/no	Symptom of weight gain
3	Dry skin	Yes/no	Symptom of dry skin
4	Humid skin	Yes/no	Symptom of humid skin
5	Warm skin	Yes/no	Symptom of warm skin
6	Tachycardia	Yes/no	Symptom of tachycardia
7	Bradycardia	Yes/no	Symptom of bradycardia

Table 5.7 Attribute table no_6

Attribute number	Attribute name	Value type	Attribute description
1	Fatigue/weakness	Yes/no	Symptom of weakness
2	Weight gain	Yes/no	Symptom of
3	Feeling cold	Yes/no	Symptom of feeling cold
4	Drier, itchier skin	Yes/no	Symptom of skin
5	Forgetfulness, dementia	Yes/no	Symptom of memory
6	Menstrual problems	Yes/no	Symptom of menstrual problems
7	Muscle cramps/joint aches	Yes/no	Symptom of cramps/aches
8	Hair loss	Yes/no	Symptom of hair loss
9	Hypersomniance	Yes/no	Symptom of excessive sleep
10	Nervousness feel	Yes/no	Symptom of nervousness
11	Swelling in front of the neck	Yes/no	Symptom of swelling
12	Any thyroid disorder/ family history	Yes/no	Anyone in family having thyroid disorder
13	Constipation	Yes/no	Symptom of constipation
14	Other glandular failure	Yes/no	Symptom of other organ failure

Table 5.8 Attribute table no_7

Attribute number	Attribute name	Value type	Attribute description
1	T4	Continuous	Thyroxine hormone
2	TSH	Continuous	Thyroid stimulating hormone

machine learning, it is written in java and it contains the tools for classification, clustering visualization, data pre-processing and association rules. WEKA is used for building and testing the data mining models. It is one of the most popular machine learning software which is developed at University of Waikato, New Zealand. The whole soft-ware is written in java. WEKA is free software under general public licenses- GNU and can be downloaded from University of Waikato website. The WEKA has collection of all state-of-the-art machine learning algorithms for modelling and analysis of data. WEKA is easy to use GUI software, however expert programmers can use command line interface for data mining tasks. WEKA also supports python scripting for advanced programmers.

Table 5.9. Attribute description

Attribute	Domain
Age	[0.01, 0.97]
Sex	[0, 1]
On_thyroxine	[0, 1]
Query_on_thyroxine	[0, 1]
On_antithyroid_medication	[0, 1]
Sick	[0, 1]
Pregnant	[0, 1]
Thyroid surgery	[0, 1]
I131 treatment	[0, 1]
Query_hypothyroid	[0, 1]
Query_hyperthyroid	[0, 1]
Lithium	[0, 1]
Goitre	[0, 1]
Tumor	[0, 1]
Hypopituitary	[0, 1]
Psych	[0, 1]
TSH	[0.0, 0.53]
T3	[0.0005, 0.18]
TT4	[0.0020, 0.6]
T4U	[0.017, 0.233]
FTI	[0.0020, 0.642]
Class	1,2,3

5.4.3 Major Classification Algorithms

The following are the major classification algorithms used in the proposed methodology.

5.4.3.1 Bagging

Bagging is one of the methods of ensemble learning. In bagging, original data set is splitted into several different data sets. Splitting of data set can be achieved with replacement or with no replacement. After splitting data set, some machine learning technique are applied on each of split data set and combine the results of each one by averaging the results or by voting.

5.4.3.2 Boosting

In boosting, the results of new models are dependent on the performance of previously built models. In boosting, some machine learning scheme are applied on original data set and look for miss classified instances, then extra weights on those misclassified instances are applied and build a new training set for producing next model. In this technique, the new model built becomes expert for misclassified instances. In the end, results are produced either by averaging the results or by voting.

5.4.3.3 LAD Tree

Logical analysis of data (LAD) tree is the class of trees which generates multi-class alternating decision tree by using the method of Logit Boost algorithm.

5.4.3.4 Logit Boost

Logit boost uses regression scheme as the base learner for performing classification. It can handle multiclass problems.

5.4.3.5 Vote

Voting predicts the outcome by combining multiple classifiers. In voting, every classifier makes a prediction on the test instance of data set and the final prediction result is that one which has more than half votes in its favour.

5.4.3.6 Decorate

Decorate is one of the most popular ensemble machine learning algorithms. Decorate can be used as a strong learner which creates a number of folds to data set and each fold of the data set is fed to the supplied base learner. In Decorate, predictions are made by averaging the results.

5.4.3.7 J48

It is the new version of C4.5. The algorithm uses divide-and-conquer strategy for achieving results and it uses pruning in order to avoid over fitting during construction of decision tree. For splitting criteria, the attribute with highest information gain is selected as root node and then tree is constructed. This process is recursed on remaining attributes.

5.4.3.8 CART

Classification and regression Tree (CART) is a tree structure that produces binary trees. In CART, according to the selected test attribute, each of the internal nodes has a pair of departing edges. There are many types of splitting criteria and impurity measures in CART.

5.4.3.9 J48 Graft

It produces grafted decision tree from J48 algorithm. J48 graft algorithm infers the decision tree by adding new nodes for the reason to minimize the errors in predication 3.

5.5 Experimental Setup

This section explains about the tools, performance metrics and tenfold crsoss validation used in assessing the model. Further, this section represents the empirical results obtained after evaluating the model.

5.5.1 Tools Used

WEKA (Waikato Environment for Knowledge Analysis) was used for building and testing the data mining models. It is one of the most popular machine learning softwares which is developed at University of Waikato, New Zealand. The whole software is written in java. WEKA is free software under general public licenses-GNU and can be downloaded from University of Waikato website. The WEKA has collection of all state-of-the-art machine learning algorithms for modeling and analysis of data. WEKA is easy to use GUI software, however expert programmers can use command line interface for data mining tasks. WEKA also supports python scripting for advanced programmers.

5.5.2 Performance Evaluation Strategies

This section explains about the performance metrics used in evaluating the performance of the model.

Table 5.10 Representation of confusion matrix

Actual	Predicted	
	Negative	Positive
Negative	TN (True Negative)	FP (False Positive)
Positive	FN (False Negative)	TP (True Positive)

5.5.2.1 Confusion Matrix

Confusion matrix is sometimes called as error matrix. It is the tool used for performance evaluation in the domain of machine learning. Confusion matrix shows the performance of an algorithm in tabular form. Confusion matrix shows the total number of correct and incorrect predictions for each class variable. Table 5.10 shows representation of confusion matrix.

5.5.2.2 Equation Used for Analysis

For the analysis of algorithms, the following equations-Accuracy, True positive rate (TPR), False positive rate (FPR), Precision, recall (or sensitivity), ROC (Receiver Operator Characteristic) Curve have been used.

a. **Accuracy**: Percentage of total number of correctly classified instances.

$$\text{accuracy} = \frac{\text{TP} + \text{TN}}{\text{TP} + \text{FP} + \text{FN} + \text{TN}}$$

b. **True positive rate**: It is the rate of total number of correctly classified instances in the given dataset.

$$\text{TPR} = \frac{\text{TP}}{\text{FN} + \text{TP}}$$

c. **False positive rate**: It is the rate of instances that are incorrect classified in the given dataset.

$$\text{FPR} = \frac{\text{FP}}{\text{TN} + \text{FP}}$$

d. **Precision**: It is the proportion of instances that truly belong to class divided by the total number of true positives and true negatives.

$$\text{precision} = \frac{\text{TP}}{\text{TP} + \text{FP}}$$

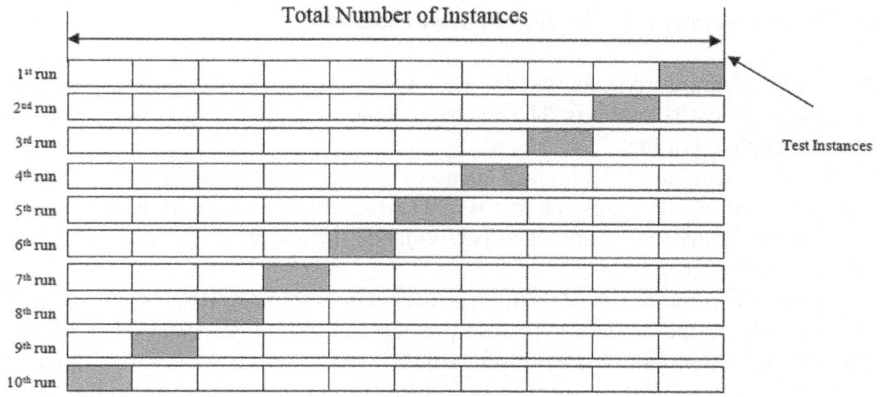

Fig. 5.1 Process ten-fold cross validation

e. **Recall**: It is the proportion of total number of instances that are true positive values.

$$recall = \frac{\mathrm{TP}}{\mathrm{FN} + \mathrm{TP}}$$

f. **ROC**: ROC shows the diagnostic ability of a classifier at various threshold values.

5.5.3 10 Fold Cross Validation

In machine learning, the trouble with the developed models is that the performance are not known until and unless testing is done on some independent data set. To tackle with the problem, cross validation method is used for calculating the performance of the model. a tenfold cross validation method is used to evaluate the deployed models. In this method a data set is divided in 10 subsets then first data set is treated as test data and remaining 9 data sets are used to fit the model. After that the model is applied to test data and same procedure is applied on each subset of divided data set. Finally, average of classification results is calculated. This process is given in Fig. 5.1.

5.5.4 Experimental Results

It represents the experimental results obtained after evaluating the proposed model.

5.5.4.1 Experiment A: Finding the Best Classifier

In this experiment, forty-two machine leaning algorithms on data set are compared and found out best 5 classifiers. The results of deployed classifiers are shown in Table 5.11 and depicted in Fig. 5.2.

Classifiers who achieved highest accuracy are bagging, boosting, J48, J48 graft and classification and regression tree (CART). tenfold cross validation method was used for validating the results. The performance measures of best classifier's are shown in Table 5.12.

Bagging classifier achieved the highest accuracy of 99.72%. 0.71 s were taken by bagging to build the model for thyroid predication. 7180 instances were correctly classified and 20 instances were misclassified.

99.72% accuracy was archived by boosting. 7180 instances were correctly classified and 20 instances were misclassified. 1.22 s were taking by bagging for building thyroid prediction model.

Table 5.11 Accuracy obtained by classifiers

S. no.	Classifier	Accuracy	S. no.	Classifier	Accuracy
1	Bagging	99.72	22	SPAARC tree	99.28
2	Boosting	99.72	23	Bayes net	99.13
3	J48	99.71	24	Random tree	98.6
4	J48 graft	99.71	25	J48 consolidated	97.19
5	CART	99.68	26	Multi layer perceptron	96.94
6	Decorate	99.67	27	Logistic regression	95.74
7	BF Tree	99.65	28	Simple logistic regression	95.65
8	Random forest	99.64	29	Naïve bayes	95.49
9	Logit boost	99.6	30	NB updateable	95.49
10	Hoeffding tree	99.58	31	Decision stump	95.27
11	REP tree	99.56	32	WISARD	95.24
12	Rotation forest	99.56	33	Dadding	95.23
13	LAD tree	99.54	34	LIB linear	93.86
14	Forest PA	99.51	35	Classification via regression	93.82
15	Logistic model tree	99.51	36	Support vector machine	93.82
16	A1DE	99.41	37	RBF network	93.51
17	A2DE	99.41	38	RBF classifier	93.19
18	CS forest	99.36	39	Stacking	92.58
19	Sys For tree	99.36	40	Stacking C	92.58
20	Functional trees	99.32	41	Vote	92.58
21	Filtered classifier	99.29	42	NB multinominal	92.57

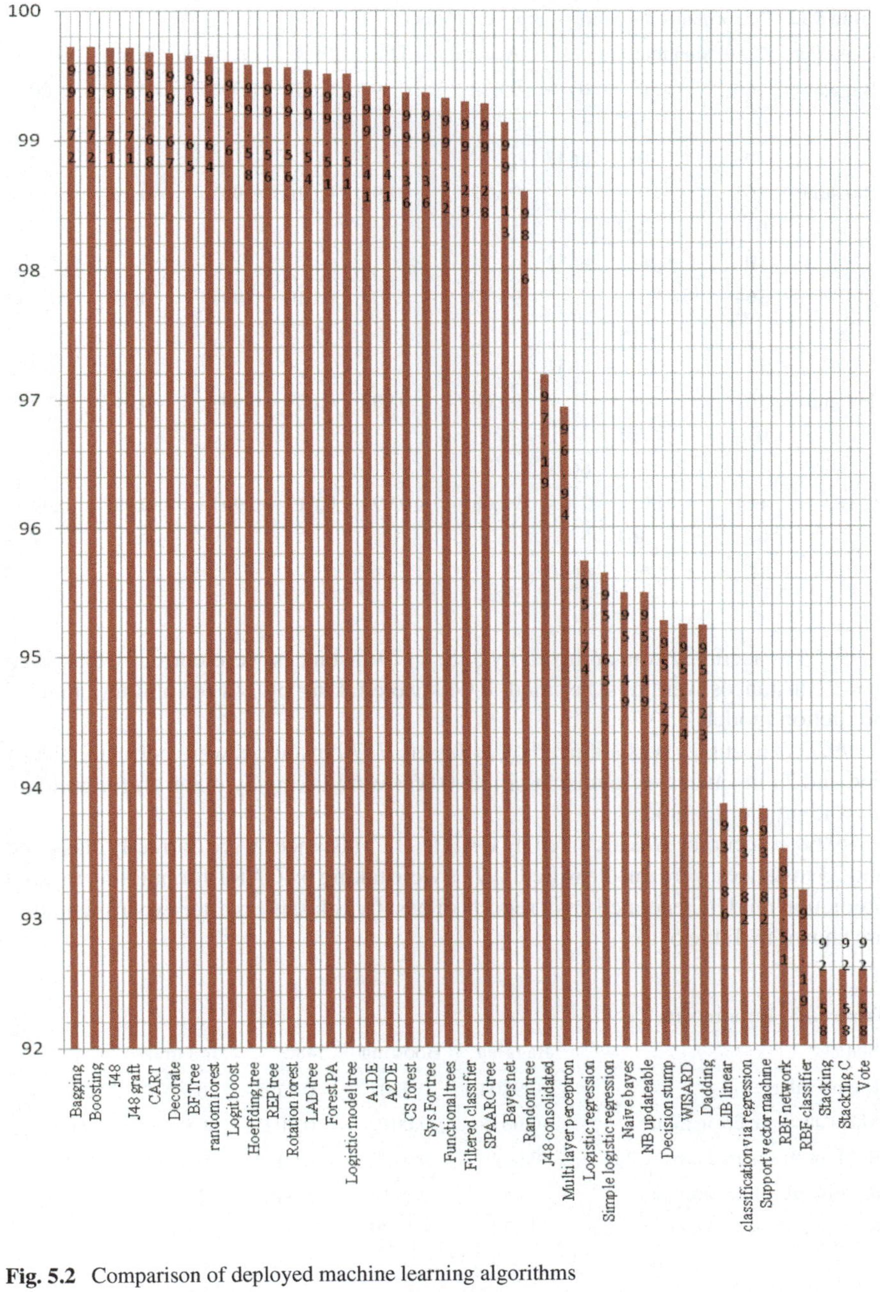

Fig. 5.2 Comparison of deployed machine learning algorithms

Table 5.12 Performance measure of top 5 classifiers

Classifier	Confusion matrix			Accuracy	TPR	FPR	Precision	Recall	ROC
Bagging	166	0	0	99.72	0.997	0.002	0.997	0.997	1.000
	0	367	1						
	10	9	6647						
Boosting	165	0	1	99.72	0.997	0.010	0.997	0.997	0.999
	0	363	5						
	10	4	6652						
J48	164	0	2	99.70	0.997	0.010	0.997	0.997	0.996
	0	364	4						
	11	7	6651						
J48 graft	165	0	2	99.68	0.997	0.009	0.997	0.997	0.995
	0	365	3						
	11	7	6648						
CART	164	0	2	99.68	0.997	0.012	0.997	0.997	0.997
	0	363	5						
	10	6	6650						

99.71% accuracy was archived by J48. 7179 instances were correctly classified and 21 instances were misclassified. 0.04 s were taking by J48 for building thyroid prediction model.

99.71% accuracy was archived by J48 graft. 7179 instances were correctly classified and 21 instances were misclassified. 0.05 s were taking by j48 graft for building thyroid prediction model.

99.68% accuracy was archived by CART. 7177 instances were correctly classified and 23 instances were misclassified. 0.72 s were taking by CART for building thyroid prediction model Generated error reports of best five classifiers after experimentation are shown in Table 5.13.

Table 5.13 Error reports

Statistic	Bagging	Boosting	J48	J48 graft	Cart
Kappa value	0.9804	0.9803	0.9793	0.9793	0.9773
Mean absolute error value	0.0033	0.0019	0.0025	0.0025	0.0027
Root mean squared error value	0.0428	0.0422	0.0432	0.0432	0.045
Relative absolute error value	3.4977	2.0212	2.646	2.646%	2.8885
Root relative squared error value	19.8327	19.5629	20.0412	20.0412	20.8587

5.5.4.2 Experiment B: Removing Outliers

Outliers are those extreme instances in dataset which deviates from the rest of dataset. Outliers can be caused in dataset by execution or measurement error. Outliers can deteriorate the performance and computational time required for building machine learning model. the outliers in data set have been removed to increase the computational time and accuracy of the model. The original KEEL data set contained 7200 instances, however after outlier elimination methods the dataset was reduced to 3802 instances disposing off 3398 instances. The total number of attributes remained same during this experimentation. Only instances are eliminated in this method not attributes. The results obtained after comparing forty-two machine learning algorithms is shown in Table 5.14 and depicted in Fig. 5.3.

Table 5.15 shows the performance measures of the top 5 classification algorithms after removing outliers in thyroid data set. Classifiers who achieved highest accuracy after outlier elimination are bagging, LAD tree, Logit Boost, J48 graft, boosting and decorate.

Table 5.14 Accuracy obtained by classifiers after outlier elimination

S. no.	Classifier	Accuracy	S. no.	Classifier	Accuracy
1	LAD tree	99.98	22	Random tree	99.77
2	Logit boost	99.94	23	Rotation forest	99.77
3	J48 graft	99.92	24	Classification via regression	99.7
4	Boosting	99.92	25	CS forest	99.69
5	Decorate	99.92	26	Decision stump	99.65
6	Vote	99.92	27	Dagging	99.64
7	Bagging	99.9	28	MLP	99.5
8	BF tree	99.9	29	j48 consolidated	99.47
9	CART	99.89	30	Logistic regression	99.32
10	J48	99.89	31	RBF network	99.29
11	LMT	99.87	32	Bayes net	99.26
12	Random forest	99.87	33	Simple logistic	99.26
13	Naïve Bayes	99.86	34	WISARD	99.16
14	SPAARC tree	99.84	35	SMO	99.11
15	Forest PA	99.84	36	RBF classifier	99.09
16	REP tree	99.82	37	Naivebayes updateable	98.88
17	Functional tree	99.82	38	Hoeffding tree	98.67
18	A1DE	99.79	39	Naivebayes multinominal	98.28
19	A2DE	99.79	40	LIB linear	97.28
20	Filtered classifier	99.79	41	Stacking	97.28
21	SYS for tree	99.77	42	Stacking C	97.26

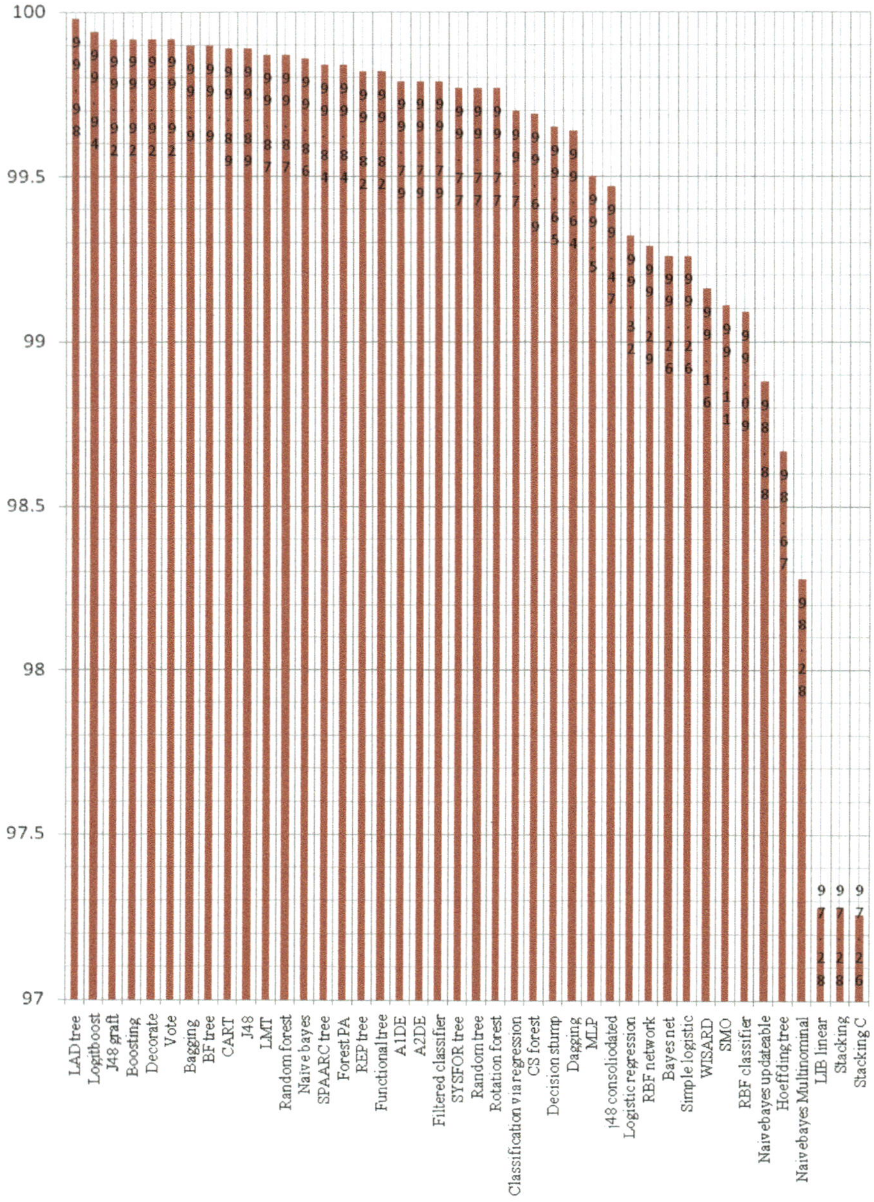

Fig. 5.3 Comparison of machine learning algorithms after outlier elimination

Table 5.15 Performance measure of top 5 classifiers after outlier elimination

Classifier	Confusion matrix			Accuracy	TPR	FPR	Precision	Recall	ROC
LAD tree	1	0	0	99.95	0.999	0.000	0.999	0.999	1.000
	1	113	0						
	0	1	3686						
Logit boost	1	0	0	99.94	0.999	0.000	0.999	0.999	1.000
	0	113	0						
	0	2	3685						
J48 graft	1	0	0	99.92	0.999	0.001	0.999	0.999	1.000
	0	114	0						
	0	2	3684						
Boosting	1	0	1	99.92	0.997	0.001	0.997	0.997	0.995
	0	114	0						
	1	0	3684						
Decorate	1	0	1	99.92	0.997	0.001	0.999	0.999	0.999
	0	114	0						
	0	1	3684						

The LAD tree classifier achieved the highest accuracy of 99.95%. 0.60 s were taken by bagging to build the model for thyroid predication. 3800 instances were correctly classified and 2 instances were misclassified.

99.94% accuracy was archived by Logit boost. 3799 instances were correctly classified and 3 instances were misclassified. 0.63 s were taking by bagging for building thyroid prediction model.

99.92% accuracy was archived by J48 graft. 3799 instances were correctly classified and 3 instances were misclassified. 0.09 s were taking by J48 for building thyroid prediction model.

99.92% accuracy was archived by boosting. 3799 instances were correctly classified and 3 instances were misclassified. 0.52 s were taking by j48 graft for building thyroid prediction model.

99.92% accuracy was archived by decorate. 3799 instances were correctly classified and 3 instances were misclassified. 0.21 s were taking by CART for building thyroid prediction model Generated error reports of best five classifiers after experimentation are shown in Table 5.16.

The comparison of machine learning algorithms before and after outlier removal is depicted in Fig. 5.4.

Table 5.16 Error reports

Statistic	LAD tree	Logit boost	J48 graft	Boosting	Decorate
Kappa value	0.9837	0.9984	0.9784	0.9787	0.9775
Mean absolute error value	0.0022	0.0016	0.0024	0.0024	0.0023
Root mean squared error value	0.0421	0.0419	0.0436	0.0471	0.0210
Relative absolute error value	3.4322	2.0101	2.545	2.654%	2.1232
Root relative squared error value	18.4352	18.7461	19.0643	19.0743	19.9380

5.6 Conclusion

In the literature review, the highest accuracy of 99.47% attained by the Amit et al. [38] using the CART method has been found. They adopted the data set from UCI with binary class values. In the research, the data set from KEEL repository is considered because it is pre-processed data with no missing values. The data set contained in KEEL has 3 class values. A complete survey on the various attributes and machine learning models used by the various researchers in the prediction of thyroid disease has also been performed. In the paper, forty-two popular machine learning classification algorithms on KEEL dataset with 7200 instances are compared to find out best five classifiers in terms of performance measures. The best five classifiers found during experimentation are Bagging, Boosting, J48, J48 Graft and CART. A highest accuracy of 99.72% has been achieved with bagging method used with J48 as the base classifier. Again, the experiment is performed after removing outliers in data set to improve the performance of the machine learning algorithm. After outlier elimination the dataset was reduced to 3802 instances, however number of attributes remained same during experimentation. Again, forty two machine learning algorithms are compared with the aim to find out how outlier removal technique improves the performance of machine learning algorithms. The best five classifiers found after elimination of outliers are LAD Tree, Logit Boost, J48graft, Boosting and Decorate with less time taken to build the prediction model before outlier elimination. In an average case, there was an increase of 1.98% of accuracy except heoffding tree as it showed decrease in accuracy by 0.91% because of under fitting. Under fitting occurs when the machine learning model shows high bias and low variance. Intuitively under fitting happens when the machine learning algorithm is unable to fit data well enough. The highest accuracy was shown by LAD tree with 99.95% after outlier removal, which is highest accuracy achieved so far in thyroid prediction.

5.7 Future Work

It is seen that all the researchers have done research on the dataset taken from UCI repository. The dataset of the thyroid disease in the UCI repository is outdated as the dataset was donated by Ross Quinlan to the University of California during his

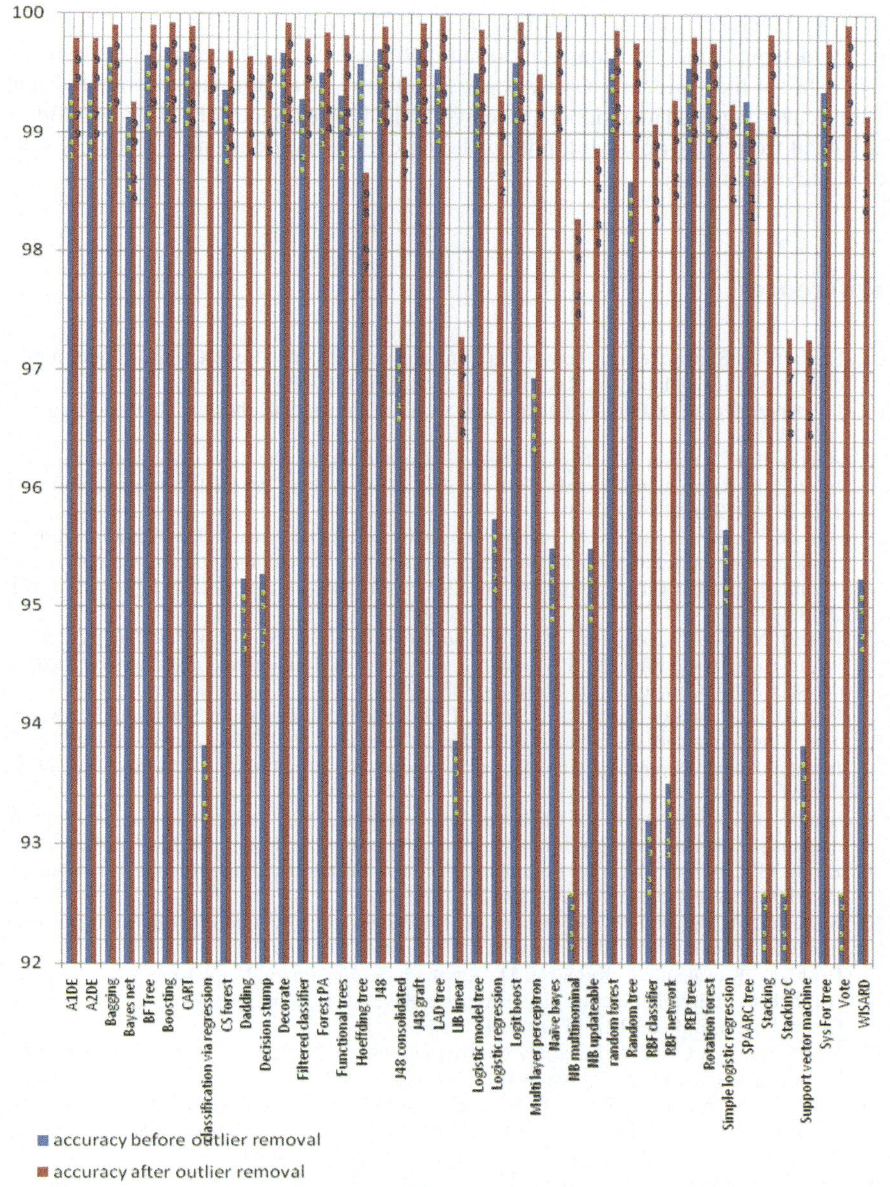

Fig. 5.4 Comparison of classifiers before and after outlier removal

visit for machine learning workshop in 1987. The data in the UCI repository has many missing values and many important pathological attributes are not present in this data set like hair fall, heart rate etc. Therefore, it is strongly recommend that there is a strong need to conduct a research in the future on the dataset that should be collected from real life having both pathological observations and serological tests of the thyroid patients.

References

1. Hayashi, Y.: Synergy effects between grafting and subdivision in Re-RX with J48 graft for the diagnosis of thyroid disease. Knowl. Based Syst. **131**, 170–182 (2017)
2. US department of health and human services office on women's health. Thyroid Disease, 9 Apr 2009
3. Agarawal, K., Dhakar, M.: Thyroid prediction system using auto associative neural network. Int. J. Adv. Res. Electr. Electron. Instrum. Eng. **3297**, 2320–3765 (2016). https://doi.org/10.15662/IJAREEIE.2017.0604008
4. Aswathi, A.K., Antony A.: An intelligent system for thyroid disease classification and diagnosis. In: Second International Conference on Inventive Communication and Computational Technologies (ICICCT), Coimbatore, pp. 1261–1264 (2018). https://doi.org/10.1109/ICICCT.2018.8473349
5. Honest, N., Patel, A.: A survey of big data analytics. Int. J. Inf. Sci. Tech. (IJIST)**6**(1/2) (2016)
6. Lavanya, D., Usha Rani, K.: Performance evaluation of decision tree classifiers on medical datasets. Int. J. Comput. Appl. **26**, 0975–8887 (2011)
7. Fayyad, U., Piatetsky-Shapiro, G., Smyth, P.: Knowledge discovery and data mining: towards a unifying framework. In: Simoudis, E., Han, J., Fayyad, U. (eds.) Proceedings of the Second International Conference on Knowledge Discovery and Data Mining. AAAI Press, pp. 82–88 (1996)
8. Sharpe, P.K., Solberg, H.E., Rootwelt, K., Yearworth, M.: Artificial neural networks in diagnosis of thyroid function from vitro laboratory tests. Clin. Chem. **39**, 2248–2253 (1993)
9. Zhang, G.P., Berardi, V.L.: An investigation of neural networks in thyroid function diagnosis. Health Care Management Science, pp. 29–37 (1998)
10. Brameier, M., Banzhaf, W.: A comparison of linear genetic programming and neural networks in medical data mining. IEEE Trans. Evol. Comput. **5**(1), 17 (2001)
11. Hoshi, K., Kawakami, J., Kumagai, M., Kasahara, S., Nishimura, N., Nakamura, H., Sato, K.: An analysis of thyroid function diagnosis using Bayesian type and SOM-type neural networks. Chem. Pharm. Bull. **53**(12), 1570–1574 (2005)
12. Temurtas, F.: A Comparative Study on Thyroid Disease Diagnosis Using Neural Networks. Selcuk University, Expert System with Application (2007)
13. Polat, K., Sahan, S., Gunes, S. (2007): A novel hybrid method based on artificial immune recognition system (AIRS) with fuzzy weighted pre-processing for thyroid disease diagnosis, pp. 1141–1147. Selcuk University, Expert System with Application
14. Saiti, F., Naini, A.A., Shoorehdeli, M.A., Teshnehlab, M.: Thyroid disease diagnosis based on genetic algorithms using PNN and SVM. In: 3rd International Conference on Bioinformatics and Biomedical Engineering, ICBBE, pp. 1–4 (2009). https://doi.org/10.1109/ICBBE.2009.5163689
15. Shariati, S., Haghighi, M.M.: Comparison of Anfis Neural Network with Several Other ANNs and Support Vector Machine for Diagnosing Hepatitis and Thyroid Diseases. In: 2010 International Conference on Computer Information Systems and Industrial Management Applications (CISIM), vol. 10, pp. 1101–1109 (2010)

16. Dogantekin, E., Dogantekin, A., Avci, D.: An expert system based on generalized discriminant analysis and wavelet support vector machine for diagnosis of thyroid diseases. Expert Syst. Appl. **38**(1), 146–150 (2011)
17. Liu, D.Y., Chen, H.L., Yang, B., Xe, Lv., Li, L.N., Liu, J.: Design of an enhanced fuzzy k-nearest neighbor classifier based computer aided diagnostic system for thyroid disease. J. Med. Syst. **36**(5), 3243–3254 (2012)
18. Khanale, P.B., Ambilwade, S.P.: A fuzzy inference system for diagnosis of Hypothyroidism. J. Artif. Intell. **4**(1), 45–54 (2011)
19. Lavanya, D., Rani, K.U.: Performance evaluation of decision tree classifiers on medical datasets. Int. J. Comput. Appl.**26** (2011). https://doi.org/10.5120/3095-4247
20. Chen, H.L., Yang, B., Wang, G., Liu, J., Chen, Y.D., Liu, D.Y.: A three-stage expert system based on support vector machines for thyroid disease diagnosis. J. Med. Syst. **36**, 1953–1963 (2012)
21. Jaganathan, P., Rajkumar, N.: An expert system for optimising thyroid disease diagnosis. Int. J. Comput. Sci. Eng. **7**(3), 232–238 (2012)
22. Margret, J., Lakshmipathi, B., Kumar, S.A.: Diagnosis of thyroid disorders using decision tree splitting rules. Int. J. Comput. Appl. **44**(8), 0975–8887 (2012)
23. Li, L.-N., Ouyang, J.H., Chen, H.-L., Liu, D.Y.: A computer aided diagnosis system for thyroid disease using extreme learning machine. J. Med. Syst. **36**(5), 3327–3337 (2012)
24. Gharehchopogh, F.S., Molany, M., Mokri, F.D.: Using artificial neural network in diagnosis of thyroid disease: a case study. Int. J. Comput. Sci. Appl. (IJCSA) **3**(4) (2013)
25. Yilmaz, K.A.Y.A.: A fast intelligent diagnosis system for thyroid diseases based on extreme learning machine. Anadolu Univ. J. Sci. Technol. A Appl. Sci. Eng. (2015). https://doi.org/10.18038/btd-a.89202
26. Rawte, V., Roy, B.: Thyroid disease diagnosis using ontology based expert system.Int. J. Eng. Res. Technol. **4**(6), 365–370 (2015)
27. Maysanjaya, I.M.D.,Nugroho, H.A., Setiawan, N.A.: A comparison of classification methods on diagnosis of thyroid diseases. In: Proceedings of International Seminar on Intelligent Technology and Its Applications (ISITIA), pp. 89–92 (2015)
28. Prerana, P.S., Khushboo T.: Predictive data mining for diagnosis of thyroid disease using neural network. Int. J. Res. Manage. Sci. Technol. (E-ISSN: 2321–3264) **3**(2) (2015)
29. Prasad, V., Rao, T.S., Babu, M.S.P.: Thyroid disease diagnosis via hybrid architecture composing rough data sets theory and machine learning algorithms. Soft Comput **20**(3), 1179–1189 (2016)
30. Razia, S., Ramanarasingarao, M., Sridhar, G.R.: A decision support system for prediction of thyroid disease-A comparison of multilayer perceptron neural network and radial basis function neural network. **80**, 544–551 (2015)
31. Taneja, S., Gupta, C., Grover, T., Tripathi, D.: Analysis of factors which contribute to thyroid disease using data mining techniques. In: International Journal of Advanced Research in Computer Science and Software Engineering, vol. 5, p. 6 (2015). ISSN:2277–128X
32. Biyouki, S.A., Turksen, I.B., Zarandi, M.H.F. (2015): Fuzzy rule-based expert system for diagnosis of thyroid disease. In: IEEE Conference on Computational Intelligence in Bioinformatics and computational Biology (CIBCB), pp. 1–7. Niagara Falls, Canada
33. Ionita, I.,Ionita, L.: Prediction of thyroid disease using data mining techniques. BRAIN. Broad Res. Artif. Intell. Neuron Sci. **7**(3), 115–124 (2016)
34. Turanoglu-Bekar, E., Ulutagay, G., Kantarci-Savas, S.: Classification of thyroid disease by using data mining models: a comparison of decision tree algorithms. Oxford J. Intell. Decis. Data Sci. **2**, 13–28 (2016). https://doi.org/10.5899/2016/ojids-00002
35. Mirza, S., Mittal, S., Zaman, M.: A review of data mining literature. Int. J. Comput. Sci. Inf. Secur. (IJCSIS) **14**, 437–442 (2016)
36. Pan, Q., Zhang, Y., Zuo, M., Xiang, L., Chen, D.: Improved ensemble classification method of thyroid disease based on random forest. In 2016 8th International Conference on Information Technology in Medicine and Education (ITME), pp. 567–571. IEEE (2016). https://doi.org/10.1109/ITME.2016.01344

37. Sundaram, N.M., Renupriya, V.: Artificial neural network classifiers for diagnosis of thyroid abnormalities. In: International Conference on Systems, Science, Control, Communication, Engineering and Technology, pp. 206–211 (2016)
38. Dewangan, A., Shrivas, A., Kumar, P.: Classification of thyroid disease with feature selection technique. Int. J. Eng. Tech. (IJET) **2**(3), 128–131 (2016). ISSN: 2395-1303
39. Dash, S., Das, M.N., Mishra, B.K.: Implementation of an optimized classification model for prediction of hypothyroid disease risks. In: 2016 International Conference on Inventive Computation Technologies (ICICT), vol. 2, pp. 1–4. IEEE (2016). https://doi.org/10.1109/INVENTIVE.2016.7824794
40. Hameed, M.A.: Artificial neural network system for thyroid diagnosis. J. Univ. Babylon **25**(2), 518–528 (2017)
41. Pavya, K., Srinivasan, B.: Feature selection algorithms to improve thyroid disease diagnosis. In 2017 International Conference on Innovations in Green Energy and Healthcare Technologies (IGEHT), pp. 1–5. IEEE (2017). https://doi.org/10.1109/IGEHT.2017.8094070
42. Umadevi, S., JeenMarseline, K.S.: Applying classification algorithms to predict thyroid disease. International Journal of Engineering Science and Computing, Int. J. Eng. Sci. Comput. **7**(10), 15118–15120 (2017)
43. Ammulu, K., Venugopal, T.: Thyroid data prediction using data classification algorithm. Int. J. Innov. Res. Sci. Technol. **4**(2), 208–212 (2017)
44. Mahurkar, K.K., Gaikwad, D.P.: Normalization using improvised K-means applied in diagnosing thyroid disease with ANN. In: 2017 International Conference on Trends in Electronics and Informatics (ICEI), Tirunelveli, pp. 579–583 (2017)
45. Shrivas, A.K., Ambastha, P.: An ensemble approach for classification of thyroid disease with feature optimization. Int. Educ. Res. J. (S.l.) **3**(5), (2017). ISSN 2454-9916
46. Gurram, D., Rao, M.N.: A comparative study of support vector machine and logistic regression for the diagnosis of thyroid dysfunction. Int. J. Eng. Technol. (S.l.) **7**(1.1), 326–328 (2017). ISSN 2227-524X
47. Jatav, S.,Sharma, V.: An algorithm for predictive data mining approach in medical diagnosis. Int. J. Comput. Sci. Inf. Technol. (IJCSIT) **10**(1) 2018
48. Turki, T.: An empirical study of machine learning algorithms for cancer identification. In: 2018 IEEE 15th International Conference on Networking, Sensing and Control (ICNSC), pp. 1–5. IEEE (2018). https://doi.org/10.1109/ICNSC.8361312
49. Deepika, M., Kalaiselvi, K.: A Empirical study on disease diagnosis using data mining techniques. In: 2018 Second International Conference on Inventive Communication and Computational Technologies (ICICCT), pp. 615–620. IEEE (2018)
50. Razia, S., Prathyusha, P.S., Krishna, N.V., Sumana, S.N.: A Comparative study of machine learning algorithms on thyroid disease prediction. Int. J. Eng. Technol. (UAE) **7**(315) (2018). https://doi.org/10.14419/ijet.v7i2.8.10432
51. Yadav, D.C., Pal, S.: To generate an ensemble model for women thyroid prediction using data mining techniques. Asian Pac. J. Cancer. Prev. **20**(4), 1275–1281 (2019)
52. Begum, A., Parkavi, A.: Prediction of thyroid disease using data mining techniques. In: 2019 5th International Conference on Advanced Computing and Communication Systems (ICACCS), Coimbatore, India, pp. 342–345 (2019). https://doi.org/10.1109/ICACCS.2019.8728320
53. Sindhya, M.K.: Effective prediction of hypothyroid using various data mining techniques, vol. 5, 2nd edn. pp. 311–317 (2020)
54. Chaubey, G., Bisen, D., Arjaria, S., Yadav, V.: Thyroid Disease Prediction Using Machine Learning Approaches. Nat. Acad. Sci. Lett. (2020).https://doi.org/10.1007/s40009-020-00979-z
55. Mir, Y.I., Mittal, S.: Thyroid disease pprediction using two tier eensemble classifier. Int. J. Adv. Sci. Technol. **29**(06), 4460–4471 (2020)
56. Mir, Y. I., Mittal, S.: Thyroid disease prediction using hybrid machine learning techniques: an effective framework. Int. J. Sci. Technol. Res. **9**(02), 2868–2874 (2020)

57. Shariati, S., Haghighi, M.M.: Comparison of anfis neural network with several other ANNs and support vector machine for diagnosing hepatitis and thyroid diseases. In: 2010 International Conference on Computer Information Systems and Industrial Management Applications (CISIM), vol. 10, pp. 1101–1109 (2010)
58. Ertugrul, O., Kaya, Y.: A detailed analysis on extreme learning machine and novel approaches based on ELM. Am. J. Comput. Sci. Eng. **1**, 43–50 (2014)
59. Hameed, M.A.: Artificial neural network system for thyroid diagnosis. J. Univ. Babylon **25**(2), 518–528 (2017)
60. Umadevi, S., JeenMarseline, K.S.: Applying classification algorithms to predict thyroid disease. Int. J. Eng. Sci. Comput. **7**(10), 15118–15120 (2017)

Chapter 6
Automated Breast Cancer Diagnosis Based on Neural Network Algorithms

Kamran Alam, Lalita Sharma, and Namarta Chopra

Abstract Breast cancer, the most common among the women, is primarily examined visually by starting with initial screening of breast and lymph nodes in armpit, dermoscopic analysis, histopathological tests and a biopsy. In India as per the ratings, 25–35% women are affected with breast cancer in every city in India. Being in a developing country like India, majority of women are dying due to breast cancer and for every 4 min women is affected with the same. Women are suffering a lot due to this curse, masses or micro calcification are the symptoms a woman can have at a previous stage, where microcalcification is mineral which gets into the breast tissue. It's quite hard to examine due to ultra-fine shapes and uncertain edges. It is being categorized into three main categories normal, malignant and Benign, which can be detected using proposed system. In proposed scheme, input images are being compared with large collection of databases with the replacement of sigmoid activation function. Probabilistic neural network is used to describe nonlinear statement limits which further leads to Bayes optimal and also all the function which bear same properties as well. Any input data or algorithm can be pointed with the four layer neural network. Standard PNN consists of input layer of N nodes, a pattern layer of m nodes, a summation layer of k node and it consists of pseudo layer L nodes, which is used for decision making which is also known as decision layer for producing output.

Keywords Probabilistic neural network · MATLAB · Breast cancer · Mammography

K. Alam (✉) · L. Sharma · N. Chopra
Amritsar College of Engineering and Technology, Amritsar, India

N. Chopra
e-mail: namartachopra@yahoo.co.in

J. Nayak et al. (eds.), *Advanced Machine Learning Approaches in Cancer Prognosis*, Intelligent Systems Reference Library 204,
https://doi.org/10.1007/978-3-030-71975-3_6

6.1 Introduction

Neural system processes in the same way as the brain does. Manmade neurons are helping hand in their structure, capable of processing more than single inputs to one common result as output. As all the neurons are in contact with each other due to set up and connection assemblies and the way they develop a working network and that very network or assembly further look for the fetched data to analyze it and to process it well. Also helps to detect whether that data and its bits are connected with one another. When there is a large quantity of data, then it looks a bit complex and sometimes one cannot observe it well. The assemblies that were made to fix and check queries about networks and probabilistic neural networks are the same. It performs its operation in steps and stages. It will observe the data and computes it to training vectors thus develop a factor which describes the relation of input data with training factor. The second step processes this data and performs the addition function of inputs of every class so as to develop main results as output which is a factor of probabilities. Mechanism of the human body is primarily based upon the formation of cells. Cells keep increasing and decreasing, it is the natural behavior of cells and meanwhile they nature the growth of the human body. Furthermore, ensures the working processes of the human body in a proper manner and they preserve the automatic working of the body as well. So, this was about standard body working process and production of cells accurately in order to perform the proper functioning of the body yet in some cases these cells, basically their production is not standard and said to be abnormal too. Abnormal in the sense that they do not grow as they supposed to be. For a human body to work properly, it requires the conservation of cells as increment and decrement as well as a genuine resemblance between working cells and dead cells. But in some cases, cells start to grow anomalously, this is an unusual state which further leads to cancer. Cancer is basically the unusuality and disorder of the cells and it can be present at any part of the body leading from the forehead to feet. It is not limited to some parts only or a particular area but it may affect the surrounding area as well. There are several kinds of cancers which can be found in the human body while breast cancer is regarded as the most concerned one. However, it is mostly found in women. The major factors for this cancer are age, genetic issue, health disorders, alcohol, and breast density. As far as determination and examination of cancer is concerned, neural networks are regards as one of the major techniques. Treatment of cancer is directly proportional to the examination of cancer and the time at which it has been detected. If the cancer is examined at preliminary stages then it is easy to cure but if it is determined at crucial stages then the chances to get properly treated decreases. A report of victim is being made by considering medical history and demographic as base and from those particular reports it has been analyzed that the victims who died with the same had the survival rates up to 30%. Though every scientist wants to make novel and efficient treatment for cancer, yet lots of resources are needed and sometimes they are not affordable. Moreover, they are time consuming. Indeed, science is working to cure or to eradicate cancer totally by analyzing the cause. So that, it cannot harm the patient more. For these cancers, neural networks are there, which bear a unique strategy to fight with cancer merely known as the updated and advanced version of computation. So, to take care the victims of lung cancer, this technology is being used. Not only in medical region but this particular methodology is currently there in different areas just because of their effectiveness and efficiency. They have capability to perform multiple tasks. From long time, science is working to find the advanced treatment for cancer. Chiou et al. [1] developed an artificial neural system with hybrid lung cancer monitoring. This further proved fruitful to increase the efficiency and particular known for their rapidness in working. There are methods to work under this category, early processing for quality of background of image and its contrast in addition to it, for to select the nodule which is under observation and merely the cause. Gutter et al. [2] came with a purely advanced technique basically for the FDG that is fluorodeoxyglucose, positron emission tomography-PET and CT—computed tomography figures which have been there for cure. Kenji et al. [3] proposed a theme understanding method with artificial neural networks. Penedo et al. [4] worked for determination of accused area in low resolution picture and developed a different artificial neural network for peaks of accuse area. Bartfay et al. [5] came with contrast of different victims from national cancer institute of Canada basically for the accuracy purpose and to measure the deadly cells in victim of lung cancer.

When the growth of cells becomes unusual then they create a tumour in the concerned party from the rapid growth of cells. It's a kind of threat to a woman as breast cancer is said to be the second major cause that is responsible for the death of a woman all over the globe [6]. According to the American cancer research study, it is found that about 266,000 numbers of occurrences of invasive breast tumour have examined and almost 63,960 numbers of mortality from the same cancer [7]. Hence there is a need to control this cancer in order to save women, who are dying every single second because of this particular disease and it demands for the very root to distinguish benign and spitefulness. However previous data and identification of this cancer bears mammography data. While the victims are rapid in race of getting this cancer, it has become a challenge for the doctors and radiologists to make the worth checkup of every single victim, also to cure them hand in hand because of limited resources and time. This very paper is basically a hope for the radiologists in movement of quick and up to the mark examination of breast cancer with the help of deep learning; relate this process to manual using WEKA on single images that are draggy on.

A survey shows that from the last few years the situation is getting drastic. From a researcher study which concludes that breast cancer in Australia for twelve years which states that in 2007 cases were 12,775 meanwhile in 2018 they increased to 18,235. This shows that victims are rapidly increasing with the passage of each single day. It was predicted that in 2018 almost 3156 would be dying in which women were the most. Women's breasts are due to lobules, ducts, nipples and fatty tissues. Lobules contain milk further transport to the nipple by ducts. Taking a standard case, immense mass is gathered in lobules and duets as well which forms tumours and later converted into cancer [8]. Once it gets initiated, it begins to flow everywhere in the body, especially the area near by the affected part to the rest of the parts as well. Then it turns into an immense harm and becomes uneasy to give a full stop to it.

With the passage of every single day, moment and year as well, the breast cancer cases are increasing and this increment with the passage of time is basically said to be "INCIDENCE". In India, in 2018, particularly there were almost 162,468 new cases of cancer and the major part to note is that all were women. Amongst which, high percentage of women were affected with breast cancer as shown in Fig. 6.1. It is not hard and fast that each patient of cancer can be cured; sometimes it turns into a deadly phase where it is hard to save lives and one dies with cancer in that year, it is said to be MORTALITY. Hence in 2018, 87,090 women patients were dead. Approximately 23.5% deaths were due to breast cancer in India amongst all the cancers and it clearly shows that one forth death among all cancers was particularly because of breast cancer in India. Figure 6.2 describes mortality rate of women due to various cancers. Breast cancer tumours can be classified into two major cases.

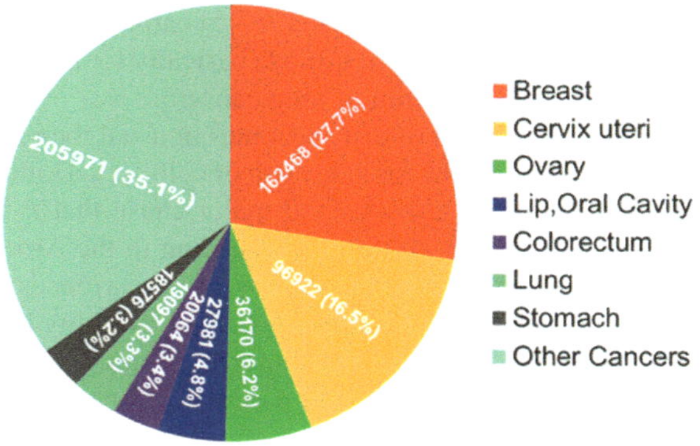

Fig. 6.1 Estimated number of new cases in 2018, India

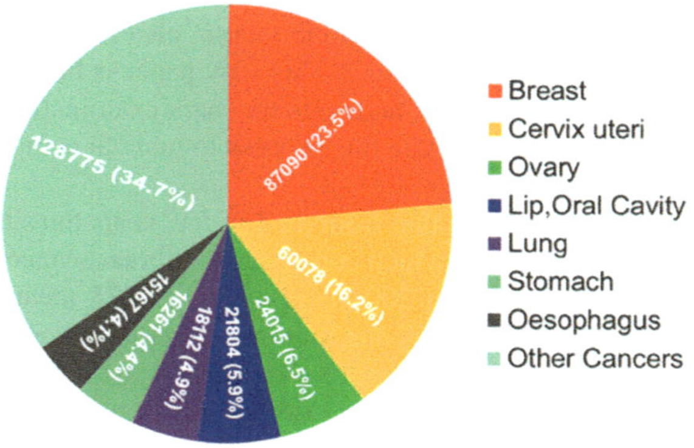

Fig. 6.2 Mortality in women due to various cancers

6.1.1 *Benign (Non-cancerous)*

It is basically non-life threatening. Yet rarely gets to cancer. An immune system is "SAC" and in usual benign tumors are distinguishable from healthy cells and hence it can be taken out from the body easily.

6.1.2 *Malignant*

It is generally dangerous due to immense growth of cells and their disordered behavior. These are the cells which flow through tissues as quickly as fire to the next area. As the nuclei of any malignant tissue are more than standard one which can further be deadly. Though cancer is always a bane to society, hence its need is overcome. If the victim would cure in an effective manner then surely lives can be saved nonetheless it merely be possible at early stages, as once it's getting spread then it may become uncontrollable. Therefore, it is said that preventions are always better than cure. So, the major necessity is to detect and examine cancer whether one is at standard stage, benign or malignant bearing tissues, so that further steps could be performed. Moreover, for the specific examination of the victim's photography is there which is really fruitful for a doctor to test patients and to find the affective area in the body as well. So taking penetration and damage as major medical photography further can be categorized in two parts which is based on noninvasive and invasive method of screening of breast cancer.

6.1.2.1 Noninvasive

The following are the different noninvasive techniques used.

Ultrasound
This technique of photography is totally based on working of ultrasonic transducers which work on the principle of SONAR i.e., Sound Navigation and Ranging. The electrode used has two functions first the high frequency sound wave is triggered or produced using PWM signal then using Echo the signal is received and thus using image processing, image can be drawn [9]. This machine is composed of a processing unit, transducer for Triggering high frequency and Echo, and a display unit in order to display 2 dimensional as well as 3 dimensional images of patients under test. Therefore, this technique is free from hazardous electromagnetic waves, chemicals, gas emission. So, it has no side effects of heating body tissues to an extent which gives rise to cancer cells.

X-rays
This technique of photography is totally based on Emission of electromagnetic radiation which was invented by roentgen in 1895 [10]. The detailed information of

breast cancer can be gathered using low dose X-ray imaging technique which is also known as mammogram imaging. Due to a sulphurous amount of electromagnetic radiation, body tissue can be heated up which can produce hydrogen peroxide in the cells which can damage the cells and hence the chances of cancer can be increased.

CAT

CAT refers to Computer Aided Tomography. It is also known as CT scan. This technique of imaging is also based on the principle of electromagnetic radiation where high intense X-ray is produced and is sent to the test object. The only difference between X-ray and CT scan is, X-ray can only be used to capture an image at 180° whereas CT scan can capture images on film at 360° means it is angular and flexible. Therefore, CT scan is used to film internal injuries and soft tissues of a subject.

MRI

MRI refers to magnetic resonance imaging and it uses non-invasive technique of imaging which is responsible for capturing 3-dimensional images of a subject under test and formulated and designed by sir marsfield and this process uses both a radio waves as well as electromagnetic radiation [11]. For image production MRI's generally take more time for image production which can be uncomfortable and uneasy. It also requires more caution for the one wearing any kind of metal, and needs extra care.

6.1.2.2 Invasive

The following is the invasive techniques used.

Histopathological image

This technique is also known as biopsy imaging. It is basically microscopic investigation and identification of a tissue. For this particular method, one requires performing several surgical methods before then the images from histopathological tissue provide histopathological images as shown in Fig. 6.3. The non-invasive method of early detection of breast cancer is shown in Fig. 6.3a, b and detection of breast cancer using Histopathological invasive method is shown in Fig. 6.3c, d and is performed by surgery.

6.2 Related Work

The examination and to conclude mammograms in a well efficient manner is an immensely hard process even for all the well-educated and highly experienced radiologists. In order to make it clearer and more understandable, methods are adopted which are explained below.

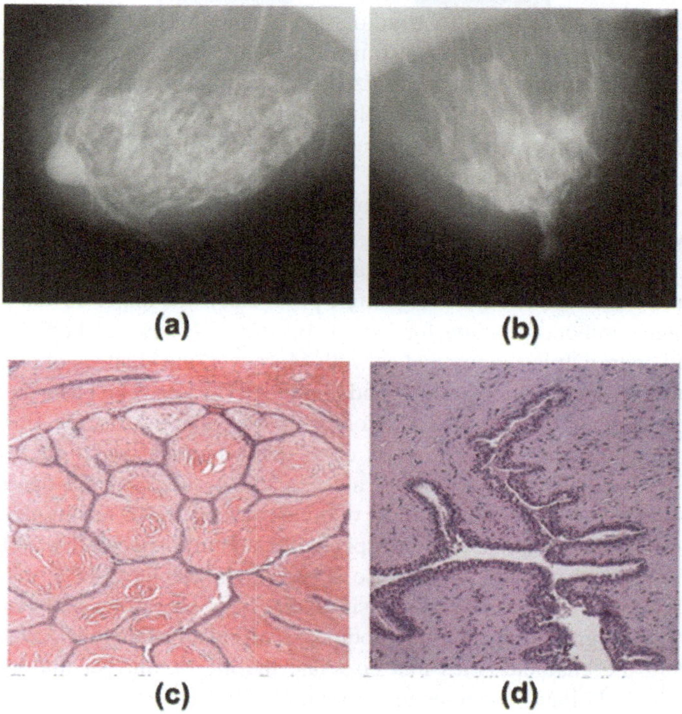

Fig. 6.3 **a**, **b** Benign,malignant mammogram images using non invasive method, **c**, **d** Histopathological benign 85% and malignant 15% using invasive method

6.2.1 CAD (Computer Aided Diagnosis)

CAD refers to computer aided diagnosis, principally works on different complicated patterns of images of test subjects for the detection of breast cancer is used for initial method of screening of mammography images. It is a low dose X-ray imaging technique in order to capture female breasts in a film. Therefore, it can be used for initial detection of breast cancer in females [12, 13]. Hence it requires sequential analysis of test images, characterization and combination of several clinical parameters which are very difficult for the health worker itself [14, 15]. This causes less efficiency and accuracy of test reports. So, a huge change of false positive and false negative is observed in the report. The combination of radiological image elucidation into the computer-based models can increase the detection accuracy of test images up to a large extent. Therefore, computer aided diagnosis can help in early detection, analysis of breast, irregularity of mammographic images, malformation of breast tumor and recognition of abnormalities can be done. Radiology basically bears two major points—the very first is usual perception as having a look over the image and the other one is cognition as into detect and analyze what is seen [16]. There are several studies which assured that radiography sometimes has abnormal behavior as it was clear there an image is, at times not reported. In order to have an exact analysis, double reading was being utilized for example- in order to capture as well as screening mammography which further led to an increment rate of detection of cancer. Being labor intensive, it is not more utilized though some exceptional cases are still there in which it is being used.

The salient point of the very CAD system is to enhance the examination of the disease by lessening the negative rating which was due to observational oversight. Instead of having more than one human as radiologist, computers are being accessed to detect and examine each and every single point that is the major advancement as it decreases the number of humans for a single operation. Likewise, it results in saving of time and energy. It is economical as well. Moreover, the chances of error are less as machines are operating everything and complexity is less. The basic motto of this system is to increase the rate of tests in order to overcome the disease. Furthermore, the required results are gained in most cases and efficiency was found more. The aim of CAD methods and techniques are exactly the same as the operation of a radiologist during case study and in case of breast cancers, CAD techniques looked at micro-calcifications and masses (both speculated and non-speculated, architectural, distortions and asymmetric). And in case of chest radiographs and CT scans, current CDA tools looked for pulmonary densities that bear some physical features like sphericity that might represent living nodules. Despite all of them, CAD techniques will point to the characteristics that co-relate the algorithm, yet findings are not there that the radiologist assumes to warrant and study upcoming reports i.e. false CAD marks. In addition to it, at times an exact positive CAD point, upon study by radiologists is declined as not assuring further study. Meanwhile that is considered to be an error, the false negative data.

6.2.2 Feature Extraction

The input images are dimensionally reduced into computerized matrix in order to process the image to get meaningful results. In order to pre-process the raw image feature extraction is executed. Furthermore, techniques can be also be used after texture analysis [17]. For illustration with ANN (Artificial Neural Network), an immense area of cases associated with benign can be exactly examined from cases of malignancies. In the year 2007 in Varela et al. [18], channel chief of iris at different scopes was there to check and detect malignant tumours on mammograms. Neural systems based on back propagation was developed to decrease false positives. For the development and detection methods of two data set in which active contour model method [19] utilized for segmentation of pre-processed images, which further bears an edge detection based active contour model methodology showing the utilization of a limp power using damping coefficient; a geometric active contour model (GAC) model as well as active contour without edges (ACWE) method. There were also the tests which used a case study of hundreds of cases from two fetching indexes;

they are mammographic image analysis society and digital index for screening mammography.

In a digitized mammogram, a pixel is being addressed by its next one and which is described with a square shaped window Wn of n × n pixels which are centered in it. Then, this very window is moved together with the image, furthermore operated for extracting the characteristics of each one and it is operated with normalization gray level values of its pixels, to get mainly zero and basic value of deviation unity. In order to get desired results. This window is operated at several methods depending upon their various characteristics extraction perspective which mainly include Gray-map, SGLDM, SFUM, sobel filters and AFUM [20]. Besides all these prewritten perspectives, AFUM obtains an attribute route which gives values according to the parameter and value. The dimensionality of the feature vector is decreased with principal component analysis (PCF). The AFUM techniques retrieve a single feature for each pixel rather than generating feature vectors which can be accessed as it is for further required classification. Feature extraction techniques are successively discussed above.

6.2.3 Gray-Map

Gray map is considered to be a simple or standard method along with PCA, gray map usually extracts any pixel immensely and is reserved as a sample, providing desired results compared to others. Feature extraction ways are generally implemented in picture processing [21, 22]. For the analyzation of above discussed methodology, two dimensional vectors are there having normalized values of gray level in window Wn. Further, all the routes or vectors with the help of PCA and reserved samples are projected towards bottom proportionality space.

6.2.4 SOBEL

A sobel filter generally is for increasing the edges of objects in image with convolution. This is also considered as the standard method. These filters bear two kernels which examine horizontal as well as vertical modification in picture. In case either two kernels are there in picture, then the result is supplementary utilized to analyze the direction as well as direction of the edge in image. In this perspective, there is only an analysis of the magnitude of the edges which results in time saving. Yet, it is firmly endangered to noise and disconnects the contour also. It basically determines the edges with three pixels wide.

6.2.5 SGLDM

There are several perspectives for health exposures and therapeutic purposes having quality and surface as foundation including SGLDM, dependence matrices and it is known as co-occurrence matrices as well [23], pattern feature [24] with more appearance properties [25]. Here it is tested with SGLDM descriptors. A subset of SGLDM descriptors is also there to describe the authenticity of this method from Haralick et al. [26]. Fractal 2nd significance distinction, correction, variation, reverse variation bit, aggregate mean, aggregate variation, aggregate randomness, randomness or entropy, contrast variation, and contrast randomness. For the determination of the spatial gray level dependence matrix descriptors, every picture first operated with standard vector quantization in order to reduce the amount of gray levels which is leading from 256 to sharp 20. Eleven figures had been extracted from 16 matrices in accordance with 4 angles (0, π4, π 2 and 3π4) and 4 distances (1–4 pixels) with 176 frameworks. Moreover, the frameworks were adapted with basic calculations with instructing set, providing a variation of almost 1.0 ending up with results in 176-dimensional vector in a bottom dimensional space with respect to PCA.

6.2.6 AFUM

Average fraction under the minimum is basically the mass detection algorithm given by health and bowyer. To make it more clear, consider any pixel pij, the fragmentation of components at a distance like r2 from the pij, which bears the bottom strength values among the components defined by centre (I, j) and radius rl is calculated. The particular calculation is the radius of r1 and r2 and the mean is described. The main merit of this algorithm specifically is that it is constant towards rotation and hence parameter training process is not required.

6.2.7 SFUM

Possessing one characteristic for each pixel like AFUM techniques assures, is merely a merit, a deduction of data can be experienced when the mean of a group of properties is calculated. To overcome it, it suggests a variation to AFUM formulae. The whole set of fractions under the minimum (SFUM) is taken into account rather than computing the average, providing a characteristic route rather than singular variant. In case the measurements of this route are more, it is lessened with respect to PCA. Then the feature vector calculated for each window Wn is reserved like samples, at the end it is clear with k-nearest neighbor rule.

The K-nearest neighbor K-NN Classification method is a firm as well as vigorous including common written characteristics and practical in shape as well as feature specifications. The main demerit frequently mentioned for the method is cost that it is uneconomical. In this work almost the next neighbor looked in KD trees are utilized to decrease the cost.

KD trees as well as search algorithms are utilized in other shape and feature testing, having drastic decrement in finding time during possessing recognition evaluations. So, to categorize with respect to standard class a conviction basis function having interval up to K-nn is there.

$$f_c = \frac{\sum_{i \varepsilon sc} \frac{1}{d(p,ni)}}{\sum_{i=1}^{k} \frac{1}{d(p,ni)}} \tag{6.1}$$

from Eq. (6.1),

fc = conviction of class c and d

(p, ni) = interval from check junction to the i-neighbor

sc = group of sub-signals of prototypes from class c with respect to k nearest neighbour as n1….nk.

Hence, the conviction of only single class cancer is determined as the threshold (T) is adjusted, a component is said to have cancer, if that conviction is more than T. Yet, in this case grouping ranges are calculated for T at various instants, rather than selecting a specific threshold, progressing a receiver operating characteristic curve and to neglect this by the same picture in trails, a standard technique is implemented which assures that when an X-ray is assessed not one, yet the another out from instructing group of similar victim.

6.2.8 Deep Learning Techniques

The standard aim of research and development is primarily to create an innovative notion to overcome breast cancer with deep learning technology followed by CAD. Then for random evaluations a deep learning rooted graph was developed which is composed of two modules namely, Risk prediction module and module based on adaptive feature identification. Prediction of risk can be also analyzed with (MLP) that is multiple layer perceptron classifier that provide a risk rate to predict growth of tumour using mammography reprehensible tumours. The DL Architecture based Computer Aided Diagnosis increment also known as CADx is used for identification and detection of benign or malignant and computation of tumour scenario avoiding imminent blunders due to improper image processing results like boundary segmentation and classification techniques vigorous features. Intersection of level set generalship by DCNNs that means deep convolutional neural network is conducted using feature representation. Multi task transfer learning technique i.e., DCNN was delivered first, along with a transfer learning associated with a single task as well. After that a DCNN technique was developed and it was further tested on (SFMs) i.e., mammograms with screen film were used to develop DCNN with multi task transfer learning tested on SFMs when results of autonomous test set were consented, then DCNN multi task exchange learning was regarded to be extensive high execution that is p is equals to 0.007 when varied using a single task transfer technique bearing DCNN. DCNN technique in image analysis suggests a simple and victorious plan specifically for positioning and scoring of histological breast related disease, decoloration of images including more than 100 illustrations, data amplification is there for expansion cordiality of classifier and at several platforms deep convolutional features were divided with openly accessible (CNN) that is convolution neural networks, where over fitting inclination and accurate augmenting is there. A well-planned distance measure was utilized for the composition of the neural system. The probability to augment the analytical accuracy was illustrated with computer-aided design index using order and DL methodologies.

6.3 Methodology

In general, a histogram is a graphical representation. It shows the distribution of data with intervals like [0, l −1] is defined by the discrete function h(rk) = nk

Where rk = kth is the intensity value and nk = number of pixels contained in image.

So, basically histogram can be regarded as digital image as well. It is standard criteria under which a histogram is separating every component with total no. of pixels present in image and can be represented as (MN).

where, M is for rows and N is for columns of image dimensions.

Hence a normalized histogram is represented as

$$P\ (rk) = nk/MN$$

For the value [k = 0,1———,l −1]

pk is an approximation of intensity level of the pixel
rk is total sum of all the components which should is unity.

Histograms are considered as the fundamentals for several formal computing processes and its utilization is to develop and advance the image and to make it more desirable. Histograms not only provide required graphical data but also the specifications including image compression and segmentation. These are easy to analyze and are economical as well which is the major function. Hence widely used. Histogram operations for intensity alteration as an initiation several figures and graphs are there like pollen images which shows mainly four intensity features consisting dark, light, low contrast and high contrast. These figures also describe the histogram resemblance to these images where the horizontal axis represents intensity values rk and likewise vertical axis shows values of hk = nk or p(rk) = nk/MN with the condition values being normalized. Hence histograms are seen graphically easily. It is seen that the dark image that the histogram constituents are gathered on low or dark side of scale and alike the histogram constituents of light images are influenced with regards to high side. Low contrast images bear limited histogram close to middle of scale.

Yet a dark and washed-out gray look is being there in case of monochrome image. At last, an extensive range is being balanced by histogram constituents in case of high contrast image and moreover distribution is a bit close to infirmity using few vertical lines which are higher than others. Inherently it can be deduced that the high contrast aspect is being possessed by the pixels of the image which have an entire range of intensity level and display gray level vastly and the net effect comes with the image which contains gray level details and much high dynamic range, which can be illustrated using block diagram in Fig. 6.4.

6.3.1 Histogram Equalization Used in Proposed System

Assume for a moment continuous intensity values where r is range [0, l −1] with r = 0 shows black

$$r = l - 1 \text{ shows white}$$

when r fulfils above conditions then further goal is on transformation that is basically intensity mapping of the form

$$s = T(r)\ 0 \leq r \leq l - 1 \tag{6.2}$$

Equation (6.2) provides output intensity (s) for each pixel in input with intensity (r).

Consider, T(r) which is monotonically increasing function in range $0 \leq r \leq l - 1$; $0 \leq T(r) \leq l - 1$ for $0 \leq r \leq l - 1$ Sometimes inverse is used

$$r = T - 1(s)\ 0 \leq s \leq l - 1 \tag{6.3}$$

Then according to Eq. (6.3), condition (a) is changed to (a'). T(r) is typically monotonically increasing time ranging from $0 \leq r \leq l - 1$.

This condition (a) demands that T(r) to be monotonically increasing with assurance that output intensity cannot be less than input values. Hence, preserving artifacts are there with reversals of intensity. Condition (b) assures that both output and input intensities are similarly in range and at last condition (a') assures the mapping from s back to r be one to one. Hence preserving obscurity for more clearness, some graphs and figures are developed which provide every important information showing that

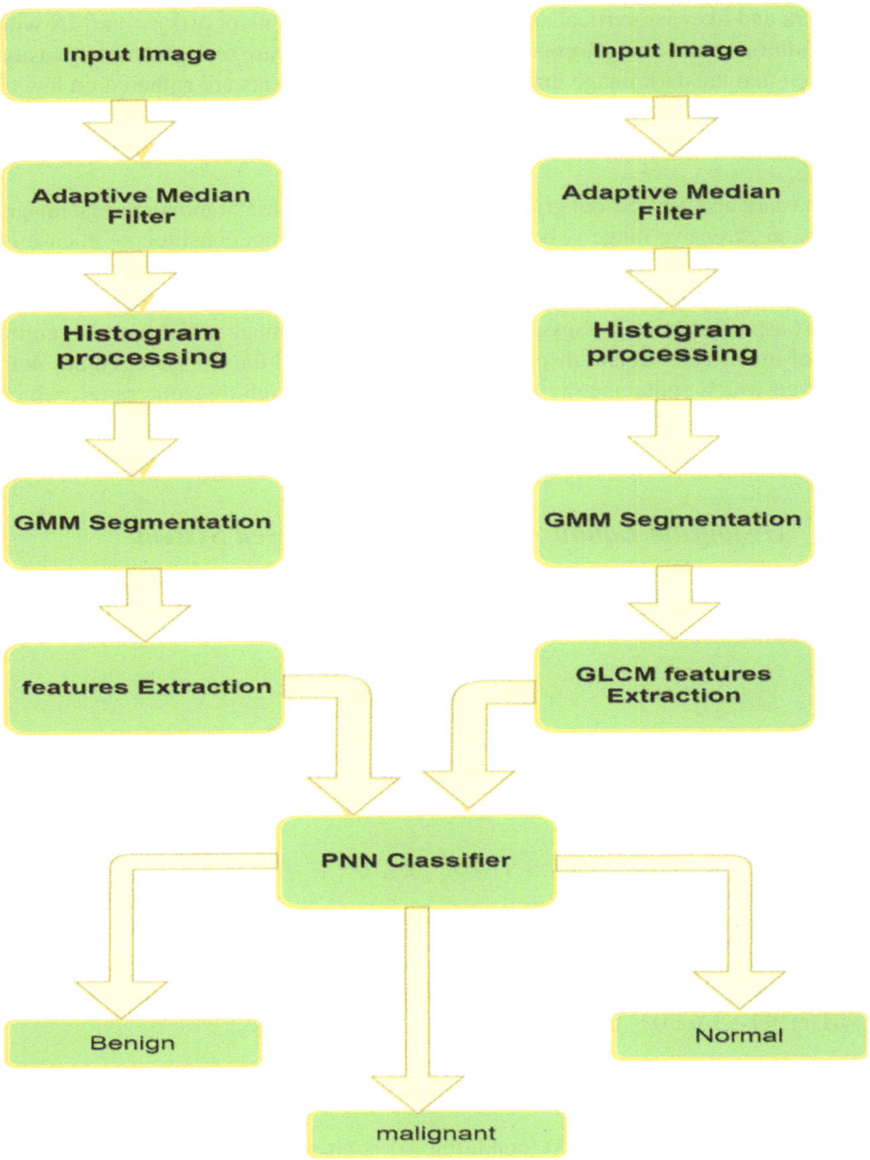

Fig. 6.4 Block diagram of proposed system

both the conditions are being fulfilled where multiple values can map to single one with both one-to-one and many-to-one mapping is operated by monotonic transformation function especially for r to s mapping. Yet, there could be an error when taking values of r specifically from mapping is envisaged if arrow's direction is being reversed and can be performed for sk inverse mapping. While sq inverse mapping is basically interval of values that basically avert from the original value recovering of r which further leads to sq. It is shown that T(r) is typically monotonic which generally assures that inverse mapping with a single value that is the mapping is one-to-one for both the directions. So, this is a somewhat theoretical method with necessary histogram operation. In actual, operations are performed with integer intensity values and if typically, monotonicity is not satisfied then there is an error in non-inverse transformation. Suppose the intensity level of an image haphazardly seen with range $[0, l-1]$. The basic method of that very varying quantity is prospect denseness factor.

Consider pr(r) represents PDFs of r and ps(s) represents PDFs of s and substandard of p shows that Pr and Ps are variable function actually. A standard conclusion from basic prospective theory is when pr(r) and T(r) are studied and T(r) is constant and differentiable up to the interval of required range then PDF of mapped value s is being attained with the standard relation

$$P_s(s) = P_r(r)\left|\frac{dr}{ds}\right| \tag{6.4}$$

Hence from Eq. (6.4), the Probability density function of output intensity variable s is represented with the Probability density function of input intensities and the transformation function used as r and s are correlated with T(r)

$$S = T(r) = (l-1)\int_0^r pr(\omega)d\omega \tag{6.5}$$

Using Eq. (6.5), ω = is integer of dummy variable and the RHS of above equation is taken as CDF that is cumulative distribution function of random variable r as PDF are generally positive as the integral of the function is the area under the function with transformation function of Eq. (6.5) fulfills condition-(a) as the area under the function is not decreasing with the increment in r. when higher limit in this equation $r = (l-1)$, the integral evaluates to unity that is the area under a Probability density function curve is unity. Therefore, the maximum value of s is $(l-1)$ and condition (b) is fulfilled. For Original image Histogram Response refer Fig. 6.5 after processing of raw image with histogram equalization the response is shown as in Fig. 6.6.

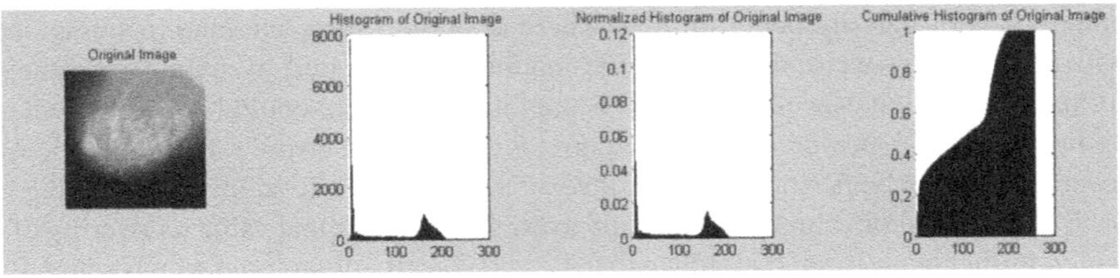

Fig. 6.5 Original image histogram response

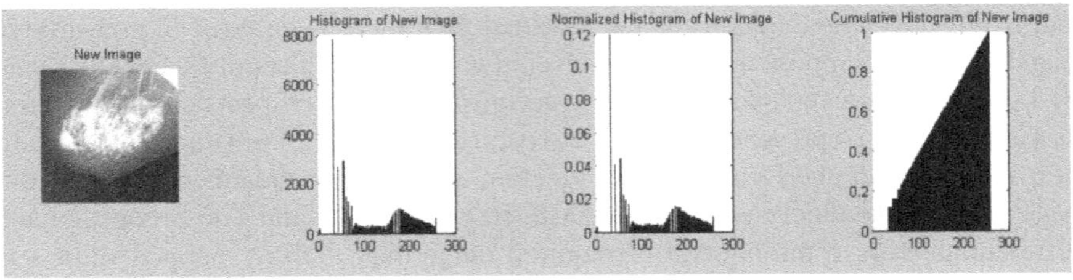

Fig. 6.6 Raw image processed using histogram equalization

6.3.2 Adaptive Median Filter

In order to operate properly the median filter as shown in Fig. 6.7, the formal density should not be more than 0.2. This filter handles impulse noise having more probabilities than others. Furthermore, these filters secure data yet non impulse noise does not. Moreover, it works in rectangular window and Sxy alike rest of filters. They increase size of Sxy as it has a modification quality which merely makes it different from other filters. The modification in size particularly in accordance with certain condition described further. One thing to note that the output obtained of the filter

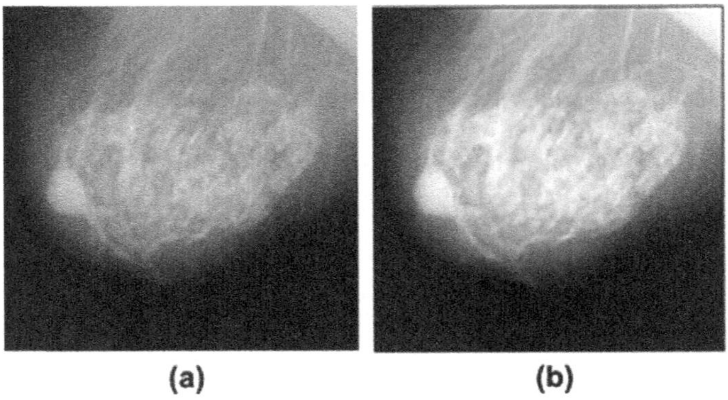

Fig. 6.7 **a** Raw mammogram, **b** Adaptive median filter

single valued which is further require to replace pixel value at (x,y), at any given instance of time, that point on which the value of Sxy is centered.

Z_{min} = when intensity value in Sxy is minimum
Z_{max} = when intensity value in Sxy is maximum
Z_{med} = is a median of intensity value in Sxy
Zxy = intensity parameter at coordinates (x, y)
S_{max} = maximum accepted size of Sxy.

The standard median algorithm technique operates in 2 steps. The representation of step A and B are given as follows

Step A:-

```
A1 = Zmed minus Zmin i.e. Zmed - Zmin
A2 = Zmed minus Zmax i.e. Zmed - Zmin
The logical operation is now operates as
If A1 is greater than zero AND A2 is greater than zero,
go to step -B
Else make an increment in size of window
If window_size is lesser and equals to Smax repeat step
A
Else output display is Zmed
```

Step B:-

```
B1 = Zxy minus Zmin; Zxy-Zmin
B2 = Zxy minus Zmax; Zxy-Zmax
If B1 is greater than zero AND B2 is lesser than zero
output Zxy
Else display output Zmed.
```

6.3.3 Hardware Implementation of Filter

In order to remove impulse noise, then to access smoothness which would not be impulsive and to lessen the distortion as well, like excessive thinning or thickening of object boundaries and meanwhile Z_{min} and Z_{max} are taken statically or graphically by algorithm and be statically impulse like noise constituents whether these are not the lowest and highest possible pixel image value. By using above values, it is clear that step A is defined when median filter output, Zmed is an impulsive that is (black or white) or not. When this very conditions Zmin is lesser than Zmed is lesser than Zmax satisfies, only when Zmed would not be impulse in nature. In this particularly study, it moved to step B and for identifying whether the point in the center of window, Zxy is the impulse element.

When condition B1 is greater than zero AND B2 is lesser than zero is true then Zmin is lesser than Zxy is lesser than Zmax which cannot be an impulsive.

Further the value of pixel is extreme and algorithms outputs the median values Zmed. Yet there is an error in standard median filter, replaces every pixel value in image with median of next one. Due to this loss of data can be faced.

6.3.3.1 Image Partition

The median filter which is the processing unit is fed with the images in a column of data in the form of (9 × 1). Therefore, for 9 columns it has to buffer the 9 cycles. Hence the Input/Output count is reduced in the filter chip to a large extent.

6.3.3.2 Image Region Filtering (Processing Unit)

Each of the subregions is computed for zmin, zmed, and zmax pixel. Partition can be buffered for 3 × 3, 5 × 5, 7 × 7, and 9 × 9 regions for 9 cycles making 9 × 9 region. The median filter output for each region is given by -'center_pixel' (data signal -'pixel_valid' (control signal). Computation of subsequent center pixels does not have any delay.

6.3.3.3 Median Filter Unit (d3 x 3)

The median filter unit is shown in Fig. 6.8.

For 3 × 3 regions, 36 comparators are required, that is four comparators of nine stages each to compute the value of min/max/median. Neighboring pixels are

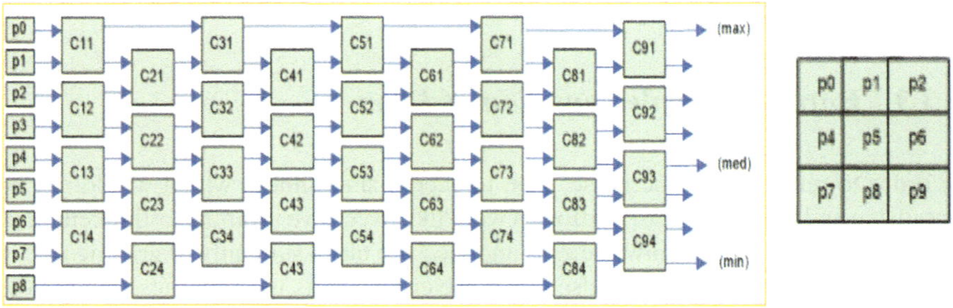

Fig. 6.8 Median filter unit

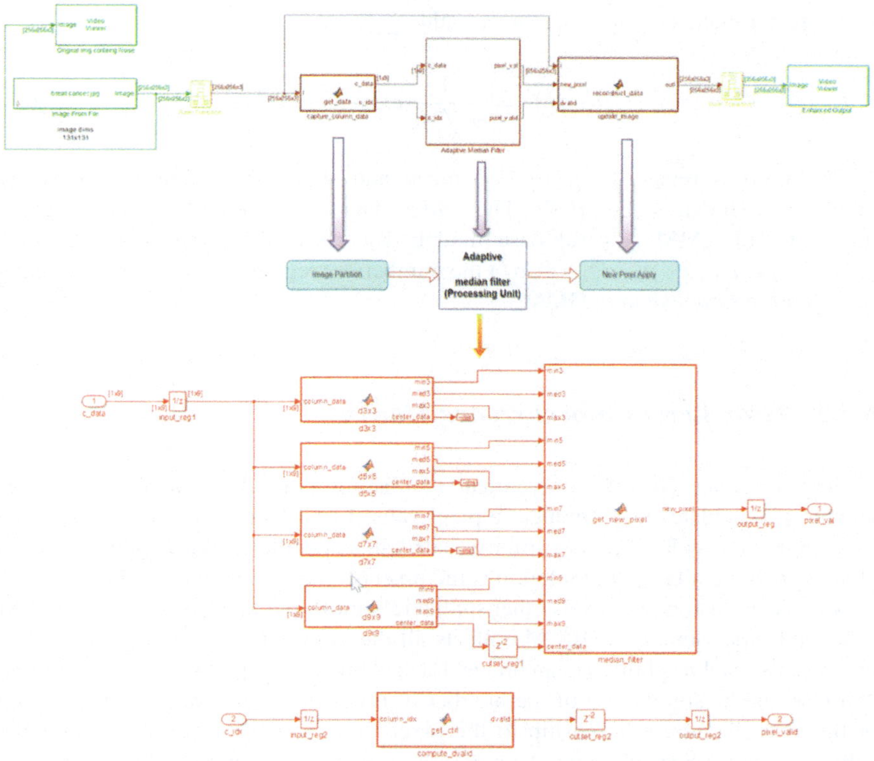

Fig. 6.9 Hardware implementation of filter

compared by computational elements. Therefore, the hardware implementation of adaptive median filter as shown in Fig. 6.9 is very resource intensive in computation.

6.3.4 Gaussian Mixture Models

Each element in the image is pixel whereas the image is a matrix. In that matrix, Pixel value is a number which has its own entity like intensity, color of image. Consider variable X which is random in nature and can take pixel values. Suppose Mixture of Gaussian distribution for probability model is described as the following Eq. (6.6).

$$f(x) = \sum_{i=1}^{k} p_i N\left(x \mid \mu_i, \sigma_i^2\right) \tag{6.6}$$

p_i Is greater than zero ($p_i > 0$), are weights $\sum_{i=1}^{k} p_i = 1$

$$N\left(\mu_i, \sigma_i^2\right)^1 = \frac{1}{\sigma\sqrt{2p_i}} exp\frac{-(x-\mu_i)^2}{2\sigma_i^2} \tag{6.7}$$

For a given image X, μ_i, σ_i are mean and standard deviation respectively of class as shown in Eq. (6.7). The lattice data are values of Pixels for given image x and GMM is pixel base model. Therefore, the parameters are $\theta = (p_1, \ldots, p_k, \mu_1 \ldots, \mu_k, \sigma_1^2, \ldots, \sigma_k^2)$ the numbers or regions can be identified using histogram of lattice data in GMM.

6.3.5 Gray Level Co-occurrence Matrix

In order to create GLCM, "graycomatrix" function is used in matlab. The "graycomatrix" calculates how frequent a pixel value I (that is gray-level) has occurred by creating a gray level co-occurrence matrix in a specific spatial relationship with element j. Generally, spatial relation is the pixel of interest and the pixel to horizontally adjacent; using two pixels other spatial relationships can also be stated. GLCM is second order statistics, GLCM collects all the information regarding pixel pairs and reveals pixel brightness in an image. Each element in (i, j) matrix in the resultant "GLCM" is the summation of the number of times pixel with value i encountered in the stated spatial relationship to the pixel value j of the input image. For the fully dynamic range of an input image, the processing requires calculating gray-level co-occurrence matrix which is prohibitive; therefore "graycomatrix" scales can be used for input image. In general, to deduce the number of intensity values in grayscale from 8 to 256, a "graycomatrix" is used for scaling. The size of the gray-level co-occurrence matrix is defined by the number of gray levels. "Graycomatrix" function has two parameters namely "NumLevels" and the "GrayLimits" which is used to control the amount of gray levels and scaling of intensity values in gray level co-occurrence matrix. The relationship between two pixels that is, reference and neighbor pixel at any instance is chosen. In order to level the pixels with the element j, it is estimated how often a pixel with gray level values encountered either diagonally, horizontally or vertically.

The directions of gray level co-occurrence matrix are:

(a) Horizontal direction (0),
(b) Vertical direction (90)

Diagonal consists of two directions

(a) top to bottom right (−135)
(b) bottom left to top right (−45).

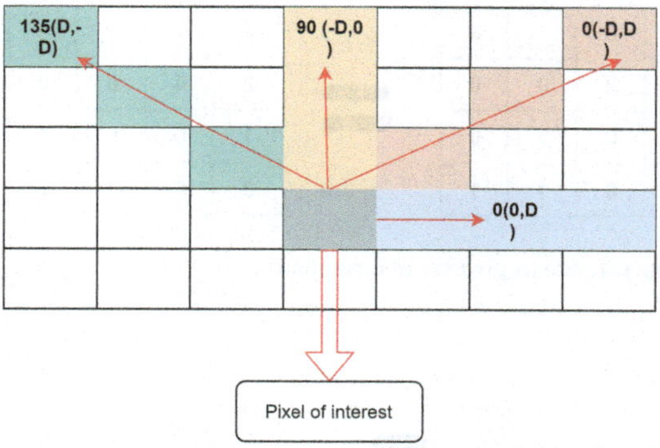

0	0	1	1
0	0	1	1
0	2	2	2
2	2	3	3

Fig. 6.10 Image pixel/Subsection

i / j	0	1	2	3
0	#(0,0)	#(0,1)	#(0,1)	#(0,3)
1	#(1,0)	#(1,1)	#(1,2)	#(1,3)
2	#(2,0)	#(2,1)	#(2,2)	#(2,3)
3	#(3,0)	#(3,1)	#(3,2)	#(3,3)

2	2	1	0
0	2	0	0
0	0	3	1
0	0	0	1

Fig. 6.11 Co-occurrence matrix for the image

They are also declared as p135 for top to bottom right, p90 for vertical, p45 for bottom left to top right and p0 for horizontal. For experiment, 8 tone input image is considered.

From Fig. 6.10, Pixel value = 0, 1, 2, 3, quantization number (N) = 4, therefore size of Co-occurrence matrix = 4 × 4, $d = 1$, $\theta =$ horizontal (zero degree).

Diagonal element represents homogenous area whereas going away from diagonal increases heterogeneity.

Considering Horizontal direction, $i_0 j_0$ in Fig. 6.10 number of times that a zero pixel is appearing with zero pixels. For $i_0 j_1$ from Fig. 6.11, it represents number of times zero pixels is appearing with one pixel in 0°. Similarly, all the elements in Fig. 6.10 is filled according to image pixels. The co-occurrence matrix is not symmetric therefore in order to make it symmetric; transpose of co-occurrence is added to the co-occurrence matrix itself. The relationship *i* to *j* is indistinguishable for the relationship *j* to *i* as shown in Fig. 6.12.

Each element in symmetric GLCM as shown in Fig. 6.13 is divided with the sum of all elements of matrix.

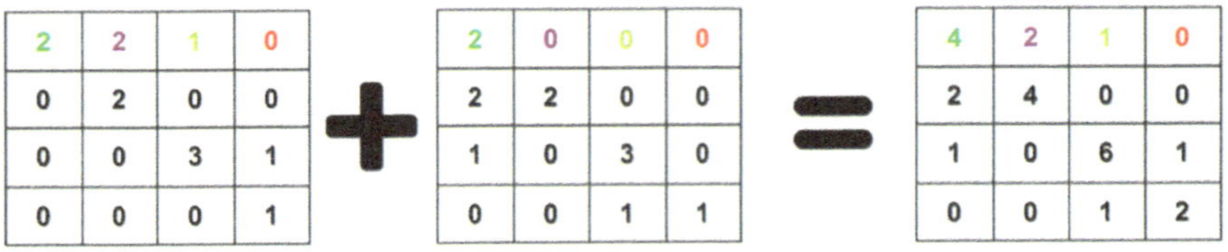

Fig. 6.12 Transpose is added with co-occurrence to give symmetric matrix

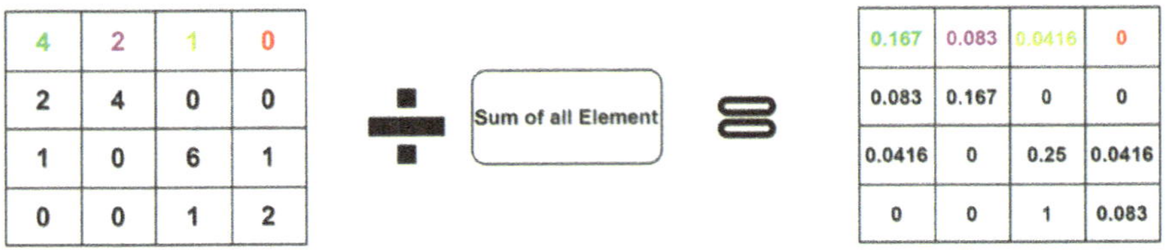

Fig. 6.13 Normalized GLCM

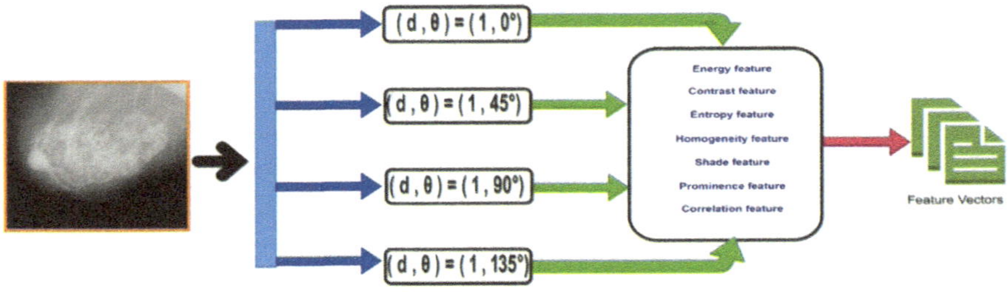

Fig. 6.14 GLCM model

From Fig. 6.14 it is clear that co-occurrence matrices can be calculated with 0°, 45°, 90° and 135° and using these angles several features of GLCM can be calculated.

6.3.6 Probabilistic Neural Network

A PNN i.e., probabilistic neural network consists of nodes with 3 layers. To understand its architecture there are several figures which describe k = 2 classes, it should be limited to number of class k. During the input process the section which is on the left has N input feature for each N nodes respectively of a feature vector, basically are said to be fan-out nodes which branch all the nodes together with one in the middle layer as all the nodes including the hidden may get the input feature vector x completely. Then all the hidden nodes are combined in parts or groups. And for each of the k classes, one part is displayed in figure. In the group for class k, Each and every hidden node correlates with the Gaussian function middle on the feature vector in accordance with the kth class as every illustration of feature vector, there is Gaussian.

6.3.7 *Working of PNN*

All of the Gaussian values for k number of class are being summed and the sum is then measured properly at the k number of class for output node at k = 1 or 2, In order to make sum factor unity then it will form a probability density function. To make it more clear, some specific notations are utilized. P illustrator feature vector {x(p): p = 1,......P} is considered as class1. Similarly, the Q illustrator feature vector {y(r): r = 1,.....R} considered as class 2. There are p nodes in the group for class 1 and so are R nodes for class 2. x(p) and y(r) are the points for class 1 and 2, for each Gaussian center where N is dimension of the vector for the input vector that is x as shown in Eqs. (6.8) and (6.9).

$$g1x = [1/\surd(2\pi 2)\ N]\exp\{-\|x - xp\|2/(22)\} \tag{6.8}$$

$$g1y = [1/\surd(2\pi 2)\ N]\exp\{-\|y - yp\|2/(22)\} \tag{6.9}$$

With the average distance between vectors which are in a same group or exemplar with each, the resultant can be one half of the distance from its nearest exemplar to the exemplar considered as shown in Eqs. (6.10) and (6.11), where f is taken as one-half.

$$f1x = [1/(2\pi 2)\ N](1/P)\ (p = 1, P)\exp\{-\|y - yp\|2/(22)\} \tag{6.10}$$

$$f2y = [1/(2\pi 2)\ N](1/Q)\ (q = 1, Q)\exp\{-\|y - yp\|2/(22)\} \tag{6.11}$$

6.3.8 *Pseudo Code for Probabilistic Neural Network*

In the pseudocode, Dim is dimension of examples training, smoothing factor is sigma, test example is an example which is needed to be classified, ver_fy[num][dim] is example of training data. Num is number of classes.

```
int Probabilistic_neural_network (int class, int num, int
dim, float sigma, float test_classified[dim], float
ver_fy[num][dim])

{

int cls_fy = -1;
float larg_new = 0;
float summation[ class ];

//it is the oputut layer which is used to compute for
each class of PDF
for ( int A=1; A<=class; A++ )
{
sumation[ A ] = 0;
// summation layer collects PDF
// from specific class of  A for each test
// NumA are from class A
for ( int i=0; i<NUMA; i++ )
{

float pro_cl = 0;
// this is pattern layer which is used to multiply the
test classifier by the weight
for ( int j=0; j<dim; j++ )
pro_cl += test_classified[j] * ver_fy[i][j];
pro_cl = ( pro_cl - 1 ) / ( sigma * sigma );
pro_cl = exp( pro_cl );
sumation[ A ] += pro_cl;
}
Summation [ A ] /= NumA;
}

for ( int A=1; A<=class; A++ )
if ( summation[ A ] > largest_new )

{
Larg_new = summation [ A ];
Cls_fy = A;
}
return cls_fy;
}
```

6.3.9 Experimental Setup

Noise from the Input image is removed by the use of Adaptive median filter, here adaptive median filter is used because it has best results among all spatial filters and it can also differentiate fine details from noise. Impulse noise affects the pixel in an image therefore adaptive median filter performs spatial processing to regulate it. Images are composed of numerous number of pixels in the proposed scheme each pixel is compared to the neighboring pixel in order to identify noise in the pixel. There is an Adjustability of neighborhood pixels, as well as there is comparison for the threshold pixel value. During the process, the pixels are labeled as impulse noise if the majority of the pixel's neighbors differ, as well as if the pixel is not structurally aligned. The median pixel value returns to the noise pixel labeled as impulse noise with neighborhood pixels that have passed noise labeling test. First input image of mammogram is located then it is converted into "grayscale" using the function rgb2gray () in matlab then adaptive median filter is applied to the gray image and then image is converted into unsigned integer 8 by applying unit8 () function in matlab. This process is called as preprocessing of image in order to enhance the quality of test image, to increase the conversion accuracy, and hence great chance of true positive and true negative. The working procedure of the proposed scheme is shown in Fig. 6.15.

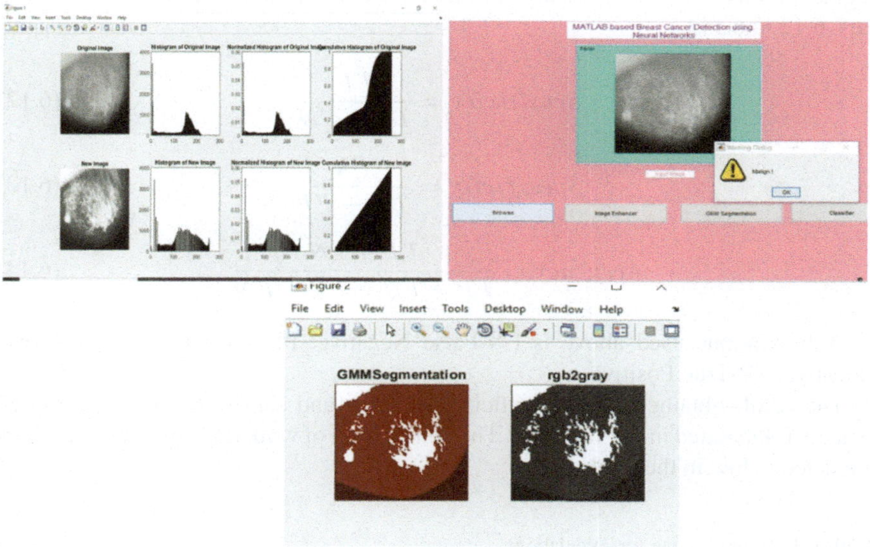

Fig. 6.15 Working of proposed system

6.3.10 Dataset

The dataset used in this research is taken from MIAS i.e. the Mammographic Image Analysis Society consisting of 322 number of digital mammograms and has 161 pairs at the resolution of 50 micron pixel edge in PGM (portable gray map) form.

6.4 Results

The proposed algorithm is applied for the process of detection as well as classification of breast cancer segmented mass from X-ray images and the accuracy of the proposed scheme is reported in Table 6.2. The proposed scheme is based on probabilistic neural network algorithm to classify mammogram images which is taken from MIAS (Mammographic Image Analysis Society) database. In order to classify normal/abnormal and benign/malignant class, two neural network models based on GLCM for classification were designed. The splitting of data is in the ratio 70% for training purpose, 15% for testing data and rest 15% for validating data. The standard deviation as well as average of the result carried out by executing the code for 100 of time in an iteration to get stable results and reported using the reference tags specified in Table 6.1. The parameters required for the diagnosis of type of breast cancer segmentation is defined by using sensitivity, specificity and accuracy as shown in Eqs. 6.12 to 6.14.

$$Sensitivity = \frac{TP}{TP + FN} \tag{6.12}$$

$$Specificity = \frac{TN}{TN + FP} \tag{6.13}$$

$$Accuracy = \frac{TP + TN}{TP + TN + FP + FN} \tag{6.14}$$

Abbreviations used above is FN-False Negative; FP-False Positive; TN-True Negative, TP-True Positive.

The result obtained from specificity, accuracy and sensitivity of the proposed scheme is tabulated in the Table 6.2. The comparison of work done by several authors are listed below in the Table 6.3.

Table 6.1 Reference tag for calculations

Algorithm tag			
Reference tag	Benign	Benign	Malignant
		Benign-Benign (TN)	Benign-malignant (FN)
	Malignant	Malignant-Benign (FP)	Malignant-malignant (TP)

Table 6.2 Results obtained from specificity, sensitivity and accuracy

Method implemented	Accuracy	Sensitivity	Specificity
Probabilistic neural network	90.8% ± 3.02	100% ± 0	93.5% ± 1.22

Table 6.3 Comparisons of work done by several authors

Author	Year	Method	Database	Accuracy	Sensitivity	Specificity
Wang et al. [27]	2013	Back propagation neural network	Stored database of breast cancer patient in Northern Taiwan	85.1%	94.83%	52.86%
Vadivel and Surendiran [28]	2013	Fuzzy rules	Digital Database for Screening Mammography	ILOR:87.76% RO:100% RL:95.45%		
Beheshti et al. [29]	2016	SVM asymmetric masses detection	Mammographic Image Analysis Society	94.01%	91.54%	97.14%
Chakraborty et al. [30]	2018	Analysis of multi-resolution of patterns of tissue	Digital Database for Screening Mammography	77.89%		
Rabidas et al. [31]	2018	Neighborhood Structural Similarity	Mini Mammographic Image Analysis Society & Digital Database for Screening Mammography	85.42%		

6.5 Conclusion

Breast cancer is in fire alarming condition and is dangerous threat to the female all over the globe which is the main cause of increment of mortality rate in women. Today's matter of concern is methods to improve the present scenario with breast cancer with proper research, diagnosis system and techniques, investigation and personal level awareness in the society we are living. Therefore, identification of breast cancer in its very early period has great importance in order to fight against breast cancer. Hence, it is necessary that early detection technology should be available for second verification of early detection of breast cancer. Here researchers all over the world come into play by developing several technique and software by which it can be analyzed, detected, and cured in early period of detection. Hence, due to human error even if physician sometimes encounter problem then the proposed software can be used to verify as the second opinion which has image enhancer and several techniques by which true positive as well as true negative can be identified. The proposed scheme classifies mammographic image into normal, Benign and malignant. Using the proposed scheme, the classifier has attained good prediction accuracy of about 90.8% ± 3.02 on mammographic X-ray dataset from MIAS i.e. Mammographic Image Analysis Society.

Acknowledgements The Authors would like to express their sincere gratitude to Amritsar Group of Colleges, Amritsar, India for providing the support to proceed on the project during research work.

References

1. Chiou, H.-L., Wu, M.-F., Liaw, Y.-C., Cheng, Y.-W., Wong, R.-H., Chen, C.-Y., Lee, H.: The presence of human papillomavirus type 16/18 DNA in blood circulation may act as a risk marker of lung cancer in Taiwan. Cancer **97**, 1558–1563 (2003). https://doi.org/10.1002/cncr.11191
2. Gutte, H., Jakobsson, D., Olofsson, F., Ohlsson, M., Valind, S., Loft, A., Edenbrandt, L., Kjær, A.: Automated interpretation of PET/CT images in patients with lung cancer. Nucl. Med. Commun. **28**(2), 79–84. https://doi.org/10.1097/MNM.0b013e328013eace
3. Suzuki, K., Armato III, S.G., Li, F., Sone, S., Doi, K.: Effect of a small number of training cases on the performance of massive training artificial neural network (MTANN) for reduction of false positives in computerized detection of lung nodules in low-dose CT. Proceedings SPIE 5032, Medical Imaging 2003: Image Processing, (15 May 2003)
4. Penedo, M.G., Carreira, M.J., Mosquera, A., Cabello, D.: Computer-aided diagnosis: a neural-network-based approach to lung nodule detection. IEEE Trans. Med. Imaging **17**(6), 872–880 (1998). https://doi.org/10.1109/42.746620
5. Bartfay, E., Mackillop, W.J., Pater, J.L.: Comparing the predictive value of neural network models to logistic regression models on the risk of death for small-cell lung cancer patients. Eur. J. Cancer Care (Engl). **15**(2), 115–124 (2006). https://doi.org/10.1111/j.1365-2354.2005.00638.x. PMID: 16643258
6. Liu, B., et al.: Fully automatic and segmentation-robust classification of breast tumors based on local texture analysis of ultrasound images. Pattern Recogn. **43**(1), 280–298
7. American Cancer Society. Breast Cancer Facts & Figures 2017–2018. Atlanta: American Cancer Society, Inc. 2017. https://www.cancer.org/research/cancer-facts-statistics/breast-cancer-facts-figures.html. Accessed Jan 2 2021
8. Skandalakis, J.E.: Embryology and anatomy of the breast. Breast Augmentation. Springer, Berlin, Heidelberg, pp. 3–24 (2009)
9. Shampo, M.A., Kyle, R.A.: Karl theodore dussik—pioneer in ultrasound. Mayo Clin. Proc. **70**(12), 1136 (1995)
10. Karatas, O.H., Toy, E.: Three-dimensional imaging techniques: a literature review. Eur. J. Dentistry **8**(1), 132–140 (2014)
11. Lakrimi, M., Thomas, A.M., Hutton, G. et al.: The principles and evolution of magnetic resonance imaging. J. Phys.: Conf. Ser. **286**(1). Article ID 012016 (2011)
12. Ciecholewski, M.: Malignant and benign mass segmentation in mammograms using active contour methods. Symmetry **9**, 277 (2017)
13. Posso, M., Carles, M., Rué, M., Puig, T., Bonfill, X.: Cost-effectiveness of double reading versus single reading of mammograms in a breast cancer screening programme. PLoS ONE **11**(7), (2016)

14. Samala, R.K., et al.: Multi-task transfer learning deep convolutional neural network: application to computer-aided diagnosis of breast cancer on mammograms. Phys. Med. Biol. **62**(23), 8894
15. Rakhlin, A., Shvets, A., Iglovikov, V., Kalinin, A.A.: Deep convolutional neural networks for breast cancer histology image analysis. Campilho, A., Karray, F., Ter Haar Romeny, B. (eds.), Image analysis and recognition. ICIAR 2018. Lecture Notes in Computer Science, vol. 10882. Springer, Chamdoi
16. Krupinski, E.A.: The future of image perception in radiology. Acad. Radiol. **10**, 1–3 (2003)
17. Chan, H.-P., et al.: Computerized classification of malignant and benign microcalcifications on mammograms: texture analysis using an artificial neural network. Phys. Med. Biol. **42**(3), 549
18. Varela, C., et al.: Computerized detection of breast masses in digitized mammograms. Comput. Biol. Med. **37**(2), 214–226
19. Ciecholewski, M.: Malignant and benign mass segmentation in mammograms using active contour methods. Symmetry **9**(11), 277
20. Heath, M.D., Bowyer, K.W.: Mass detection by relative image intensity. In: Proceedings of the 5th International Workshop on Digital Mammography (IWDM-2000), pp. 219–225. Medical Physics Publishing (2000)
21. Llobet, R., Perez-Cortes, J.C.: Breast cancer detection in digitized mammograms using non-parametric methods. In: Proceedings of the 2nd International Conference on Advances in Biomedical Signal and Information Processing (MEDSIP), vol. 1, pp. 281–287, Sliema, Malta (2004)
22. Llobet, R., Toselli, A.H., Perez-Cortes, J.C., Juan,A.: Computer-aided prostate cancer detection in ultrasonographic images. In: Proceedings of the 1st Iberian Conference on Pattern Recognition and Image Analysis (IbPRIA), vol. 1, pp. 411–419, Puerto de Andratx (Mallorca, Spain) (2003)
23. Landeweerd, G., Gelsema, E.: The use of nuclear texture parameters in the automatic analysis of leukocytes. Pattern Recogn. **10**, 57–61 (1978)
24. Chen, C-C., DaPonte, J.S., Fox, M.D.: Fractal feature analysis and classification in medical imaging. IEEE Trans. Med. Imaging **8**(2), 133–142
25. Insana, M., et al.: Analysis of ultrasound image texture via generalized rician statistics. Opt. Eng. **25**, 743–748 (1986)
26. Haralick, R.M., et al.: Textural features for image classification. IEEE Trans. SMC **3**(6), 610–621 (1973)
27. Wang, T., Cheng, C., Chiu, H. (eds.): Predicting post-treat-ment survivability of patients with breast cancer using Artificial Neural Network methods. 35th Annual International Conference of the IEEE Engineering in Medicine and Biology Society (EMBC); 2013 Jul 3–7; Osaka, Japan IEEE. https://doi.org/10.1109/embc.2013.6609744
28. Vadivel, A., Surendiran, B.: A fuzzy rule-based approach for characterization of mammogram masses into BI-RADS shape categories. Comput. Biol. Med. **43**(4), 259–267 (2013). https://doi.org/10.1016/j.compbiomed.2013.01.004. PMID:23414779
29. Beheshti, S.M.A., Noubari, H.A., Fatemizadeh, E., Khalili, M.: Classification of abnormalities in mammograms by new asymmetric fractal features. Biocybern. Biomed. Eng. **36**(1), 56–65 (2016). https://doi.org/10.1016/j.bbe.2015.07.002
30. Chakraborty, J., Midya, A., Rabidas, R.: Computer-aided detection and diagnosis of mammographic masses using multi-resolution analysis of oriented tissue patterns. Expert Syst. Appl. **99**, 168–179 (2018). https://doi.org/10.1016/j.eswa.2018.01.010
31. Rabidas, R., Midya, A., Chakraborty, J.: Neighborhood structural similarity mapping for the classification of masses in mammograms. IEEE J. Biomed. Health Inform. **22**(3), 826–834 (2018). https://doi.org/10.1109/JBHI.2017.2715021. PMID: 28622679

Part II
Prediction of Cancer Susceptibility

Chapter 7
Feature Extraction and Classification of Colon Cancer Using a Hybrid Approach of Supervised and Unsupervised Learning

Joydev Ghosh, Amitesh Kumar Sharma, and Sahil Tomar

Abstract The demand for research in the medical field is growing at a very rapid rate which can be seen in the unprecedented progress of COVID19 medication and detection development which take a lot of time and effort. But due to recent advancement of Machine Learning and Artificial Intelligence (i.e. ML/AI) in the medical field, it has been observed that the time frame for the development of such medications and detection has reduced a lot. This chapter paves the way for such demand by combining two basic ML techniques involving unsupervised and supervised learning. Since the occurrence of Colon Cancer is somewhat rare and complex, available Colon Cancer data sets are still underdeveloped and the Colon Cancer data set that is present is complex. The data set also has very less number of samples. To resolve this problem of fewer data and to get the most relevant information from the available data set, our research involves an oversampling method on the original data with preserving of the basic nature of the data set which is followed by the clustering of the data using K-Medoid clustering, Girvan-Newman clustering and Mahalanobis distance-based clustering for multivariate data. Once the same set of samples are predicted using the clustering, we are extrapolating the data based on the clusters formed using a statistical approach. To reduce complex processing and remove the irrelevant features with the intent of cleaning the data set, we are applying a correlation-based approach for feature selection and then Principal Component Analysis (PCA) has been applied for dimensionality reduction. The final set of features thus obtained is then fed into an Artificial Neural Network for the classification of the Colon Cancer. The result of the experiment shows that the methodology proposed has a better accuracy than the available approaches which proves the effectiveness of our proposed method.

J. Ghosh (✉) · A. K. Sharma · S. Tomar
Central Research Laboratory, Bharat Electronics Limited, Bengaluru, India
e-mail: joydevghosh@bel.co.in; ghoshjoydev.123@gmail.com

A. K. Sharma
e-mail: amiteshks@bel.co.in

S. Tomar
e-mail: sahiltomar@bel.co.in

J. Nayak et al. (eds.), *Advanced Machine Learning Approaches in Cancer Prognosis*, Intelligent Systems Reference Library 204,
https://doi.org/10.1007/978-3-030-71975-3_7

Keywords Colon cancer · Clustering · Dimensionality reduction · Artificial neural network · Principal component analysis · Feature extraction

7.1 Introduction

Colon Cancer has now became the world's third most common cancer with 104610 new cases registered for the year 2020 in United States [1, 2]. With mortality rate as high as the fourth highest in the world, it is still one of the most fatal cancer known to the mankind. With all the medical advancements and technologies, the mortality rate has decreased from the past but this changes in the numbers are not that significant. One of the major reason for this to happen is the inability to detect the cancer at its early stage. Colon Cancer, which develops mostly from the polyps, has very little or no signs or symptoms. As a result, a regular check-up needs to be done. The diagnosis of the Colon Cancer is usually done with the method of colonoscopy [3, 4]. The procedure of colonoscopy is done by inserting a tube inside the colon of the patient with a camera attached to the tip of the tube which is then visually analysed for the detection of the cancer. The major drawback in this procedure is that the detection of the malignant depends on the naked eye visual estimation. Due to which the small tumor size are often neglected by the naked eye thus preventing from early detection of the malignancy. To mark colon biopsy using Hematoxylin and Eosin [5] technique is the basic key step for leading the treatment and verifying the diagnosis of malignancy. The old traditional approaches for cancer detection become very tedious and laborious job. So, for faster diagnosis with better accuracy speed is also a major part of the treatment. Now a days, due to high computational power, speed and storage capability computer visions draw a lot focus on it. Various modern deep neural network [6, 7], convolutional networks [8] models and different improved image processing techniques [9–11] has been proposed to improve the malignancy detection with faster accuracy. To detect the tumors at there early stages and for proper treatments, better features selection from the images and classification is required. Due to the high complexity of the process of reproducing the structural information of high dimensional biological data into functional genomics [12] has been replaced by the microarray technology [13]. This technology helps the researchers from different domains like biology and chemistry for understanding the genes expression profile. The condition of patients is also considered in this technology. Selection of highly informative genes from thousand of genes is the major part of the cancer classification and detection as these genes are correlated with various respective diseases [14, 15]. A high number of features of the available datasets creates challenges for the researchers with the high dimentionality. To remove these challenges features selection techniques play a important role and helps to acquire prior knowledge for cancer classification. The entire process of classification becomes very complex and tedious due to some irrelevant, redundant features [16, 17]. The process of removing significant number of irrelevant features [18–20] improve the performance of classification models with proper learning. There are mainly two segments of classification and statistical analysis namely, features selection is the first segment and classification is the final one [21]. The classification procedure is improved by reducing the dimensions in feature selection using various methods. Unsupervised learning methods [22] as well as supervised learning methods [23, 24] can be implemented for features selection from the primary data. For feature selection Genetic algorithm (GA) based approaches [25–27] are also employed in various works. Besides the feature selection procedures different clustering methods are also implemented by clustering similar features from the raw data.

In our proposed method, we are addressing this problem of the scarcity of the data in the data set using various unsupervised learning methods. For this, we are using three different clustering algorithms for clustering the similar characteristics data and then we are increasing the number of data along the best cluster selected using the value of Dunn Index. This allows to increase the data along with keeping the characteristics of the data. Also, for selection of the relevant features from the set of 2000 features, we are using a correlation graph based approach followed by PCA. With the increased data with the relevant features, we are classifying the data for the prediction of Colon Cancer using an Artificial Neural Network (ANN). The final accuracy revealed promising results suggesting its efficiency for both the test data as well as real time data.

7.2 Realted Work

In prior works, several research papers has claimed promising results in the detection of the Colon Cancer from the image using different Machine Learning and Deep Learning methods. Jiao et al. [28] proposed Colon Cancer detection method, which has used various permutations of major 18 features including textural features derived from the grey level co-occurrence matrix (GLCM) and then a Support Vector Machine (SVM) based classifier [29, 30] is being used for the classification giving a precision level of 96.67%. In another work, Peyret et al. [31] proposed a method of evaluation using text based features along with different classifiers accompanied with the PCA for dimensionality reduction. Many works has also been done using different Colon Cancer data sets. As done by Shapcott et al. [32] which uses a Deep Learning based cancer cell identification algorithm and random sampling model for detection of Colon Cancer on diagnostic images data fetched from The Cancer Genome Atlas (TCGA) repository. Although there is a high accuracy in test data for all the prior works, this methods failed to perform well in real-time scenario. The major reason behind this is the presence of huge number of irrelevant features and less sample data in the train data set. Bychkov et al. [33] proposed a method that includes a combination of Convolution Neural Network (CNN) and Recurrent Neural Network (RNN) to predict colorectal cancer disease based on samples of images of tumour tissue samples in his paper. Whereas, Ramalingam et al. [34] used a probabilistic neural network approach for dataset classification. Sirinukunwattana [35] proposed a Spatially Constrained Convolutional Neural Network (SC-CNN) to perform nucleus detection in his paper. He also proposed the use of Neighboring Ensemble Predictor (NEP) coupled with CNN to more accurately predict the class label of detected cell nuclei to classify nuclei for on colorectal adenocarcinoma images. In the paper "Deep Learning Models for Histopathological Classification of Gastric and Colonic Epithelial Tumours", Iizuka et al. [36] proposed deep learning models to classify colon and epithelial tumours (adenocarcinoma and adenoma) of stomach. A trained CNN based architecture for each organ was used to classify a tile into one of three labels: adenocarcinoma, adenoma, and non-neoplastic. Also, RNN and Max pooling approaches were used for the final classification. In the paper "RCCNet: An Efficient Convolutional Neural Network for Histological Routine Colon Cancer Nuclei Classification", Shabbeer Basha et al. [37] claimed to proposed an efficient convolutional neural network based classification model RCCNet to classify Colon Cancer images build and optimized for histological low-resolution patches. In this paper, we have proposed a method for Colon Cancer detection based on clustering and feature extraction methodology and using Artificial Neural Network for final classification.

7.3 Contribution

The contributions of this work is highlighted below in few steps.

- In this research work, we first reduce the dimension of the original dataset and then the processed data with reduced features has been used to train Artificial Neural Network (ANN) based classifier.
- To minimize the complexity of dimension reduction we have first employed three popular clustering algorithms, namely K-medoid clustering, Girvan Newman clustering and Mahalanobis distance based clustering to assemble similar characteristics data and then identify the best clusters among the all other clusters using Dunn Index.
- Here, Adaptive Synthetic Sampling method has been incorporated before the feature selection as the samples of the available dataset is not enough to train a ANN based cancer classifier. This method helps to increase data for the best selected clusters without losing the characteristics of the given data.
- After preprocessing of the data, we have considered Pearson's Correlation and PCA for removing highly correlated and redundant features in features selection phase.
- Finally, the data with reduced features is fed into the proposed ANN based classifier with single hidden layer.
- In this work, we have also considered some state-of-art colon cancer classifiers for comparative study with the help of different performance analysis like accuracy measurements, ROC curve and also statistical analysis like Wilcoxon Rank-Sum Test. This comparative study proves that the proposed classifier is the most effective classifier.

7.4 Summary

The remaining work has been organised as follows: The entire proposed methodology of this work is demonstrated in Sect. 7.6. Section 7.7 explains the experimental results with the comparative study and lastly, we have concluded our work with some future scope in Sect. 7.8.

7.5 Material and Proposed Methodology

This section describes the data extrapolation the proposed feature selection methods and the classification model in details. The entire work flow has been depicted in Fig. 7.1 as block diagram representation whereas Fig. 7.2 represents the flow diagram of the proposed methodology. The dataset details and the tools that has been used in this experiment are also defined in this section.

7.5.1 Dataset

Recently, the cancer is considered as one of the most dangerous diseases concerning all over in the world. Information seekers and researchers are continuously looking for the fastest and accurate classification method to lighten the issue of the cancer

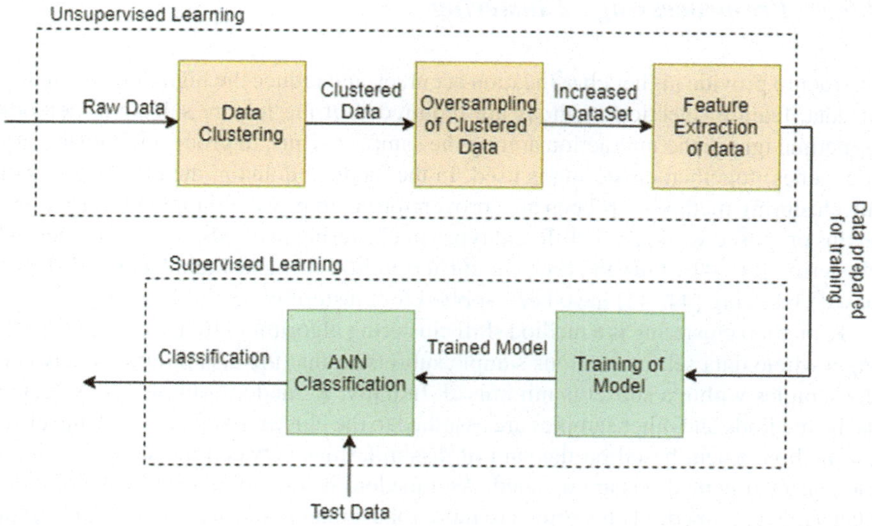

Fig. 7.1 Flowchart of the proposed system

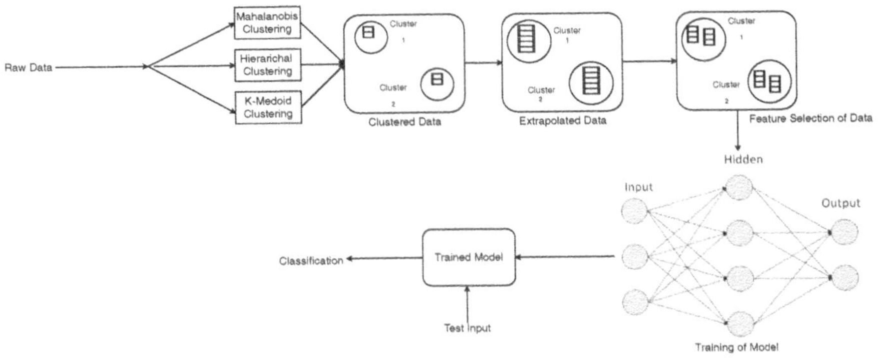

Fig. 7.2 Work flow of the proposed classifier

detection. Thus, to achieve the accuracy of classification the medical science community is still working in various directions. Colon Cancer is one kind of cancer disease which is considered as third ranked and a major leading cause of mortality among men and women [38]. In this experiment, Colon Cancer microarray dataset is used to distinguish cancer from normal samples for getting an initial result. This dataset is publicly available at http://genomics-pubs.princeton.edu/oncology/affydata/index.html [39]. The dataset consists of 2000 attributes and 62 instances with 2 classes whereby there are 22 normal, and 40 cancer samples.

7.5.2 Pre-processing : Clustering

In order to provide higher classification accuracy and reduce the high dimensionality of data, feature selection methods are required. But the feature selection methods sometime ignore the interaction among the samples. Thus, to group similar samples (i.e. genes) together, clustering is used. In the medical domain, the effectiveness of the clustering methods has been also proven for inherently overlapping information. In this proposed work, three different types of clustering methods, namely K-medoid clustering [40, 41], Girvan Newman clustering [42, 43] and Mahalanobis distance based clustering [44, 45] have been applied for clustering the similar genes.

K-mediod clustering is a mediod shift clustering algorithm [46] used for partitioning a whole data set into various sample subsets so that the dissimilarities between the samples within a subset is minimised. Initially, *K* random samples are selected as the mediods and other samples are assigned to the cluster associated with the closest mediod. Then, based on the sum of dissimilarities between the samples within the clusters the mediods are updated. As a medoid is less influenced by the outliers than a mean, K-mediod clustering are more robust than K-mean clustering in case of occurrence of outliers and noise. Hierarchical Girvan Newman clustering is a community detection clustering where the communities are derived from the original constructed graph by removing edges with the highest betweenness centrality [47]. Here the betweenness centrality is the multivariate centrality for the samples of the Colon Cancer data set which has been used in the experiment. Betweenness centrality is recalculated after edge removal in every iteration. Instead of constructing a measure to find most central samples within the community this clustering mainly focus on the most likely edges within the community. Finally, this clustering gives a Dendrogram [48] as the graph separated by several communities with successive edge removal. The Mahalanobis distance [49] based clustering is used to find the distance of different multi-variate points. The Mahalanobis distance refers to the distance between a point y and the distribution of the data. The reason behind the selection of Mahalanobis distance metric over the famous Euclidean metric is that the euclidean distance deals with the point to point distance where as Mahalanobis distance deals with point to distribution distance. The Mahalanobis Distance (i.e. D_y) is calculated using Eq. (7.1).

$$D_y = \sqrt{(y - y_m)^T.COV^{-1}(y - y_m)} \quad (7.1)$$

where y is the vector of points in the data, y_m is the mean vector of the observation, COV^{-1} is the inverse Co-variance Matrix of independent data. After calculating the Mahalanobis distance of the each observation from the distribution, multiple clusters are formed based on the threshold value.

7.5.3 Clustering Validation

The gene clusters are obtained after validating the generated clusters with the help of Dunn index [50, 51]. The clustered data is used for evaluation of final result whereas for the evaluation of internal metric, Dunn index has been used. Dunn index identifies the sets of clusters with high compactness [52] (i.e. small variance) within the clusters and high inter-cluster separation [53] (i.e. the variance within the cluster is lower as compared to the means of different clusters). Clustering is better when the Dunn index value is higher. In this work, a threshold value for the Dunn index has been set up experimentally to identify well clustered gene. After applying the clustering methods, Dunn index(i.e. DI) is calculated to determine which cluster (C_k) has better Dunn index value using Eq. (7.2).

$$DI_k = \frac{\min_{1 \le k' \le c, k \ne k'} \delta(C_k, C'_k)}{\max_k \Delta(C_k)} \quad (7.2)$$

where $\delta(C_k, C'_k)$ is a measure of the inter-cluster distance between cluster C_k and C'_k and $\Delta(C_k)$ is a measure of the within-cluster distance (which is also called the diameter of the cluster (i.e. C_k)).

Further, the higher number of genes from the representative clusters have been chosen for the stage of feature selection. Finally, the best clusters with higher Dunn index values for every clustering methods are further used for feature selection.

7.5.4 Oversampling: Adaptive Synthetic Sampling

The publicly available colon dataset which is used in this experiment is highly imbalanced dataset. For any classifier it is very important to have sufficient and balanced data for training the model. For Colon Cancer the available dataset has only 22 normal, and 40 cancer samples which is very much insufficient to train our proposed classifier model. The main bottleneck of dealing with imbalance dataset is that one class samples dominate another class sample which resulting a highly underfitted model where the model is not able to succesfully classify the class having less number of samples. Sometimes it may also happen the trained model suffers from high variance and low bias condition (i.e., overfitting) due to the imbalance data. To avoid the overfitting and underfitting problem caused by the imbalanced data we have applied Adaptive Synthetic sampling (ADASYN) technique [54, 55]. More synthetic data is generated for the minority class by applying this oversampling technique according to the density distributions of minority class considering one cluster at a time. Random oversampling just increases the likelihood of occurring overfitting by replicating the minority class examples. ADASYN considers the K-nearest neighbors of each minority instance and the new points are generated at the same distance from each minority points. Also to generate new synthetic samples, the class ratio of the minority and majority instances has been taken into consideration. The entire procedure of ADASYN is elaborated in the following steps:

Step 1: Let, C_t be the training dataset with l samples $= \{a_i, b_i\}$, $\forall i = 1, 2, \dots l$ where a_i is the N dimensional feature vector and b_i is the corresponding class label.

Step 2: Let, l_m and l_M be the number of minority and majority class samples respectively, such that $l_m \leq l_M$ and $l_m + l_M = l$.

Step 3: Degree of Imbalance, $I = l_m / l_M$ has been calculated.

Step 4: If $I < I_t$ (where, I_t is the preset maximum tolerated imbalance threshold. In our experiment we took 0.6) then:

(a) The number of synthetic samples to be generated from the minority class G_m has been calculated using Eq. (7.3), where β is the balance level of the synthetic generated samples. $\beta = 1$ indicates that there is a total balance between two classes and we have considered the value as 1.

$$G_m = |l_M - l_m| \times \beta \tag{7.3}$$

(b) Based on Euclidean distance [56] (i.e. α_i) the k-nearest neighbors [57] has been found for each $a_i \in$ minority samples and calculate the ratio r_i as $r_i = \alpha_i / k$.

(c) The ratio (r_i) has been normalised as $r_{n_i} = r_i / \sum_{i=1}^{l} r_i$ and now r_{n_i} is a density distribution $\forall i = 1, 2, \ldots l$.
(d) For each minority class data example a_i, generate g_{m_i} synthetic data using Eq. (7.4).

$$g_{m_i} = r_{n_i} \times G_m \tag{7.4}$$

Here we have also implemented the step 4 for both minority and majority classes to increase overall sample size. This technique also helped us to increase overall sample size for this experiment which indirectly accelerated the training procedure for classification.

7.5.5 Feature Selection

Feature Selection has been useful in selection of informative samples and in removal of non-informative samples so that the high dimensionality that has little or no role in the process of classification has been reduced. Also, the selection of the features helps the classification algorithm with a clean and reduced data to form the relation between the input and the output which leads to better accuracy. As a part of the feature selection in the proposed methodology we are using two popular methods.

1. Selection of the related features based on correlation matrix. In this section we have used Pearson's Correlation [58] to form a matrix that depicts the correlation among the features. Based on the result of the matrix, we are selecting the features with correlation value between −0.5 to +0.5. The reason being that the Pearson correlation gives values between −1 to +1 and more the values tends to fall towards −1 or +1, indicates that the features are either highly negatively correlated or positively correlated. Based on this, the range between −0.5 to +0.5 can be considered as the range where the features are most likely to be uncorrelated and have their own significance in determining the nature of the cancer. Let, $F_i = \{f_{i1}, f_{i2}, f_{i3} \ldots f_{iN}\}$ $\forall i = 1, 2, \ldots M$ be a set of features where, N is the total number of features present in the colon data set (i.e. 2000) and M is the number of samples obtained from the pre-processed data set after clustering. Thus, the correlation coefficient matrix $correlation\_coefficient$ is obtained which looks like.

$$correlation\_coefficient = \left[\begin{array}{c|cccc} & f_1 & f_2 & \cdots & f_N \\ \hline f_1 & w_{11} & w_{12} & \cdots & w_{1N} \\ f_2 & w_{21} & w_{22} & \cdots & w_{2N} \\ \vdots & \vdots & & \ddots & \\ f_N & w_{n1} & w_{n2} & & w_{NN} \end{array}\right]$$

Correlation coefficient for the feature f_{ij} (i.e. jth feature of the ith sample) and f_{ik} (i.e. kth feature of the ith sample) is calculated as Eq. (7.5).

$$W_i(f_{ij}, f_{ik}) = \frac{\sum_{l=1}^{N}(f_{ij_l} - \overline{f_{ij}})(f_{ik_l}) - \overline{f_{ik}})}{\sqrt{\sum_{l=1}^{N}(f_{ij} - \overline{f_{ij_l}})^2(f_{ik} - \overline{f_{ik_l}}))^2}} \tag{7.5}$$

So, the calculation of correlation of each of the given features with every other has been based on a threshold range −0.5 to +0.5 features have been removed from the features set as those are considered as the highly correlated features. After removing the highly correlated features, we are left with **X** number of features.

2. Principal Component Analysis(PCA): Once, we get the uncorrelated features, next step that we are using in our proposed methodology is the method of Dimensionality reduction based on PCA [59]. The idea behind using the PCA is to form a new set of features from the remaining once so that each of the new features contains a glimpse of all the previous features. Applying PCA, provides us with the new set of features based on the Eigen Values and Eigen Vectors [60]. In PCA, a symmetric (XxX) Covariance Matrix (X is the number of reduced features set) for the already reduced features has been calculated. This matrix has been used to find the Eigen Vectors corresponding to the reduced features with their Eigen Values. This will be obtained by the following:

$$\begin{bmatrix} VAR(f_1) & COV(f_1, f_2) & \dots COV(f_1, f_X) \\ COV(f_2, f_1) & VAR(f_2) & \dots COV(f_2, f_X) \\ \vdots & \ddots & \vdots \\ COV(f_X, f_1) & COV(f_X, f_2) \dots & VAR(f_X) \end{bmatrix} \begin{bmatrix} v_1 \\ v_2 \\ \vdots \\ v_X \end{bmatrix}' = \begin{bmatrix} \lambda_1 \\ \lambda_2 \\ \vdots \\ \lambda_X \end{bmatrix} \begin{bmatrix} v_1 \\ v_2 \\ \vdots \\ v_X \end{bmatrix}$$

Once this new set of features are generated, we are sorting the features based in descending order based on the Eigen values and then we are selection top **K** features as our final output.

7.5.6 Classification

For classification, we have used Artificial Neural Network (ANN) [61]. Artificial Neural Network has been designed as a replication of human brain where the function of the neurons of the human brain is replicated by the nodes of the neural network. An ANN are further divided into three parts, namely, the input layer, hidden layer and the output layer. The training of the Artificial Neural Network involves primarily of two steps i.e. The forward pass for the finding the patterns and pass the information from the input layer to the output layer through the hidden layers. The next step known as Back propagation, is the method to adjust the weights of the neural network based on the error calculated at the output layer. In the Colon Cancer classification problem, we are using $Sigmoidfunction$ to classify the output into two classes, namely, Cancer present denoted by $ClassID1$ and Cancer not present denoted by $ClassID2$. For calculation of the error, $Crossentropylossfunction$ [62] has been used. To update

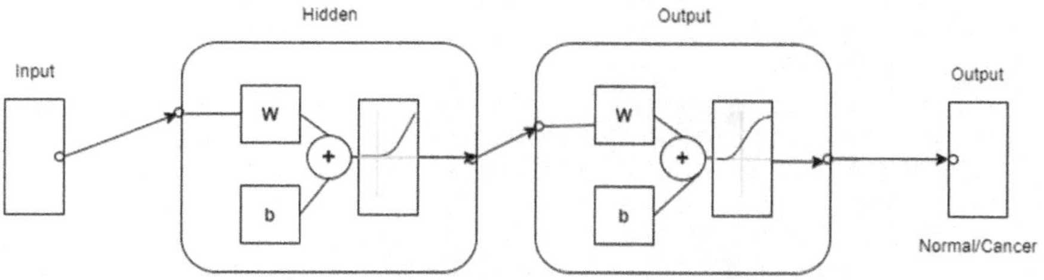

Fig. 7.3 Basic Architecture of the proposed ANN

the weights of the neural network, *AdamOptimizer* [63] has been used because of its Adaptive Learning Rate and Weight updation mechanisms. After the feature selection, the number of nodes in the Input Layers in Neural Network has chosen to be 20, where each node takes each of the extracted features as an input. Also, the number of hidden layers that we have chosen for our Neural Network is 1. The hyper parameters has to be chosen using hit-and-trial method based on the accuracy where hyper parameters consists of the number of hidden layers and number of nodes present in the network. For the evaluation of number of hidden layers and number of nodes in those hidden layers, we have used the rule which was proposed in [64]. According to the proposed Rule of thumb, the selection of number of nodes in the hidden layer can be done based on the following criteria:

(1) The number of hidden neurons selected for the model should lie in the range between the size of the input layer and the size of the output layer.
(2) The number of hidden neurons selected for model should be 2/3rd of the combined addition of input size and the output size.
(3) The number of hidden layer neurons selected for the model should be at least as large as twice the numbers of neurons in the input layer.

Finally the output layer consists of 2 nodes for the two classes mentioned earlier. As a part of other Hyper-parameter tuning, which involves the learning rate for the classifier we have finalised the Learning Rate as 0.001. With the higher learning rate, the chances to miss the global optima is high and for very small learning rate, the time and the resource utilization is very high. This is the reason behind choosing a moderate learning rate as this gives the model a better flexibility to learn the patterns in the data set. Also ReLu(Rectified Linear Unit) is chosen as the activation function for the non-output layers [65] because of its simplicity and it's effectiveness in the case of vanishing gradient problem. The basic blocks of our proposed ANN Classifier architecture is represented in Fig. 7.3 and the graphical representation of a traditional ANN is shown in Fig. 7.4. In these figures W stands for the assigned weight and b stands for the bias of the ANN classifier. The entire process of the proposed classifier is represented in Fig. 7.5.

Once, the architecture of the neural network has been decided, we have trained the model on our pre-processed data set for an iteration of 500. The finally trained model, with all the updated weights is then used for the testing of the test data. The outline

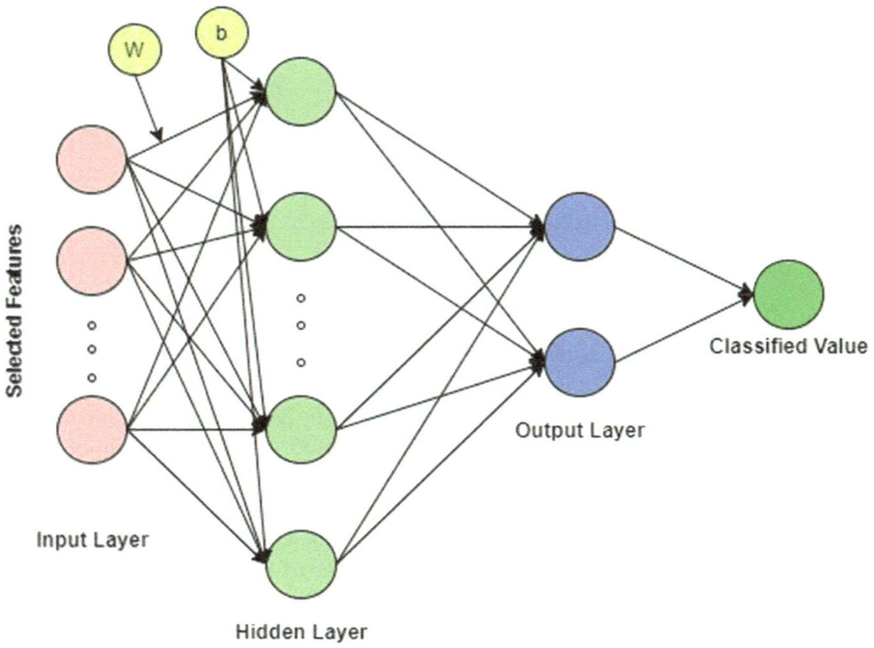

Fig. 7.4 Graphical representation of ANN

of our proposed classifier is given in Algorithms 1 and 2. Algorithm 1 describes the outline of the features selection technique which has been proposed in our work and Algorithm 2 describes the entire proposed classification methods step by step.

7.6 Experimental Results

The proposed algorithm tested by using Colon Cancer dataset to classify Colon Cancer with the initial result after feature selection. This experiment have been independently run for 50 times on HP PC with Pentium core i7 processor with 64-bit Windows 10. For doing matrix operations, we have used numpy library. For implementing machine learning algorithms the sklearn library of Python 3.6 has been used. Table 7.1 shows the experiment results. The dataset which we have considered divided into three groups. For training we have used 70% of the sample data and 15% of the sample data have been used for both validation and testing. Figure 7.6 shows that gradient is 0.0012982 at epoch 500 at training phase. In this proposed work, the validation performance is 0.0005430 at epoch 500 and and at that point of the cross-entropy, the error was almost zero. The performance analysis of ANN based on cross-entropy is shown in Fig. 7.7. The experiment has five results with

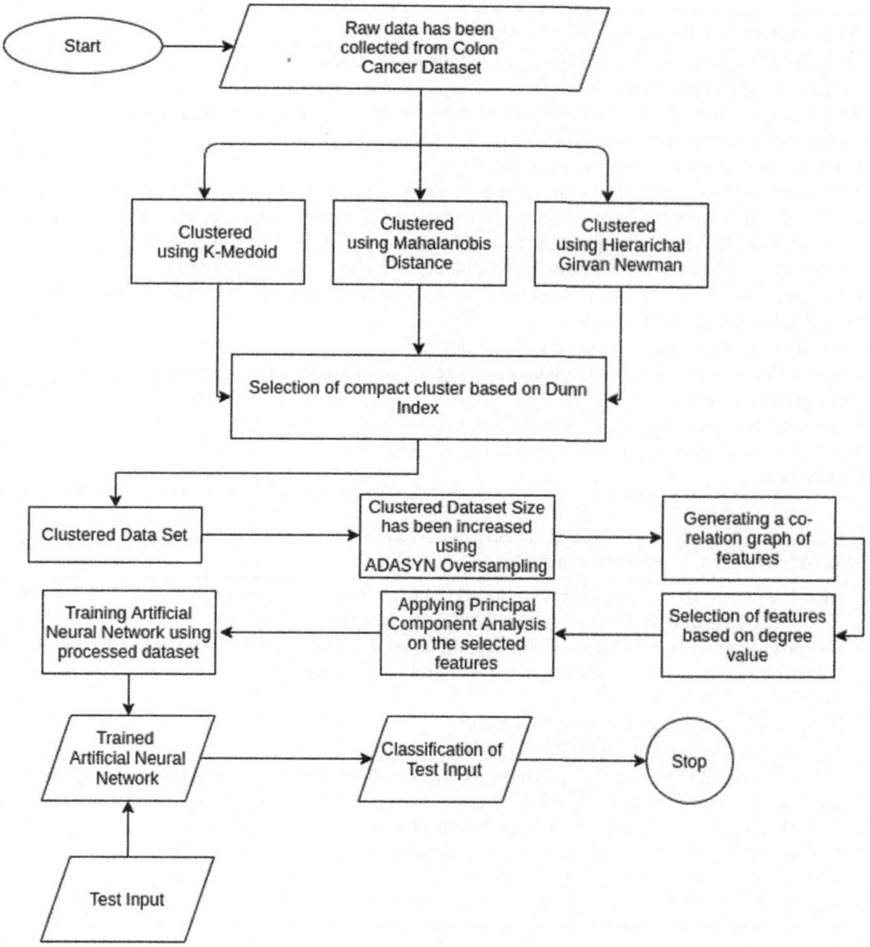

Fig. 7.5 Flow diagram of the proposed classifier

Cross-Entropy, Percent of Error, and Classification Accuracy Percent and the best value is marked by bold face. The results have been compared with some state of the art methods based on the accuracy in Table 7.2.

For the calculation of Accuracy(A), first relative error(R) is calculated, where R is the ratio between the number of samples classified wrongly and the total number of samples using Eqs. (7.6) and (7.7). Now, Accuracy is calculated as the difference between 1 and relative error (RER) multiplied by 100.

Algorithm 1: FEATURES SELECTION

Input: F= Raw Colon Dataset, $Feature\_Values$ = Feature Values.
Output: Selected Features E

Clustering of the raw data using K-medoid clustering, Girvan newman clustering and multivariate clustering using Mahalanobis distance;
Select the best cluster using DUNN index;
Extrapolate the data on each clusters individually using oversampling and stored in F';
Construct a NxN correlation_coefficient matrix for N features by computing the Pearson's Correlation between every possible pair of features i.e $(f_{ij}, f_{ik})\ \forall i = 1, 2, \ldots M \in F'$ using Eq. (7.5) based on Feature_Values, where M is the number of samples;
Considering all features in F', find the features with high correlation coefficient based on a threshold range -0.5 to $+0.5$;
Highly correlated features are removed from F';
Apply PCA on the selected features using eigen vectors representation where the vectors are feature vector;
Arrange the features $\in F'$ in descending order of their eigen values;
Take first K features from the sorted list and put those in the Extracted Features list E;
return E.

Algorithm 2: CLASSIFICATION

Input: F'= Modified Dataset with reduced features, $Target\_Classes$ = Target Class labels, L= Learning Rate, $Network$ = Untrained Network.
Output: Trained Neural Network for classification $Trained_NeuralNetwork$

Receive input $Network$ with a hidden layer and output layer with two $Target\_Classes$ (i.e. Standard and Colon Cancer);
Receive the input samples with F' features;
Initialise the weights of input $Network$;
Apply the weights on Adam gradient based optimization algorithm with stochastic algorithm;
Update the weights with the learning rate L;
Classify the samples using ReLu activation function at the output layer;
The output $Trained_Neural_Network$ is generated for classification of Colon Cancer after the convergence;
return $Trained_NeuralNetwork$.

Table 7.1 Experimental results

No of experiments	Cross-entropy (CE)	Error percentage (%RE)	Classification accuracy (%)
10	5.023	3.303	96.7
100	4.567	3.102	96.9
300	**3.018**	**1.401**	**98.60**
500	3.101	1.780	98.30

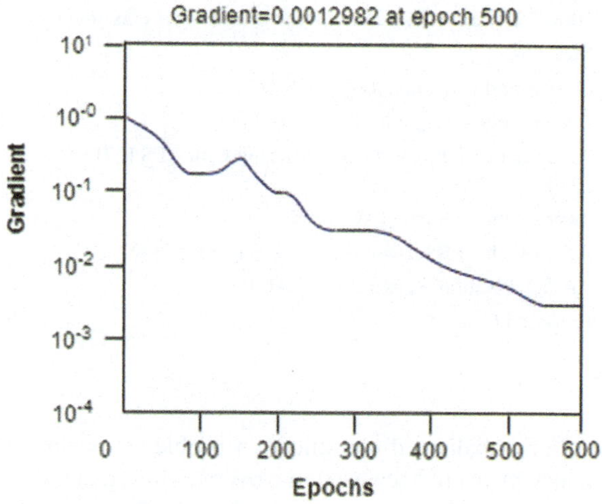

Fig. 7.6 Gradient at epochs

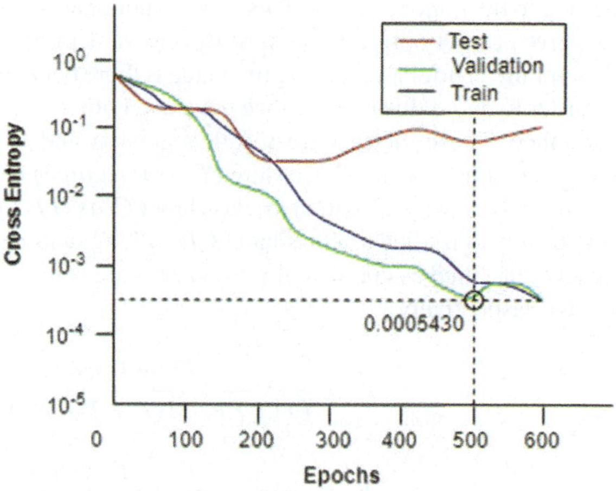

Fig. 7.7 ANN cross entropy performance

$$A = (1 - RER) * 100 \tag{7.6}$$

$$RER = \frac{|actual\_type - predicted\_type|}{actual\_type} \tag{7.7}$$

where $actual\_type$ is the target class label and $predicted\_type$ is the actual predicted class label of the trained multilayer perceptron model.

In Table 7.2, the best accuracy values for all state-of-art classifiers and our proposed classifier are listed and the best value is marked by bold face. This result shows how much effective the proposed method is and also shows the accuracy of this proposed method.

Table 7.2 Performance comparison with other classifiers

Methods	Classification accuracy (%)
Garzón and González [66] (GC)	88.71
k-means clustering with Inf-FS [67] (KC)	90.18
Agglomerative hierarchical clustering with CFS [67] (HCFS)	80.35
Agnes with CFS [67] (ACFS)	82.14
Agnes with CFS (classifier: Naïve Bayes) [67] (NCFS)	85.79
Artificial Neural Network [68] (AC)	98.40
Proposed Classifier (PC)	**98.60**

For imbalanced classification problems, accuracy is inappropriate as a performance measure because of the overwhelming of the number of samples in the minority class. The main reason behind this problem is the large number of samples which belong to the majority class. This problem indicates that even an inappropriate model can give correct output in most of the cases, achieving an accuracy exceeding 90% depending on how severe this imbalance is there between minority and majority class. In order to avoid this problem we have used other metrics to evaluate our model performance. These metrics are recall, precision and F-Measure metrics [69]. Recall (R), Precision (P) and F-Measure ($F - Measure$) based on the True Positive classification (i.e. truly classified as class label $ClassID1$), False Negative classification (i.e. falsely classified as class label $ClassID2$) and False Positive classification (i.e. falsely classified as class label $ClassID1$) are calculated using Eqs. (7.8), (7.9), and (7.10), respectively.

$$R = \frac{True\,Positive}{True\,Positive + False\,Negative} \tag{7.8}$$

$$P = \frac{True\,Positive}{True\,Positive + False\,Positive} \tag{7.9}$$

$$F - Measure = \frac{2 * Recall * Precision}{Recall + Precision} \tag{7.10}$$

Precision quantifies the total number of predicted cancer samples with respect to the predicted. Recall value quantifies the total number of predicted cancer samples with respect to the all actual cancer samples. The harmonic mean of Precision and Recall is F-Measure. F-Measure balances both Precision and Recall values. The performance of the proposed methodology for Colon Cancer classifier based on the Recall Precision and F-Measure is shown by Table 7.3. From this table it is also observed that the F-Measure value for our proposed classifier is highest which is

Table 7.3 Performance analysis for colon cancer classifiers

Classifier	Recall	Precision	F-Measure
GC	0.752	0.956	0.842
KC	0.812	0.912	0.859
HCFS	0.780	0.758	0.769
ACFS	0.700	0.930	0.800
NCFS	0.880	0.752	0.811
AC	0.910	0.892	0.901
Proposed Classifier (PC)	0.968	0.994	**0.981**

almost closed to accuracy value as we considered the oversampling to handle the problem of imbalance Colon Cancer dataset. This proves the effectiveness of our proposed classifier.

7.6.1 Statistical Analysis

For statistical analysis of our proposed approach with other state of art classifiers we have performed Wilcoxon Rank-Sum Test [70, 71] (Non-parameterized). It has been assumed that variance is same for the datasets and independent samples have been used in this test. 10-fold cross validation methodology [72] has been used for these statistical tests. After performing the Wilcoxon Rank-Sum Test on the proposed approach, p-value is calculated. After calculation of p-value, a significance level of p-value (i.e. critical value: α) ≥ 0.05 implies that the proposed classifier method can not be considered as statistically significantly different. If the obtained p-value is below the critical level then the null hypothesis [73] selected is rejected. To consider both precision and recall, the statistical analysis is done based on F-measure. The possible pair wise comparisons with our classifier and other considering state-of-art classifiers are shown in Table 7.4. The calculated p-values (maximum calculated p-value = 0.0028) are always less than α (i.e. $\leq$0.05), which indicates the rejection of null hypothesis has been observed from this table. In Table 7.4 the best results are marked by bold faces. This result emphasise that the proposed Colon Cancer classifier can be considered as statistically significant. It is also noted that we have checked the p-values for all the given features where p-values for selected features are always $<$0.05 which implies rejection of null hypothesis and the statistical significance of those features.

Table 7.4 p-value comparison for colon cancer classifier

Classifier	GC	KC	HCFS	ACFS	NCFS	AC
PC	1.8063e-04	2.4480e-04	1.7861e-04	**0.0028**	1.8063e-04	2.4480e-04

7.6.2 Performance Comparison Using Receiver Operating Characteristic Curve

The proposed work is also compared by constructing Receiver Operating Characteristics (ROC) curve [74, 75] with other state-of-art classifiers for evaluating the performance. The evaluation is based on an confusion matrix [76] given in Table 7.5.

In Table 7.5, 'True' stands for the number of samples of the dataset classified as $ClassID1$ (i.e. Cancer present) and 'False' stands for the number of samples of the data classified as $ClassID2$ (i.e. Cancer not present). Here, u indicates the total number of samples of the dataset truly classified as $ClassID1$, v indicates the total number of samples of the dataset truly classified as $ClassID2$, w is the total number of samples of the dataset classified as $ClassID1$ with actual class label $ClassID2$ and x is the total number of samples of the dataset classified as $ClassID2$ with actual class label $ClassID1$. From Table 7.5, we can calculate the True Positive Rate (TPR) and False Positive Rate (FPR) for the proposed classifier using Eqs. (7.11) and (7.12), respectively.

$$TPR = \frac{u}{u+v} \quad (7.11) \qquad FPR = \frac{w}{w+x} \quad (7.12)$$

The False Positive Rate (FR) and the True Positive Rate (TR) is represented by the X-axis and Y-axis in a ROC curve. The 'ideal' point is indicated by the top left bend of the ROC plotting. At this top left bend, the value of FR is zero and value of TR is one. It implies that accuracy will be better when area under the curve is large and vice versa. Ideally, it is recommended to minimize the FR while maximizing the TR. So, the steepness present in the ROC plotting is a crucial aspect. ROC curve for Classification Colon Cancer dataset is demonstrated in Figs. 7.8, 7.9, 7.10 and 7.11 for training, validation, test and overall performance analysis based on Tables 7.6, 7.7, 7.8 and 7.9. From Figs. 7.8, 7.9, 7.10 and 7.11, it is observed that the Area

Table 7.5 Confusion matrix for classification

Actual	Predicted	
	True	Flase
True	u	v
False	w	x

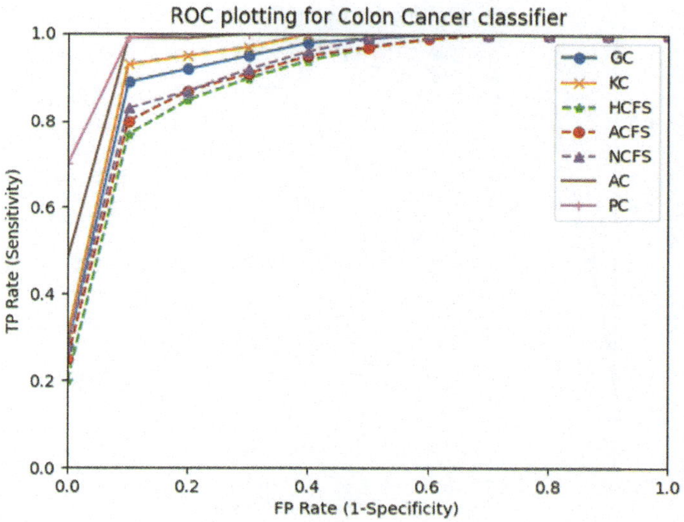

Fig. 7.8 Training ROC plotting for colon cancer classifiers

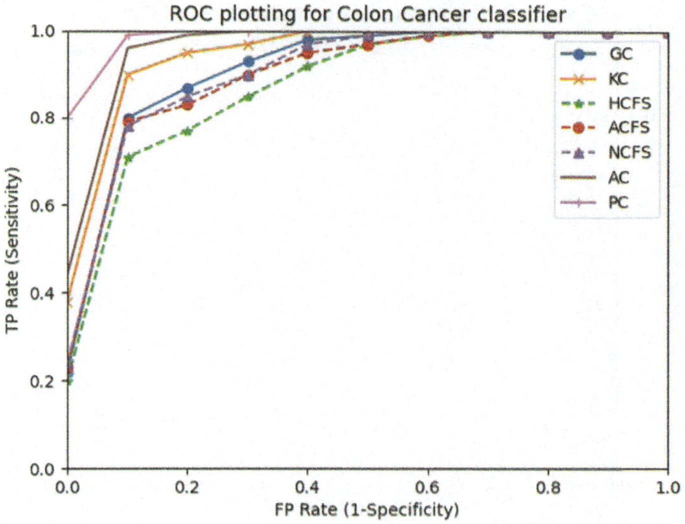

Fig. 7.9 Validation ROC plotting for colon cancer classifiers

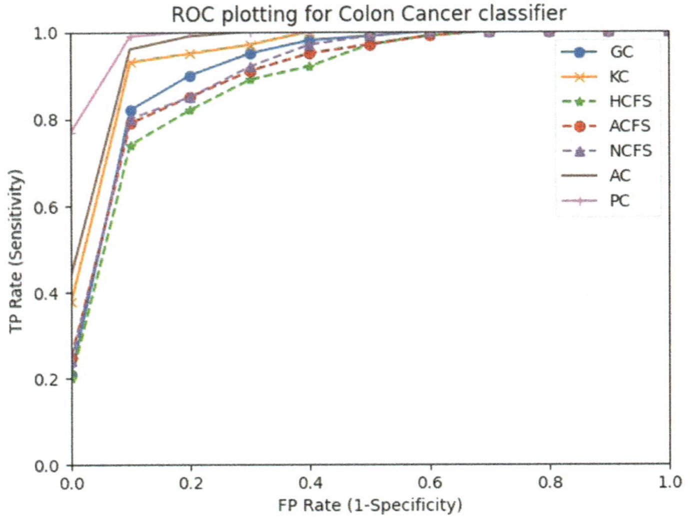

Fig. 7.10 Testing ROC plotting for colon cancer classifiers

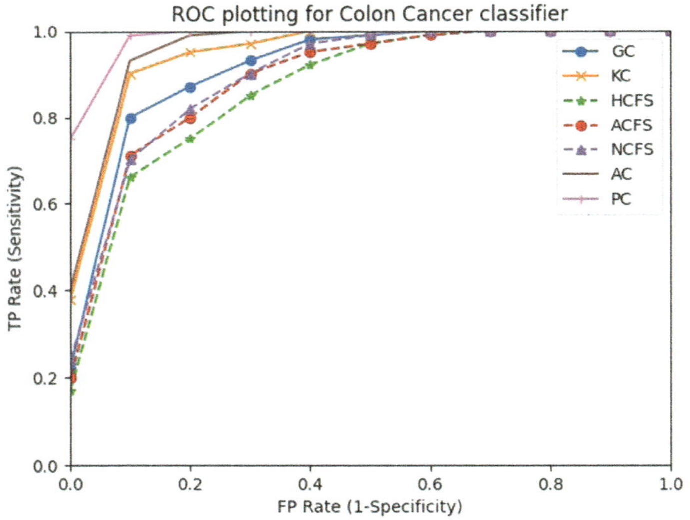

Fig. 7.11 Overall ROC plotting for colon cancer classifiers

Table 7.6 Training confusion matrix

Actual	Predicted	
	True (%)	Flase (%)
True	33.9	0.0
False	0.0	66.1

Table 7.7 Validation confusion matrix

Actual	Predicted	
	True (%)	Flase (%)
True	33.1	0.0
False	0.0	66.9

Table 7.8 Test confusion matrix

Actual	Predicted	
	True (%)	Flase (%)
True	44.1	10.9
False	0.0	45.0

Table 7.9 Overall confusion matrix

Actual	Predicted	
	True (%)	Flase (%)
True	35.4	1.4
False	0.0	63.2

Under Curve for the proposed classifier is higher than other considered classification techniques, though the ROC for AC, and KC are very closed to that of PC.

7.7 Conclusion

This paper aimed at the feature selection of relevant features from a feature set of 2000 features and also extrapolation of the samples. The approach used for the oversampling of the data ensures that the newly extrapolated data maintain the characteristics of the overall data set. Also, the feature reduction techniques reduced the number of features to 20 from 2000, thus removing all the unwanted correlated features. The accuracy achieved showed to be quite impressive and can be used in the real time prediction scenario. For the future scope of this paper, much deeper neural networks can be used to increase the efficiency even more. Also, a data set with more number of cancer data can be used for better understanding of the patterns in the data set thus improving the accuracy.

References

1. Siegel, R.L., Miller, K.D., Goding Sauer, A., Fedewa, S.A., Butterly, L.F., Anderson, J.C., Cercek, A., Smith, R.A., Jemal, A.: Colorectal cancer statistics. A Cancer J. Clin, CA (2020)
2. Haggar, F.A., Boushey, R.P.: Colorectal cancer epidemiology: incidence, mortality, survival, and risk factors. Clin. Colon Rectal Surg. **22**(4), 191 (2009)
3. Phillips, K.A., Liang, S.-Y., Ladabaum, U., Haas, J., Kerlikowske, K., Lieberman, D., Hiatt, R., Nagamine, M., Van Bebber, S.L.: Trends in colonoscopy for colorectal cancer screening. Med. Care, 160–167 (2007)
4. Walsh, J.M.E., Terdiman, J.P.: Colorectal cancer screening: scientific review. JAMA **289**(10), 1288–1296 (2003)
5. Fischer, A.H., Jacobson, K.A., Rose, J., Zeller, J.: Hematoxylin and eosin staining of tissue and cell sections. Cold Spring Harbor Protocols **2008**(5), pdb–prot4986 (2008)
6. Teare, P., Fishman, M., Benzaquen, O., Toledano, E., Elnekave, E.: Malignancy detection on mammography using dual deep convolutional neural networks and genetically discovered false color input enhancement. J. Digital Imaging **30**(4), 499–505 (2017)
7. Monirul Kabir, Md., Monirul Islam, Md., Murase, K.: A new wrapper feature selection approach using neural network. Neurocomputing **73**(16–18), 3273–3283 (2010)
8. Tekchandani, H., Verma, S., Londhe, N.D.: Mediastinal lymph node malignancy detection in computed tomography images using fully convolutional network. Biocybern. Biomed. Eng. **40**(1), 187–199 (2020)
9. Chekkoury, A., Khurd, P., Ni, J., Bahlmann, C., Kamen, A., Patel, A., Grady, L., Singh, M., Groher, MNavab, N. et al.: Automated malignancy detection in breast histopathological images. In: Medical Imaging 2012: Computer-Aided Diagnosis, vol. 8315, page 831515. International Society for Optics and Photonics (2012)
10. Kurmi, Y., Chaurasia, V., Ganesh, N.: Tumor malignancy detection using histopathology imaging. J. Med. Imaging Radiat. Sci. **50**(4), 514–528 (2019)
11. Reed, W.M., Lee, W.B., Cawson, J.N., Brennan, P.C.: Malignancy detection in digital mammograms: important reader characteristics and required case numbers. Acad. Radiol. **17**(11), 1409–1413 (2010)
12. Kelly, D.L., Rizzino, A.: Dna microarray analyses of genes regulated during the differentiation of embryonic stem cells. Molecu. Reprod. Dev.: Incorp. Gamete Res. **56**(2), 113–123 (2000)
13. Moorthy, K., Mohamad, M.S.: Random forest for gene selection and microarray data classification. In: Knowledge Technology Week, pp. 174–183. Springer (2011)
14. Mohamad, M.S., Omatu, M.S., Deris, S., Misman, M.F., Yoshioka, M.: Selecting informative genes from microarray data by using hybrid methods for cancer classification. Artif. Life Robot. **13**(2), 414–417 (2009)
15. Tarek, S., Abd Elwahab, R., Shoman, M.: Cancer classification ensemble system based on gene expression profiles. In: 2016 5th International Conference on Electronic Devices, Systems and Applications (ICEDSA), pp. 1–4. IEEE (2016)
16. John, G.H., Kohavi, R., Pfleger, K.: Irrelevant features and the subset selection problem. In: Machine Learning Proceedings 1994, pp. 121–129. Elsevier (1994)
17. Elkhani, N., Muniyandi, R.C.: Membrane computing to model feature selection of microarray cancer data. Proc. ASE BigData Soc. Inform. **2015**, 1–9 (2015)
18. Koller, D., Sahami, M.: Toward optimal feature selection. Technical report, Stanford InfoLab (1996)

19. Kohavi, R., Sommerfield, D.: Feature subset selection using the wrapper method: overfitting and dynamic search space topology. In: KDD, pp. 192–197 (1995)
20. Das, S.N., Mathew, M., Vijayaraghavan, P.K.: An approach for optimal feature subset selection using a new term weighting scheme and mutual information. Int. J. Adv. Sci. Eng. Inform. Technol. **1**(3), 273–278 (2011)
21. Sarkar, I.N., Planet, P.J., Bael, T.E., Stanley, S.E., Siddall, M., DeSalle, R., Figurski, D.H.: Characteristic attributes in cancer microarrays. J. Biomed. Inform. **35**(2), 111–122 (2002)
22. Park, M.S., Choi, J.Y.: Theoretical analysis on feature extraction capability of class-augmented pca. Pattern Recogn. **42**(11), 2353–2362 (2009)
23. Song, L., Smola, A., Gretton, A., Borgwardt, K.M., Bedo, J.: Supervised feature selection via dependence estimation. In: Proceedings of the 24th International Conference on Machine Learning, pp. 823–830 (2007)
24. Ang, J.C., Mirzal, A., Haron, H., Nuzly Abdull Hamed, H.: Supervised, unsupervised, and semi-supervised feature selection: a review on gene selection. IEEE/ACM Trans. Comput. Biol. Bioinform. **13**(5), 971–989 (2015)
25. Salem, H., Attiya, G., El-Fishawy, N.: Classification of human cancer diseases by gene expression profiles. Appl. Soft Comput. **50**, 124–134 (2017)
26. Chen, M., Ludwig, S.A.: Fuzzy decision tree using soft discretization and a genetic algorithm based feature selection method. In: 2013 World Congress on Nature and Biologically Inspired Computing, pp. 238–244. IEEE (2013)
27. Xi, M., Sun, J., Liu, L., Fan, F., Wu, F.: Cancer feature selection and classification using a binary quantum-behaved particle swarm optimization and support vector machine. Comput. Math Methods Med (2016)
28. Jiao, L., Chen, Q., Li, S., Xu, Y.: Colon cancer detection using whole slide histopathological images. In: World Congress on Medical Physics and Biomedical Engineering May 26–31, 2012, Beijing, China, pp. 1283–1286. Springer (2013)
29. Qiao, Y.H., Liu, J.L., Zhang, C.G., Xu, X.H., Zeng, Y.J.: Svm classification of human intergenic and gene sequences. Math. Biosci. **195**(2), 168–178 (2005)
30. Burges, C.J.C.: A tutorial on support vector machines for pattern recognition. Data Mining Knowl. Discov. **2**(2), 121–167 (1998)
31. Peyret, R., Bouridane, A., Al-Maadeed, S.A., Kunhoth, S., Khelifi, F.: Texture analysis for colorectal tumour biopsies using multispectral imagery. In: 2015 37th Annual International Conference of the IEEE Engineering in Medicine and Biology Society (EMBC), pp. 7218–7221. IEEE (2015)
32. Shapcott, M., Hewitt, K.J., Rajpoot, N.: Deep learning with sampling in colon cancer histology. Front. Bioeng. Biotechnol. **7**, 52 (2019)
33. Bychkov, D., Linder, N., Turkki, R., Nordling, S., Kovanen, P.E., Verrill, C., Walliander, M., Lundin, M., Haglund, C., Lundin, J.: Deep learning based tissue analysis predicts outcome in colorectal cancer. Scientific Reports **8**(1), 1–11 (2018)
34. Srinivasa, R.P., Sujatha, R.: Analysis of colon cancer dataset using k-means based algorithms and see5 algorithms. Int. J. Comput. Sci. Technol. **2**, 482–484 (2011)
35. Sirinukunwattana, K., Ahmed Raza, S.E., Tsang, Y.-W., Snead, D.R.J., Cree, I.A., Rajpoot, N.M.: Locality sensitive deep learning for detection and classification of nuclei in routine colon cancer histology images. IEEE Trans. Med. Imaging **35**(5), 1196–1206 (2016)
36. Iizuka, O., Kanavati, F., Kato, K., Rambeau, M., Arihiro, K., Tsuneki, M.: Deep learning models for histopathological classification of gastric and colonic epithelial tumours. Scientific Reports **10**(1), 1–11 (2020)
37. Shabbeer Basha, S.H., Ghosh, S., Babu, K.K., Dubey, S.R., Pulabaigari, V., Mukherjee, S.: Rccnet: an efficient convolutional neural network for histological routine colon cancer nuclei classification. In: 2018 15th International Conference on Control, Automation, Robotics and Vision (ICARCV), pp. 1222–1227. IEEE (2018)
38. Redmond, J., Vanderpool, R., McClung, R.: Effectively communicating colorectal cancer screening information to primary care providers: application for state, tribe or territory comprehensive cancer control coalitions. Amer. J. Health Educ. **43**(4), 194–201 (2012)

39. Alon, U., Barkai, N., Notterman, D.A., Gish, K., Ybarra, S., Mack, D., Levine, A.J.: Broad patterns of gene expression revealed by clustering analysis of tumor and normal colon tissues probed by oligonucleotide arrays. Proc. Natl Acad. Sci. **96**(12), 6745–6750 (1999)
40. Vora, P., Oza, B., et al.: A survey on k-mean clustering and particle swarm optimization. Int. J. Sci. Modern Eng. **1**(3), 24–26 (2013)
41. Kaur, N.K., Kaur, U., Singh, D.: K-medoid clustering algorithm-a review. Int. J. Comput. Appl. Technol. (IJCAT) **1**(1), 2349–1841 (2014)
42. Bolla, M.: Penalized versions of the newman-girvan modularity and their relation to normalized cuts and k-means clustering. Phys. Rev. E **84**(1) (2011)
43. Despalatović, L., Vojković, T., Vukicevic, D.: Community structure in networks: girvan-newman algorithm improvement. In: 2014 37th international convention on information and communication technology, electronics and microelectronics (MIPRO, pp. 997–1002. IEEE (2014)
44. Xiang, S., Nie, F., Zhang, C.: Learning a mahalanobis distance metric for data clustering and classification. Pattern Recogn. **41**(12), 3600–3612 (2008)
45. Zhao, X., Li, Yu., Zhao, Q.: Mahalanobis distance based on fuzzy clustering algorithm for image segmentation. Digital Signal Process. **43**, 8–16 (2015)
46. Gilani, Z., Rao, N.I.: Fast block clustering based optimized adaptive mediod shift. In: International Conference on Computer Analysis of Images and Patterns, pp. 435–443. Springer (2009)
47. Bader, D.A., Kintali, S., Madduri, S., Mihail, M.: Approximating betweenness centrality. In: International Workshop on Algorithms and Models for the Web-Graph, pp. 124–137. Springer (2007)
48. Phipps, J.B.: Dendrogram topology. Systematic Zoology **20**(3), 306–308 (1971)
49. De Maesschalck, R., Jouan-Rimbaud, D., Massart, D.L.: The mahalanobis distance. Chemometrics Intell. Lab. Syst. **50**(1), 1–18 (2000)
50. Misuraca, M., Spano, M., Balbi, S.: Bms: an improved dunn index for document clustering validation. Commun. Stat.-Theory Methods **48**(20), 5036–5049 (2019)
51. Bezdek, J.C., Pal, N.R.: Cluster validation with generalized dunn's indices. In: Proceedings 1995 Second New Zealand International Two-Stream Conference on Artificial Neural Networks and Expert Systems, pp. 190–193. IEEE (1995)
52. Pérez-Suárez, A., Martínez-Trinidad, J., Carrasco-Ochoa, J.A., Medina-Pagola, J.E.: An algorithm based on density and compactness for dynamic overlapping clustering. Pattern Recogn. **46**(11), 3040–3055 (2013)
53. Sitao, Wu, Chow, T.W.S.: Clustering of the self-organizing map using a clustering validity index based on inter-cluster and intra-cluster density. Pattern Recogn. **37**(2), 175–188 (2004)
54. He, H., Bai, Y., Garcia, E.A., Li, S.: Adasyn: Adaptive synthetic sampling approach for imbalanced learning. In: 2008 IEEE International Joint Conference on Neural Networks (IEEE World Congress on Computational Intelligence), pp. 1322–1328. IEEE (2008)
55. Tang, B., He, H.: Kerneladasyn: kernel based adaptive synthetic data generation for imbalanced learning. In: 2015 IEEE Congress on Evolutionary Computation (CEC), pp. 664–671. IEEE (2015)
56. Danielsson, P.-E.: Euclidean distance mapping. Comput. Graph. Image Process. **14**(3), 227–248 (1980)
57. Kozma. L.: k-nearest neighbors algorithm (knn). Helsinki University of Technology (2008)
58. Sedgwick, P.: Pearson's correlation coefficient. BMJ **345**, (2012)
59. Karamizadeh, S., Abdullah, S.M., Manaf, A.A., Zamani, M., Hooman, A.: An overview of principal component analysis. J. Signal Inform. Process. **4**(3B), 173 (2013)
60. Balci K., Atalay, V: Pca for gender estimation: Which eigenvectors contribute? In: Object Recognition Supported by User Interaction for Service Robots, vol. 3, pp. 363–366. IEEE (2002)
61. Taud, H, Mas, J.F.: Multilayer perceptron (mlp). In: Geomatic Approaches for Modeling Land Change Scenarios, pp. 451–455. Springer (2018)

62. Zhang, Z., Sabuncu, M.: Generalized cross entropy loss for training deep neural networks with noisy labels. In; Advances in Neural Information Processing Systems, pp. 8778–8788 (2018)
63. Zhang, Z.: Improved adam optimizer for deep neural networks. In: 2018 IEEE/ACM 26th International Symposium on Quality of Service (IWQoS), pp. 1–2. IEEE (2018)
64. Gardner, M.W., Dorling, S.R.: Artificial neural networks (the multilayer perceptron)-a review of applications in the atmospheric sciences. Atmosph. Environ. **32**(14–15), 2627–2636 (1998)
65. Maas, A.L., Hannun, A.Y., Ng, A.Y.: Rectifier nonlinearities improve neural network acoustic models. In: Proceedings ICML, vol. 30, p. 3 (2013)
66. Castellanos Garzón, J.A., Ramos González, J., et al.: A gene selection approach based on clustering for classification tasks in colon cancer (2015)
67. Nies, H.W., Daud, K.M., Remli, M.A., Mohamad, M.S., Deris, S., Omatu, S., Kasim, S., Sulong, G.: Classification of colorectal cancer using clustering and feature selection approaches. In: International Conference on Practical Applications of Computational Biology and Bioinformatics, pp. 58–65. Springer (2017)
68. Rahman, Md.A., Muniyandi, R.C.: Feature selection from colon cancer dataset for cancer classification using artificial neural network. Int. J. Adv. Sci. Eng. Inf. Technol **8**(4–2), 1387 (2018)
69. Burduk. R.: Classification performance metric for imbalance data based on recall and selectivity normalized in class labels. arXiv preprint arXiv:2006.13319 (2020)
70. Saha, S., Seal, D.B., Ghosh, A., Dey, K.N.: A novel gene ranking method using wilcoxon rank sum test and genetic algorithm. Int. J. Bioinform. Res. Appl. **12**(3), 263–279 (2016)
71. Liao, C., Li, K.N., Luo, Z.: Gene selection using wilcoxon rank sum test and support vector machine for cancer classification. In: International Conference on Computational and Information Science, pp. 57–66. Springer (2006)
72. Zhang, P.: Model selection via multifold cross validation. Ann Stat. pp. 299–313 (1993)
73. Anderson, D.R., Burnham, K.P., Thompson,W.L.: Null hypothesis testing: problems, prevalence, and an alternative. J. Wildlife Manag. pp. 912–923 (2000)
74. Yonelinas, A.P.: Receiver-operating characteristics in recognition memory: evidence for a dual-process model. J. Exp. Psychol.: Learn. Memory Cognit. **20**(6), 1341 (1994)
75. Streiner, D.L., Cairney, J.: What's under the roc? an introduction to receiver operating characteristics curves. Canadian J. Psych. **52**(2), 121–128 (2007)
76. Townsend, J.T.: Theoretical analysis of an alphabetic confusion matrix. Percept. Psychophys. **9**(1), 40–50 (1971)

Chapter 8
Automatic Detection of Tumor Cell in Brain MRI Using Rough-Fuzzy Feature Selection with Support Vector Machine and Morphological Operation

Amiya Halder and Apurba Sarkar

Abstract Brain cancer is occurred due to the abnormal growing of brain cells forming tumors. These tumors may grow double in size in just 25 days. If these tumors are not identified in the initial stage a patient may die within half of a year. The detection of these brain tumors need an automatic technique to help medical practitioners. This chapter presents an automatic technique to segregate brain magnetic resonance imaging (MRI) images as abnormal, in the presence of a brain tumor or as normal in the absence of a tumor and then detect the regions of abnormal tumor cells. The exact cancerous cells from these images are then extracted. The proposed algorithm is completed using two steps. Initially, a set of statistical features are produced, and then the most important features are selected using the Rough-Kernelized Fuzzy C-Means (RKFCM) algorithm. The important features are used for accurately identifying brain MRI images containing abnormal cells. After the feature selection, classify the images into two groups, namely, tumor affected and tumor-free using Support Vector Machine (SVM). In the second step, tumor affected regions in brain tumor images are detected and then segmented out from the scanned image applying a rough set-based KFCM algorithm. Then, extract the exact tumor region from images using thresholding and morphological operations. The proposed method is tested on different benchmark data sets such as BRATS2013, Harvard, and real-patient MRI brain images from M. R. Bangur Hospital for validation. From the observation, it is clearly noticed that the proposed method provides better result in terms of accuracy, specificity, and sensitivity than exiting methods.

Keywords MRI images · Rough set theory · KFCM · Thresholding · Morphological operation

---

A. Halder (✉)
Department of CSE, STCET, 4-D. H. Road, Kidderpore, Kolkata 700023, India

A. Sarkar
Department of CST, IIEST, Shibpur, Howrah 711103, India

J. Nayak et al. (eds.), *Advanced Machine Learning Approaches in Cancer Prognosis*, Intelligent Systems Reference Library 204,
https://doi.org/10.1007/978-3-030-71975-3_8

8.1 Introduction

A brain tumor is a mass of abnormal cells within the brain that are produced due to the uncontrolled proliferation of cells that cause cancer in the human brain. It develops from the brain cells near the membrane or meninges of the brain. Normally, brain tumors are separated by two categories: malignant and benign. Malignant cells are also known as cancerous tumors and benign are non-cancerous tumors. Malignant tumors are the most dangerous form of the tumor and which is the cause of a huge number of fatalities each year in the world. Based on severity [1], the malignant tumors are broadly classified into grade I, grade II, grade III, and grade IV. Among all the tumors, Gliomas are grade I type brain tumors which is less fatal and have a high survival rate. Grade IV type tumor is a more aggressive and most dangerous malignant tumor, and its survival span is limited to one to two years. If these brain tumor tissues are identified and detected in very early stages, then proper treatment can be planned and as a result, the survival rate of brain a tumor affected patient are increased.

The aim of this chapter is to classify brain tumor images and present efficient segmentation algorithms that would automatically and accurately segment the brain MRI images and identify, detect, and extract exact brain tumor cells. This would help the radiologists and doctors to diagnose brain tumors or various injuries in the brain and plan the treatment as soon as possible.

A lot of techniques have been published for brain tumor classification, identification, detection, and extraction using supervised, unsupervised, region growing, active contour, support vector machine, or morphological techniques [2–12]. Many of them work well but are time consuming whereas other methods are unable to properly classify, detect, or extract tumor cells. This chapter presents an efficient algorithm using unsupervised techniques that runs sequentially step by step. At first, different statistical texture features are extracted from brain MRI images. Then the features are reduced using the Rough-kernelized fuzzy C means clustering algorithm. After that, images are classified as tumor affected or tumor free using a support vector machine. Finally, the tumor cells are extracted from tumor affected image using the combination of RKFCM based segmentation method, thresholding technique, and morphological operations.

The rest of the chapter is organized as follows. Section 8.2 briefly discusses earlier work on this particular and related problems. Section 8.3 explain the details of the proposed method. Section 8.4 describes the experimental results. Finally, Sect. 8.5 concludes the chapter with possible future directions.

8.2 Literature Study

In this section, various existing brain MRI medical image classification and segmentation techniques are discussed. Earlier days domain expertises were used to manually classify and segment brain abnormalities. This approach is very time consuming and error prone meaning that this manual process may misclassify some of the images. To overcome this problem various automated techniques have been proposed from time to time by various researchers. Some of them are briefly explained below.

Corso et al. [13] proposed an automatic efficient segmentation method for multilevel brain tumor segmentation using affinity-based segmentation and generative model-based approaches, it also uses a Bayesian model based classification method. This method detects and segments brain tumor and edema from MR brain images. Zacharaki et al. [14] have suggested a classification method for brain tumor images using texture and shape-based features. It also uses a support vector machine. El-Dahshan et al. [15] published a hybrid technique for the classification of the MR images using discrete wavelet transformation, principal component analysis (PCA), back propagation artificial neural network (FP-ANN), and k-nearest neighbor (k-NN). Zhang et al. [16] presented an automated classification technique of MR brain images using a neural network (NN). First, it calculates image features using wavelet transform and then reduce the dimensions of features using PCA. After that, classify the image using NN with a scaled conjugate gradient (SCG).

Anitha et al. [17] presented a brain tumor segmentation and classification system using adaptive pillar K-means algorithm, DWT, self-organizing map neural network and K-nearest neighbour techniques. Amin et al. [18] presented an automatic distinctive brain tumor detection and classification approach that easily differentiates non-cancerous and cancerous images. According to this method, for the segmentation of lesions of brain images, at first, the image is transformed into Lab color space, then K-means clustering is to be applied. After that texture, shape, and intensity-based features set are extracted for every applicant lesion. In the following step, SVM classifier is used for different cross-validations.

Khan et al. [19] have published an automated brain tumor detection, extraction, and classification technique using marker-based watershed segmentation method and multilevel priority features selection. Halder and Dobe [20, 21] proposed brain tumor detection algorithms using fuzzy feature selection and Support Vector Machine. In this technique, at first, a set of features were generated using the statistical features selection technique. Then, the important features are selected using FCM or rough set based K-means algorithm. After that, SVM is used to classify whether the MRI scan images are tumor-free or tumor affected. Also, various other segmentation, feature extraction, and classification methods have been presented over the last few years. Arasi et al. [22] presented a classification technique using soft computing methods. This method uses the genetic optimized median filter, hierarchical fuzzy clustering algorithm, gray level co-occurrence matrix (GLCM) method, and Lion Optimized Boosting SVM model. Pareek et al. [23] presented a tumor classification and calculation of tumor area from MRI images using GLCM feature extraction, DWT, and Kernel SVM (KSVM). Islam et al. [24] have proposed a detection and classification algorithm of brain MRI images based on multilevel segmentation with Convolutional Neural Network (MLS-CNN). Tiwari et al. [25] have presented a methodical literature review on brain tumor classification and segmentation from MR images using deep learning techniques, meta heuristic techniques, and hybrid methods.

8.3 Proposed Method

This section includes our proposed model for the classification, detection, and extraction of the exactly affected areas from brain MRI images. This method is divided into different sequential steps as follows.

1. Data set creation.
2. Feature extraction.
3. Feature selection.
4. Tumor classification.
5. Tumor detection and extraction.

The proposed technique is displayed in Fig. 8.1 in the form of a block diagram to comprehend the flow of steps of the proposed method.

8.3.1 Data Set Creation

This kind of automatic model requires huge data sets to understand how well the system performs. In this case, the data set consists of MR images containing both normal and abnormal brain cells. Different freely available MR image databases are used for the classification, training and testing of SVM, detection, and extraction of tumor affected region in the brain while building the system. MR image data set have been collected from different research organizations like Harvard, BRATS2013, etc. Also, a data set of real patient data have been collected from M. R. Bangur Hospital, Kolkata. All data sets are focused normally on color formats. Due to the difficulty in handling color images, MRI images are converted to gray level images with pixel intensity from 0 to 255. This conversion helped to generate GLCM for different feature calculations.

8.3.2 Feature Set Extraction

An image is defined by the intensity values of all the pixels in the image. To process a whole image for classification all pixels are required to process which costs a huge time. To reduce the time, we extract certain features from each brain MRI image that represent the essential information about a normal and abnormal image. Alternatively, these features assist us to represent an image accurately. For these reasons, the features set are used as input to the classifier for image classification. In proposed method, we have calculated different texture-based statistical features for classification. These features classify the brain MRI images in white matter, gray matter, cerebrospinal fluid, and tumor region.

Let us consider the image $\xi(\nu, \omega)$ of size $M \times N$ and γ_n is the gray levels. $\rho(\upsilon, \beta)$ is the normalized value of the row υ and column β for GLCM. GLCM measures

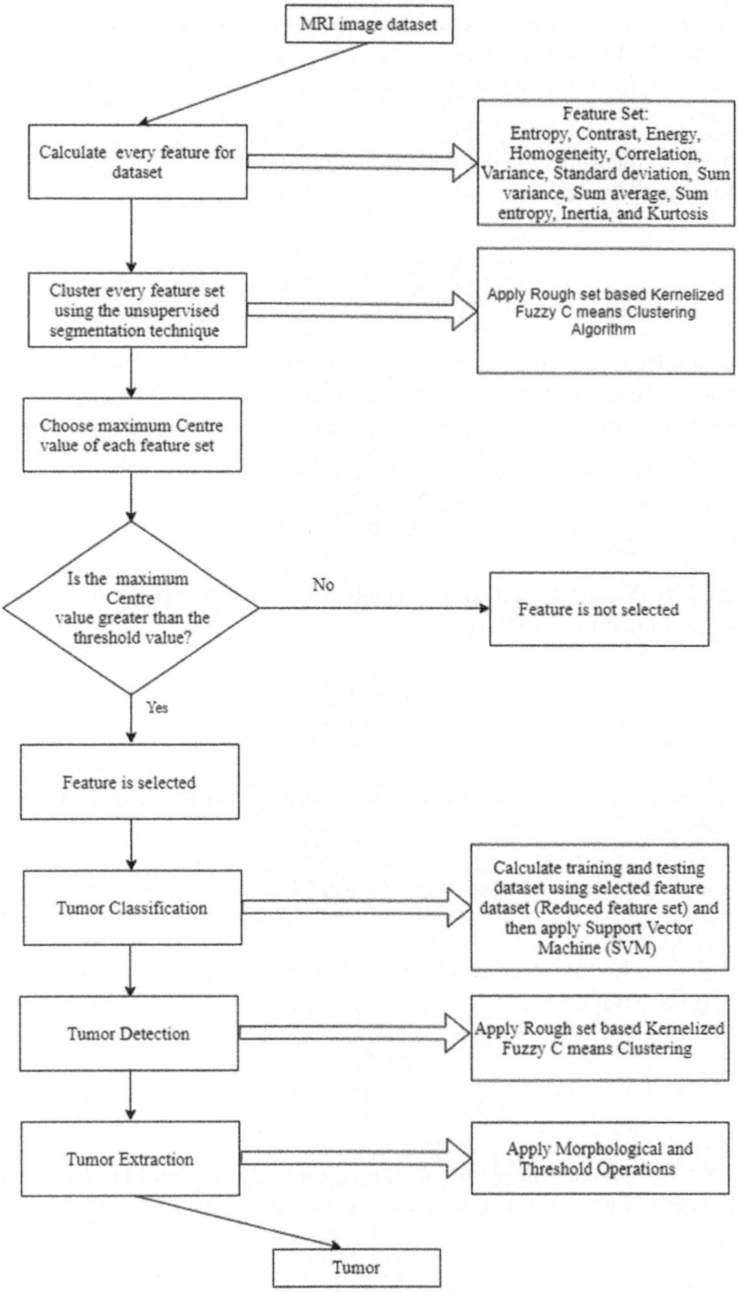

Fig. 8.1 Block diagram of the proposed algorithm framework

the variation in intensity at the pixel of interest that calculates the texture feature. An example of GLCM calculation is shown in Fig. 8.2. In proposed algorithm, we have used the following features set to exactly separate between the two classes of images:

1. Entropy: It measures the disorder of an image (Eq. 8.1). Complex texture tends to have high entropy.

$$I_{entropy} = \sum_{\upsilon=0}^{\gamma_{n-1}} \sum_{\beta=0}^{\gamma_{n-1}} (\rho(\upsilon, \beta) * log_2(\rho(\upsilon, \beta))). \tag{8.1}$$

2. Contrast: Contrast is the dissimilarity between the uppermost and smallest values of the continuous set of pixels and calculates the spatial frequency of an image and different moments of GLCM (Eq. 8.2).

$$I_{contrast} = \sum_{\upsilon=0}^{\gamma_{n-1}} \sum_{\beta=0}^{\gamma_{n-1}} (\upsilon - \beta)^2 * \rho(\upsilon, \beta). \tag{8.2}$$

3. Energy: It measures the textural equality i.e. pixel pair replication and detects disorder in texture (Eq. 8.3).

$$I_{energy} = \sum_{\upsilon=0}^{\gamma_{n-1}} \sum_{\beta=0}^{\gamma_{n-1}} \rho(\upsilon, \beta)^2. \tag{8.3}$$

4. Homogeneity: It calculates the closeness of the scattering elements in the GLCM (Eq. 8.4).

$$I_{homogeneity} = \sum_{\upsilon=0}^{\gamma_{n-1}} \sum_{\beta=0}^{\gamma_{n-1}} \frac{\rho(\upsilon, \beta)}{(1 + (\upsilon - \beta)^2)}. \tag{8.4}$$

5. Correlation: It represents the similarity between the present pixel and its neighbour pixels (Eq. 8.5).

$$I_{correlation} = \frac{1}{av_p av_p} \sum_{\upsilon=0}^{\gamma_{n-1}} \sum_{\beta=0}^{\gamma_{n-1}} \upsilon * \beta * \rho(\upsilon, \beta)^2 - sm_q sm_q. \tag{8.5}$$

   where sm_q, sm_q are means of $\rho(\upsilon)$, $\rho(\beta)$ and av_p, av_p are standard deviations.
6. Variance: It determines heterogeneity among the pixels (Eq. 8.6).

$$I_{varince} = \sum_{\upsilon=0}^{\gamma_{n-1}} (\upsilon - sm_q) * \rho(\upsilon). \tag{8.6}$$

   where sm_q is average of pixel values $\rho(\upsilon)$.

GLCM Calculation:

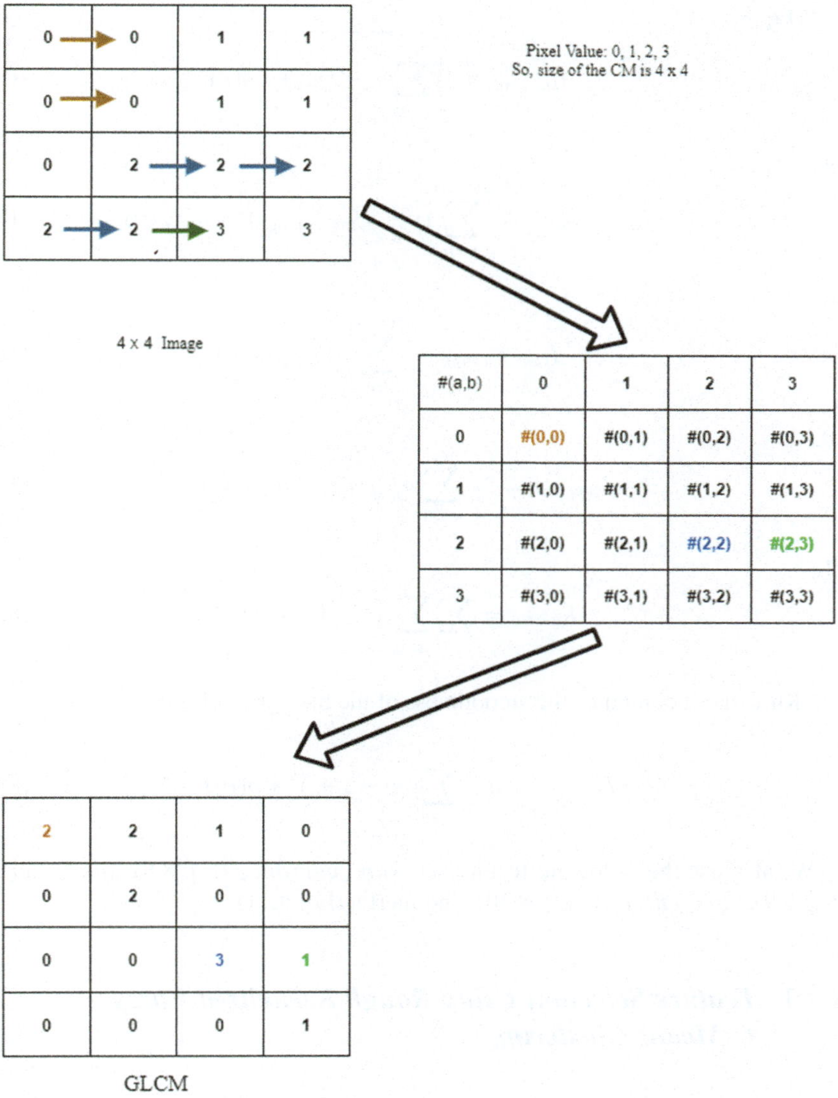

Fig. 8.2 An example of GLCM calculation on 4 × 4 image segment

7. Standard deviation: It calculates the difference of values from the average value (Eq. 8.7).

$$I_{std\_dev} = \sqrt{\sum_{\upsilon=0}^{\gamma_{n-1}} (\upsilon - sm_q) * \rho(\upsilon)}. \tag{8.7}$$

8.

$$I_{sum\_variance} = \sum_{\upsilon=0}^{2(\gamma_{n-1})} (\upsilon - I_{sum\_entropy})^2 * \rho_{q+p}(\upsilon). \tag{8.8}$$

9.

$$I_{sum\_average} = \sum_{\upsilon=0}^{2(\gamma_{n-1})} \upsilon * \rho_{q+p}(\upsilon). \tag{8.9}$$

10.

$$I_{sum\_entropy} = \sum_{\upsilon=0}^{\gamma_{n-1}} \rho_{q+p}(\upsilon) * log(\rho_{q+p}(\upsilon)). \tag{8.10}$$

11.

$$I_{inertia} = \sum_{\upsilon=0}^{\gamma_{n-1}} \sum_{\beta=0}^{\gamma_{n-1}} (\upsilon - \beta)^2 * \rho(\upsilon, \beta). \tag{8.11}$$

12. Kurtosis: It computes the smoothness of the histogram (Eq. 8.12).

$$I_{kurtosis} = a^{-4} \sum_{\upsilon=0}^{\gamma_{n-1}} ((\upsilon - sm_q)^4 * \rho(\upsilon)) - 3. \tag{8.12}$$

We also use the following feature sets $sum\_variance$ (Eq. 8.8), $sum\_average$ (Eq. 8.9), $sum\_entropy$ (Eq. 8.10), and inertia (Eq. 8.11).

8.3.3 Feature Selection Using Rough Kernelized Fuzzy C-Means Clustering

The normal and tumor affected brain MR images can be described using the above-calculated feature sets and it is easily applied to differentiate between them. There may be some features that are redundant and if the size of the data set is huge the execution time as well as the time to access the data will be very high. An innovative Rough set based Kernelized FCM clustering algorithm (RKFCM) is used to remove the redundancy of the feature set. It is a hybrid technique using rough set theory and kernelized FCM clustering method. KFCM is an unsupervised clustering method and it depends on kernel induced distance function. It has also enhanced its robustness in the noise. However, it fails to eliminate the uncertainty and vagueness of the clustering method. Rough-set theory is a new concept that is easily handling with incompleteness, vagueness, and uncertainty. Rough set with the KFCM algorithm has removed the uncertainty of the clustering by introducing the higher and lower estimation of rough set theory. Hence in this method, all the features data are contributed in clustering keep away from clustering errors. The proposed RKFCM method is applied to the feature set for the selection of the important features leaving out the redundant features. It is used individually for each feature set and clusters the feature data. Detailed information about important features selection from the features set using RKFCM method is presented in Fig. 8.3. For this proposed method, one criterion is used for feature selection: if the calculated maximum centroid value of each feature set is larger than the threshold value, then the feature is selected. In proposed method, threshold is calculated using the average feature value of a set of normal brain MR images (in our experiment, threshold is computed using the average feature of 10 normal brain MR images). The Rough Kernelized fuzzy C-mean algorithm is shown in Algorithm 1.

Algorithm 1 RKFCM clustering algorithm

//Number of data N $\{q_1, q_2, .., q_N\}$ and centroids $\{\vartheta_1, \vartheta_2, ..\vartheta_c\}$ and $\tau_{j\nu}$ is the membership value of j_{th} cluster and ν_{th} data value and $j \neq k$

// $\overline{\chi}(\vartheta_j)$ and $\underline{\chi}(\vartheta_j)$ are the lower and upper approximations of cluster ϑ_j

for $\nu = 1, .., N$ **do**

  $P = max_{1 \le j \le c}(\tau_{j\nu})$

  $R = max_{1 \le k \le c}(\tau_{k\nu})$

  if $(P - R) < threshold$ **then**

    $q_\nu \in \overline{\chi}(\vartheta_j)$ and $q_\nu \in \underline{\chi}(\vartheta_j)$

  else

    $q_\nu \in \overline{\chi}(\vartheta_j)$ and $q_\nu \in \overline{\chi}(\vartheta_k)$

  end if

end for

//Centroid calculation:

for $k = 1, .., c$ **do**

  if $\underline{\chi}(\vartheta_k) \neq 0$ and $(\overline{\chi}(\vartheta_k) - \underline{\chi}(\vartheta_k) = 0)$ **then**

    $\vartheta_k = \frac{\sum_{\nu=1}^{N} \tau_{k\nu}^m * q_\nu * \kappa(q_\nu, \vartheta_k)}{\sum_{\nu=1}^{N} \tau_{k\nu}^m * \kappa(q_\nu, \vartheta_k)}, \forall q_\nu \in \underline{\chi}(\vartheta_k)$

  else

    if $\underline{\chi}(\vartheta_i) = 0$ and $(\overline{\chi}(\vartheta_i) - \underline{\chi}(\vartheta_i)) \neq 0$ **then**

      $\vartheta_k = \frac{\sum_{\nu=1}^{N} \tau_{k\nu}^m * q_\nu * \kappa(q_\nu, \vartheta_k)}{\sum_{\nu=1}^{N} \tau_{k\nu}^m * \kappa(q_\nu, \vartheta_k)}, \forall q_\nu \in (\overline{\chi}(\vartheta_k) - \underline{\chi}(\vartheta_k))$

    else

      $\vartheta_k = \omega_{lo}\vartheta_1 + \omega_{up}\vartheta_2$, where $\{0 \le \omega_{lo} \le 0.5$ and $\omega_{up} = 1 - \omega_{lo}\}$

      $\vartheta_1 = \frac{\sum_{\nu=1}^{N} \tau_{k\nu}^m * q_\nu * \kappa(q_\nu, \vartheta_k)}{\sum_{\nu=1}^{N} \tau_{k\nu}^m * \kappa(q_\nu, \vartheta_k)}, \forall q_\nu \in (\overline{\chi}(\vartheta_k) - \underline{\chi}(\vartheta_k))$

      $\vartheta_2 = \frac{\sum_{\nu=1}^{N} \tau_{k\nu}^m * q_\nu * \kappa(q_\nu, \vartheta_k)}{\sum_{\nu=1}^{N} \tau_{k\nu}^m * \kappa(q_\nu, \vartheta_k)}, \forall q_\nu \in \underline{\chi}(\vartheta_k)$

    end if

  end if

  $\tau_{k\nu} = \frac{(1-\kappa(q_\nu, \vartheta_k))^{-\frac{1}{m-1}}}{\sum_{j=1}^{c}(1-\kappa(q_\nu, \vartheta_j))^{-\frac{1}{m-1}}}$

end for

Fig. 8.3 Block diagram for important feature selection

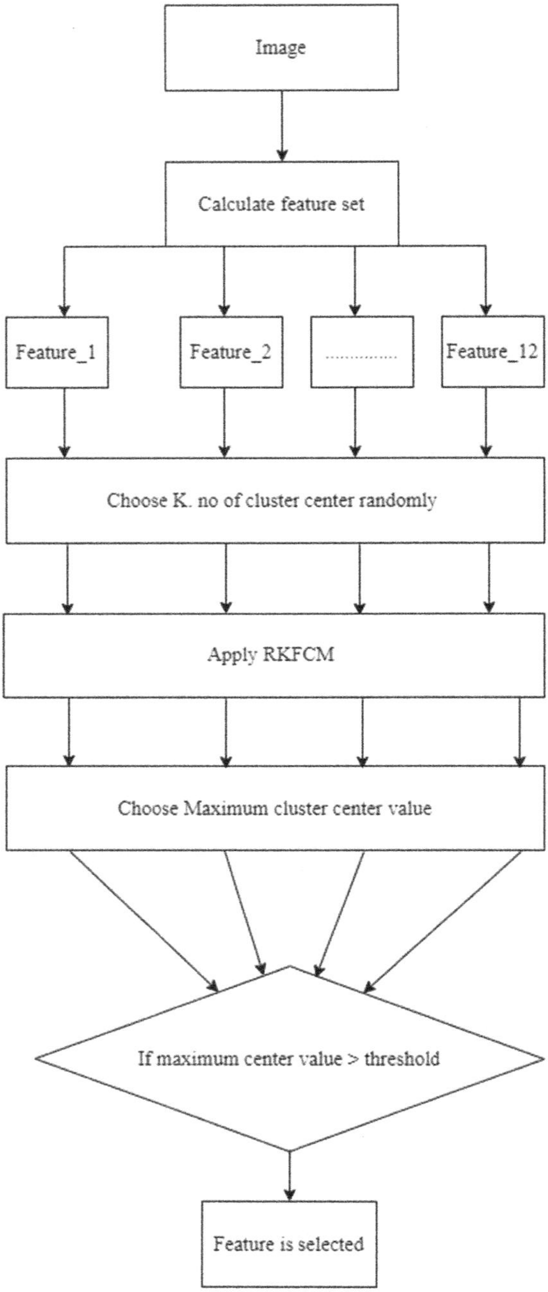

8.3.4 Tumor Classification Using SVM

This section presents the classification of cancerous cell and non-cancerous cell using SVM. After the feature is selected by a rough set based KFCM algorithm, the SVM is used for the classification of the images. Several other classifiers have been studied and it has been observed that SVM is one of the most effective classifiers and suitable for this work. The SVM classifier is based on the concept of the decision boundary or hyperplane. A set of points or objects that are linearly separable are separated using a line or decision boundaries. The equation (Eq. 8.13) of the decision boundary or hyperplane is given by

$$\vec{\varphi}.\vec{\gamma} + z = 0 \tag{8.13}$$

where $\vec{\varphi}$, $\vec{\gamma}$ and z denote the weight vector, feature vector and the bias value respectively. The margin of separation is identified by the difference between the hyperplane and the closest data point for a given weight vector $\vec{\varphi}$ and bias z. The best choice of the SVM is the maximal margin that is the particular hyperplane for which the margin of separation is maximized. For positive and negative points classification, the Eqs. 8.14 and 8.15 are used.

$$\vec{\varphi}.\vec{\gamma} + z = 1 \tag{8.14}$$

$$\vec{\varphi}.\vec{\gamma} + z = -1 \tag{8.15}$$

For non-linearly separable data points, the linear SVM classifier does not give accurate classification results. It gives higher misclassification accuracy. So, these are not directly separable. In this case, the kernel function is used for mapping lower dimensional feature space to higher dimension feature space. Then using hyperplane, these data points are classified using the classifier. A kernel function is defined as the dot product of two feature vectors in feature space (Eq. 8.16):

$$K(x_a, x_b) = \phi(x_a)\phi(x_b) \tag{8.16}$$

In the proposed algorithm, a Gaussian kernel or the kernel corresponding to the radial basis functions(RBF) is used. The most widely used RBF is the Gaussian function which is given below (Eq. 8.17),

$$K(x_a, x_b) = exp(-\frac{||x_a - x_b||^2}{2\sigma^2}) \tag{8.17}$$

where $\sigma > 0$. In SVM, the support vectors are generally training samples that extract to find the optimal plane.

8.3.5 *Tumor Detection and Extraction*

A brain MRI scan image is captured using an MRI scan system and then this image goes through the above classification approach. If the cancerous tumor cell is identified then the tumor cell is detected and extracted from the MRI image. This section discusses the detection and accurate extraction of cancerous tumor cells using global thresholding, segmentation algorithm, and morphological operation.

8.3.5.1 Preprocessing

Brain MRI images are captured by the radiology technique that uses magnetism, radio waves, radio frequency coil, etc. During acquisition, the quality of the brain MR image gets degraded in terms of intensity inhomogeneity and irregularities. Along with it, noise are also introduced in the image. These factors pose difficulty in the segmentation, detection, and extraction brain tumor tissue accurately. To get rid of these irregularities and noises, it requires some kind of preprocessing techniques like adjustments of contrast using enhancement technique and removal of the unwanted portion of the detected brain tumor. For this purpose, an adaptive contrast enhancement technique and a skull stripping method have been applied to these images.

8.3.5.2 Segmentation of Brain Tumor Image

In the general medical image, segmentation is challenging work because it changes from time to time, patient to patient in the same portion's image of the body, and brain MRI image segmentation is an even more challenging job. Lot of research has been done on this particular problem e.g. [26–31]. These algorithms on these work mainly depend on thresholding, region growing, edge detection, active contour, and clustering-based methods. From all these algorithms, it is clearly noticed that supervised and unsupervised clustering methods are most suitable for brain MRI segmentation. It has also been observed that FCM, KFCM, RFCM, Spatial Kernelized FCM (SKFCM) based clustering techniques automatically remove the noises and inhomogeneity. In the proposed algorithm, we present a rough set based Kernelized Fuzzy-C means clustering algorithm for segmentation which is robust towards the noise. It is also used to eliminate the uncertainty and vagueness of the clustering method and it does so by introducing the higher and lower estimation of rough set theory. We have already described the RKFCM algorithm in the previous section. Generally, a brain MRI image contains a range of intensity values. Surprisingly, after preprocessing, all ranges of the intensity values (256 different values for an 8-bit image) still remain in the brain image. Under this situation, it turns out to be difficult to distinguish the tumor cell from the other portion of the brain image.

To tackle this problem, brain images are segmented using the optimal number of clusters that are suggested by Turi [32] for accurate extraction of tumor cells from MRI images.

8.3.5.3 Thresholding

Segmentation is the most important technique by which the brain MRI image is segmented to segregate different regions like tumor, white matter, gray matter, background, etc. In this work, after the segmentation, isolate the brain tumor cell from the background using optimal thresholding followed by morphological operations. Binary image $B_n(\nu, \omega)$ is obtained by the thresholding techniques is described by the equation:

$$B_n(\nu, \omega) = \begin{cases} 0 \quad if & \xi(\nu, \omega) \leq \varphi \\ 255 \; if & \xi(\nu, \omega) > \varphi \end{cases}$$

where φ indicates the threshold value. To find the best φ, we used the global thresholding method. This operation helps to locate the tumor region and also helps in extracting it from the image.

8.3.5.4 Morphological Operations

By applying the thresholding technique the produced image of the tumor contains some noisy spots. This noisy spot is then further filtered out by the morphological operations. Morphology is widely used in the field of Biology and it tells about the shape and structure of different animals and different plants and so on. Basic morphological operations are applied using a structuring element (also known as the kernel). It has been observed that the proposed RKFCM based method is able to successfully extract out the accurate tumor from brain MRI images. The block diagram of the extraction of tumor from brain MRI images is shown in Fig. 8.4.

8.4 Experimental Results

Cancerous and non-cancerous brain MRI images give less information about tumor identification. This information focuses more on the size, shape, and texture of the tumor. The accurate classification depends on the predominant feature set. An attempt is made to progress a classification system based on statistical features. In this view, the estimation of this method critically recommended the following: Rough kernelized FCM achieves a better solution for tumor classification of MR images compared to other methods. It removes the redundant features and selects the most important features to classify the MRI images. This technique only selects four(4) important features among twelve (12) statistical features.

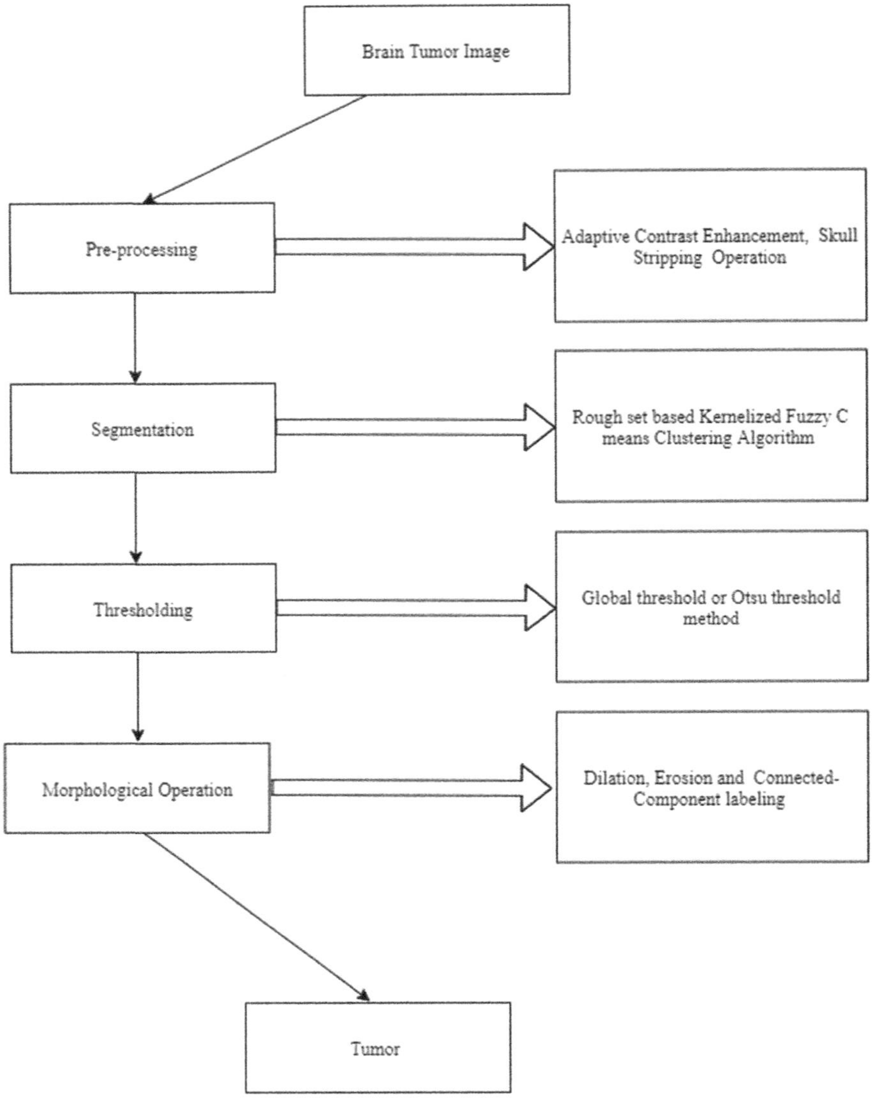

Fig. 8.4 Block diagram of the tumor extraction method

This section exhibits the performance of the proposed method on two benchmark data sets, Harvard and BRATS2013, and one real patient data set collected from M. R. Bangur Hospital in Kolkata. The results of the proposed method on the classification and extraction of brain MRI images are presented. The testing of the results has been done in two parts. In the first part, some brain MRI images from the Harvard data set and BRATS2013 data set are used. All the images are downloaded from cites [33, 34]. In the second part, real patient brain MRI images that are collected from M. R. Bangur Hospital in Kolkata have been tested. Detailed information on the collected data set is tabulated in Table 8.1. Also, training and testing data set for the classification, we have shown the data set in Table 8.2.

The comparative performance of the proposed algorithm is reported with respect to accuracy(f_{acc}), sensitivity(f_{sen}), specificity(f_{sp}), and area under the ROC curve (f_{AUC}). Equations 8.18–8.21 are used to calculate f_{acc}, f_{sen}, f_{sp}, and f_{AUC}. Tumor brain MRI images designate True Positive (X_P). True Negative (X_N) indicates the tumor free images. False Positive (W_P) points to the wrong detection of tumor free images. Tumor images are detected as tumor free images that are denoted as False Negative (W_N). The classification rate of the three data sets are tabulated in Table 8.3.

$$f_{acc} = \frac{X_P + X_N}{X_P + X_N + W_P + W_N} \tag{8.18}$$

$$f_{sen} = \frac{X_P}{X_P + W_N} \tag{8.19}$$

$$f_{sp} = \frac{X_N}{X_N + W_P} \tag{8.20}$$

$$f_{AUC} = \frac{1}{2} \times [\frac{X_P}{X_P + W_N} + \frac{X_N}{X_N + W_P}] \tag{8.21}$$

Table 8.1 Collected tumor and non-tumor data set from Harvard, BRATS2013 and real patient data set from M. R. Bangur Hospital

	Normal image	Tumor image	Total
Harvard	44	72	116
BRATS2013	58	76	134
M. R. Bangur Hospital	34	39	73

Table 8.2 Training and testing sample of different data sets

Datset	Training images		Testing images	
	Normal	Abnormal	Normal	Abnormal
Harvard	36	38	8	34
BRATS2013	34	40	24	36
M. R. Bangur Hospital	20	18	14	21

Table 8.3 Classification rates for the proposed method

Datset	T_P	T_N	F_P	F_N
Harvard	34	7	0	1
BRATS2013	35	23	1	1
M. R. Bangur Hospital	20	13	1	1

(1) *Results on Simulated Harvard and BRATS2013 data set*: To analyze the performance of the proposed technique on the Harvard data set, the experimental results for classification and segmentation of cancerous cells with different existing techniques like Discrete Wavelet Transformation (DWT) with Support Vector Machine (SOM) [35], DWT with SVM with linear kernel [35], DWT with PCA and ANN [15], SOM with FKM [36], SOM with fuzzy K means (FKM) [36], FCM, R-kmeans, KFCM, and MLS-CNN [24] are compared. For the experiment, 116 T2-type brain MRI images from Harvard dataset in which 44 normal images and 72 images with tumor are used. A few samples of T2-type brain MRI images with normal, Glioma, Metastatic bronchogenic carcinoma, Meningioma, and Sarcoma are shown in Fig. 8.5. The classification results of these above methods are shown in Table 8.4. From the tested results, it is noticed that the performance of the proposed system is superior as compared to previous methods.

Five different existing methods: Multifractal Detrended Fluctuation Analysis (MFDFA) [37], SVM Random Forest Classifier DWT [38], FCM, R-kmeans, KFCM methods, and the proposed method are applied on BRATS2013 benchmark data set for the comparison of classification results. BRATS2013 data set consists of 134 T1-type brain MRI images in which 76 with tumor and 58 tumor free images. The proposed technique successfully classifies the tumor images that are shown in Table 8.5. The results of Tables 8.4 and 8.5 indicate that the overall performance of the proposed system is better as compared to the five previous methods. Figure 8.6 displays samples of T1-type brain MRI images from the BRATS2013 data set.

(2) *Results on Real Brain MR Images*: After verifying the tested results on the above two benchmark data sets, the proposed method is applied to real patient data set which is collected from M. R. Bangur Hospital. The parameters f_{acc}, f_{sen}, f_{sp}, and f_{AUC} are calculated and shown in Table 8.6 which are very satisfactory. Some samples of T1-type brain MRI images are shown in Fig. 8.7.

Also, results of the segmentation accuracy have been compiled for the extraction of the brain tumor region. The segmentation accuracy (f_{acc}) and sensitivity (f_{sen}) are computed for the proposed method on Harvard, BRATS 2013 data sets. The results of f_{acc} and f_{sen} are shown in Tables 8.7 and 8.8. The average f_{acc} and f_{sen} value of the Harvard data set is 95.09% and 93.37% respectively. The highest f_{acc} value is 96.44% and f_{sen} is 94.85%. Also, the overall average f_{acc} and f_{sen} value of the BRATS2013 data set are 95.38% and 93.61% respectively. The ground truth image of the real patient data set is collected from the radiologist of the Hospital. A few numerical f_{acc} and f_{sen} results are shown in Table 8.9. The overall average f_{acc} and

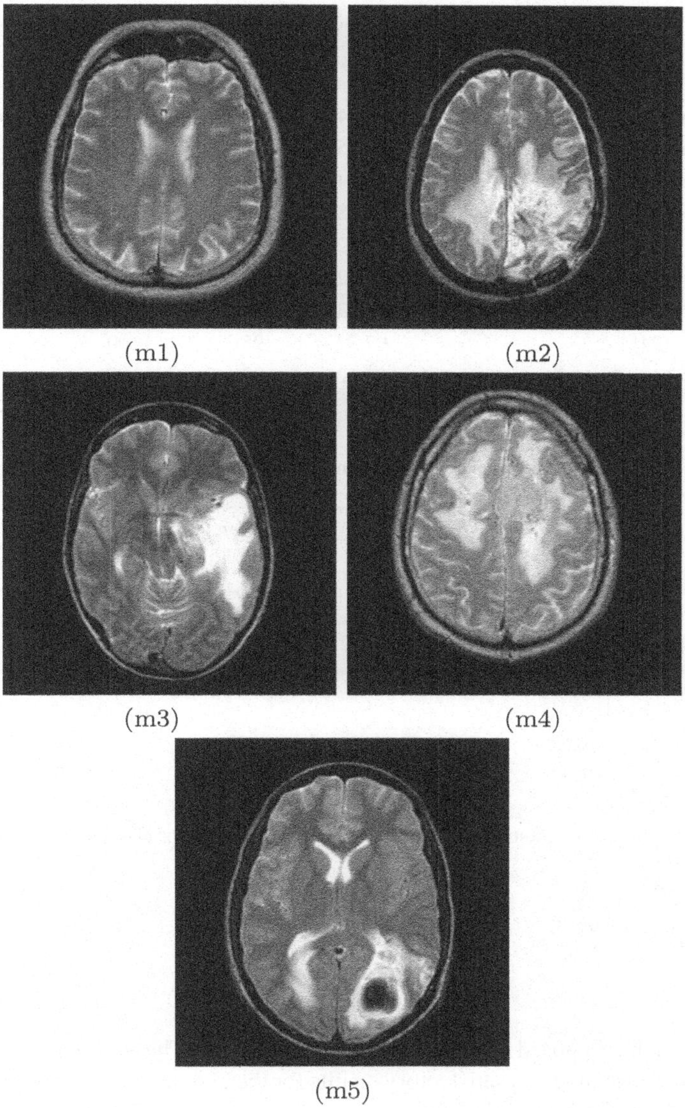

Fig. 8.5 Sample T2-weighted MRI brain images collected from Harvard dataset: (m1) Normal brain image (m2) Glioma (m3) Metastatic bronchogenic carcioma (m4) Meningioma (m5) Sarcoma

Table 8.4 f_{acc}, f_{sen}, f_{sp}, and f_{AUC} value on tumor and non-tumor classification results on Harvard data set

Methods	f_{acc}	f_{sen}	f_{sp}	f_{AUC}
DWT with SOM [35]	94.34	95.83	80	87.92
DWT with SVM and linear kernel [35]	96.15	97.83	83.33	90.58
DWT with PCA and ANN [15]	97.14	98.33	90	94.17
SOM and FKM [36]	96.18	95.10	92.50	96.23
FCM	93.02	97.05	77.77	87.41
R-kmeans	93.02	97.05	77.77	87.41
KFCM	95.23	97.05	87.50	92.27
MLS-CNN [24]	97.37	95	100	97.5
Prop. Method	97.62	97.14	100	98.57

Table 8.5 f_{acc}, f_{sen}, f_{sp}, and f_{AUC} values on tumor and non-tumor classification results on BRATS2013 data set

Methods	f_{acc}	f_{sen}	f_{sp}	f_{AUC}
FCM	78.67	82.93	73.53	78.23
R-kmeans	74.67	82.93	64.71	73.82
KFCM	74.67	82.93	64.71	73.82
MFDFA [37]	86.70	86.05	87.50	86.77
SVM with DWT [38]	95	100	90	94.93
Prop. Method	96.67	97.22	95.83	96.53

Table 8.6 f_{acc}, f_{sen}, f_{sp}, and f_{AUC} values on tumor and non-tumor classification results on real patient data set Z

Methods	f_{acc}	f_{sen}	f_{sp}	f_{AUC}
Prop. Method	94.29	95.24	92.86	94.05

f_{sen} value of the proposed method is 93.75% and 91.87%. The overall performance of the proposed system gives satisfactory results for the classification and segmentation of different types of brain MRI images.

After the classification and segmentation, the tumor is successfully extracted from brain images using our proposed method. The extracted tumor region are displayed in Figs. 8.8, 8.9 and 8.10. It is noticed from all the tabulated results and output figures that the proposed method presents very acceptable results.

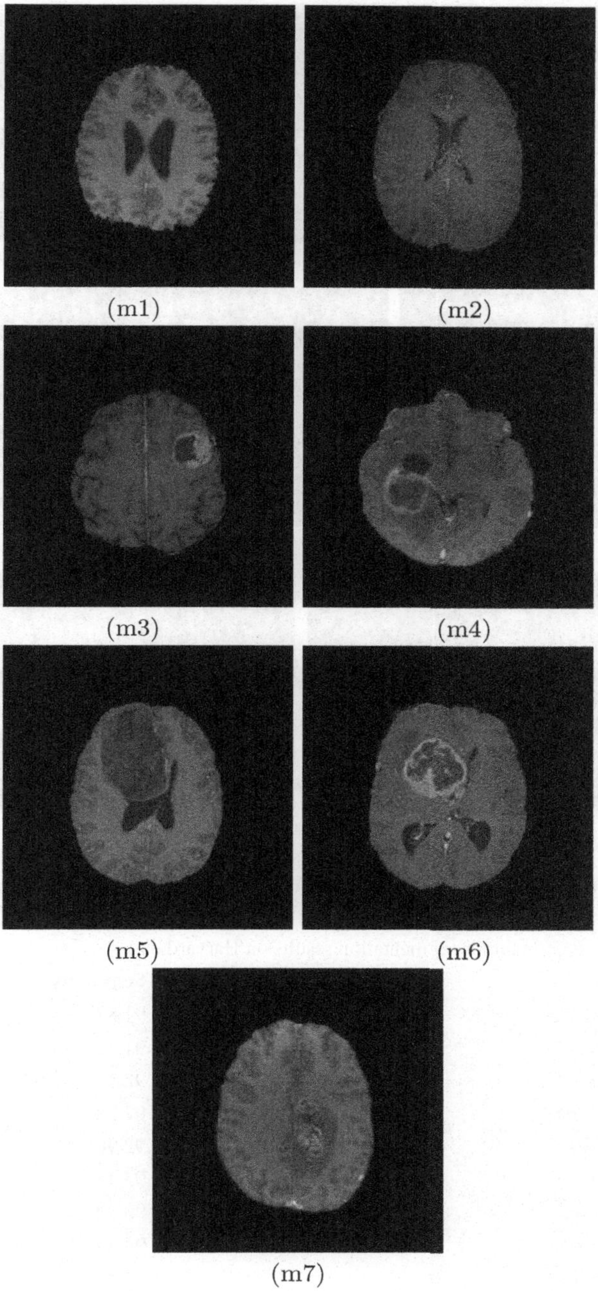

Fig. 8.6 Samples of T2-weighted MRI brain images collected from BRATS2013 data set

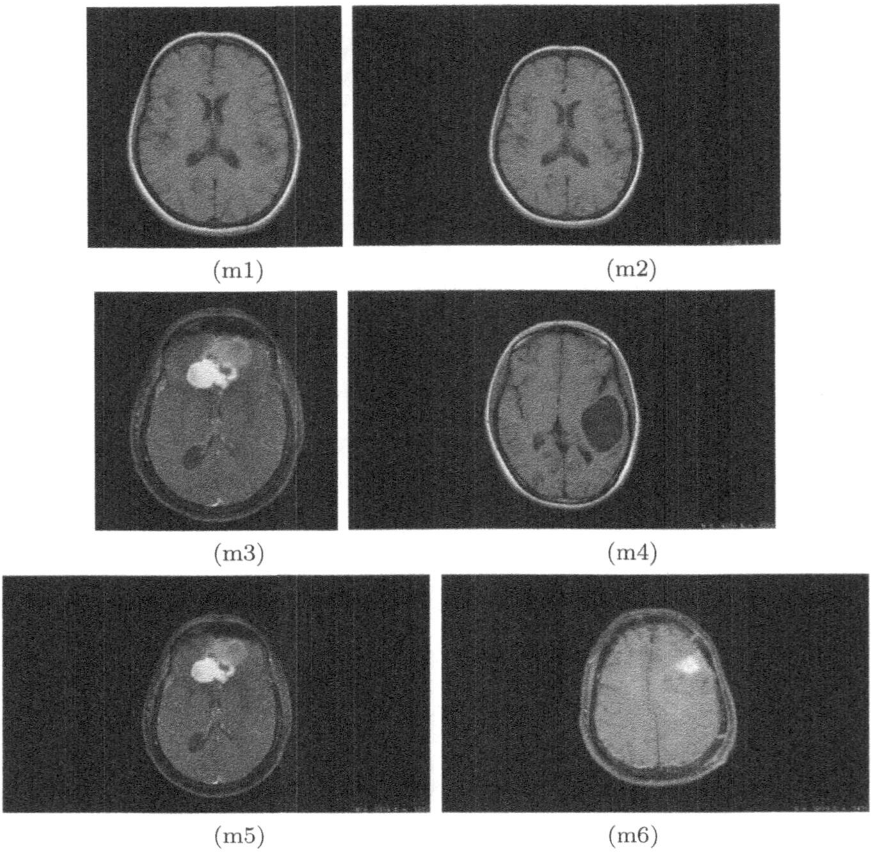

Fig. 8.7 Samples of T2-weighted MRI brain images collected from the real patient data set

Table 8.7 f_{acc}, f_{sen} on tumor segmentation results on Harvard data set

$Image\_number$	Accuracy	Sensitivity
$Harvard\_Image1$	93.18	91.87
$Harvard\_Image2$	93.69	91.89
$Harvard\_Image3$	94.88	92.52
$Harvard\_Image4$	94.67	92.88
$Harvard\_Image5$	94.78	92.90
$Harvard\_Image6$	95.84	93.75
$Harvard\_Image7$	95.56	93.79
$Harvard\_Image8$	96.44	94.45
$Harvard\_Image9$	96.32	94.85
$Harvard\_Image10$	95.61	94.83

Table 8.8 f_{acc} and f_{sen} tumor segmentation results on BRATS2013 data set

$Image\_number$	Accuracy	Sensitivity
$Brats\_Image1$	96.09	94.78
$Brats\_Image2$	95.00	93.19
$Brats\_Image3$	95.39	93.52
$Brats\_Image4$	94.76	92.88
$Brats\_Image5$	94.92	92.90
$Brats\_Image6$	95.65	93.75
$Brats\_Image7$	94.89	92.79
$Brats\_Image8$	96.06	94.45
$Brats\_Image9$	96.0	94.85
$Brats\_Image10$	95.09	93.03

Table 8.9 Real patient images on tumor segmentation results on M. R. Bangur data set

$Image\_number$	Accuracy	Sensitivity
$Image1$	92.77	90.56
$Image2$	92.32	90.23
$Image3$	93.78	91.56
$Image4$	93.	91.88
$Image5$	93.78	91.87
$Image6$	94.42	92.75
$Image7$	94.89	92.79
$Image8$	94.35	92.45
$Image9$	94.23	92.35
$Image10$	94.00	92.33

8.5 Conclusion

A novel automated system for the classification and extraction of tumor in brain MR images is proposed in this chapter. The proposed algorithm uses texture based statistical features that are extracted using a new reduction approach. The most significant part of this work is the use of the RKFCM clustering method that selects important features reducing redundancy. The RKFCM method is also applied to the MRI images for segmentation. In both cases, it has been observed that the algorithm gives superior results. In the experiment, both T1 and T2 types of brain MRI images are tested. The testing is performed on three data sets like Harvard, BRATS 2013, and real patient data set.

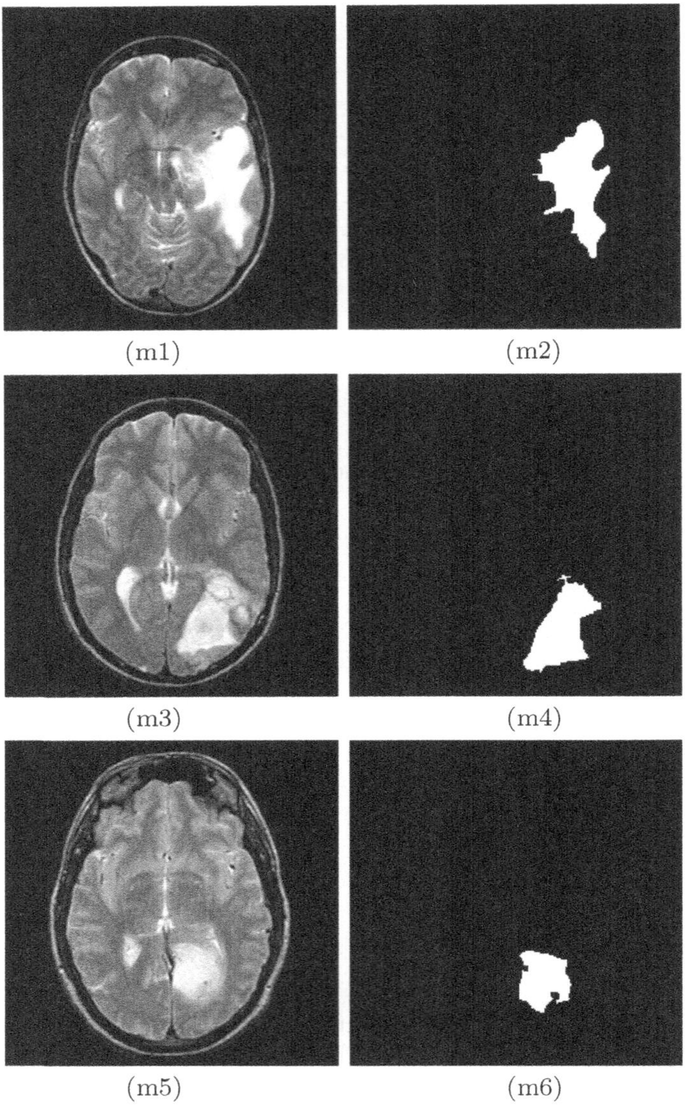

Fig. 8.8 Samples of T2-weighted MRI brain images collected from Harvard data set

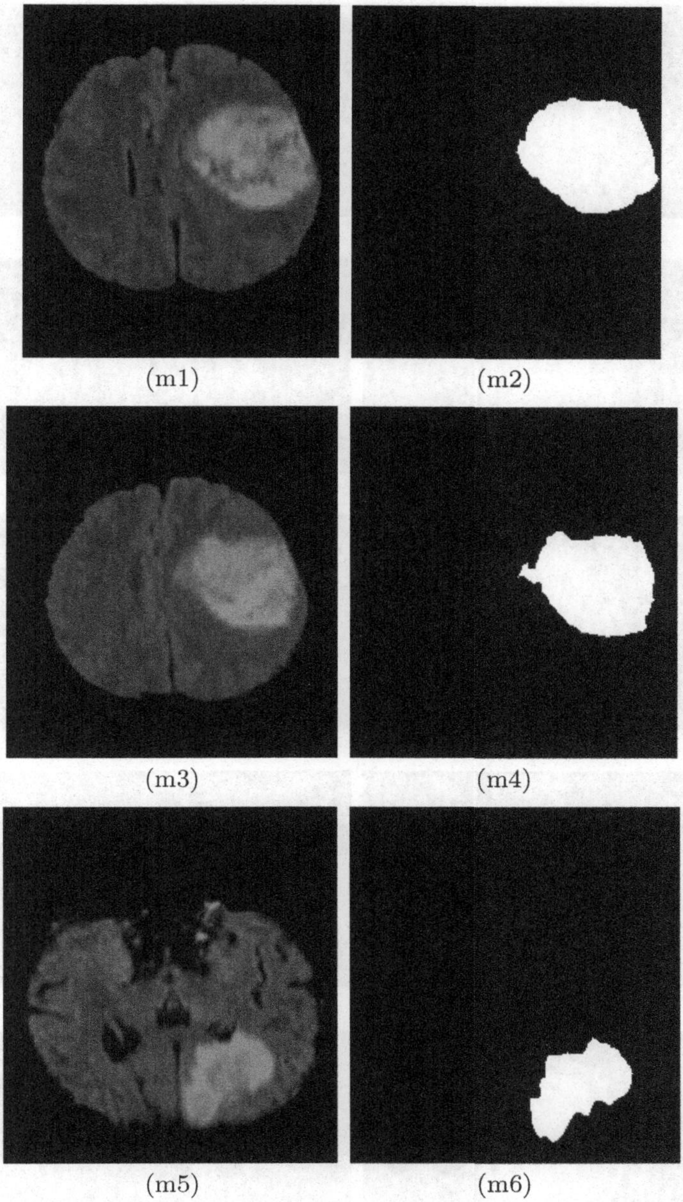

Fig. 8.9 Sample T2-weighted MRI brain images collected from BRATS2013 data set

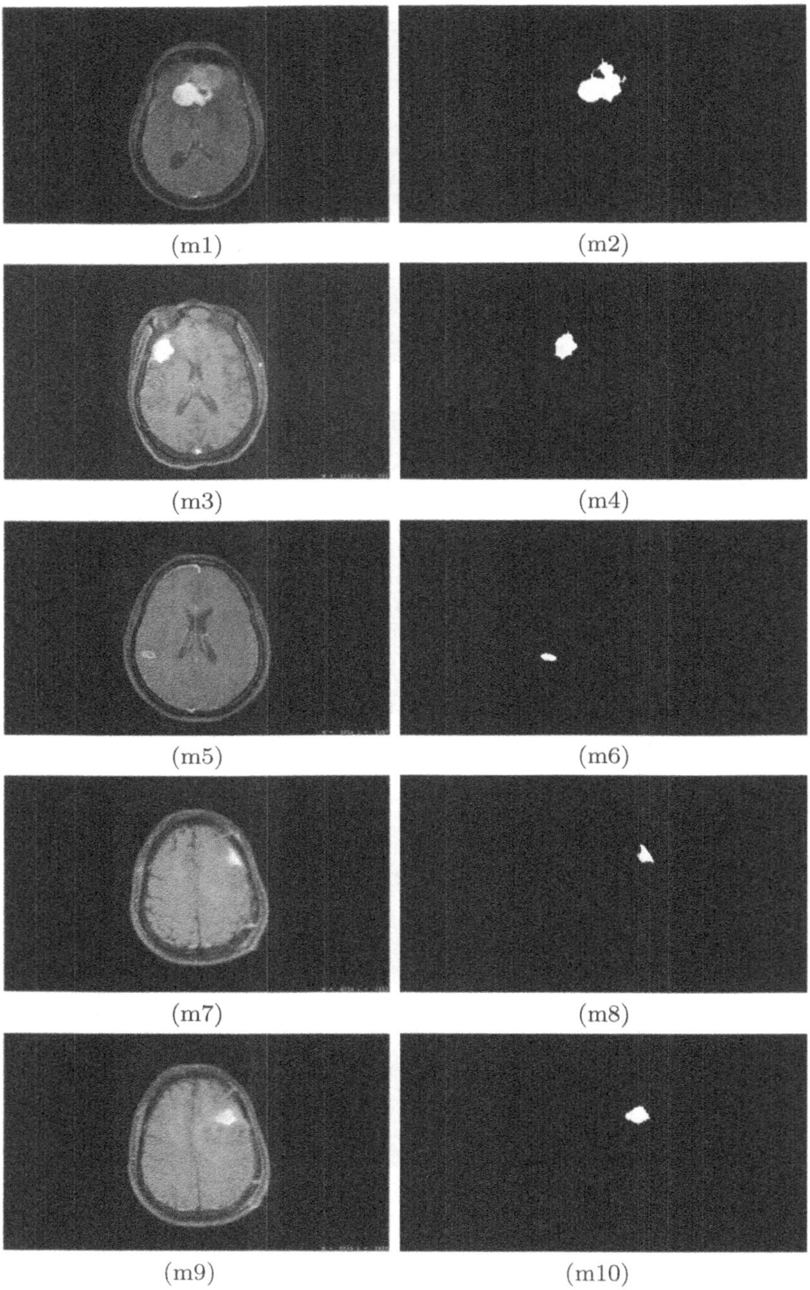

Fig. 8.10 Sample T2-weighted MRI brain images collected from real patient data set

In the recent past, machine learning and deep learning model has exposed a lot of interest in medical imaging. As a future work deep learning technique may be used to see if it improves system accuracy and also help to build a more robust and efficient system. Also, in the future, a system may be developed that can automatically and accurately detect different grades (I, II, III, and IV) of the cancer cells.

References

1. Rajasekaran, K.A., Gounder, C.C.: Advanced Brain Tumour Segmentation from MRI Images, pp. 83–108. Basic Physical Principles and Clinical Applications, High-Resolution Neuroimaging (2018)
2. Louis, D.N., Perry, A., Reifenberger et al.: The 2016 World Health Organization classification of tumors of the central nervous system: a summary. Acta Neuropathologica **131**, 803–820 (2016)
3. Gerig, G., Jomier, M., Chakos, M.: Valmet: a new validation tool for assessing and improving 3D object segmentation. Proceedings in International Conference on Medical Image Computing and Computer-Assisted Intervention, pp. 516–523 (2001)
4. Prastawa, M., Bullitt, E., Ho, S., Gerig, G.: Robust estimation for brain tumor segmentation. Proceedings in International Conference on Medical Image Computing and Computer-Assisted Intervention, pp. 530–537 (2003)
5. Devos, A., Lukas, L., Suykens, et al.: Classification of brain tumours using short echo time 1H MR spectra. J. Magn. Reson. **170**(1), 164–175 (2004)
6. Zach, L., Guez, D., Last, et al.: Delayed contrast extravasation MRI for depicting tumor and non-tumoral tissues in primary and metastatic brain tumors. PloS One **7**(12) (2012)
7. Nabizadeh, N., John, N., Wright, C.: Histogram-based gravitational optimization algorithm on single MR modality for automatic brain lesion detection and segmentation. Expert Syst. Applic. **41**(17), 7820–7836 (2014)
8. Abdel-Maksoud, E., Elmogy, M., Al-Awadi, R.: Brain tumor segmentation based on a hybrid clustering technique. Egyptian Inform. J. **16**(1), 71–81 (2015)
9. Menze, B.H., Jakab, A., Bauer, S., et al.: The multimodal brain tumor image segmentation benchmark (BRATS). IEEE Trans. Med. Imaging **34**(10), 1993–2024 (2014)
10. Nabizadeh, N., Kubat, M.: Brain tumors detection and segmentation in MR images: gabor wavelet vs. statistical features. Comput. Electr. Eng. **45**, 286–301 (2015)
11. Hasan, A.M., Meziane, F., Aspin, R., Jalab, H.A.: Segmentation of brain tumors in MRI images using three-dimensional active contour without edge. Symmetry **8**(11), 132–143 (2016)
12. Subashini, M.M., Sahoo, S.K., Sunil, V., Easwaran, S.: A non-invasive methodology for the grade identification of astrocytoma using image processing and artificial intelligence techniques. Expert Syst. Appl. **43**, 186–196 (2016)
13. Corso, J.J., Sharon, E., Dube, et al.: Efficient multilevel brain tumor segmentation with integrated bayesian model classification. IEEE Trans. Med. Imaging **27**(5), 629–640 (2008)
14. Zacharaki, E.I., Wang, S., Chawla, et al.: Classification of brain tumor type and grade using MRI texture and shape in a machine learning scheme. Magn Reson Med: Offic J Int Soc Magn Reson Med **62**(2), 1609–1618 (2009)
15. El-Dahshan, E.-S.A., Hosny, T., Salem, A.-B.M.: Hybrid intelligent techniques for MRI brain images classification. Digital Signal Process. **20**(2), 433–441 (2010)
16. Zhang, Y., Dong, Z., Wu, L., Wang, S.: A hybrid method for MRI brain image classification. Expert Syst. Appl. **38**(8), 10049–10053 (2011)
17. Anitha, V., Murugavalli, S.: Brain tumour classification using two-tier classifier with adaptive segmentation technique. IET Comput. Vis. **10**(1), 9–17 (2016)

18. Amin, J., et al.: A distinctive approach in brain tumor detection and classification using MRI. Pattern Recogn. Lett. (2017). https://doi.org/10.1016/j.patrec.2017.10.036
19. Khan, M.A., et al.: Brain tumor detection and classification: a framework of marker-based watershed algorithm and multilevel priority features selection. Microscopy Res. Technique **82**(6), 909–922 (2019)
20. Halder, A., Dobe, O.: Detection of tumor in brain MRI using fuzzy feature selection and support vector machine. Proceedings in International Conference on Advances in Computing, Communications and Informatics, pp. 1919–1923 (2016)
21. Halder, A., Dobe, O.: Rough K-means and support vector machine based brain tumor detection. Proceedings in International Conference on Advances in Computing, Communications and Informatics, pp. 116–120 (2017)
22. Islam, R., Imran, et al.: Detection and classification of brain tumor based on multilevel segmentation with convolutional neural network. J. Biomed. Sci. Eng. **13**(4), 45–53 (2020)
23. Arasi, P., Rupa, E., Suganthi, M.: A clinical support system for brain tumor classification using soft computing techniques. J. Med. Syst. **43**(5), 144–154 (2019)
24. Gupta, T., Manocha et al.: Tumor classification and segmentation of MR brain images (2017). arXiv preprint arXiv:1710.11309
25. Pareek, M., Jha, C.K., Mukherjee, S.: Brain Tumor Classification from MRI Images and Calculation of Tumor Area, pp. 73–83. Theories and Applications, Soft Computing (2020)
26. Singh, C., Bala, A.: A transform-based fast fuzzy C-means approach for high brain MRI segmentation accuracy. Appl. Soft Comput. **76**, 156–173 (2019)
27. Turi, R.H.: Clustering-Based Color Image Segmentation, Ph.D Thesis, Monash University (2001)
28. Menze et al.: The multimodal brain tumor image segmentation benchmark (BRATS).IEEE Trans. Med. Imaging (2014)
29. Summers, D.: Harvard Whole Brain Atlas: www. med. harvard. edu/AANLIB/home. html. J. Neurol. Neurosur. Psychiatry **74**(3), 288 (2003)
30. Chaplot, S., Patnaik, L.M., Jagannathan, N.R.: Classification of magnetic resonance brain images using wavelets as input to support vector machine and neural network. Biomed. Signal Process. Control **1**(1), 86–92 (2006)
31. Vishnuvarthanan, G., Rajasekaran, et al.: An unsupervised learning method with a clustering approach for tumor identification and tissue segmentation in magnetic resonance brain images. Appl. Soft Comput. **38**, 190–212 (2016)
32. Reza, Syed, M.S., Mays, R., Iftekharuddin, K.M.: Multi-fractal detrended texture feature for brain tumor classification. Med. Imaging 2015: Comput. Aided Diagnosis **9414**, 941410 (2015)
33. Adhikari, S.K., et al.: Conditional spatial fuzzy C-means clustering algorithm for segmentation of MRI images. Appl. Soft Comput. **34**, 758–769 (2015)
34. Namburu, A.: Soft fuzzy rough set-based MR brain image segmentation. Appl. Soft Comput. **54**, 456–466 (2017)
35. Tiwari, A., Srivastava, S., Pant, M.: Brain tumor segmentation and classification from magnetic resonance images: Review of selected methods from 2014 to 2019. Pattern Recogn. Lett. **131**, 244–260 (2020)
36. Pham, D.L., Prince, J.L.: Adaptive fuzzy segmentation of magnetic resonance images. IEEE Trans. Med. Imaging **18**(9), 737–752 (1999)
37. Ahmed, M.N., et al.: A modified fuzzy c-means algorithm for bias field estimation and segmentation of MRI data. IEEE Trans. Med. Imaging **21**(3), 193–199 (2002)
38. Krinidis, S., Chatzis, V.: A robust fuzzy local information C-means clustering algorithm. IEEE Trans. Image Process. **19**(5), 1328–1337 (2010)

Chapter 9
Overlapping Oral Epithelial Cells Segmentation: Voronoi-Based Hybrid Active Contour Model

Shreya Adhikary, Ranjan Rashmi Paul, Mrinal Mandal, Santi Prasad Maity, and Ananya Barui

Abstract Oral cancer is a major healthcare problem and accounts for approximately 40% of cancer risk. It is evident that the detection of oral cancer at an early stage can markedly improve the survival rate. Though several invasive 'gold standard' methods continue to be practiced clinically, non-invasive detection modalities look promising for early oral cancer risk assessment. Exfoliative cytology is one such method in which the desquamated cells are collected from the oral epithelium and examined under microscope. However, the main challenge in automated quantification arises here on the formation of cellular clump during the smear preparation. In this chapter, the role of computational advances in segmentation of overlapping cells is illustrated. A computational model, based on Voronoi-based hybrid active contour method, is proposed for segmenting the overlapping oral epithelial cells.

Keywords Oral cancer · Voronoi-based hybrid active contour model · Pap smear

9.1 Introduction

According to the report of World Health Organization (WHO), approximately 657000 new cases of oral cancers are diagnosed worldwide per annum [2]. The increasing habit of tobacco smoking/chewing is one of the most prominent risk factors for the development of oral cancer. Moreover, delay in the detection method makes

S. Adhikary · S. P. Maity · A. Barui (✉)
Indian Institute of Engineering Science and Technology, Shibpur, Howrah, India

S. P. Maity
e-mail: santipmaity@it.iiests.ac.in

R. R. Paul
Department of Oral and Dental Sciences, Kolkata and Guru Nanak Institute of Dental Sciences and Research, JIS University, Kolkata, India

M. Mandal
University of Alberta, Edmonton, Canada
e-mail: mmandal@ualberta.ca

J. Nayak et al. (eds.), *Advanced Machine Learning Approaches in Cancer Prognosis*, Intelligent Systems Reference Library 204,
https://doi.org/10.1007/978-3-030-71975-3_9

the situation more aggravated and enhances cancer related death. According to the National cancer control and registration program, the prevalence of oral cancer in India among different cancer types is significant, as represented in Fig. 9.1 [21].

Studies have shown that early detection of oral cancer can reduce the mortality rate [30]. In this regard, rapid, cytology-based screening methods are gaining popularity due to their non-invasiveness and for the scope of early cancer risk detection. In cytology-based method, the abnormal cells are detected from the population of the normal cells and for this, incorporation of suitable computational model is necessary for improving the detection accuracy [35].

Cytology is widely used as a diagnostic tool in which the stained slides are visualized under light microscope. The most common staining practice in cancer cytology is Papanicolaou (Pap) staining test. However, this method includes an extensive staining process and involvement of technical expert. Furthermore, the erroneous interpretation on pap stained data often delays the diagnosis process. To overcome this problem, interpretation of the unstained cellular images using computer aided system becomes a viable alternative for the detection of cellular abnormality [5]. Amongst the label-free microscopy methods, phase contrast (PhC) mode is the most popularly employed process for imaging the unstained cells. However, the PhC images suffer from an unclear 'halo effect' and 'shade-off' effects which suppress the information from the cellular boundary [25]. Autofluorescence imaging (AF) is another approach for early cancer diagnosis, which detects the change in cellular autofluorescence status during pathological manifestation due to an altered accumulation of the different cellular metabolites. The autofluoresence signatures are acquired through fluorescence mode of microscope. Similar to PhC, AF images also suffer from poor boundary information of cells and nucleus [15]. To address the above-mentioned limitations, researchers are now employing differential interference contrast (DIC) microscopy as lable-free imaging modality for cytological imaging. DIC provides

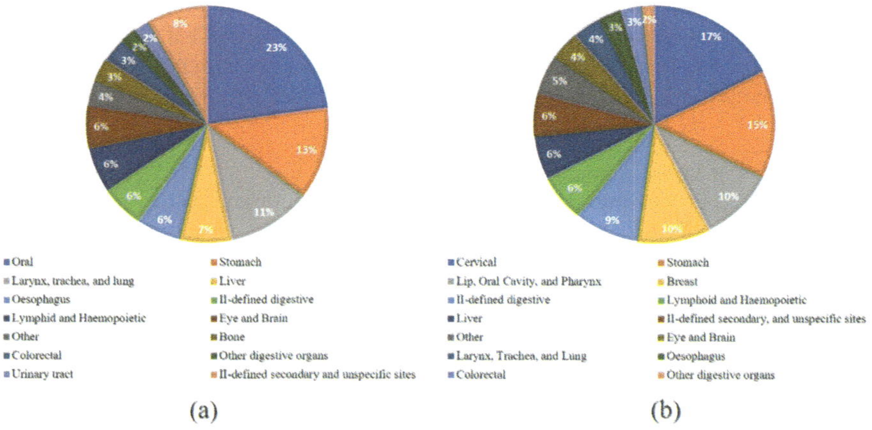

Fig. 9.1 Position and rate of oral cancer in **a** male and **b** female [21] in India

both phase and amplitude information of transparent objects-like cells [12]. In DIC, a pseudo-three-dimensional image information is obtained which provide the distinct cellular features with distinguishable boundaries. The advantages and the disadvantages of different imaging methodology for cytological screening are discussed in Table 9.1.

In the area of biomedical imaging, quantitative analysis has been applied to upgrade the diagnostic accuracy. Digital pathology has developed an option to the advancement on quantitative analysis, especially in the direction of cancer screening. In cytology-based studies, the recent research trend has been shifted towards the computer aided diagnosis (CAD) which detects the cytological alterations from the microscopy images for early risk detection [29]. The CAD system includes different processing stages like pre-processing, segmentation, feature extraction and classification. In cytology-based method, cellular overlapping is one of the important tasks

Table 9.1 Different screening methods for cytological analysis

Methodology for cancer screening	Description	Advantages	Remarks
Pap smear test	It yields polychromatic transparent staining reaction with certain nuclear and cytoplasmic features Clearly distinguish between cell components	It has reduced the rate of incidence of cancer by 70% in developed countries	Excessive staining procedure Needs expertise Excessive requirement of ethanol Needs more time
PhC	An alternative unstained method of Pap test Quality of images based on contrast which is captured through the phase information of the cells	Cells can be examined without any need of staining or fixation	Suffers from 'halo' and 'shade off' effects
AF	Cells are captured by its natural pigmentation without any external staining	Staining process is not required Metabolic features can be captured	Captures low contrast images Unclear boundary of nucleus
DIC	Advantageous method of transparent cells by inspecting the refraction of several components of cells Can retrieve phase and amplitude information.	Examine the cells in their natural state Gives the greater depth of focus Producing the monochromatic image Cell areas appear with greater details No need to stain the cells No 'halo' effect occurs	Heightened regions of shadow and light may add corruption in the image in some cases.

which prevents the appropriate cell segmentation and hence also affects the detection of cellular abnormality [26]. Several approaches have been employed by different research groups for segmentation of the overlapping cells [17, 27, 40]. In present study, the DIC images of oral epithelial cells are obtained at 20X magnification. Voronoi-based hybrid active contours model is applied for segmenting the isolated, slightly touched as well as overlapped cells.

The present scenario shows many cytological analyses, among which Pap is a conventional method. However, it has several limitations. To overcome these limitations the developed method is based on DIC imaging on oral cells, can be achieved by label-free DIC microscopy. DIC microscopy is used to capture the phase objects. Phase objects are almost transparent objects with a refractive index differences to the neighbouring medium. In this respect, segmentation of cell and nucleus is a critical and challenging task and there are certain factors such as, noise, low contrast and sudden intensity variation that may affect segmentation process. DIC image has intensity variation termed as image inhomogeneity which is mostly occurs due to the spatial variation. As best of the knowledge, there are few literatures available related to DIC oral cell. Therefore, oral cell segmentation in label-free quantitative image analysis is essential.

In this scenario, active contours model (ACM) is one of the most commonly used segmentation methods over last two decades. The working principle of ACM is to evolve a planar curve defined by two main constrains: external and internal energies. Moreover, the ACM formulation depends on the image type; therefore, it can be identified as: edge-based and region-based ACM. However, traditional ACM is less sensitive to the boundary of the objectswhereas, edge-based ACM can improve the results of boundary detection on the specified objects. Moreover, GVF-ACM can segment the cells from the background accurately. Another ACM is CV model which detects the boundary of object without involving the edges [3]. However, it cannot segment complex images with intensity variation, whereas, study on region-based ACM by local energy fitting model can segment the objects accurately [14]. However, it has some computational complexity due to convolution operation. Another study by two local ACMs based hybrid segmentation method can establish the contour curves towards the boundaries of desired objects [32]. However, due to limited global information some image related information may be lost. Another study on shape-based ACM specifically for 3 dimensional images was developed [10]. However, shape-based information was needed; as a result, computational complexity might have increased. Therefore, a hybrid ACM model was developed to overcome the above-mentioned limitations. In this respect, first model is applied for the segmentation of foreground from complex background and second model is for the segmentation of nucleus.

Voronoi diagram creates polygons due to intensity variation values using information from the vertices of the external boundary of Delaunay triangulations. Another study by Zhang et al. [40] depicted how Voronoi diagram helped to detect the initial cell region mainly based on optical translucency. However, light transmission model is inappropriate for DIC overlapping cell segmentation. Therefore, in this study,

Voronoi diagram can be drawn with the help of centroids of the nuclei to approximate the cell regions in cellular cluster. Afterwards, the boundaries are accurately specified by the edge-based ACM.

The contributions of this study are as follows:

- Edge based method facilitates in segmenting the target object with the help of gradient vector flow active contour model (GVF-ACM). This process is important to detect the boundaries of target cells from complex background in fast and reliable manner. GVF snake has higher capture range and robust convergence ability and sensitive to the boundary compared to traditional snake model.
- This paper introduces an approach to detect and characterize the cellular nucleus from complex background and cellular cluster. The improved CV model enhances the segmentation efficiency than traditional CV model. After several iterations, the noise could progressively dissolve.
- Combination of GVF-ACM and improved CV model is implemented in the present study for nucleus segmentation.
- Voronoi diagram makes the region of cell in a more specific way to determine the initial boundary of individual cell from cellular cluster.

The outcomes of this proposed model are

I. The GVF model is more sensitive to the boundary concavities than traditional models, as a result initial segmentation is more accurate than any other snake model,
II. Due to smoothness constrain of image pixels under and over segmentation problem could be reduced in the nucleus segmentation step,
III. Voronoi diagram gives the discretization of the approximation of the cell region uniquely.

Section-wise organization of this article is as follows: Sect. 9.2 presents the related works on the cytological analysis of cancer. Section 9.3 defines the materials, and Sect. 9.4 presents the proposed method. Next Sect. 9.5 is furnished for the experimental results. Finally, Sect. 9.6 makes the summary and some future research works.

9.2 Related Works

This section describes about the cytological analysis of oral cancer and related work performed on the cytological analysis of oral cancer.

9.2.1 *Cytological Analysis on Oral Cancer*

Exfoliative cytology is an efficient tool for evaluating the malignant transformation in oral cavity. The cytological diagnosis of the oral lesions, specifically to differentiate the benign lesions from malignant ones, is crucial for the treatment as well as for clinical research including the study of early diagnosis. Different methodologies are available in the area of oral cancer screening which are listed below.

9.2.1.1 Analysis of Pap Smeared Images

It describes about the Pap smear test and the processing of the Pap images.

Imaging modality of Pap smear test
The Pap smear is clinical 'gold standard' for cancer detection which uses the bright field imaging method [1]. Components of the cells are allowed to see by the light absorption in stain, pigmentation, and dense areas. However, weakly stained area shows low contrast and resolution due to the blurry appearance. Hence, lengthy staining procedure needs a constant expertise.

Processing of the cytological Pap images
A computer assisted analysis was developed for Pap smear test as oral cancer diagnosis [19]. The cell nuclei were detected by the fractal-based method by means of the Triangular Prism Method. Selection of the proper color subspace, from digital Pap smear test, was investigated. The green channels of the Pap images were specified for the best results. As the fractal dimension is inadequate for the classification, therefore, this procedure was constructed by two-sections, where, an improved separation was gained in cell nuclei in any cytoplasmic index.

Another study showed segmentation, object detection and image classification models using deep learning approaches [31]. Nuclei detection and localization were furnished by faster region based convolutional neural network (R-CNN) through the detection of binary object. The ResNet 34 achieved an improved performance on classification of the abnormal nuclei with an accuracy of 0.88 and F_1 score of 0.86. Therefore, these above-mentioned models were used in a combination for the localization and the classification of the nucleus for an early oral cancer screening. Automated classification model was established by Wang et al. [33], where the conventional classification model was employed on cell segmentation. Due to debris, an impurity, an accurate segmentation may be hampered, therefore, to overcome this problem an adaptive pruning deep transfer learning method was developed. The accuracy of this method was 98% and the method is further used as resourceful tool for detecting the cervical cancer. Another study by Win et al. [36] showed a screening system for computer-based detection of cervical cancer. In their method cell segmentation and nucleus detection was done by using iterative method and overlapping cells were detached by using a marker-control watershed method. The classification result shows 98.27% accuracy for the two-classes and 94.09% accuracy on the five-classes.

This predictable model deeply depended heavily on accurate nucleus segmentation. In [42], a novel Instance Relation Network was employed for the overlapping cell segmentation by investigating instance relation interaction. Specifically, the Instance Relation Module was applied to build up the cell association matrix for extracting information among individual cell. However, performance of these methods was not tested on the other type of dataset.

9.2.1.2 Analysis of PhC Images

It describes about the capturing of PhC images and the processing of the PhC images.

Imaging modality for capturing PhC images
Heterogeneous optical transparent samples usually reduce the visible quality due to out of focus. Therefore, non-homogeneity can't be seen properly and it produces some focal points and lines. The maximum intensity is required to study the sample in label-free PhC microscopy [8]. This powerful tool produces the images with contrast on optical absorption, scattering and thickness revealing properties. However, two most usual effects detected in PhC images are namely, the halo and the shade-off effects. These are basically surrounded by the samples and the medium. These effects are further emphasized by the optical path difference variations.

Processing of the cytological PhC images
Flight et al. [7] presented a study related to the quantitative assessment of the oral cell numbers in monolayer cells. The work suggests a technique for assessing the maximum contrast deviations of defocusing phase contrast microscopy using the morphological operations. However, inherent image artifacts, detected by thresholding-based segmentation approaches make it inadequate to recognize the cells. The technique suggests the usage of the morphological dilation to allocate the contrast in cells just as estimated for segmentation by implying a threshold value. K-means clustering is later employed to increase the accuracy by eliminating the artifacts present in segmentation. However, the result can be improved using supervised classification techniques.

Another study showed segmentation accuracy through filter size selection for accurately confirming the number of segmented areas corresponding to the number of cells present in the image [6]. The intelligent imaging approach was evaluated by choosing the filter size for detecting the cells using discrete mereotopology. However, this procedure requires stained cell samples and the method needs to be performed for determining the optimal filter parameters.

In another study, Suberi et al. [27] showed dendritic cell segmentation from the overlapping peripheral blood mononuclear cell. It is a challenging task due to two major effects of PhC images i.e., shade-off and halo effects. For improving the performance of dendritic cell classification, pre-processing, enhancement was required. At first, local contrast thresholding had been employed in pre-processing stage. Still, results had suffered from low performance towards identification. Therefore, a hybrid sigma was used in Gaussian kernel filtering with the local adaptive thresholding through the AND operator. Subsequently, to remove the halo area, a post-processing was applied through morphological operations. The results showed the improved performance 76%, 93.3% and 99.5% of precision, recall and accuracy, respectively.

9.2.1.3 Analysis of AF Images

It describes about the fluorescence and the processing of the AF images.

Imaging modality of fluorescence
An optical microscope captures images through fluorescence without involving any scattering, absorption on the sample. Autofluorescence is the natural emission of light on the samples without using any fluorescent markers. However, this modality generates the images with very low contrast and unclear nucleus boundary.

Processing of the cytological AF images
Roblyer et al. [22] showed a study for detection and explanation of the oral neoplastic lesions by assessing the usage of quantitative autofluorescence imaging. This objective based method can be used for classification of the regions of interest with the value of 100% and 91.4% as sensitivity and specificity, respectively. This procedure can explain the occurrence and degree of neoplastic lesions and evaluate the outcomes associated with the cellular assessment. Thus, the quantitative autofluorescence imaging may deliver a non-invasive procedure for advanced screening of the oral cancers and the precancers.

Gamarra et al. [9] showed a segmentation process by novel split and merge (SM) watershed method. This appropriate method was developed for cell separation towards cell characterization for multipart studies, like, virus infection analysis. Initially, a Marker-controlled watershed algorithm was applied for extracting the cells. This preliminary resultant image was generally used as the input to the two-stage algorithm. The SM-watershed method was used to cut out the cells individually. The split method detects the overlapping cells using some features such as, area and solidity of cells, and afterwards, the distance transform was designed to employ the watershed method. The merge method used the area and eccentricity to categorize the over segmented areas and employed morphological operations to remove the separations. The results obtained from the SM-watershed method showed high accuracy and aim proved balance between over and under segmentation. Additionally, this procedure evaluated the irregular shape of the objects. Though, the SM-watershed is a well-performed method to identify the cells, moreover, advanced study is required to indicate the missed cells.

9.2.1.4 Analysis of DIC Images

It describes about the capturing of DIC images and the processing of the DIC images.

Imaging modality of DIC
This optical mode of the microscope captures unstained images with enhanced contrast. It is an advantageous method on refraction difference by different components of sample without halo and shade off effects. This system can be easily incorporated in bright field microscope.

Processing of the cytological DIC images
As per our knowledge, few studies are available in DIC oral cell analysis. As our work is generally based on DIC, hence, all types of DIC related studies are considered here.

A study was shown by Dey et al. [5] where the isolated oral cell segmentation was achieved by using GVF-ACM. This study represents a method for cancer screening at early stage based on cytological features. For assessing the cellular abnormalities, the selected cytological features of oral cells were classified with the non-smoker group and pre-cancer groups using support vector machine (SVM). Accuracy of the classification is 85.71% with 80% sensitivity and 88.89% specificity. However, the nucleus boundary was not properly detected through this method. Another study showed a novel non-invasive process for early cancer screening in smokers by validating cytological features from autofluorescence images [24]. Fuzzy trend analysis was used for assessing the risk factors among smokers, whereas, the risk assessment showed a positive correlation for early cancer risk factors of 0.86 during smoking habit.

Another study by Young et al. [39] addressed more flexible shape modelling for semi-transparent objects. Segmentation of cells in DIC images by template matching is a crucial task due to inhomogeneity, such as, a cell illumination effect. Cell size and orientation of cells cause additional difficulties. The template construction was developed for different kinds of cell, and ineffective automatic technique was developed for cell counting and sizing. However, in such case templates can be demonstrated by integrating information from corresponding bright field images that means DIC does not solely address the cell.

In 2008, Wojtas et al. [37] developed a segmentation algorithm for DIC foveal retina images. An algorithm was established for automatically defining the locations and boundaries of cones through foveal retina DIC images. The robust method required nominal user input, and achieved 90%–95% accuracy. The algorithm may be modified to identify the cones and rods in peripheral samples or to analyse other epithelial cell layers. This study is mostly applicable for normal retinal images; still it needs more advanced study for diseased one.

Another study by Ronneberger et al. [23] showed u-net architecture for segmentation of DIC and PhC images with accurate segmentation results. In this scenario, another study addressed for image segmentation of cellular cluster based on deep learning and watershed method. However, these methods involve steps with computational complex and time consuming. Moreover, the specificity and sensitivity of these studies were not reported.

Another study by Kuijper et al. [13] described a method for segmentation of the DIC yeast cell images. Traditional PDE-based methods were developed for automatic segmentation, while this algorithm does not achieve improved performance on clustered cells. Therefore, DIC images cover a phase gradient, which should be eliminated first. After removing the gradient, individual cell centers were found. However, the daughter cells were not segmented properly due to clustering and ambiguous boundaries.

In this context, Chen et al. [4] showed a novel segmentation method for DIC red blood cell implanted with local complex phase information and shape prior. Based on the generalized framework for individual surfaces, a multifaceted local phase-based edge indicator function was presented to change the conventional gradient based edge detector for feature acquisition. This is an important factor for the development of the surface. However, this method was not suitable for complex studies.

Bacterial cells were identified by Obara, where Otsu's thresholding method was employed for segmentation [18]. This work was outlined for DIC images to reproduce spatiotemporal maps of proteins. The DIC was applied for working with minor levels of photobleaching and producing advanced resolution maps. This process was acceptable for the high throughput analysis of a smaller number of bacterial proteins. However, this method is not applicable for highly overlapping cells.

9.2.2 Related Works on This Present Work

All the above-mentioned methods possess some limitations and cellular image segmentation is a critical issue due to inhomogeneous intensity, noise and blurred boundaries. Therefore, active contour models (ACM) have become very popular from almost two decades. A few studies are considered for selecting our present study irrespective of oral DIC image segmentation.

Chan-Vese model is an improved active contours model without edges to detect the objects, based on curve converged techniques [3]. Another method of Mumford-Shah functional is for segmentation with the help of level sets. This model can determine the objects without defined gradient boundaries. It minimizes the functional energy which may be applicable for a specific problem of the nominal divider solution. In the level set design, the problem becomes a 'mean-curvature flow'-like developing the active contour curve, which is converged onto the expected boundary. Though, the converged term is independent of the gradient. Therefore, the initial curve can be wherever in the image, and final contours are automatically detected. It achieves good segmentation for many medical images, however it failed to segment complex problems.

In this context, Zhang et al. [41] showed an enhanced ordinary differential equation method based on region-based ACM for segmentation of images. The paper is enhanced by presenting gradient of images to Chan Vese model, because gradient of images can reproduce the characteristic of all contours in images. This model can detect objects whose boundaries are interior contours. However, it was unable to segment the images with heterogeneous intensity.

Wang et al. [34] proposed hybrid segmentation method by integrating two local ACMs. In this paper, a novel region-based active contour model was established. This model was constructed on two different local fitted images was projected by creating a novel local hybrid image fitting energy, which was minimalized in a variational level set technique. This is the converging of contour curves toward the chosen boundaries. The model was assessed and linked with several active contour models to segment synthetic and real images with different intensity. However, due to the limited global information, some significant image information may be lost.

Zhang et al. [40] showed Voronoi diagram with level set optimization model for Pap image segmentation. This segmentation method was developed with the help of spatial relationship of the non-overlapping and overlapping areas as well as Overlapping Translucency Light Transmission Model. The spatial relationship represented the overlapping area pinpoints in the ground of the non-overlapping areas, reproduced the overlapping area which could be accurately expanded by the exact non-overlapping areas. After eliminating the background by threshold technique, a segmentation method by using mean shift and watershed was implemented to split up the overlapping cells into different segment relating to the comparison of their colours. Firstly, this method created the initial segmentation of non-overlapping areas with respect to the Voronoi diagram and further improved by using the initial cell overlapping matrix based on the spatial relationship. However, this light transmission-based model was not appropriate for segmenting the overlapping cells of DIC images on the basis of peripheral intensity difference in foreground and background.

9.3 Materials

This section describes the process of sample collection and preparation and the process of acquisition of images from microscopic slides and the generation of database.

9.3.1 Sample Collection and Preparation

Clinical oral samples were composed from the different study groups: (i) fit volunteers' absence of any smoking habit (n = 8), (ii) fit volunteers with habit of tobacco smoking (n = 2), clinically confirmed (iii) pre-cancer (PC) patients (n = 5), and (iv) oral squamous cell carcinoma (OSCC) patients (n = 4). All the samples were collected under the informed written consent of patients. Healthy volunteers were selected with no previous record of smoking, chewing tobacco, consuming alcohol and oral lesions free cavities. The volunteers with habit of tobacco smoking were selected on the basis on any kind of smoking, however, does not have the habit of chewing tobacco and oral lesions free cavities. The persons were advised to not consume food, water, and any kind of tobacco before one hour and to clean the oral cavity properly with distilled water earlier to oral cell collection. The cells were gathered from buccal mucosa via a spatula and store in in a phosphate buffered saline (PBS). Subsequently, samples centrifuged at 1500 rpm in ambient temperature. The supernatant was removed and the cell pellet was cleaned with the help of PBS 4 times (each of them for 3 min only). Lastly, the cell pellet was smeared onto the glass slide and put it under microscopic inspection.

9.3.2 *Image Acquisition from Microscopic Slides and Generation of Database*

Cell images were captured under Nikon Eclipse inverted microscope (Eclipse M449 E, Japan) in DIC mode at magnification of 20X. Sample under different FOVs were taken by CCD camera, attached to the microscope. The dataset consists of 190 images at different FOVs. Two groups were nominated from dataset (i) 201 isolated cells and (ii) 163 clumped cells consisting of slightly-touched and highly overlapped cells. The ground truth images of different study groups were generated by the medical practitioner from the cell images.

The proposed work implements a robust model based on DIC imaging modality to segment and localizes the abnormality in oral cavity. An automated method was employed for segmenting the oral cells of DIC images. In this present work, isolated, slightly touched and overlapped cells were segmented for further characterizing the cells.

9.4 Proposed Method

The functioning of the proposed methodology is described below.

9.4.1 *Pre-processing*

In the path of overlapping cell segmentation, pre-processing is the foremost step to reduce noise and enhance contrast. As the noise present in microscopic images is unknown, the widely used filters namely median filter [16], Wiener filter, and Gaussian filter [38] were employed for noise reduction. Median filter is extensively used in pre-processing techniques; it conserves edges while eliminating noise. The aim of the median filter is to undergo the pixel entry wise, and replacing entry one by one with the median of neighbour. The robust median filters are generally used as smoothers for noise reduction.

The aim of the Wiener filter is to filter out the noise, which has distorted a signal. This statistical approach is designed for a desired frequency response. The Wiener filter works from a different angle. Wiener filters are characterized by the following: it has mainly three parts, namely assumption, requirement and performance criteria. Assumption specifies signal and noise as spectral characteristics, requirement ensures the filter is taking place physically, and performance criteria define for minimizing the mean-square error.

In this paper, most commonly used method like low pass Gaussian filter is used for noise elimination in microscopy images. Gaussian filter smooths the noise by blurring it. The Gaussian filter gives higher significance to the pixels near the edges. This filter smooths the noise by its blurring effect. Normal distribution is an adequate in weight distribution model. Through the graphical representation, normal distribution of the Gaussian model looks like a bell-shaped curve that means the closer to the centre, the greater is the value. These three denoised filters were applied on the DIC oral cell images and based on the results final the denoised filter was selected.

The second step of the pre-processing is to enhance the cellular region of microscopic images for obtaining high contrast towards segmentation. Enhancement technique is also required for low resolution image, which enhances the cellular region. In this paper, CLAHE technique was used for improving contrast. This technique is a modified technique of HE, however, it captures the minute details of edges and corners while HE does not. In this work, CLAHE is implemented on all neighbourhood pixels and transformation function is resulted. Three enhancement techniques were evaluated by applying on the denoised images, including contrast stretching, HE and CLAHE. Finally, based on results, CLAHE was selected. The pre-processing steps are shown in Fig. 9.2.

To evaluate the possible methods in analyzing the pre-processed oral cell images, four stepped approach has been performed including the initial segmentation, debris removal, nucleus segmentation, and overlapping cell segmentation. These four approaches are described below.

9.4.2 Initial Segmentation

For initial segmentation, GVF, an extended and well-defined technique of ACM was used. Before applying GVF-ACM, Canny edge detector was used to find out the edge information. The traditional ACM has the limitation of low convergence performance on the contour for irregular boundaries, while the GVF has been used as an energy constraint to define the contour flow [20]. The flow diagram of the initial segmentation is depicted in Fig. 9.3.

This GVF model represents the boundaries of the foreground along with the highlighted cell regions in the DIC images. Initial segmentation method segmented

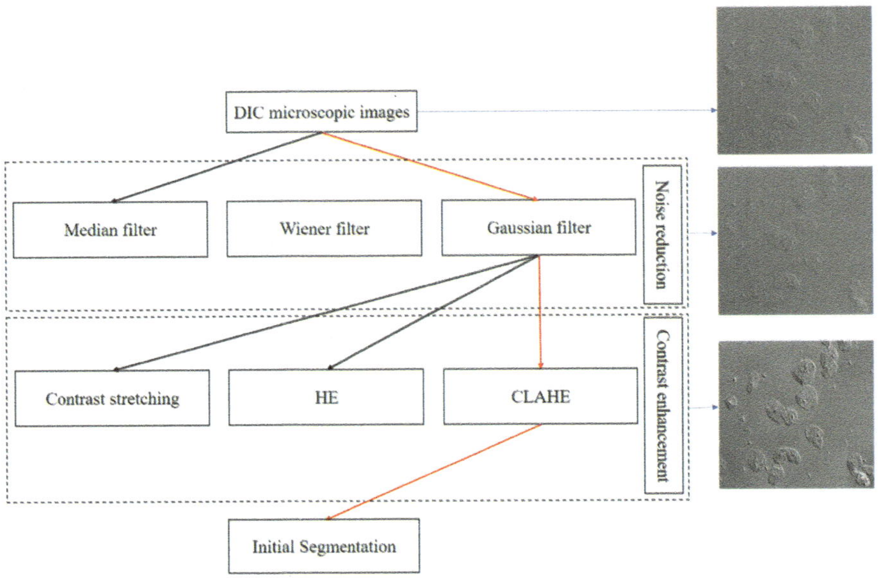

Fig. 9.2 Pre-processing of the images

the cellular region containing some unwanted particles like debris. To eliminate the debris, an algorithm of debris removal is needed which is described in the next subsection.

9.4.3 Debris Removal

The aim of this present subsection is to construct a method for removing the debris from the initial segmentation result, since the images are combined with the unwanted particles. This approach was based on elimination scheme, where the objects of distinguishable features from the initial segmentation are removed [38]. In the initial step of this method, the objects were thresholded based on their areas. Furthermore, the objects were accessed based on the textural analysis. This analysis can quantify the variation in surface intensity or patterns. Textural analysis may be well suited for monitoring and characterizing the abnormality. One of the most convenient approaches of the textural analysis is the statistical approach.

This method characterizes the texture with some non-predetermined properties that establish the relations between the gray-level of an image. Further, the second order statistical features for the textural analysis result from the co-occurrence matrix. In this article, energy and entropy were used for the textural analysis of debris and the cell region. By considering the three features, namely area, energy, and entropy,

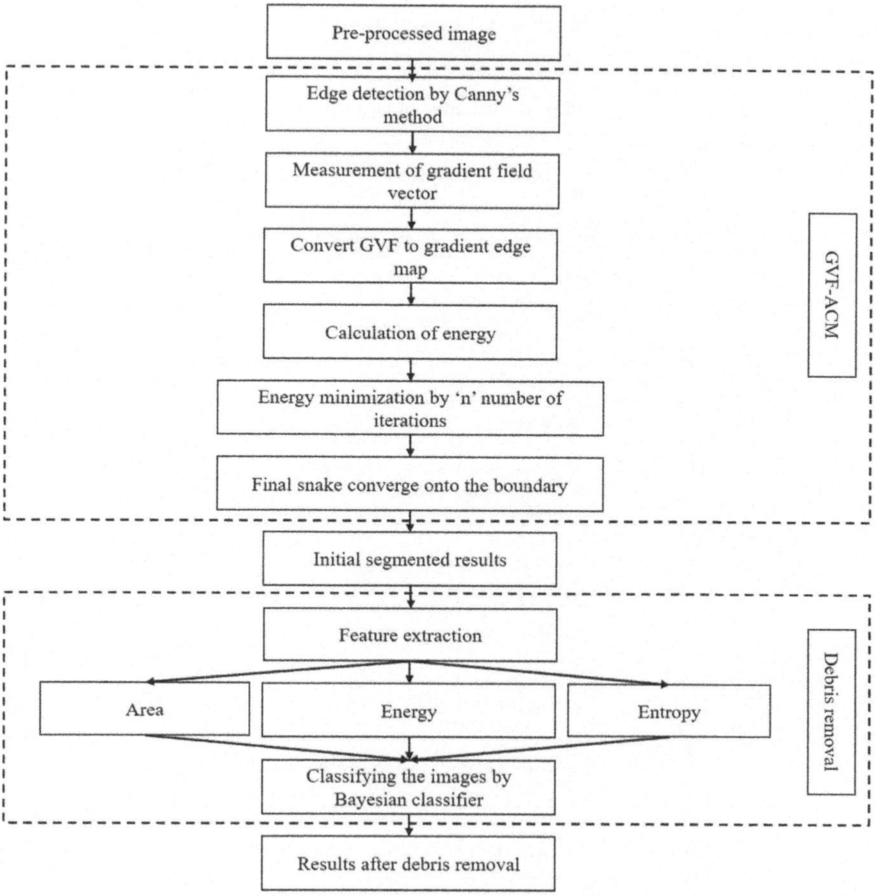

Fig. 9.3 Flow diagram of initial segmentation and debris removal

Bayesian classifier had been used to differentiate the debris and the cells. The overall procedure for debris removal is shown in Fig. 9.3.

9.4.4 Nucleus Segmentation

The purpose of this stage is to detect the location of every nucleus in the initial segmented debris-free images and segment out the nucleus area. It includes two consecutive stages: the morphological reconstruction [38] and the improved C-V model. The enhanced image segmentation procedure was primarily constructed through morphological reconstruction.

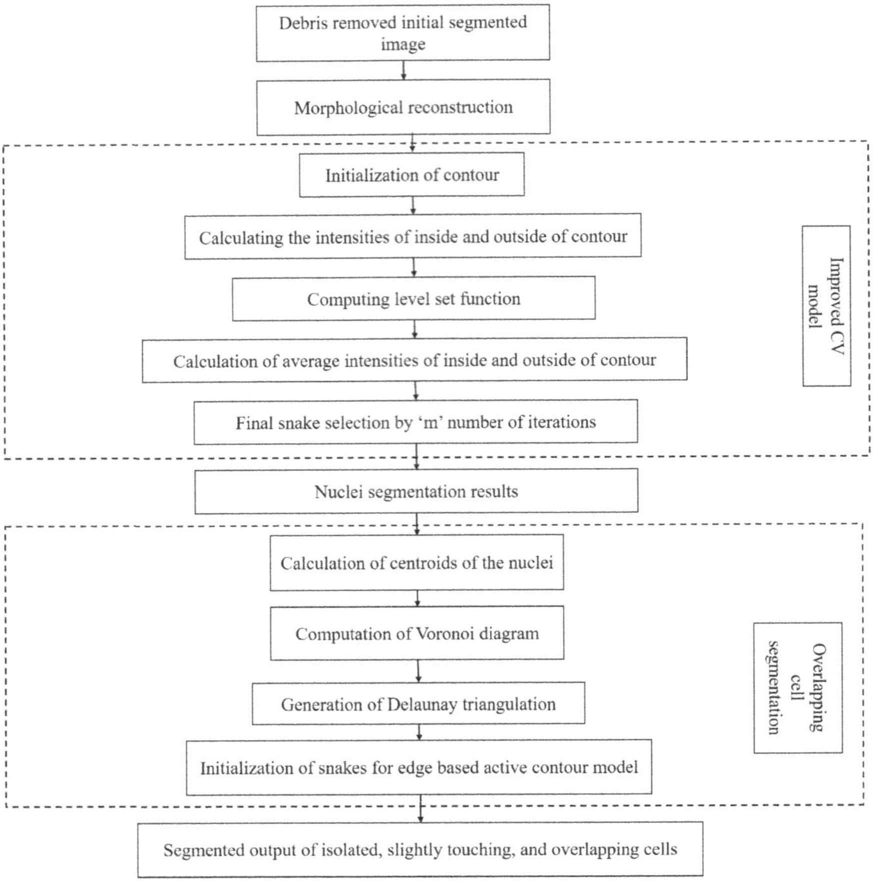

Fig. 9.4 Graphical flow representation of nucleus segmentation and overlapping cell segmentation

The objective is to extract the nuclei which are highlighted more than the background cytoplasm. Initial contour started from the bottom left corner and after 3000 iterations the evolving curve is converged to the nuclear boundaries. The procedure for nucleus segmentation is shown in Fig. 9.4.

9.4.5 Overlapping Cell Segmentation

After the nucleus segmentation, the centroids of each nucleus were calculated—they are the fundamental to determine the cellular mass individually from the overlapping condition. By the centroids as the centres of Voronoi diagram, Delaunay triangles were constructed which helped to find out the initial boundary of each cell. In other words, the cell images are partitioned into different convex polygons such that each Voronoi polygon covers at least one nucleus [40].

With the help of ground truth images, the maximum cell radius was calculated. By the radius, the circles were drawn on the cell region and initiated as the initial contour of ACM. After certain iteration it was converged into the cell boundary and the cells were separated out from each other. The Voronoi diagram representation is depicted in Fig. 9.4.

9.5 Experimental Results

Evaluation of the noise reduction filters were assessed by peak signal to noise ratio (PSNR) and contrast enhancement techniques were evaluated by structural similarity matrix (SSIM).

9.5.1 Performance Evaluation

The following are the performance metrics used in evaluating the efficiency of the system.

9.5.1.1 Psnr

PSNR is used to specify the image quality [11]. It is represented as shown in Eq. (9.1).

$$\text{PSNR} = 10 \log_{10} \frac{255^2}{\text{MSE}} \tag{9.1}$$

here, mean square error (MSE) estimates the unobserved quantity i.e., noise component. 255 is the maximum possible intensity value of gray scale image.

9.5.1.2 SSIM

SSIM is used to inspect the similarity between images [11]. SSIM of the reference image (r) and pre-processed image (p) is defined as shown in Eq. (9.2).

$$\text{SSIM} = \frac{(2i_r i_p + l_1)(2s_r + l_2)}{(i_r^2 + i_p^2 + l_1)(s_r^2 + s_p^2 + l_2)} \tag{9.2}$$

where, i_r and i_p are for the mean intensities of the reference and pre-processed images, respectively. The l_1 and l_2 are representing the luminance constant and contrast constant, respectively. The s_r and s_p are the standard deviations of the reference image and pre-processed image.

9.5.1.3 Quantitative Measures

To investigate the performance of approached segmentation, the quantitative measures: sensitivity (SE), specificity (SP), precision (PR), accuracy (AC) [28] and dice coefficient (DC) [43] are used. These are defined as shown in Eqs. (9.3) to (9.7).

$$SE = \frac{TP}{TP + FN} \tag{9.3}$$

$$SP = \frac{TN}{TN + FP} \tag{9.4}$$

$$PR = \frac{TP}{TP + FP} \tag{9.5}$$

$$AC = \frac{TP + TN}{TP + TN + FP + FN} \tag{9.6}$$

where, true positive (TP) accepts object pixels correctly, true negative (TN) rejects the non-object pixels correctly, false positive (FP) accepts object pixels incorrectly, and false negative (FN) rejects non-object pixels incorrectly. All measures are evaluated with respect to ground truth image.

$$DC = 2\frac{|G \cap S|}{|G| + |S|} \tag{9.7}$$

here, G and S represent the ground truth images and corresponding segmented images, respectively. The sign $\cap$ signifies the intersection.

9.5.2 Experimental Results of Overall Cell Segmentation

Image pre-processing stage performs an efficient representation though noise reduction and the contrast enhancement. Microscopic images suffer from noise, therefore, the use of proper noise removal and contrast enhancement process become important in the pre-processing stage. To analyse the image quality, PSNR and SSIM values were calculated to access noise reduction and contrast enhancement technique. For denoising the images, three filters were used, namely the median, the Wiener, and the Gaussian filter while for contrast enhancement the methods like, contrast stretching, HE, and CLAHE were used. On the basis of PSNR values obtained after each filtering. Gaussian filter was finally selected to do the denoising of the images. CLAHE method was selected as it did the best contrast enhancement technique due to its SSIM values obtained. The values of the PSNR and SSIM for each filter and techniques are depicted in Tables 9.2 and 9.3.

For DIC oral cell segmentation, the gradient vector field had been evaluated at first. The GVF diminishes the energy functions. To initialize the contour, the normalized gradient field random points were nominated. From the position of minimum energy, the contour converges onto the object boundary after'n' number of iterations. Figure 9.5 shows an image with initial segmentation along with debris removal. In one of the studies related to DIC [5] showed a segmentation method for isolated DIC oral cell by GVF-ACM. However, nucleus was not precisely segmented. To avoid this limitation, additionally improved C-V model was employed in this present study.

At first, morphological reconstruction was employed. This technique employed with structuring element, which was associated with the corresponding neighbourhood of pixels. The opening and the closing operations were employed on the initial segmented debris removed images. The nucleus has rough boundary; there may be chance of false nucleus detection. The morphological reconstruction removed these uneven assemblies, and highlight the nucleus. The contour was converged and enhanced by the average intensities of the inner and the outer contours on the nuclei boundaries. It was employed for governing over the smoothness of the contours near attaining the converged result. In this procedure, the energy function concerning the external and the internal energy was fundamentally to the contour construction to get the information of boundary. By'm' number of iterations which is 3000 the nuclei were identified. Three nuclei detected image is shown in the Fig. 9.6. After initial segmentation and nuclei detection, the single cells were isolated from the overlapping cells. The next step was applied for the slightly-touching or overlapping cells present in the cell images.

The centroid of nucleus was detected as the preliminary points for identifying individual cell. By selecting the centroids, Voronoi diagram was dividing the plane in the overlapping cells from one to another cell into convex polygons by individual

Table 9.2 Comparisons of denoised filters

Denoised filters	PSNR value (dB)
Median Filter	34.12
Wiener filter	41.85
Gaussian filter	47.10

Table 9.3 Comparisons of contrast enhancement techniques

Contrast enhancement techniques	SSIM value
Contrast Stretching	0.91
HE	0.94
CLAHE	0.98

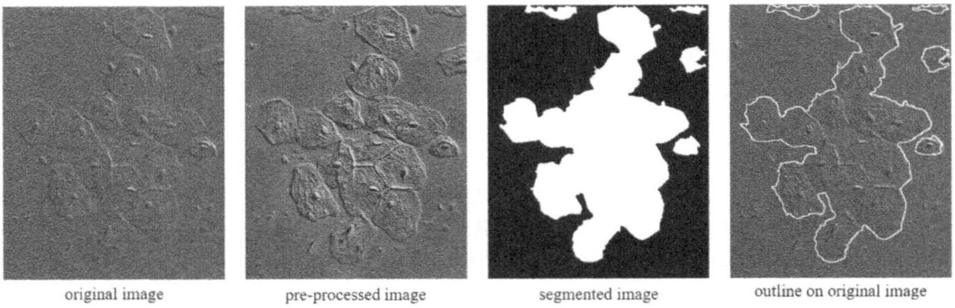

Fig. 9.5 Debris removed initial segmented image

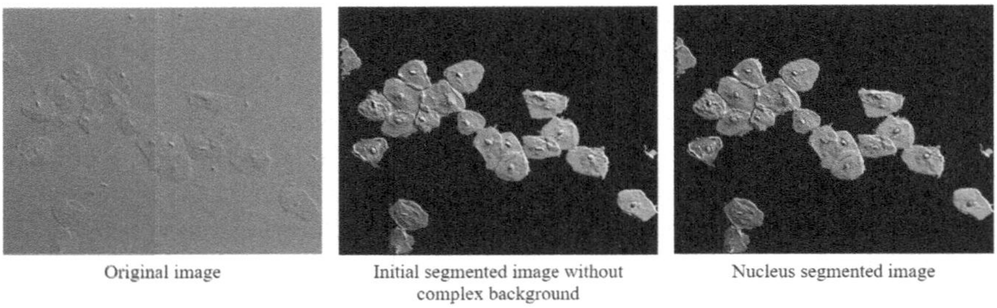

Fig. 9.6 Nucleus segmented image

section. In order to split the individual cytoplasmic mass in cellular cluster, it has been considered that the nuclei are the inputs to position the lines in equal distance. Subsequently, the image was partitioned into several polygons as each polygon contains at least one nucleus. The average radius of cell composed from the ground truth images and superimposed with the cell segregated image. This was employed for dividing the cell mass distinctly. Then the ACM was fitted out the outcomes of this segmentation of individual cell region. Demonstrative segmentation of the overlapping cell images along with the detected nuclei are depicted in Fig. 9.7.

9.5.3 Segmentation Performance Assessment

The results of the proposed method were applied on DIC oral cell dataset. Performance of the results, was evaluated using the ground truths, which then spotted by the medical practitioner on the DIC image dataset. The performance of the proposed segmentation process is assessed by five statistical parameters, namely SP, SE, AC, PR, and DC in this study.

This segmentation method is mainly concentrated on overlapping cells; therefore, overlapping ratio is a key factor. The overlapping area was indicated by the

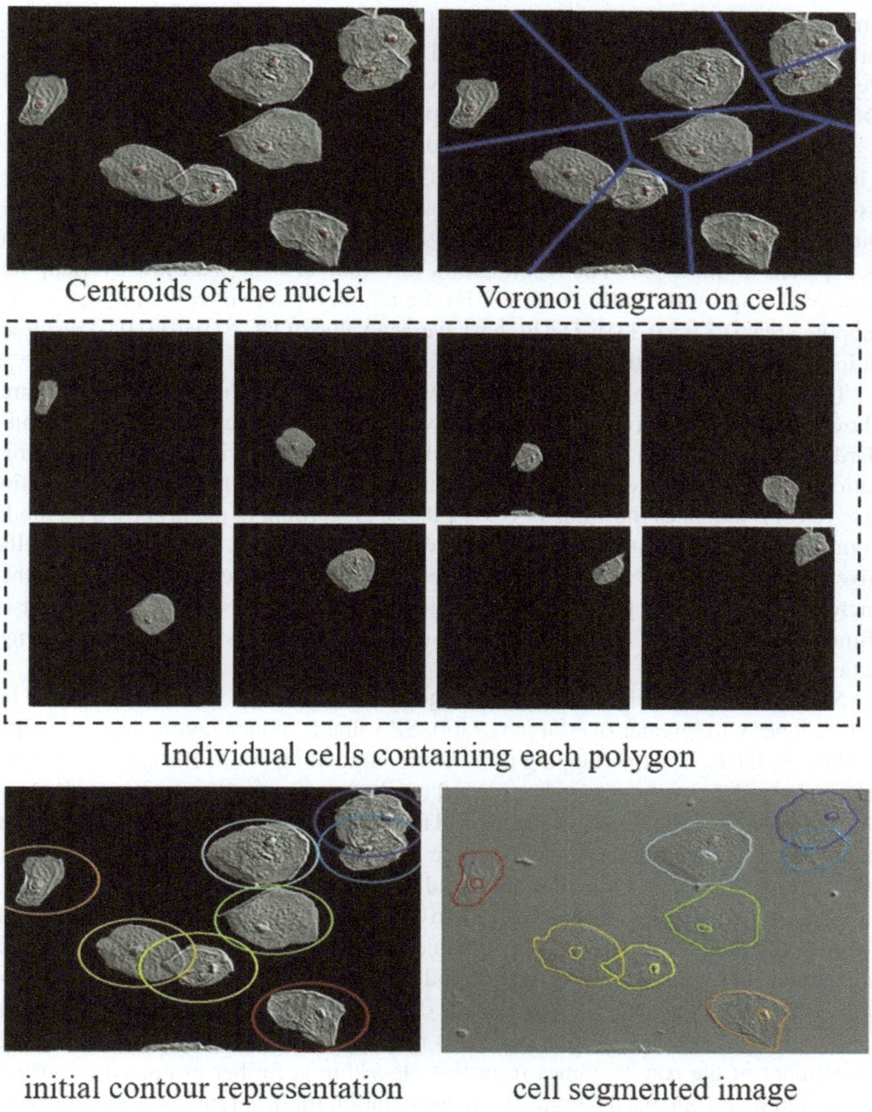

Fig. 9.7 Overlapping cell segmentation

overlapped area of two or more cells with respect to each and individual cell. This overlapping ratio varies from 0 to 1. The evaluation of the cell segmentation was typically concentrated with a specific range, i.e., 0.1, 0.2, 0.3, 0.4, 0.5, are considered. Constructed on the overlapping ratio, the process was separated in five sub-regions like [0–0.1], [0.1–0.2], [0.2–0.3], [0.3–0.4], [0.4–0.5]. Performance evaluation of segmentation on cell and nucleus were assessed individually with the help of marked ground truth images. Images with size of 1024 × 1024 were selected for this algorithm. In this study, fit volunteer, PC, and OSCC oral cell images were collected. Performance of the segmentation efficiency is directed and characterised in terms of DC, SE, SP, PR, and AC values which help in four matrices TP, TN, FP and FN.

The proposed segmentation model yielded a stable result at different DC values. The procedure was originated with less overlapping ratio of 0. Subsequently exceeding the ratio of 1, the DC value was reduced. In this study, the overlapping ratio from 0 to 0.5 was considered to establish the improved results, which is depicted in Table 9.4. The result shows low number cells with low overlapping area gives improved results (0.96(±0.01)) than high number of cell with high overlapping area (0.87(±0.23)). The highest average value of DC (0.94(±0.03)) resulted at low overlapping ratio of [0 0.1].

The proposed segmentation method was assessed in terms of SE. Literature showed the good performance is achieved with the mean value above 93% and standard deviation 2% [34]. This study showed the average value is 0.95 at overlapping ratio of [0 0.5]. Additionally, for large number of cells, the low overlapping ratio (i.e. [0 0.1]) indicates the value of 0.97(±0.03). According to the proposed method, significant cell segmentation is noticed at different SE values. Less number of cells gives an improved SE value which reduced as the cell number enhances. With the increase in the overlapping ratio with a greater number of cells, SE value is also diminished. Outcomes show an improved segmentation results up to 0.5 overlapping ratio.

Non-overlapping cells show the average value of SP $\approx$ 1. With the increase in cell number with greater overlapping ratio, SP value is reduced with an mean value of 0.97 (± 0.07). The overlapping ratio SP for large number of cells is 0.95(±0.11). The proposed process delivered improved results for the overlapping ratio of below 0.5. The average PR values were increased towards the low overlapping ratio in most of the involved cell numbers. The average value of PR for the overlapping ratio of [0.4 0.5] is 0.89(±0.09), which is increased as 0.92(±0.05) in low overlapping ratio.

The AC is fluctuating in between 0.91 to 0.95. Aimed at a high number of cells and overlapping ratio the AC reduces by its value. Existing study specifies that this model is effective for segmentation in less time and is convenient too. In the nucleus segmentation, this technique shows PR of 0.91 ± 0.05, respectively. Although insignificant false detected nucleus is also noticed this may be due to intensity fluctuation. The assessment of the results comes from this algorithm is further evaluated by visual plots. Figure 9.8. shows the graphical representation for different evaluation metrics (DC, SE, SP, PR, and AC) with overlapping ratio. It shows the values of evaluation metrics are decreased with the increasing overlapping ratio towards 0.5.

The assessment of the result for the proposed segmentation method is also studied by visual inspection of the results in light of clinical interpretation. The cell masses were segment out from the background and morphological reconstruction suppresses the region other than nuclei. This further supports the nucleus segmentation. Through the improved C-V model, the borders of the nuclei were assessed. The overlapping appearances between the fit volunteer and PC made the cancer screening method imprecise. Digital pathology helps in cancer diagnosis through automated algorithm.

Table 9.4 Overall cell segmentation results on the basis of number of cells with respect to DC, SE, SP (mean and standard deviation in parenthesis)

No. of cells	Overlapping ratio ε [0, 0.1]	Overlapping ratio ε [0.1, 0.2]	Overlapping ratio ε [0.2, 0.3]	Overlapping ratio ε [0.3, 0.4]	Overlapping ratio ε [0.4, 0.5]
2	DC = 0.96(0.01), SE = 0.99(0.00), SP = 1(0.00), PR = 0.95(0.02), AC = 0.98(0.01)	DC = 0.95(0.02), SE = 0.99(0.01), SP = 1(0.00), PR = 0.94(0.04), AC = 0.98(0.04)	DC = 0.94(0.02), SE = 0.99(0.03), SP = 1(0.03), PR = 0.94(0.02), AC = 0.98(0.02)	DC = 0.93(0.02), SE = 0.97(0.03), SP = 1(0.03), PR = 0.94(0.07), AC = 0.97(0.03)	DC = 0.92(0.02), SE = 0.96(0.03), SP = 0.99(0.03), PR = 0.93(0.05), AC = 0.96(0.05)
3	DC = 0.96(0.02), SE = 0.99(0.01), SP = 1(0.00), PR = 0.96(0.03), AC = 0.98(0.03)	DC = 0.94(0.06), SE = 0.98(0.03), SP = 1(0.00), PR = 0.95(0.08), AC = 0.97(0.05)	DC = 0.93(0.10), SE = 0.98(0.11), SP = 1(0.09), PR = 0.94(0.04), AC = 0.97(0.02)	DC = 0.92(0.10), SE = 0.96(0.11), SP = 0.99(0.09), PR = 0.94(0.03), AC = 0.96(0.08)	DC = 0.91(0.10), SE = 0.95(0.09), SP = 0.99(0.05), PR = 0.93(0.09), AC = 0.95(0.10)
4	DC = 0.96(0.04), SE = 0.98(0.04), SP = 1(0.00), PR = 0.94(0.06), AC = 0.97(0.02)	DC = 0.94(0.08), SE = 0.98(0.09), SP = 1(0.00), PR = 0.94(0.11), AC = 0.96(0.05)	DC = 0.92(0.12), SE = 0.98(0.16), SP = 1(0.05), PR = 0.93(0.10), AC = 0.96(0.07)	DC = 0.92(0.12), SE = 0.95(0.16), SP = 0.99(0.05), PR = 0.92(0.08), AC = 0.95(0.08)	DC = 0.91(0.12), SE = 0.93(0.16), SP = 0.98(0.05), PR = 0.92(0.06), AC = 0.93(0.06)
5	DC = 0.95(0.01), SE = 0.98(0.01), SP = 1(0.00), PR = 0.93(0.04), AC = 0.96(0.09)	DC = 0.93(0.03), SE = 0.97(0.10), SP = 1(0.00), PR = 0.92(0.04), AC = 0.95(0.05)	DC = 0.92(0.09), SE = 0.97(0.09), SP = 0.99(0.10), PR = 0.92(0.09), AC = 0.95(0.13)	DC = 0.91(0.09), SE = 0.95(0.21), SP = 0.98(0.10), PR = 0.92(0.11), AC = 0.94(0.07)	DC = 0.90(0.09), SE = 0.93(0.21), SP = 0.98(0.10), PR = 0.89(0.08), AC = 0.92(0.08)
6	DC = 0.95(0.03), SE = 0.97(0.06), SP = 1(0.00), PR = 0.93(0.07), AC = 0.95(0.14)	DC = 0.93(0.10), SE = 0.96(0.06), SP = 1(0.00), PR = 0.92(0.04), AC = 0.94(0.02)	DC = 0.91(0.07), SE = 0.96(0.04), SP = 0.98(0.13), PR = 0.92(0.03), AC = 0.93(0.15)	DC = 0.91(0.01), SE = 0.93(0.04), SP = 0.98(0.03), PR = 0.90(0.02), AC = 0.95(0.07)	DC = 0.90(0.10), SE = 0.92(0.04), SP = 0.97(0.03), PR = 0.90(0.12), AC = 0.91(0.04)

(continued)

Table 9.4 (continued)

No. of cells	Overlapping ratio ε [0, 0.1]	Overlapping ratio ε [0.1, 0.2]	Overlapping ratio ε [0.2, 0.3]	Overlapping ratio ε [0.3, 0.4]	Overlapping ratio ε [0.4, 0.5]
7	DC = 0.94(0.04), SE = 0.95(0.05), SP = 1(0.00), PR = 0.91(0.02), AC = 0.95(0.04)	DC = 0.92(0.11), SE = 0.96(0.10), SP = 1(0.00), PR = 0.90(0.09), AC = 0.93(0.05)	DC = 0.91(0.15), SE = 0.96(0.06), SP = 0.98(0.11), PR = 0.92(0.08), AC = 0.94(0.04)	DC = 0.91(0.15), SE = 0.93(0.06), SP = 0.98(0.11), PR = 0.89(0.09), AC = 0.92(0.08)	DC = 0.89(0.15), SE = 0.91(0.06), SP = 0.96(0.09), PR = 0.88(0.22), AC = 0.92(0.11)
8	DC = 0.93(0.06), SE = 0.97(0.03), SP = 1(0.00), PR = 0.90(0.05), AC = 0.95(0.09)	DC = 0.92(0.06), SE = 0.96(0.09), SP = 0.99(0.00), PR = 0.89(0.07), AC = 0.94(0.06)	DC = 0.91(0.01), SE = 0.94(0.19), SP = 0.97(0.16), PR = 0.89(0.09), AC = 0.92(0.13)	DC = 0.90(0.13), SE = 0.93(0.10), SP = 0.97(0.06), PR = 0.86(0.03), AC = 0.90(0.09)	DC = 0.88(0.13), SE = 0.91(0.10), SP = 0.96(0.02), PR = 0.89(0.06), AC = 0.91(0.13)
9	DC = 0.93(0.05), SE = 0.97(0.02), SP = 1(0.00), PR = 0.91(0.06), AC = 0.93(0.11)	DC = 0.92(0.09), SE = 0.96(0.11), SP = 0.98(0.00), PR = 0.90(0.11), AC = 0.91(0.09)	DC = 0.90(0.09), SE = 0.93(0.10), SP = 0.97(0.07), PR = 0.87(0.13), AC = 0.91(0.09)	DC = 0.90(0.09), SE = 0.92(0.18), SP = 0.96(0.07), PR = 0.89(0.11), AC = 0.89(0.06)	DC = 0.88(0.09), SE = 0.90(0.18), SP = 0.95(0.07), PR = 0.88(0.17), AC = 0.89(0.09)
10	DC = 0.92(0.03), SE = 0.96(0.05), SP = 0.99(0.00), PR = 0.90(0.11), AC = 0.91(0.05)	DC = 0.91(0.10), SE = 0.95(0.16), SP = 0.98(0.02), PR = 0.90(0.06), AC = 0.90(0.09)	DC = 0.89(0.02), SE = 0.93(0.10), SP = 0.96(0.10), PR = 0.88(0.12), AC = 0.92(0.04)	DC = 0.88(0.02), SE = 0.92(0.10), SP = 0.96(0.12), PR = 0.87(0.11), AC = 0.90(0.06)	DC = 0.87(0.23), SE = 0.90(0.10), SP = 0.95(0.11), PR = 0.85(0.13), AC = 0.88(0.11)
Average	DC = 0.94(0.03), SE = 0.97(0.03), SP = 0.99(0.00), PR = 0.92(0.05), AC = 0.95(0.05)	DC = 0.92(0.07), SE = 0.96(0.08), SP = 0.99(0.00), PR = 0.91(0.07), AC = 0.94(0.05)	DC = 0.91(0.07), SE = 0.96(0.09), SP = 0.98(0.09), PR = 0.91(0.07), AC = 0.94(0.08)	DC = 0.90(0.08), SE = 0.94(0.11), SP = 0.97(0.08), PR = 0.90(0.07), AC = 0.93(0.06)	DC = 0.89(0.09), SE = 0.92(0.10), SP = 0.97(0.07), PR = 0.89(0.10), AC = 0.91(0.08)

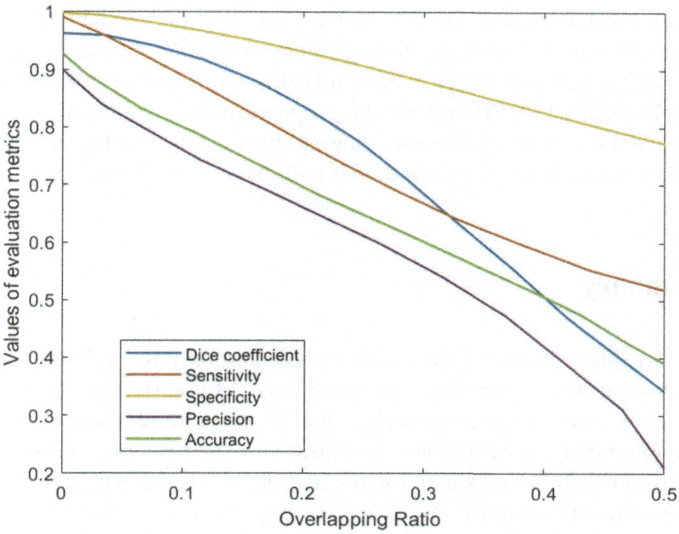

Fig. 9.8 Plot of evaluation metrics versus overlapping ratio for DC, SE, SP, PR and AC

Cell images contain complex background (viz. mucus, debris, broken cells etc.) which affect the results of the segmentation. The proposed methodology estimated the cell and the nucleus boundaries in overlapping cells. This model supported to make an automated segmentation method with high accuracy and protects from under and over segmentation problem. The overlapping cell with low overlapping ratio made the segmentation accuracy more than 0.93, while high overlapping cells may suffer under segmentation, specifically with more than 0.5 overlapping ratio.

To overcome the present problems of overlapping segmentation illustrated above, this study presents an automated algorithm to the segmentation of cell and nucleus. This segmentation performance and efficiency were also validated through the extensive experiments above. Initially, for noise reduction, low pass Gaussian filter was implemented and CLAHE contrast enhancement method was applied to solve the pixel unevenness, which further helped for defining the boundary characteristic of each object. The boundary information of the concerned area was subjected to the high-level features dilated by the active contour. This method for segmentation could be seen in Dey et al. [5] which combine the snake model, with their simple combination of high-level features and the minimum energy choosing methods. However, this method was only selected for isolated single cell and nucleus. The images were next used for nuclei detection and segmentation. By the above-mentioned method the nucleus was also detected, whereas the nucleus boundary suffers from the over segmentation problem. Then the task was to consider every closed contour that recognized this object, closed by the inner and the outer contours through improved C-V model. The increased numbers of contours are chosen so that the object is distinguished by discretising the bounding contours. Each contour is spaced on the points of the object which represents its smoothness, depending upon the application. The level set method was also implemented by a study, which showed their non-clustered mother cells were only segmented. The small cells were not clearly segmented due to the unclear boundary [13]. Therefore, the proposed model was constructed through the initial region selection via Voronoi diagram for the non-overlapping area of cell, then the ACM was applied to get smoother boundary on each cell.

9.6 Summary

The proposed study shows a segmentation algorithm on DIC oral cell images. The label-free, non-invasive screening procedure is vital for early screening of the oral cancer. To assess the cancer at an early stage, an accurate segmentation is needed. The overlapping cell segmentation is important for the detection of oral cancer by analyzing the abnormalities. Manual segmentation of cell needs time to evaluate and existing Pap smear test requires excessive staining procedure. To avoid such limitations, the present study shows a segmentation method of the overlapping oral cells from DIC images without staining. Therefore, the present study reports a segmentation algorithm for the isolated, slightly touching and overlapping cells. There is still some scope for improvement of the segmenting accuracy for the high overlapping cells. Our future work will address the following: (i) to evaluate the segmentation algorithm more accurately, (ii) feature extraction and suitable feature selection for gaining high rate of classification, (iii) make a suitable automated algorithm for an early oral cancer diagnosis, (iv) to validate the result in medical diagnosis by taking the help of medical practitioners for developing an automated system for an early cancer diagnosis.

References

1. Boone, J.D., Erickson, B.K., Huh, W.K.: New insights into cervical cancer screening. J. Gynecol. Oncol. **23**, 282–287 (2012)
2. Bray, F., Ferlay, J., Soerjomataram, I., Siegel, R.L., Torre, L.A., Jemal, A.: Global cancer statistics 2018: GLOBOCAN estimates of incidence and mortality worldwide for 36 cancers in 185 countries. CA Cancer J. Clin. **68**, 394–424 (2018)
3. Chan, T.F., Vese, L.A.: Active contours without edges. IEEE Trans. Image Process. **10**, 266–277 (2001)
4. Chen, T., Zhang, Y., Wang, C., Qu, Z., Wang, F., Syeda-Mahmood, T.: Complex local phase based subjective surfaces (CLAPSS) and its application to DIC red blood cell image segmentation. Neurocomputing **99**, 98–110 (2013)
5. Dey, S., Sarkar, R., Chatterjee, K., Datta, P., Barui, A., Maity, S.P.: Pre-cancer risk assessment in habitual smokers from DIC images of oral exfoliative cells using active contour and SVM analysis. Tissue Cell **49**, 296–306 (2017)
6. Flight, R., Landini, G., Styles, I., Shelton, R., Milward, M., Cooper, P.: Automated optimisation of cell segmentation parameters in phase contrast using discrete mereotopology. Proceedings 19th Conference Medicine Image Understanding Analysis, pp. 126–131 (2015)

7. Flight, R., Landini, G., Styles, I.B., Shelton, R., Milward, M., Cooper, P.: Semi-automated cell counting in phase contrast images of epithelial monolayers. Proceedings 18th Annual Conference Medicine Image Understanding Analysis Egham, UK, pp. 241–246 (2014)
8. Galeana, A., Porras-Aguilar, R.: Real-time label-free microscopy with adjustable phase-contrast. Opt. Express **28**, 27524 (2020)
9. Gamarra, M., Zurek, E., Jair, H., Hurtado, L.: Split and merge watershed: a two-step method for cell segmentation in fluorescence microscopy images. Biomed. Signal Process. Control **53**, (2019)
10. Gloger, O., Tönnies, K., Bülow, R., Völzke, H.: Automatized spleen segmentation in non-contrast-enhanced MR volume data using subject-specific shape priors. Phys. Med. Biol. **62**, 5861–5883 (2017)
11. Horé, A., Ziou, D.: Image quality metrics: PSNR vs. SSIM. Proceedings International Conference Pattern Recognit, pp. 2366–2369 (2010)
12. Kim, M., Choi, Y., Fang-Yen, C., Sung, Y., Kim, K., Dasari, R.R., Feld, M.S., Choi, W.: Three-dimensional differential interference contrast microscopy using synthetic aperture imaging. J. Biomed. Opt. **17**, (2012)
13. Kuijper, A., Heise, B.: An automatic cell segmentation method for differential interference contrast microscopy. Proceedings International Conference Pattern Recognition (2008)
14. Lankton, S., Tannenbaum, A.: Localizing region-based active contours. IEEE Trans. Image Process. **17**, 2029–2039 (2008)
15. Ljosa, V., Carpenter, A.E.: Introduction to the quantitative analysis of two-dimensional fluorescence microscopy images for cell-based screening. PLoS Comput. Biol. **5**, 1–19 (2009)
16. Mihailova, A., Georgieva, V.: Comparative analysis of various filters for noise reduction in MRI abdominal images. Int. J. Inf. Technol. Knowl. **10** (2016)
17. Nosrati, M.S., Hamarneh, G.: Segmentation of overlapping cervical cells: A variational method with star-shape prior. In: Proccedings on IEEE 12th International Symposium on Biomedical Imaging (ISBI), pp. 186–189. IEEE (2015)
18. Obara, B., Roberts, M.A.J., Armitage, J.P., Grau, V.: Bacterial cell identification in differential interference contrast microscopy images. BMC Bioinformatics **14**, 134 (2013)
19. Oszutowska-Mazurek, D., Mazurek, P., Sycz, K., Waker-Wójciuk, G.: Estimation of fractal dimension according to optical density of cell nuclei in Papanicolaou smears. In: Information Technologies in Biomedicine, pp. 456–463 (2012)
20. Plissiti, M.E., Nikou, C., Charchanti, A.: Accurate localization of cell nuclei in PAP smear images using gradient vector flow deformable models. In: Proceedings on Third International Conference on Bio-inspired Systems and Signal Processing, pp. 284–289 (2010)
21. Rath, G., Gandhi, A.: National cancer control and registration program in India. Indian J. Med. Paediatr. Oncol. **35**, 288 (2014)
22. Roblyer, D., Kurachi, C., Stepanek, V., Williams, M.D., El-Naggar, A.K., Lee, J.J., Gillenwater, A.M., Richards-Kortum, R.: Objective detection and delineation of oral neoplasia using autofluorescence imaging. Cancer Prev. Res. **2**, 423–431 (2009)
23. Ronneberger, O., Fischer, P., Brox, T.: U-net: Convolutional networks for biomedical image segmentation. Lect. Notes Comput. Sci. (including Subser. Lect. Notes Artif. Intell. Lect. Notes Bioinformatics). vol. 9351, pp. 234–241 (2015)
24. Sarkar, R., Dey, S., Pal, M., Paul, R.R., Chatterjee, J., RoyChaudhuri, C., Barui, A.: Risk prediction for oral potentially malignant disorders using fuzzy analysis of cytomorphological and autofluorescence alterations in habitual smokers. Futur. Oncol. **13**, 499–511 (2017)
25. Shade-Off and Halo Phase Contrast Artifacts Shade—Off and Halo Phase Contrast Artifacts, 1–4 (2017)
26. Song, Y., Tan, E.-L., Jiang, X., Cheng, J.-Z., Ni, D., Chen, S., Lei, B., Wang, T.: Accurate cervical cell segmentation from overlapping clumps in pap smear images. IEEE Trans. Med. Imaging **36**, 288–300 (2017)
27. Suberi, A.A.M., Zakaria, W.N.W., Tomari, R., Lim, K.P.: Optimization of overlapping dendritic cell segmentation in phase contrast microscopy images. In: Proccedings on IEEE-EMBS Conference on Biomedical Engineering and Sciences, pp. 246–250 (2016)

28. Tareef, A., Song, Y., Huang, H., Feng, D., Chen, M., Wang, Y., Cai, W.: Multi-pass fast Watershed for accurate segmentation of overlapping cervical cells. IEEE Trans. Med. Imaging **37**, 2044–2059 (2018)
29. Ulaganathan, G., Niazi, K.T.M., Srinivasan, S., Balaji, V.R., Manikandan, D., Hameed, K.A.S., B.A.: A clinicopathological study of various oral cancer diagnostic techniques. Asian J. Pharm. Clin. Res. **7**, 1–5 (2017)
30. Van der Waal, I.: Are we able to reduce the mortality and morbidity of oral cancer; some considerations. Med. Oral Patol. Oral y Cir. Bucal. **18**, e33–e37 (2013)
31. Victoria Matias, A., Cerentini, A., Buschetto Macarini, L.A., Atkinson Amorim, J.G., Perozzo Daltoe, F., Von Wangenheim, A.: Segmentation, detection and classification of cell nuclei on oral cytology samples stained with papanicolaou. Proc. IEEE Symp. Comput. Med. Syst. **7**, 53–58 (2020)
32. Wang, L., Chang, Y., Wang, H., Wu, Z., Pu, J., Yang, X.: An active contour model based on local fitted images for image segmentation. Inf. Sci. (Ny) **418–419**, 61–73 (2017)
33. Wang, P., Wang, J., Li, Y., Li, L., Zhang, H.: Adaptive pruning of transfer learned deep convolutional neural network for classification of cervical Pap smear images. IEEE Access. **8**, 50674–50683 (2020)
34. Wang, P., Wang, L., Li, Y., Song, Q., Lv, S., Hu, X.: Automatic cell nuclei segmentation and classification of cervical Pap smear images. Biomed. Signal Process. Control **48**, 93–103 (2019)
35. Wang, X., Yang, J., Wei, C., Zhou, G., Wu, L., Gao, Q., He, X., Shi, J., Mei, Y., Liu, Y., Shi, X., Wu, F., Luo, J., Guo, Y., Zhou, Q., Yin, J., Hu, T., Lin, M., Liang, Z., Zhou, H.: A personalized computational model predicts cancer risk level of oral potentially malignant disorders and its web application for promotion of non-invasive screening. J. Oral Pathol. Med. **49**, 417–426 (2020)
36. Win, K.P., Kitjaidure, Y., Hamamoto, K., Aung, T.M.: Computer-assisted screening for cervical cancer using digital image processing of pap smear images. Appl. Sci. **10** (2020)
37. Wojtas, D.H., Wu, B., Ahnelt, P.K., Bones, P.J., Millane, R.P.: Automated analysis of differential interference contrast microscopy images of the foveal cone mosaic. J. Opt. Soc. Am. A **25**, 1181 (2008)
38. Wu, Y., Peng, X., Ruan, K., Hu, Z.: Improved image segmentation method based on morphological reconstruction. Multimed. Tools Appl. **76**, 19781–19793 (2017)
39. Young, D., Gray, A.J.: Template construction and matching for identification of cells in differential interference contrast microscope images. Proceedings IEEE Southwest Symposium Image Anal. Interpret, pp. 238–243 (1998)
40. Zhang, J., Hu, Z., Han, G., He, X.: Segmentation of overlapping cells in cervical smears based on spatial relationship and overlapping translucency light transmission model. Pattern Recognit. **60**, 286–295 (2016)
41. Zhang, N., Zhang, J., Shi, R.: An improved chan-vese model for medical image segmentation. proc. int. conf. comput. Sci. Softw. Eng. CSSE 2008. **1**, 864–867 (2008)
42. Zhou, Y., Chen, H., Xu, J., Dou, Q., Heng, P.A.: IRNet: Instance relation network for overlapping cervical cell segmentation. Lect. Notes Comput. Sci. (including Subser. Lect. Notes Artif. Intell. Lect. Notes Bioinformatics). vol. 11764 LNCS, 640–648 (2019)
43. Zou, K.H., Warfield, S.K., Bharatha, A., Tempany, C.M.C., Kaus, M.R., Haker, S.J., Wells, W.M., Jolesz, F.A., Kikinis, R.: Statistical validation of image segmentation quality based on a spatial overlap index1. Acad. Radiol. **11**, 178–189 (2004)

Chapter 10
In Silico Modeling of Anticancer Drugs: Recent Advances

Smriti Sharma and Vinayak Bhatia

Abstract Cancer is one of the leading causes of death globally and the number of cancer patients is increasing. The highly complex nature of this disease and non-specificity of anti-cancer drugs is a major issue in the treatment of cancer. The advent of high-speed processing units and sophisticated molecular modeling software has completely altered the landscape of drug discovery in cancer research. This review focuses on the importance and latest advances of in silico modeling for the design of new and potent anti-cancer drugs. Though in silico methods have transformed the growth and design of small molecule anti-cancer drugs, but acquired resistance and intra-tumor heterogeneity are still challenges for which solutions need to be sought. Also, there is a shift from the 'One Ligand-One Target' approach to the 'Multi Target Drug Ligands' (MTDL)' approach for drug design for treating cancer.

Keywords In-silico · Computational · Anti-cancer drugs · SBDD · LBDD · Virtual screening

10.1 Introduction

There are lot of problems being faced by pharmaceutical companies and it is becoming increasingly tough for them to sustain novel drug discovery programs [1, 2]. There are many reasons for this trend: first is the prohibitive cost (estimated at around $2.6 billion) to develop a single drug [3, 4]; then the huge investment of time as the complete process of drug discovery takes around 14 years [5]; according to a rough estimate from phase I to FDA approval, only 15 percent of the compounds make it, rest are rejected [6]. Because of all these reasons, gradually, the trend is to shift towards in-silico medicine [7–14]. This is true for anti-cancer compounds

S. Sharma (✉)
Department of Chemistry, Miranda House, University of Delhi, New Delhi, India
e-mail: smriti.sharma@mirandahouse.ac.in

V. Bhatia
ICARE Eye Hospital and Postgraduate Institute, Noida, India
e-mail: drvinayak@icarehospital.org

J. Nayak et al. (eds.), *Advanced Machine Learning Approaches in Cancer Prognosis*, Intelligent Systems Reference Library 204,
https://doi.org/10.1007/978-3-030-71975-3_10

also. In–silico design and development of drugs has been used almost for all known drug targets like G Protein-Coupled Receptors like, Dopamine D3 Receptor [15], Endothelin A Receptor [16], Kinases [17–19], Retinoic Acid Receptor [20], NPY5 Receptor [21], Muscarinic M3 Receptor [22, 23], Nuclear Receptors like Thyroid Hormone Receptor [24], Proteases [25–27], Urotensin II Receptor (GPR14) [28], Hydrolases [29, 30], α_{1A} Adrenergic Receptor [31], Oxidases/Reductases [32, 33], Neurokinin-1 Receptor [34], T-Type selective Ca^{2+} channel [35], Protein-protein and protein-RNA interactions [36–39], Purinergic A2A Receptor [40], Melanin-Concentrating Hormone Type 1 Receptor [41], Kv1.5 Potassium Channel [42], shaker K^{+} Channel [43] and many more [44–53]. Cancer is the second leading cause of death globally and the number of cancer patients is increasing. According to World Health Organisation (WHO) website, cancer leads to approximately 9.6 million deaths in 2018. It is estimated that around 1 in 6 deaths is due to cancer out of which seventy percent occur in low- and middle-income countries. The five major behavioural and dietary risks such as absence of physical activity, little fruit and vegetable intake, high body mass index, tobacco and alcohol use are responsible for about one-thirds of the deaths. Out of these, tobacco usage is the most significant risk factor for cancer causing around twenty two percent of cancer deaths. In low and middle-income countries, infections like hepatitis and human papilloma virus (HPV) lead to about twenty five percent of cancer cases. The most important problem is late stage presentation and inaccessible diagnosis and treatment.

There are different approaches to treat cancer. Table 10.1 summarizes these strategies. The discovery and design of novel anti-cancer drugs has many problems. The first and foremost being the highly complex nature of the disease having multiple genetic drivers and lot of variation among the tumors, which makes characterizing and defining the target very difficult. Another major issue is the lack of selectivity of the anti-cancer drugs. Anti-cancer drugs generally are not selective for the tumor and have loads of side effects. Increasing the specificity and selectivity of a drug for tumor is a major challenge in anti-cancer drug discovery. Because of these issues, the success rate for oncology drugs is low in spite of extensive research efforts in this field.

To overcome the challenges in anti-cancer drug discovery, in silico component of drug discovery is being explored at a very large scale. Due to strides in genomics and protein structures, computational techniques are the frontrunners at every phase of the drug design for cancer [55]. The improvement of new anticancer medications ends up being an exceptionally intricate, expensive and tedious procedure. CADDD is getting progressively significant due to less investment in assets, and time.

10.2 Drug Design for Anti-cancer Drugs

This section describes the drug design process of anti-cancer drugs.

Table 10.1 Different approaches to treat cancer [54]

S. no.	Methodology	Targeted route	Mechanism
1	Traditional cytotoxics	Metabolism	Decreasing vital metabolites
		Replication/cytokinesis	Interfering with DNA synthesis, cell division
2	Transformation	Apoptosis	Initiation of apoptosis pathways
		Signalling	Interfering with signal transduction, response
		Invasion/metastasis	Stop the spread of tumour
3	Neocytotoxics	Protein turnover	Constrain protein degradation
		Epigenetics	Remodelling chromatin, DNA methylation
		Stress response	Interfering with cellular stress buffering
4	Host	Angiogenesis	Interfering with blood supply of tumour
		Tumour-associated membrane proteins	Antibody-directed cytotoxicity
5	Immortalization	Senescence	Stimulation of senescence

10.2.1 Drug Discovery Cycle

Recognizing a suitable drug target is the first step in drug discovery. After this, the process of hit identification and lead discovery starts, where a lot of compounds are vetted to classify a small molecule that can act as a biological therapeutic drug. The several screening approaches used include: focused or knowledge-based screening, High throughput screening, structural aided drug design, fragment screening, physiological screening, NMR screening and virtual screening. Screening gives a series of compounds that have encouraging drug like properties and one or two compounds from the series are selected as 'lead candidate'. Around 250 out of 10000 compounds are considered for preclinical studies [56] which involves in vitro and in vivo experiments. If the results are favourable, it is allowed to initiate the process of human clinical trials of that drug [46, 47]. Figure 10.1 depicts the distinct stages of drug discovery life cycle. The stages of drug discovery can therefore be summarized as.

- Identifying the hit using virtual screening
- Hit-to-lead optimization
- Optimization of other pharmaceutical properties.

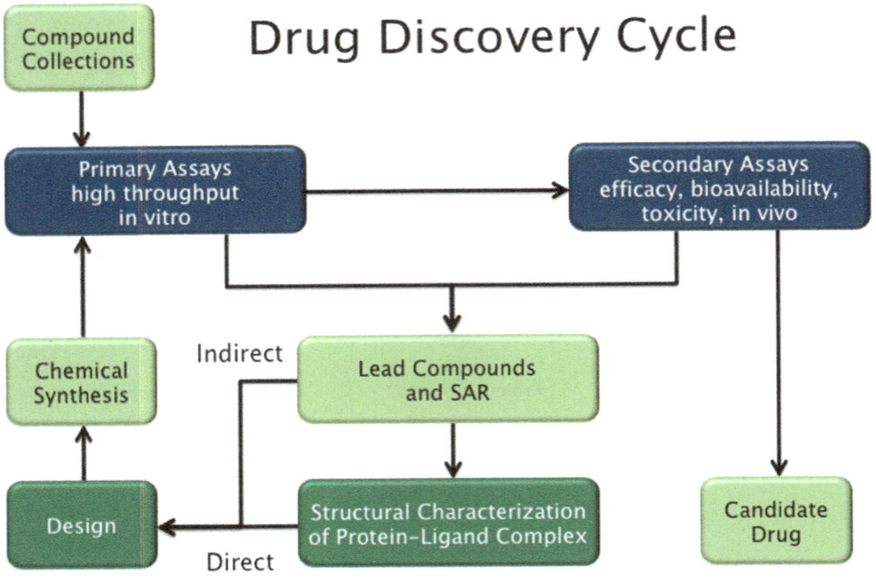

Fig. 10.1 Drug discovery cycle [57]

10.2.2 In Silico Approaches for Drug Design

These days almost all major discoveries in nanotechnology, polymers and drug design and development have a component of in silico methods [7, 8, 14, 58–66]. Computer aided drug designing (CADD) is becoming very popular as it saves money and time [9–13, 15–22, 24–28, 31–43, 50, 67–72].The various methods for CADD include: quantitative structure activity relationship (QSAR) [47, 73, 74], pharmacophore mapping [75], molecular docking [76], homology modeling [77] and virtual screening [78, 79].

The prime aim of computer aided drug design is to find out which compounds will bind with the target and what would be the strength of the binding. A ligand is bonded to the drug target how strongly is determined by molecular dynamics [80] and molecular mechanics calculations. These calculations which are based on ab initio, density functional theory, semi-empirical methods can estimate the conformational changes that occur in the target upon binding of the small molecule or ligand to it.

Apart from quantum mechanical methods, knowledge-based scoring function based on machine learning, linear regression and neural nets can also predict binding affinity. Theoretically, we should be able to calculate the highest binding affinity of a compound among a list of compounds and that compound should be sent for synthesis. Actual picture, is however, not that simple. Computational methods are very good to provide us with a direction but they mostly work on approximations and estimations, therefore, the process of designing a lead compound on computer followed by its synthesis and testing is repeated several times and finally an optimal drug is released into the market. However, still, CADD is an extremely important tool as it accelerates the process of drug discovery.

Drug design is categorised into two types.

I. Ligand-based drug design
II. Structure-based drug design.

10.2.2.1 Ligand-Based Drug Design

As the name suggests, this type of drug design is based on the ligand and is also referred to as indirect drug design [81]. It is based on the analysis of prior information and knowledge of other molecules binding to the drug target one is designing drugs for. Based on this knowledge, a rough estimate of significant structural features responsible binding of molecules to the drug target can be generated. This is called pharmacophore model as shown in Fig. 10.2. It is a better technique than just relying on a solitary reference structure.

Another approach in ligand based drug design is using quantitative structure activity relationship (QSAR) [82]. QSAR modelling methods include comparative molecular field analysis (CoMFA) [83] and comparative molecular similarity index analysis (CoMSIA)[84] and similarity searching [85–88]. Here also, calculated properties of a large number of molecules are correlated with their biological properties. This leads to the generation of QSAR modes which can predict the activities of novel compounds.

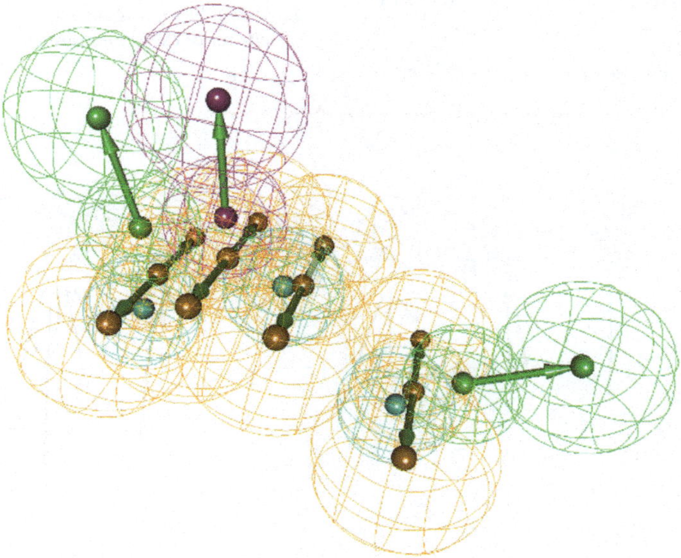

Fig. 10.2 An example of a pharmacophore model [89]

10.2.3 Structure-Based Drug Design

Structure-based drug design is also called direct drug design. It is based on the 3-D structure of a drug target and the ligand. Techniques like NMR spectroscopy or X-ray crystallography are used to find out the structure. Homology modelling is used in the cases when the structure of the drug target is not known. There are primarily three main approaches that are used in structure based drug design: The first being virtual screening in which large databases containing 3-D structures of small molecules or ligands are searched for those ligands that fit the active site of the receptor using docking [90, 91]. Second approach is the 'de novo' approach in which within the active or binding pocket the ligand is designed by assembling individual atoms or molecular fragments of the ligands in a sequential manner. This leads to design of novel ligands that are not there in the databases. The flowchart of a common clustering analysis for structure-based drug design is depicted in Fig. 10.3.

Third approach is to suggest new analogues by optimizing the already known ligands. Carbonic anhydrase inhibitor Dorzolamide, was the first drug to be developed by structure based drug design. The results of a structure based drug design endeavour would be as good as the 3-D structure that is obtained from X-ray crystallography or NMR spectroscopy. Other examples of structure based drug design include: Cimetidine, the prototypical H2-receptor antagonist; zolpidem and zopiclone which are nonbenzodiazepines, enfuvirtide, a peptide HIV entry inhibitor, raltegravir, an HIV integrase inhibitor, zanamivir, an antiviral drug; some atypical

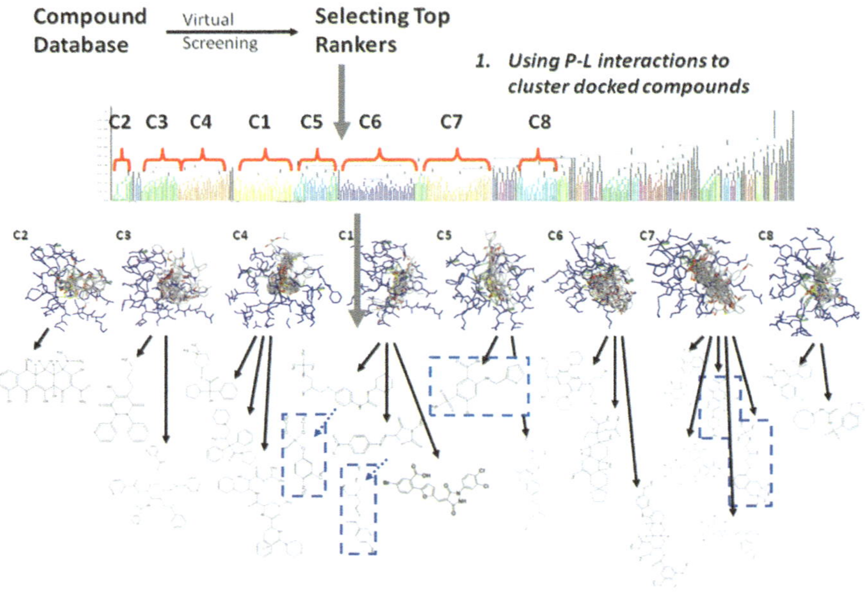

Fig. 10.3 Flowchart of a common clustering analysis for structure-based drug design [92]

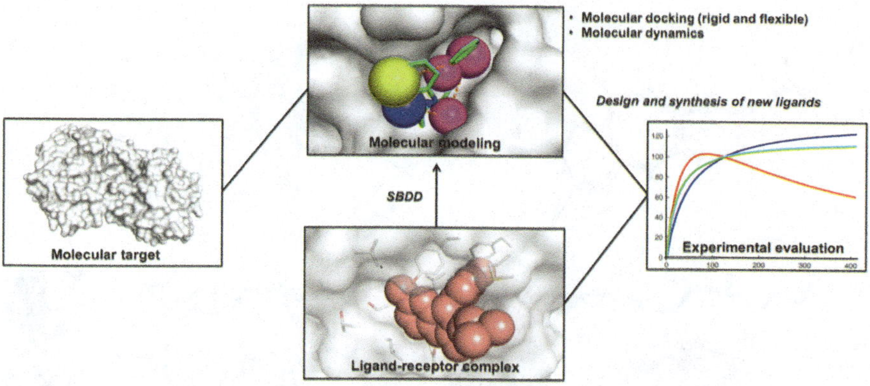

Fig. 10.4 Summary of SBDD [93]

antipsychotics, selective COX-2 inhibitors, NSAIDs and SSRIs (selective serotonin reuptake inhibitors), a class of antidepressants. With respect to cancer, imatinib, a tyrosine kinase inhibitor aimed specially for the bcr-abl fusion protein that is typical for Philadelphia chromosome-positive leukaemia's (chronic myelogenous leukaemia and occasionally acute lymphocytic leukaemia). Was developed using structure based drug design. The advantage with Imatinib is its ability to distinguish between non-cancer and cancerous cells. This is where other traditional drugs for cancer fail. In the Fig. 10.4 [93], the process of structure-based drug design (SBDD) methods is described.

As explained, structure based drug design is heavily dependent on molecular docking, which can be performed in two ways as shown in Fig. 10.5. First is the matching method which describes the protein and the ligand as complementary surfaces and second is the calculation of ligand-protein pairwise interaction energies [94, 95].

10.2.4 Virtual Screening

As explained in the earlier section, Virtual screening (VS) (Fig. 10.6) is used to search databases of small molecules to find ligands suitable for binding to the drug target. There is two type of virtual screening: Ligand based virtual screening (LBVS) and Structure based virtual screening (SBVS).

To put simply, virtual screening is automatic evaluation of very large libraries of compounds using computer programming. Basically the massive chemical universe of over 10^{60} plausible compounds have to be filtered according to the requisite criterion. Exploration of the whole chemical space is a theoretical problem but practically virtual screening strategies focus on the design and optimization of targeted combinatorial libraries and enrichment of accessible libraries. VS selects

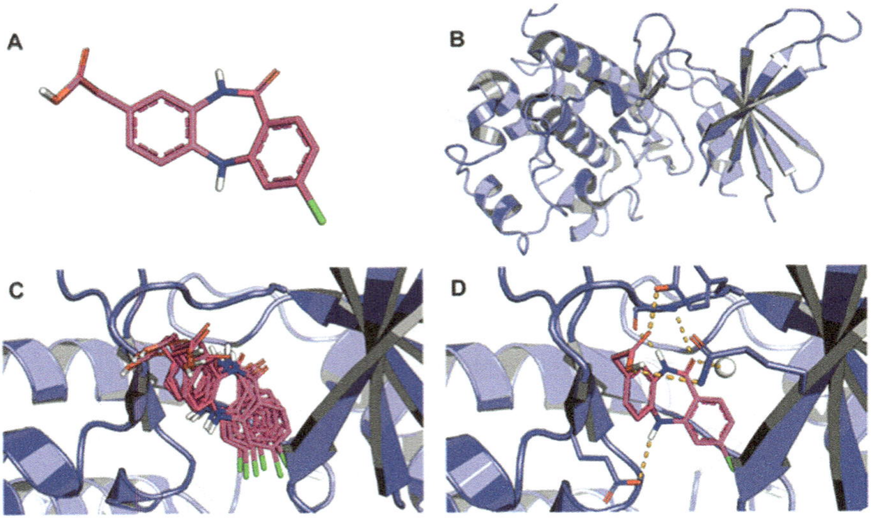

Fig. 10.5 Molecular docking process: **a** Optimization of ligand structure; **b** Optimization of the receptor structure; **c** docking of the ligand onto the receptor; **d** Identification of the best possible binding conformation [93]

in-house database compounds, screens them and chooses compounds that can be purchased or can be synthesized.

It is getting increasingly popular as it gives a fast and cheap substitute to high-throughput screening. It is of two types: Ligand-based drug design and Structure-based drug design as shown in Fig. 10.7. In Ligand-based Virtual screening, pharmacophore modelling and 2D chemical similarity analysis methods are used and in Structure-based virtual screening docking of candidate ligands into a protein target is done followed by applying a scoring function to find out best orientation of the ligand.

In some cases, the 3-D structure of the target protein is not available, for instance, if the protein structures are resolved in the apo form or with G-protein-coupled receptor (GPCR) targets. In this case, ligand based VS methods are used that utilize the information from known active ligands to identify and optimize leads because even if one does not know target protein structure, there is knowledge of the set of ligands showing activity against the target, so novel ligand/drug molecules can be designed by comparing the similarities between known active ligands and the candidate ligand. The success of the LBVS method depends upon a dependable scoring method and an effective measure of similarity generally classified as molecular fields and shapes and pharmacophores. An effective scoring method would be able to differentiate between active and inactive compounds in a large library of compounds.

Another approach to VS is structure-based. In structure based virtual screening, 3D structure of the biological target protein is utilized to study the fundamental molecular interactions between ligands and proteins. It is quick and cost-effective.

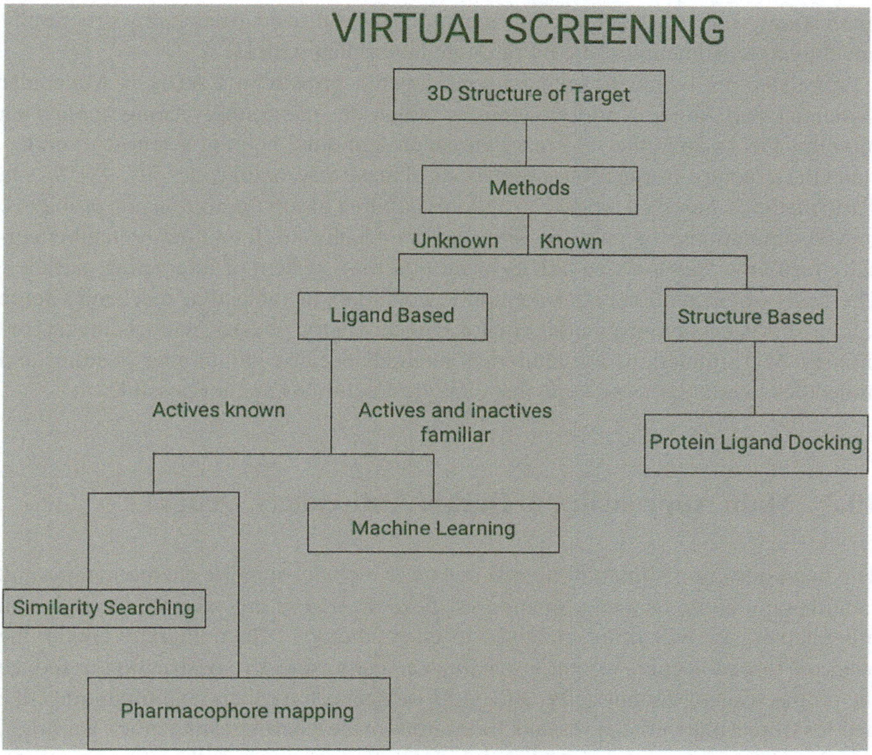

Fig. 10.6 Flow chart of virtual screening [96]

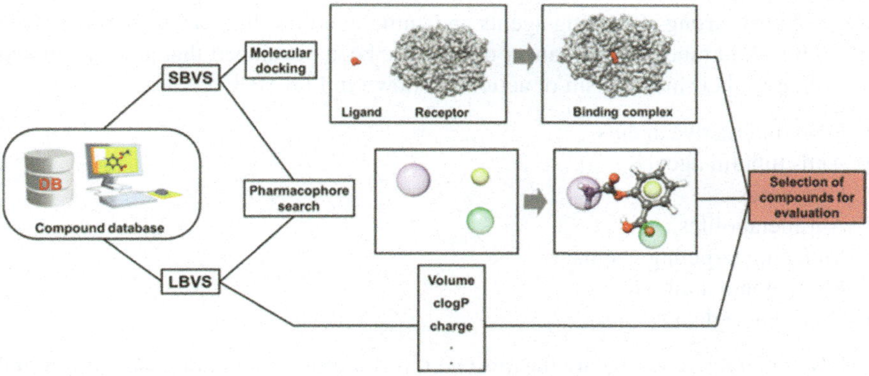

Fig. 10.7 The SBVS and LBVS methods [93]

Interestingly, the 3-D structure of the receptor can be utilized in designing structurally novel ligands. Sometimes, the hit rates are better than with HTS.

Another area which is seeing unprecedented growth in CADD is Molecular Dynamics and Monte Carlo simulations which are increasingly being applied on proteins, DNAs and other bio-macromolecules, and are helping scientist to understand the structure-to-function associations of these macromolecules [97, 98]. Monte Carlo methods, based on repetitive random sampling to solve deterministic problems. In MD simulations, the paths of atoms and molecules are found out by mathematically resolving Newton's equations of motion for a system of interacting particles. The basis of calculations are interatomic potentials or molecular mechanics force fields. This is becoming a matter of choice in chemistry, physics, nanochemistry and biology. MD simulations use numerical methods because the number of atoms and molecules interacting is so large that analytical solutions are not possible.

10.3 Main Approaches to Design Anti-cancer Drugs

The main lines of treatment followed in cancer include: surgery, chemotherapy, and radiotherapy alone or a combination of these three. For the sake of discussion in this chapter, we will limit ourselves to chemotherapy. Chemotherapy entails the usage of low-molecular-weight drugs that can cause selective destruction or reduce the propagation of tumour cells. But cytotoxic agents have their own limitations like hair loss, bone marrow suppression, lacerations in the gastrointestinal tract, vomiting, and sometimes a cancer does not shrink even after treatment with cytotoxic agents. The cytotoxic agents do not show specificity towards cancerous cells meaning they affect both cancer and healthy cells alike. Initial chemotherapeutic agents include the usage of very strong alkylating agents and antimetabolites like nitrogen mustards in the 1940s. A number of anti-cancer drugs have been developed that are categorised according to their mechanism of action as shown in Fig. 10.8.

- DNA-interactive agents
- Anti- tubulin agents
- Hormones
- Antimetabolites
- Molecule targeting agents
- Monoclonal antibodies
- Other biological agents.

DNA interactive agents are the most significant drugs out of anticancer drugs and can act through various mechanisms: For instance drugs like dacarbazine, procarbazine and temozolomide that are alkylating agents that alkylate DNA bases in the major or minor grooves, Or anthracyclines like epirubicin, doxorubicin and compounds like actinomycin-D and mitoxantrone that cause intercalation by binding between base pairs, bleomycin which cleaves DNA and leads to strand scission at the binding site, platinum complexes like cisplatin, carboplatin, oxaliplatin and

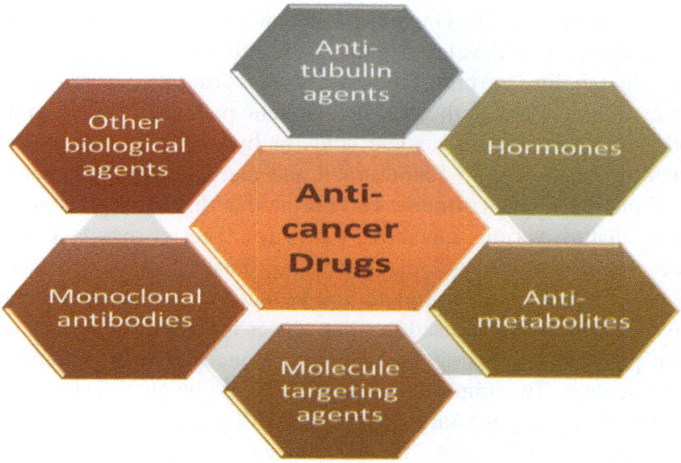

Fig. 10.8 Therapeutic approaches for designing anti-cancer drugs

nitrogen mustards like ifosfamide, cyclophosphamide and nitrosurea, compounds like thiotepa and busulfan that cause crosslinkage of DNA, etoposide and irinotecan compounds that inhibit the topoisomerase which is responsible for the cleavage, annealing, and topological state of DNA. The following Table 10.2 displays different types of anti-cancer drugs, their mechanism and examples.

Table 10.2 Different types of anti-cancer drugs, their mechanism and examples [54]

Type of drug	Examples	Mechanism of action
Alkylating/cross-linking agents	Cisplatin, Endoxan, cyclophosphamide	Damage DNA leading to cell-death
Monoclonal antibodies	Herceptin, Zevalin	Targets cancerous cells expressing specific antigen
Mitosis inhibitors	Taxol	Targets microtubules dynamics
Antitumour antibiotics	Doxorubicin, Etoposide	Bind DNA to prevent DNA and/or RNA synthesis
Antimetabolites	Methotrexate, 5-fluorouracil	Interferes in cell proliferation
Steroid hormones	Flutamide, Tamoxifen	Blocks hormone and steroid dependent tumor growth
Signal-transduction agents	Tarceva, LY900003, Gleevec, Iressa	Modulate communication between cells
Angiogenesis inhibitors	Avastin	Blocks blood-vessel formation
Histone-deacetylase inhibitors	SAHA	Hamers the transcription of genes
Telomerase inhibitors	BIBR1532	Affect telomere maintenance

Antitubulin agents include vinca alkaloids and taxanes that disrupt the microtubule aspects like spindle development or disassembly so nucleus cannot divide and cell dies. Antimetabolites are one of the earliest class drugs discovered to treat cancer. They work by interacting with the vital biosynthetic pathways. They can work either by disrupting the synthesis of nucleic acids or by interfering with crucial enzymatic routes of metabolism. 5-Fluorouracil and mercaptopurine are characteristic examples of analogues of pyrimidine and purine that disturb nucleic acid synthesis methotrexate, disturb various metabolic pathways. Thesed rugs lack in the specificity aspect that is why latest research is being done in the area of antibodies or molecular targeting agents [99]. In addition to that, other approaches that improve the selective toxicity of drugs used to treat cancer include interference with signal transduction pathways, downregulation of proto-oncogenes and interference with tumour angiogenesis. Two important examples should be quoted here: one is of the drug trastuzumab (Herceptin), targeting the ERBB2 receptor and second is imatinib (Glivec) targeting the BCR–ABL oncogene that show great specificity but still lot needs to be achieved and cytotoxic drugs still are the main course of action while treating cancer [100–102].

10.4 Some Important Examples of In-Silico Design in Anti-cancer Drugs

In this section, some of the seminal studies that used in silico and computational methods to design anti-cancer drugs will be discussed. For instance, identifying p53 upregulated modulator of apoptosis (PUMA) inhibitors by pharmacophore modeling is a seminal study in this field [103]. Another very good example where pharmacophore modelling was applied successfully is to identify prospective inhibitors against the HER2 protein's kinase domain by 3D-QSAR dependent pharmacophore search. Human epidermal growth factor receptors are associated with various types of cancers and are categorised by abnormal signal transduction. They include EGFR (ErbB1), HER2 (ErbB2, HER2/neu), HER3 (ErbB3), and HER4 (ErbB4). Out of all these, HER2 is connected with breast cancer which is why it is extensively studied as a drug target for breast cancer.

Hypol, a pharmacophore model having four main characteristics was created. Test set method Fischer's randomization, and the decoy test method were used for the validation of this model. After screening of the natural compounds database (UNPD), 33 compounds were identified and their molecular docking with the active site of the protein was performed. MD simuation of the compounds having highest scores was performed. It resulted in the identification of two promising leads Hit1 and Hit2 against HER2 [104]. Another interesting study reports that powerful and effective 'microtubule destabilizing agents' can be rationally designed as there is a structural basis of it. This is very promising as it opens up possibilities for the design of next-generation antibody–drug conjugates (ADCs) to treat cancer. The active protein filaments accumulated from tubulin subunits are called microtubules and are very important for cell division. The approach to stop or reduce the rate of cell proliferation by destabilizing microtubules is a very successful strategy to treat cancer Therefore, such ligands that can affect the dynamics of microtubules are a sought after class of compounds as anti-cancer drugs. In this case, X-ray crystallography was used to analyse three independent drugs that are known to disrupt the dynamics of microtubules. The analysis showed a novel tubulin-binding site for these three drugs. This discovery of a new site for these ligands make their mechanism of action different from the traditional microtubule assembly inhibitors. One more interesting finding was the fact that main interactions of these three ligands with tubulin were almost comparable due to which a common pharmacophore can be defined for them [105]. Moreover, the structural basis for the interface of antimitotic agents with tubulin has been greatly investigated with in silico methods [106]. In addition to that, molecular docking has been employed in lot of investigations to identify the binding modes of varied colchicine site inhibitors which was later converted to a robust structure-based pharmacophore which helped us in better appreciation of the binding interactions [106, 107]. In Fig. 10.9, it is shown that α and β tubulin associates to form α-β-heterodimer. This dimer then arranges in a head to tail manner to form the microtubule [108].

In addition to that, another interesting strategy to treat cancer is the inhibition of zinc-dependent histone deacetylase 8. Histone deacetylases is a significant therapeutic target to treat cancer as genome wide hypo-acetylation of it leads to many cancers. It is no surprise that the drugs that can act as histone deacetylases (HDAC) inhibitors can be used to treat various cancers. But the problem is the adverse effects of using HDAC inhibitors such as myocardium damage and bone marrow depression. Therefore, the design and development of HDAC inhibitors that are type specific is a big area of cancer research. The structure of the HDAC8 protein is shown in Fig. 10.10. Ligand based pharmacophore modelling has been used in a major way to meet this challenge of identify novel ligands that can act as HDAC inhibitors without any of the side effects.

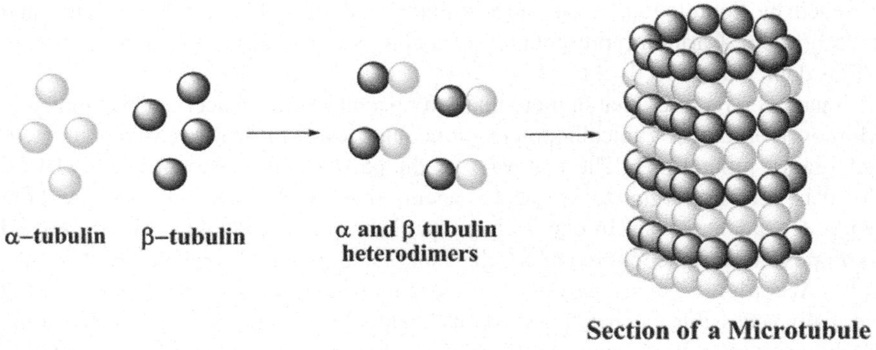

Fig. 10.9 Formation of a microtubule [109]

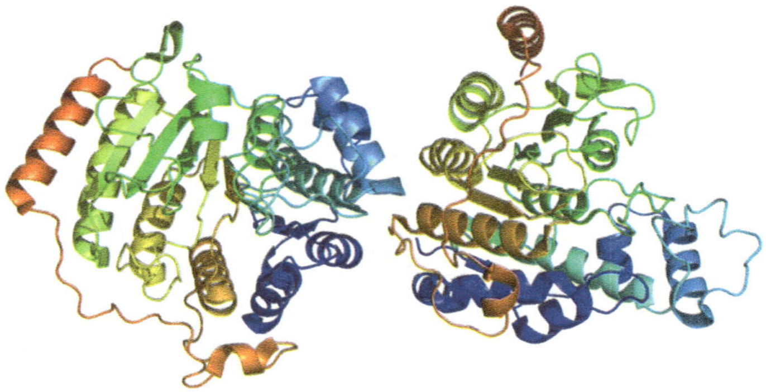

Fig. 10.10 Structure of the HDAC8 protein [110]

For instance, in a study concerning HDAC8, molecular docking experiments were performed and the best conformations of the resulting training set of compounds were used to generate a pharmacophore model which showed great correlation between predicted and experimental activities. The pharmacophore model was validated through Fischer randomization.

After validation, it was searched in a database as a 3D query to find new scaffolds that can act as inhibitors of HDAC8 resulting in 568 compounds. The molecular docking of the selected compounds into the binding site of HDAC8 gave 3 final leads. That can be used for HDAC8 inhibitor design [111]. Moreover, a pharmacophore model with a set of seventy compounds from 3 different classes and 2 subclasses to design type-specific HDAC inhibitors has been proposed. The proposed model has been authenticated by docking the selected compound into active site of HDAC8 [112, 113].

Tumor protein p53 is a very important proteins in multicellular vertebrates as it helps in prevention of cancer and is thus referred to as tumor suppressor. It also is known to conserve stability by preventing the mutation of the genome and thus referred as "the guardian of the genome". It is actually any isoform of a protein encoded by homologous genes in a number of entities like TP53 (humans) and Trp53 (mice). Cartoon representation of a complex between DNA and the protein p53 is depicted in Fig. 10.11.

It has been reported that in more than fifty percent of the cancers, p53 is mutated. Moreover, otherwise clinically potent antineoplastic agents do not have much potential against mutant p53. The pathways of the p53 protein is shown in Fig. 10.12. So, it is very important to search for agents that can lead to cell death without being dependent on p53.In one such study, electrophilic prostaglandins were used to propose a pharmacophore and mechanism of action hypothesis to solve this difficulty. According to their analysis, "a cross-conjugated, unsaturated dienone with 2 sterically accessible electrophilic carbons" that is responsible for the activity of the inhibitors of ubiquitin isopeptidases which can lead to death of the cell without being dependent on p53. Shikoccin (a diterpene), dibenzylideneacetone, and curcumin

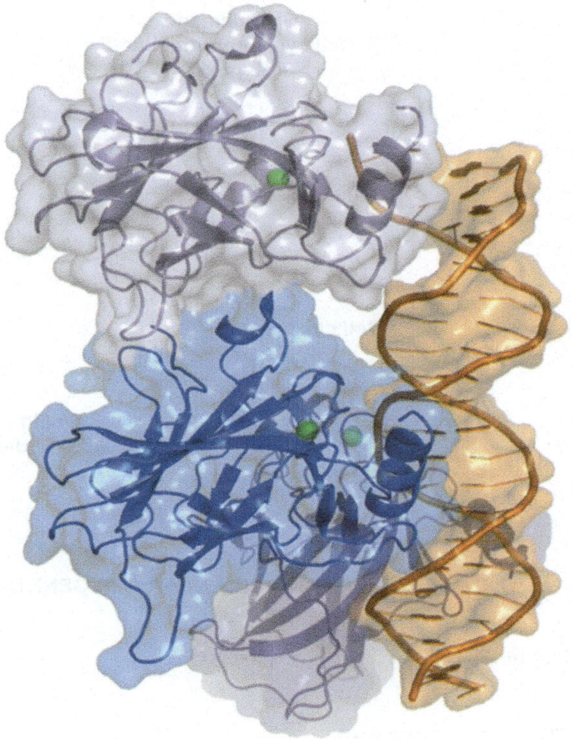

Fig. 10.11 Cartoon representation of a complex between DNA and the protein p53 [114, 115]

fulfilled this hypothesis. p53-independent cell death initiated by inhibition of the proteasome pathway can help design molecular targets appropriate for antineoplastic drug discovery [116].

Another important anti-cancer drug that has been extensively studied by in silico methods cisplatin. Or instance, the interaction of cisplatin with human serum transferrin (Tf) was studied using molecular dynamic simulations. The results indicated that cisplatin can inhabit portion of both the iron (iii)- and carbonate-binding sites in the C-terminal hemisphere of human serum transferrin (Tf). This indicates that iron (III) binding to the active site of C-terminal lobe is restricted because cisplatin binds with it. However, cisplatin does not seem to affect the N-terminal lobe active site [118].

CXC chemokine receptor 2 (CXCR2) plays an important role in metastasis of cancer. In silico design has been very successful in identifying novel CXCR2 antagonists [119]. In addition to that, development of PD-1/PD-L1 inhibitors is attracting lot of attention of researchers due to importance of immunotherapy in anti-cancer drug design. But there are challenges towards the development of small molecules and peptides as inhibitors. Here, pharmacophore modelling is proving to be of great help [120].

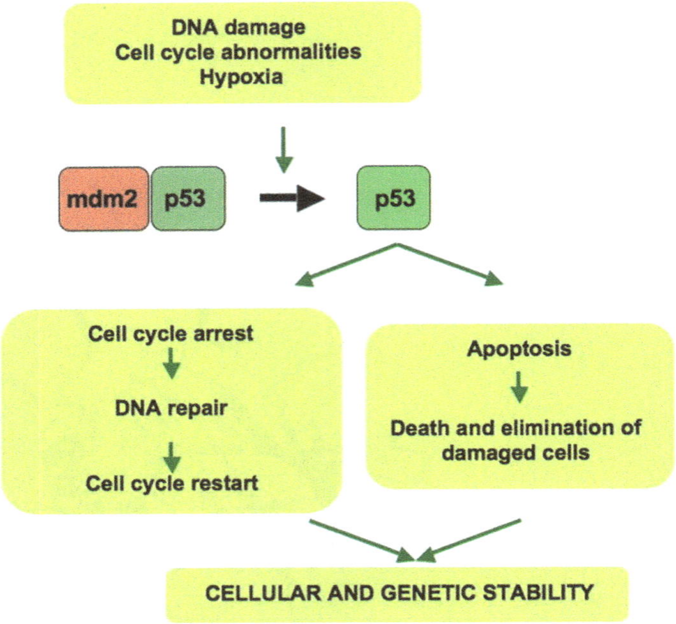

Fig. 10.12 Pathways of the p53 protein [117]

10.5 Conclusion

In silico methods are increasingly being used to meet the huge demand for novel, affordable and target- specific anti-cancer drugs. That has been made possible due to the advancement in the computational methods and corresponding exponential increase in computer hardware. Now, the traditional trial and error methodology for generating a suitable lead is giving way to screening of large number of compounds to select leads. This has been aided availability of databases that contain 3-D structures of numerous target proteins and millions of ligands. So there is a shift from the 'One Ligand-One Target' approach to the 'Multi Target Drug Ligands' (MTDL)' approach for drug design for treating cancer.

In silico methods have revolutionised the development and design of small molecule cancer drugs, but acquired resistance and intra-tumor heterogeneity are still challenges for which solutions need to be sought. The trend of in silico investigations for designing novel anti-cancer drugs will be on the rise in the future.

Acknowledgements The authors are thankful to their respective institutions for moral and administrative support.

Conflict of interest: The authors declare no competing interests.

References

1. Mcardel, S., Program, I.: Bench to Bedside : The Drug Development Pipeline Introduction
2. Lindsley, C.W.: Pharmacoeconomics and the medicinal chemist. ACS Med. Chem. Lett. **5**(10), 1066–1068 (2014)
3. Dimasi, J.A., Grabowski, H.G., Hansen, R.W.: Innovation in the pharmaceutical industry: New estimates of R & D costs. J. Health Econ. **47**, 20–33 (2016). https://doi.org/10.1016/j.jhealeco.2016.01.012
4. Lindsley, C.W.: New statistics on the cost of new drug development and the trouble with CNS drugs. ACS Chem. Neurosci. **5**, 1142 (2014). https://doi.org/10.1021/cn500298z
5. Paul, S.M., et al.: How to improve R&D productivity: the pharmaceutical industry's grand challenge. Nat. Rev. Drug. Discov. **9**, 203–214 (2010). https://doi.org/10.1038/nrd3078
6. Hay, M., Thomas, D.W., Craighead, J.L., Economides, C., Rosenthal, J.: Clinical development success rates for investigational drugs. Nat. Biotechnol. **32**(1), 40–50 (2014)
7. Zhao, Q., Yu, H., Ji, M., Zhao, Y., Chen, X.: Computational model development of drug-target interaction prediction: a review. Curr. Protein Pept. Sci., pp. 492–494 (2019). https://doi.org/10.2174/1389203720666190123164310
8. Kapetanovic, I.M.: Computer-aided drug discovery and development (CADDD): In silico -chemico-biological approach. Chem. Biol. Interact. **171**, 165–176 (2008). https://doi.org/10.1016/j.cbi.2006.12.006
9. Kumar, N., Hendriks, B.S., Janes, K.A., De Graaf, D., Lauffenburger, D.A.: Applying computational modeling to drug discovery and development. Drug Discov. Today **11**(17), 806–811 (2006). https://doi.org/10.1016/j.drudis.2006.07.010
10. Hann, M.M., Oprea, T.I.: Pursuing the leadlikeness concept in pharmaceutical research. Curr. Opin. Chem. Biol. **8**, 255–263 (2004). https://doi.org/10.1016/j.cbpa.2004.04.003
11. Roche, O., Guba, W.: Computational chemistry as an integral component of lead generation. Mini-Rev. Med. Chem. **5**, 677–683 (2005)
12. Horrobin, D.F.: Innovation in the pharmaceutical industry. J. R. Soc. Med. **93**, 341–345 (2000)
13. Tang, Y., Zhu, W., Chen, K., Jiang, H.: New technologies in computer-aided drug design: Toward target identification and new chemical entity discovery. Drug Discov. Today Technol. **3**(3), 307–313 (2006). https://doi.org/10.1016/j.ddtec.2006.09.004
14. Congreve, M., Murray, C.W., Blundell, T.L.: Structural biology and drug discovery. Drug Discov. Today, **10**(13) (2005)
15. Varady, J., et al.: Molecular modeling of the three-dimensional structure of Dopamine 3 (D3) subtype receptor: discovery of novel and potent d3 ligands through a hybrid pharmacophore- and structure-based database searching approach Judith. J. Med. Chem. **46**, 4377–4392 (2003)
16. R.J.A.W., Astles, P.C., Brown, T.J., Harris, N.V., Harper, M.F., McCarthy, C., Porter, B., Smith, C.: Selective endothelin A receptor antagonists. 2. Discovery and structure-activity relationships of 5-ketopentanoic acid derivatives. Eur. J. Med. Chem. **32**(6), 515–522 (1997)
17. Forino, M., Jung, D., Easton, J.B., Houghton, P.J., Pellecchia, M.: Virtual docking approaches to protein kinase B inhibition. J. Med. Chem. **48**, 2278–2281 (2005)
18. Peng, H., Huang, N., Qi, J., Xie, P., Xu, C.: Identification of novel inhibitors of BCR-ABL tyrosine kinase via virtual screening. Bioorg. Med. Chem. Lett. **13**, 3693–3699 (2003). https://doi.org/10.1016/j.bmcl.2003.08.014
19. Lyne, P.D., Kenny, P.W., Cosgrove, D.A., Deng, C., Zabludoff, S., Wendoloski, J.J.: Identification of compounds with nanomolar binding affinity for checkpoint Kinase-1 using knowledge-based virtual screening. J. Med. Chem. **47**, 1962–1968 (2004)
20. Schapira, M., Raaka, B.M., Samuels, H.H., Abagyan, R.: In silico discovery of novel Retinoic Acid Receptor agonist structures. BMC Struct. Biol. **1**(1), 1–7 (2001)
21. Guba, W., Neidhart, W., Nettekoven, M.: Novel and potent NPY5 receptor antagonists derived from virtual screening and iterative parallel chemistry design. Bioorg. Med. Chem. Lett. **15**, 1599–1603 (2005). https://doi.org/10.1016/j.bmcl.2005.01.063

22. Marriott, D.P., Dougall, I.G., Meghani, P., Liu, Y., Flower, D.R.: Lead generation using Pharmacophore mapping and three-dimensional database searching: application to Muscarinic M 3 receptor antagonists. J. Med. Chem. **42**, 3210–3216 (1999)
23. Sharma, S., Bhatia, V.: Treatment of Type 2 Diabetes mellitus (T2DM): Can GLP-1 Receptor Agonists fill in the gaps? Chem. Biol. Lett. **7**(4), 215–224 (2020)
24. Schapira, M. et al.: Discovery of diverse thyroid hormone receptor antagonists by high-throughput docking. PNAS **100**(12), 7354–7359 兩 (2003)
25. Desai, P.V., Patny, A., Sabnis, Y., Tekwani, B., Gut, J., Rosenthal, P.: Identification of novel parasitic cysteine protease inhibitors using virtual screening. 1. The ChemBridge database. J. Med. Chem. **47**, 6609–6615 (2004)
26. Lam, P.Y.S., et al.: Cyclic HIV Protease Inhibitors: Synthesis, Conformational Analysis, P2/P2′ Structure—activity relationship, and molecular recognition of cyclic ureas. J. Med. Chem. **39**, 3514–3525 (1996)
27. Haque, T.S., et al.: Potent, low-molecular-weight non-peptide inhibitors of malarial aspartyl protease Plasmepsin II. J. Med. Chem. **42**, 1428–1440 (1999)
28. Flohr, S., Kurz, M., Kostenis, E., Brkovich, A., Fournier, A., Klabunde, T.: Identification of Nonpeptidic Urotensin II Receptor antagonists by virtual screening based on a Pharmacophore model derived from structure—activity relationships and nuclear magnetic resonance studies on Urotensin II. J. Med. Chem. **45**, 1799–1805 (2002)
29. Doman, T.N., et al.: Molecular docking and high-throughput screening for novel inhibitors of protein tyrosine Phosphatase-1B. J. Med. Chem. **45**, 2213–2221 (2002). https://doi.org/10.1021/jm010548w
30. Krier, M.: Design of small-sized libraries by combinatorial assembly of linkers and functional groups to a given scaffold: application to the structure-based optimization of a Phosphodiesterase 4 Inhibitor. J. Med. Chem. **48**, 3816–3822 (2005)
31. Evers, A., Thomas, K.: Structure-based drug discovery using GPCR homology modeling: successful virtual screening for antagonists of the alpha 1A adrenergic receptor. J. Med. Chem. **48**(4), 1088–1097 (2005)
32. Rastelli, G., Ferrari, A.M., Costantino, L., Gamberini, M.C.: Discovery of new inhibitors of aldose reductase from molecular docking and database screening. Bioorg. Med. Chem. **10**, 1437–1450 (2002)
33. Kraemer, O., Hazemann, I., Podjarny, A.D., Klebe, G.: Virtual Screening For Inhibitors Of Human Aldose Reductase. Proteins Struct. Funct. Bioinforma. **55**, 814–823 (2004). https://doi.org/10.1002/prot.20057
34. Evers, A., Klebe, G.: Successful virtual screening for a submicromolar antagonist of the neurokinin-1 receptor based on a ligand-supported homology model. J. Med. Chem. **47**(22), 5381–5392 (2004)
35. Liu, X., Yu, H., Zhao, X., Huang, X.: Molecular simulations study of novel with a high selectivity for Cav3.1 calcium channel. Protein Sci. **24**, 1737–1747 (2015). https://doi.org/10.1002/pro.2763
36. Hue, M., Riffle, M., Vert, J., Noble, W.S.: Large-scale prediction of protein-protein interactions from structures. BMC Bioinforma. **11**(1–9), 2010 (2010)
37. Chung, C., Hann, M.M.: Targeting Protein—Protein interactions perspective detection and analysis of PPIs. In: Renaud, J.P. (Ed.) Structural Biology in Drug Discovery, pp. 479–502 (2020)
38. Phulen, S. et al.: In-silico homology assisted identification of inhibitor of RNA binding against 2019-nCoV N- protein (N terminal domain). J. Biomol. Struct. Dyn., 1–11 (2020). https://doi.org/10.1080/07391102.2020.1753580
39. Bell, D.R., Weber, J.K., Yin, W., Huynh, T., Duan, W., Zhou, R.: In silico design and validation of high-affinity RNA aptamers targeting epithelial cellular adhesion molecule dimers. PNAS **21**, 1–8 (2020). https://doi.org/10.1073/pnas.1913242117
40. Schneider, G., Nettekoven, M., Ag, F.H.R., Di V, P., Generation, L.: Ligand-based combinatorial design of selective Purinergic Receptor (A 2A) antagonists using self-organizing maps. J. Comb. Chem. **5**, 233–237 (2003)

41. Lavrador, K., Murphy, B., Saunders, J., Struthers, S., Wang, X., Williams, J.: A screening library for peptide activated G-Protein coupled receptors. 1. The test set. J. Med. Chem. **47**, 6864–6874 (2004)
42. Peukert, S., et al.: Pharmacophore-based search, synthesis, and biological evaluation of anthranilic amides as novel blockers of the Kv1. 5 channel. Bioorg. Med. Chem. Lett. **14**, 2823–2827 (2004). https://doi.org/10.1016/j.bmcl.2004.03.057
43. Liu, H. et al.: Structure-based discovery of potassium channel blockers from natural products : virtual screening and electrophysiological assay testing. Chem. Biol. **10**, 1103–1113 (2003). Doi: 10.1016/j
44. Baxter, K., et al.: An end to the myth: there is no drug development pipeline Kristin. Sci. Transl. Med. **5**(171), 6–10 (2013)
45. Naci, H., Carter, A., Mossialos, E.: Why the drug development pipeline is not delivering better medicines. BMJ **5542**(October), 1–4 (2015). https://doi.org/10.1136/bmj.h5542
46. Hughes, J.P., Rees, S., Kalindjian, S.B., Philpott, K.L.: Principles of early drug discovery. Br. J. Pharmacol. **162**, 1239–1249 (2011). https://doi.org/10.1111/j.1476-5381.2010.01127.x
47. Niranjan, D., Gill, S., Shrivastava, D., Jain, A., Agrawal, O.P.: Quantitative structure activity relationships in computer aided drug design: a review. J. Drug Deliv. Ther. **9**(3), 645–649 (2019)
48. Sliwoski, G.R., Meiler, J., Lowe, E.W.: Computational methods in drug discovery prediction of protein structure and ensembles from limited experimental data view project antibody modeling, antibody design and antigen-antibody interactions view project. Comput. Methods Drug Discov. **66**(1), 334–395 (2014). https://doi.org/10.1124/pr.112.007336
49. Becker, O.M. et al.: An integrated in Silico 3D model-driven discovery of a novel, potent, and selective Amidosulfonamide 5-HT1A Agonist (PRX-00023) for the treatment of anxiety and depression. J. Med. Chem. **49**, 3116–3135 (2006)
50. Singh, J., et al.: Successful Shape-based virtual screening: the discovery of a potent inhibitor of the Type I TGFβ receptor kinase (TβRI). Bioorg. Med. Chem. Lett. **13**, 4355–4359 (2003). https://doi.org/10.1016/j.bmcl.2003.09.028
51. Santos, R., et al.: A comprehensive map of molecular drug targets. Nat. Publ. Gr. **16**(1), 19–34 (2016). https://doi.org/10.1038/nrd.2016.230
52. Zhang, L., Tan, J., Han, D., Zhu, H.: From machine learning to deep learning: progress in machine intelligence for rational drug discovery. Drug Discov. Today **22**(11), 1680–1685 (2017). https://doi.org/10.1016/j.drudis.2017.08.010
53. Roy, K. (Ed.): computational modeling of drugs against alzheimer' s disease. Neuromethods (2018)
54. Hellman, K.: Anticancer drugs. Chem. Br. **8**(2), 69–72 (1972)
55. Dai, S.X., et al.: In silico identification of anti-cancer compounds and plants from traditional Chinese medicine database. Sci. Rep. **6**(April), 1–11 (2016). https://doi.org/10.1038/srep25462
56. Bhogal, N., Balls, M.: Translation of new technologies: from basic research to drug discovery and development. Curr. Drug Discov. Technol. **5**, 250–262 (2008)
57. Boghog, "Schematic diagram of drug discovery cycle," Creative Commons Attribution-Share Alike 4.0 International license. https://commons.wikimedia.org/wiki/File:Drug_discovery_cycle.svg (2015)
58. Sharma, S., Bhatia, V.: Phytochemicals for drug discovery in alzheimer's disease. In silico advances. Curr. Pharm. Des. **27**, 1–13 (2021). https://doi.org/10.2174/138161282666620092 8161721
59. Sharma, S., Bhatia, V.: Nanoscale Drug delivery systems for glaucoma: experimental and in silico advances. Curr. Top. Med. Chem. **20**, 1–11 (2020). https://doi.org/10.2174/156802662 0666200922114210
60. Bicerano, J.: Computational Modeling of Polymers (1992)
61. Cao, B., et al.: How to optimize materials and devices via design of experiments and machine learning: demonstration using organic photovoltaics. ACS Nano **12**(8), 7434–7444 (2018). https://doi.org/10.1021/acsnano.8b04726

62. Xiang, T.X., Anderson, B.D.: Liposomal drug transport: a molecular perspective from molecular dynamics simulations in lipid bilayers. Adv. Drug Deliv. Rev. **58**(12–13), 1357–1378 (2006). https://doi.org/10.1016/j.addr.2006.09.002
63. Leelananda, S.P., Lindert, S.: Computational methods in drug discovery. Beilstein J. Org. Chem. **12**, 2694–2718 (2016). https://doi.org/10.3762/bjoc.12.267
64. Kakkar, R., Sharma, S., Badhani, B.: Density functional study of functionalization of carbon nanotubes with Carbenes. **2**(4), 434–449 (2014). https://doi.org/10.13179/canchemtrans.2014.02.04.0132
65. Johnson, A.: Modeling molecules: computational nanotechnology as a knowledge community. Perspect. Sci. **17**(2), 144–173 (2009). https://doi.org/10.1162/posc.2009.17.2.144
66. Kakkar, R., Sharma, S.: DFT study of interactions of Carbenes with boron nitride nanotubes. **1**(1), 9–20 (2011)
67. Prajapat Lalita, B.R.S., Jadon, G., Kishor, A.: A review on computer added drug design. Int. J. Pharm. Erud. **3**(3), 53–58 (2019)
68. Haddish-Berhane, N., Rickus, J.L., Haghighi, K.: The role of multiscale computational approaches for rational design of conventional and nanoparticle oral drug delivery systems. Int. J. Nanomedicine **2**(3), 315–331 (2007)
69. Jennings, A., Tennant, M.: Discovery strategies in a pharmaceutical setting: The application of computational techniques. Expert Opin. Drug Discov. **1**(7), 709–721 (2006). https://doi.org/10.1517/17460441.1.7.709
70. Maas, J., Kamm, W., Hauck, G.: An integrated early formulation strategy—From hit evaluation to preclinical candidate profiling. Eur. J. Pharm. Biopharm. **66**(1), 1–10 (2007). https://doi.org/10.1016/j.ejpb.2006.09.011
71. Sawyer, J.S., et al.: Synthesis and activity of New Aryl- and Heteroaryl-substituted pyrazole inhibitors of the transforming growth factor-β Type I receptor kinase domain J. J. Med. Chem. Chem. **46**(19), 11–14 (2003)
72. Sharma, S., Bhatia, V.: 'Drug Design of GLP-1 receptor agonists: importance of. Curr. Pharm. Des. (2020)
73. Taylor, P., Dearden, J.C., Cronin, M.T.D., Kaiser, K.L.E.: How not to develop a quantitative structure—activity or structure—property relationship (QSAR/ QSPR). In: SAR and QSAR in Environmental Research, no. 20, pp. 241–266 (2009)
74. Smriti Sharma, V.B.: Recent trends in QSAR in modelling of drug-protein and protein-protein interactions. Comb. Chem. High Throughput Screen., vol. in press (2020). https://doi.org/10.7868/s0869565216210155
75. Polanski, J.: Self-organizing neural networks for pharmacophore mapping. Adv. Drug Deliv. Rev. **55**, 1149–1162 (2003)
76. Pagadala, N.S., Syed, K., Tuszynski, J.: Software for molecular docking: a review. Biophys. Rev. **9**, 91–102 (2017). https://doi.org/10.1007/s12551-016-0247-1
77. Cavasotto, C.N., Phatak, S.S.: Homology modeling in drug discovery : current trends and applications. Drug Discov. Today ? **14**, 676–683 (2009). https://doi.org/10.1016/j.drudis.2009.04.006
78. Geppert, H., Vogt, M.: current trends in ligand-based virtual screening: molecular representations, data mining methods, new application areas, and performance evaluation. J. Chem. Inf. Model. **50**, 205–216 (2010)
79. Sharma, S., Bhatia, V.: Appraisal of the role of In silico Methods in Pyrazole based drug design. Mini-Rev. Med. Chem. **20**(1) (2020). https://doi.org/10.2174/1389557520666200901184146
80. Paquet, E., Viktor, H.L., Simulations, M.C.: Molecular dynamics, monte carlo simulations, and Langevin dynamics : a computational review **2015** (2015). https://doi.org/10.1155/2015/183918
81. Eckert, H.: Molecular similarity analysis in virtual screening: foundations, limitations and novel approaches. Drug Discov. Today **12**, 225–233 (2007). https://doi.org/10.1016/j.drudis.2007.01.011

82. Dudek, A.Z.: Computational methods in developing quantitative structure-activity relationships (QSAR): a review. Comb. Chem. High Throughput Screen. **9**, 213–228 (2006)
83. Clark, M., Iii, R.D.C., Jones, D.M., Patterson, D.E., Simeroth, P.E.: Comparative molecular field analysis (CoMFA). 2. toward its use with 3d-structural databases. Tetrahedron Comput. Methodol. **3**(1), 47–59 (1990)
84. Malathi, K., Ramaiah, S.: Bioinformatics approaches for new drug discovery: a review. Biotechnol. Genet. Eng. Rev. **34**(2), 243–260 (2018). https://doi.org/10.1080/02648725.2018.1502984
85. Chem, M.: MedChemComm computational ligand-based rational design : role of conformational sampling and force fields in model development †, pp. 356–370 (2011).https://doi.org/10.1039/c1md00044f
86. Lionta, E., Spyrou, G., Vassilatis, D.K., Cournia, Z.: Structure-Based Virtual Screening for Drug Discovery : Principles, Applications and Recent Advances, pp. 1923–1938 (2014)
87. Lavecchia, Z., Di Giovanni, C.: Virtual Screening Strategies in Drug Discovery : A Critical Review, pp. 2839–2860 (2013)
88. Caporuscio, F., Tafi, A.: Pharmacophore Modelling : A Forty Year Old Approach and its Modern Synergies, pp. 2543–2553 (2011)
89. Dcirovic, "An example of a pharmacophore model," Creative Commons CC-Zero. https://commons.wikimedia.org/wiki/File:PharmacophoreModel_example.svg.2011
90. Chaudhary, K.K., Mishra, N.: A Review on Molecular Docking : Novel Tool for Drug Discovery, vol. 4, pp. 1–4 (2016)
91. Yuriev, E., Ramsland, P.A.: Latest developments in molecular docking : 2010–2011 in review, pp. 215–239 (2013). https://doi.org/10.1002/jmr.2266
92. Markkobo, "Flowchart of a Common Clustering Analysis for Structure-Based Drug Design," GNU Free Documentation License; https://en.wikipedia.org/wiki/File:Wiki_Clustering.png Description. (2010)
93. Ferreira, L.G., Santos, R.N., Oliva, G., Andricopulo, A.D.: Molecular docking and structure-based drug design strategies. Molecules **20**, 13384–13421 (2015). https://doi.org/10.3390/molecules200713384
94. Oshiro, C. et al.: Performance of 3D-Database Molecular Docking Studies into Homology Models, pp. 764–767 (2004). https://doi.org/10.1021/jm0300781
95. Polanski, J.: Receptor dependent multidimensional QSAR for modeling drug—receptor interactions. Curr. Med. Chemsitry **16**, 3243–3257 (2009)
96. Gyasi111, "Flow Chart of Virtual Screening," Creative Commons Attribution-Share Alike 4.0 International license. https://en.wikipedia.org/wiki/File:FlowChart.png (2018)
97. Huang, H. et al.: Journal of the Taiwan Institute of chemical engineers current developments of computer-aided drug design **41**, 623–635 (2010). https://doi.org/10.1016/j.jtice.2010.03.017
98. Press, D.: Molecular dynamics simulations: advances and applications. Adv. Appl. Bioinforma. Chem. **8**, 37–47 (2015)
99. Nussbaumer, S., Bonnabry, P., Veuthey, J.L., Fleury-Souverain, S.: Analysis of anticancer drugs: A review. Talanta **85**(5), 2265–2289 (2011). https://doi.org/10.1016/j.talanta.2011.08.034
100. Allen, T.M.: Ligand-targeted therapeutics in anticancer therapy. Nat. Rev. Cancer **2**(10), 750–763 (2002). https://doi.org/10.1038/nrc903
101. Carter, P.: Improving the efficacy of antibody-based cancer therapies. Nat. Rev. Cancer **1**(2), 118–129 (2001). https://doi.org/10.1007/s00259-004-1627-5
102. Huston, J.S., Georgeb, A.J.T.: Engineered antibodies take center stage. Hum. Antibodies **10**(3–4), 127–142 (2001). https://doi.org/10.3233/hab-2001-103-405
103. Prada-gracia, D., Huerta-yépez, S., Moreno-vargas, L.M.: Application of computational methods for anticancer drug discovery, design, and optimization. Boletín Médico del Hosp. Infant. México (English Ed., vol. 73, no. 6, pp. 411–423 (2017). https://doi.org/10.1016/j.bmhime.2017.11.040
104. Rampogu, S., et al.: Targeting natural compounds against HER2 kinase domain as potential anticancer drugs applying pharmacophore based molecular modelling approaches. Comput. Biol. Chem. **74**, 327–338 (2018). https://doi.org/10.1016/j.compbiolchem.2018.04.002

105. Prota, A.E., et al.: A new tubulin-binding site and pharmacophore for microtubule-destabilizing anticancer drugs. Proc. Natl. Acad. Sci. U. S. A. **111**(38), 13817–13821 (2014). https://doi.org/10.1073/pnas.1408124111
106. Kim, D.Y., et al.: Design and biological evaluation of novel tubulin inhibitors as antimitotic agents using a pharmacophore binding model with tubulin. J. Med. Chem. **49**(19), 5664–5670 (2006). https://doi.org/10.1021/jm050761i
107. Chiang, Y.K., et al.: Generation of ligand-based pharmacophore model and virtual screening for identification of novel tubulin inhibitors with potent anticancer activity. J. Med. Chem. **52**(14), 4221–4233 (2009). https://doi.org/10.1021/jm801649y
108. Jordan, M.A., Wilson, L.: Microtubules As a Target for anticancer drugs. Nat. Rev. Cancer **4**(April), 253–265 (2004). https://doi.org/10.1038/nrl317
109. Group6-3, "Formation of a microtubule," Creative Commons Attribution-Share Alike 3.0 Unported license; https://en.wikipedia.org/wiki/File:Formation_of_Microtubule.png (2011)
110. Emw, "Structure of the HDAC8 protein. Based on PyMOL rendering of PDB 1t64.," Creative Commons Attribution-Share Alike 3.0 Unported license. https://commons.wikimedia.org/wiki/File:Protein_HDAC8_PDB_1t64.png (2009)
111. Sundarapandian, T., Shalini, J., Sugunadevi, S., Woo, L.K.: Docking-enabled pharmacophore model for histone deacetylase 8 inhibitors and its application in anti-cancer drug discovery. J. Mol. Graph. Model. **29**(3), 382–395 (2010). https://doi.org/10.1016/j.jmgm.2010.07.007
112. Noureen, N., Kalsoom, S., Rashid, H.: Ligand based pharmacophore modelling of anticancer histone deacetylase inhibitors. African J. Biotechnol. **9**(25), 3923–3931 (2010). https://doi.org/10.5897/ajb2010.000-3268
113. Pajeva, I.K., Wiese, M.: Pharmacophore model of drugs involved in P-glycoprotein multidrug resistance: Explanation of structural variety (hypothesis). J. Med. Chem. **45**(26), 5671–5686 (2002). https://doi.org/10.1021/jm020941h
114. Splettstoesser, T.: "Cartoon representation of a complex between DNA and the protein p 53," Creative Commons Attribution-Share Alike 3.0 Unported license. https://commons.wikimedia.org/wiki/File:P53.pngCartoon (2006)
115. Cho, Y., Gorina, S., Jeffrey, P.D., Pavietich, N.P.: Crystal structure of a p 53 tumor understanding tumorigenic mutations Ppoweh. Science (80) **265**(5170), 346–355 (1994)
116. Mullally, J.E., Fitzpatrick, F.A.: Pharmacophore model for novel inhibitors of ubiquitin isopeptidases that induce p53-independent cell death. Mol. Pharmacol. **62**(2), 351–358 (2002). https://doi.org/10.1124/mol.62.2.351
117. Soussi, T.: "Pathways of the p 53 protein," The copyright holder of this work, release this work into the public domain. https://en.wikipedia.org/wiki/File:P53_pathways.jpg (2007)
118. Khalaila, I., Allardyce, C.S., Verma, C.S., Dyson, P.J.: A mass spectrometric and molecular modelling study of cisplatin binding to transferrin. ChemBioChem **6**(10), 1788–1795 (2005). https://doi.org/10.1002/cbic.200500067
119. Che, J., et al.: Ligand-based pharmacophore model for the discovery of novel CXCR2 antagonists as anti-cancer metastatic agents. R. Soc. Open Sci. **5**(7), 1–11 (2018). https://doi.org/10.1098/rsos.180176
120. Mejías, C., Guirola, O.: Pharmacophore model of immunocheckpoint protein PD-L1 by cosolvent molecular dynamics simulations. J. Mol. Graph. Model. **91**, 105–111 (2019). https://doi.org/10.1016/j.jmgm.2019.06.001

Chapter 11
Two Dimensional and Gesture Based Medical Visualization Interface and Image Processing Methodologies to Aid and Diagnose of Lung Cancer

C. Gopala Krishnan, A. H. Nishan, Theerthagiri Prasannavenkatesan, I. Jeena Jacob, and G. Komarasamy

Abstract This work aims to implement specific image processing methodologies to aid the appropriate diagnosis of lung cancer and provide a sterile environment for interacting with the medical data in operation theatre during treatment. Computer Tomography (CT) gives a good resolution axial slice image of the lung. The tumor's raw CT data analysis is quite impossible as the tumor's pixel characteristics would be approximately matching its neighboring pixels. Thus, a basic preprocessing algorithm is required to differentiate target from the background. It is processed with level set segmentation to extract tumor from the sequentially acquired multiple slices. The segmented output of each slice provides the geometric feature of the tumor. As the tumor size and shape in segmented portions are irregular, it seems appropriate to reconstruct a three-dimensional representation of 2D images for tumors' qualitative information. The volume reconstruction using the ray casting method has been applied to render the volume of tumors from a segmented stack of 2D slices. Then touch-less, computer-aided, gesture-based control of the medical images was attained using Kinect sensor, which is the best tool for human-computer interaction to maintain a sterile environment. The paper elaborates on the gestures, which is employed to interact with the medical images such as selection, drag, and swipe gesture. The selection gesture is used to open and close individual medical images. The drag gesture was used to view the patient data along with the slice image. The swipe

C. Gopala Krishnan (✉) · T. Prasannavenkatesan · I. Jeena Jacob · G. Komarasamy
Department of Computer Science and Engineering, GITAM School of Technology, GITAM University, Bengaluru, India
e-mail: gchandra@gitam.edu

T. Prasannavenkatesan
e-mail: vprasann@gitam.edu

I. Jeena Jacob
e-mail: ijacob@gitam.edu

A. H. Nishan
Department of Computer Science and Engineering, Francis Xavier Engineering College, Tirunelveli, India

J. Nayak et al. (eds.), *Advanced Machine Learning Approaches in Cancer Prognosis*, Intelligent Systems Reference Library 204,
https://doi.org/10.1007/978-3-030-71975-3_11

gesture used to view various medical data sets like 2D slices, tumor irregularity in segmented slices.

Keywords Computed tomography · Image segmentation · Kinect · Lung cancer · Volume rendering

11.1 Introduction

The prevailing threat in the world is due to cancer. To enable early diagnosis, the efforts are made to establish tumor diagnosis. The detection of lung cancer becomes challenging when the target is attached to blood vessels or surrounded by a similar intensity structure like the pleural wall [1]. Thus, the detection of the extent of lung cancer through segmentation is important for volumetric analysis. The visualization of lung cancer is important for diagnosis based on its shape and its integrity to the surrounding [2].

The uncontrolled growth of abnormal cells causes lung cancer. The abnormal cells won't ever change again back to a healthy tissue. Those abnormal cells divide and multiply speedily into an enormous number of abnormal cells which leads to cancer or to cause tumors. The stagnant tumors are known as "benign tumors". Malignant tumors spread through blood or from the vascular system. If once affected by the cancerous cells, it is very difficult to recover them from it completely. There are so many types of cancers and those were seemed to be treated with similar methods [3].

The American Cancer Society has projected 1.74 million new cancer cases and 0.61 million cancer deaths within the year 2018 [4]. During early days, diagnosis remains essential for survival. X-radiation (CT) scan images are for diagnosis and to differentiate malign cancers from benign. However, these ways need extremely sure-handed radiologists. United Nations agency do not seem to be on the market, notably to the folks of remote and impoverished regions [3, 4].

There was a high risk while examining the scan images manually. So, Detection systems will facilitate the radiologists within the diagnosing and reduce false reports' speed. Digital image process techniques are accustomed to find the nodules, type, size, and options from CT scans. The medical image process has extensively and more applied to style professional support systems to design diverse diseases, e.g., inflammatory disease detection, parasite detection, carcinoma detection, and rehabilitation. A significant quantity of analysis is being exhausted from the first Carcinoma Designation victimization CAD systems. The automatic systems requirement arises attributable to the data character—CT scans—used in carcinoma designation. A respiratory organ CT scan contains typically quite 250 pictures per scan. Examining this in-depth dataset for every patient is a complicated, long, and tedious medical specialist task [5].

Moreover, the character of nodules that decide a patient's fate is brutal, as their form and size vary from slice to slice. Typically, they are hooked up to alternative pneumonic structures, like vessels or bronchioles. The color within which they seem on CT scans may take issue. These factors augment the quality of distinctive them. However, identical parts, once recognized, facilitate researchers in shaping the course of their methodology. An elementary step in respiratory organ nodules detection is the correct respiratory organ segmentation from the CT image. For this purpose, various techniques are planned for economic respiratory organ segmentation. Some algorithms need a couple of seed pixels on the lungs region within the image. So, utilize region-growing techniques to phase the lungs. The algorithmic program extracts the chest out of complete CT pictures employing a region-growing algorithmic program taking four seed points as input. The identical technique was accustomed to phase the lungs from the chest [5]. Makaju et al. [5], additionally use a region-growing algorithmic program for respiratory organ segmentation. They use the middle picture element of the slice as a seed. The tactic segments are the nodules with the help of the radiologists. The technique planned divides the chest CT scan into four classes: respiratory organ wall, parenchyma, bronchioles, and nodules.

The active contour technique is employed to phase lungs from the CT pictures. Various ways within the literature use nodule intensity or color thresholds to find nodules in CT pictures. The CT image are preprocessed with a bi-histogram exploit to enhance its sharpness. The resultant image with threshold is processed to get corresponding parts. And picture element values of those metameric regions are passed as alternatives to fuzzy intellectual system for nodule detection. A rule-based technique for respiratory organ segmentation is developed. Nodule size is employed to find potential nodule regions. The algorithms are threshold-based methods for classifying respiratory organ nodule [4–7].

The 3D data provided by many imaging modalities are just the rendering of the whole anatomical surface, where the target to be treated will be hidden. One of the most common visualization methods is direct volume rendering as the classification of an object is possible through volume rendering in contrast to the surface rendering. The main parameter to be concentrated in volume reconstruction is that the rendered volume should be view-dependent. The generated triangle mesh of the surface extracted from 2D slices is visible from all viewpoints [8]. This paper proposes a simple approach called ray casting to obtain the 3D reconstruction from multiple 2D lung carcinoma images that address the issue due to view-dependent by occlusion culling. The second main advantage of ray casting is that it produces high-quality surface from the 2D slices and thus increases the internal resolution and classification of objects.

A precise diagnosis of a tumor is essential in the case of abolishing the tumor through surgery. The surgical planning desires a sterile environment to interact with the patient's medical record during surgery. Today computer technology is growing in the field of hospitals. This technology must be used safely to prevent serious fatal errors that could lead to potentially fatal events. Keyboards and mice are the theoretical methods of human-computer interaction today. Unfortunately, one of the most common forms of transmission from one person to another is doctors and nurses' critical monitoring units, including computer keyboards and mice.

The distributed interactive tool aimed at surgical planning is the kinect camera. Kinect is a motion sensor device produced by Microsoft which is used to create a touch-less, computer-aided, gesture-based control of the medical images in the operation theatre [9]. The hand gestures captured by kinect were transformed into computational value to control the medical data. Kinect replaces mice and keyboard functions by providing a touchless gesture-based control of medical images, thus helping surgeons locate the tumor effectively [9]. So that neither surgeon nor technician needs to touch and interact with the computer in the operation theatre.

11.2 Image Processing Methodologies for Lung Cancer

Vijh et al. [10] had developed a WOA_SVM in order to automate the lung cancer diagnosis system [10]. This method intends to determine normal or abnormalities of the lung CT image. A whale optimization algorithm has been developed for optimal feature selection and to achieve the precise construction of the results with robust model. Sunil Kumar et al. [11] developed a region growing algorithm for lung segmentation technique to separate the lung nodule from the lung lobe for better accuracy in lung nodules segmentation. The method was able to distribute lung components with high precision (77%).

Prabin et al. [12] conveyed that lung images' automatic segmentation increases as the CC-based region grows. The contextual clustering was proved to have better results than the manual seed point region growing method. Cruz et al. [13] reported that the data have a distinct and complementary nature of the combination of geometry and visual properties. Kaur et al. [14] had analyzed the importance of the early detection of lung cancer and through the preaching of the triggering images. Molina et al. [15] developed a machine learning method to identify a defined set of hand gestures using depth charts.

Chourmouzios et al. [16] designed an imaging procedure on selected anisotropic diffusion parameters. It explains the parameters of the anisotropic diffusion for better enhancement of images. Gallo et al. [17] had introduced an open-source system for uncontrolled and highly interactive research of medical images. Pedro et al. [18] had used the connecting sensors to discover detection points for analysis of human body movements. Staub et al. [19] had discussed on robot assistants that are mainly used to perform autonomous activities in minimally invasive surgery and to increase the complexity of tele presence systems.

11.3 Proposed Methodology

The paper's main objective is to acquire multiple gestures from human using Kinect motion sensor and interrelate with the 2D medical images (to diagnose Lung Cancer), segmented tumor slices, 3D volume as shown in Fig. 11.1. Based on the gestures, the proposed work, aims to manipulate and control the medical image and the visualization model. Rotation can be done by pointing at the starting and to drag towards

Fig. 11.1 3D volume

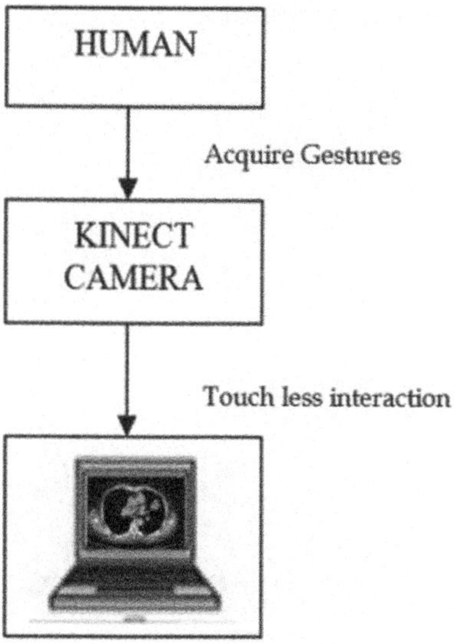

the direction needed. Other actions, like holding and turning the object, can also be done. There are two zooming options, i.e., zoom in and zoom out. To zoom in, the user has to use two fingers to bring them closer that are far away in the distance to enlarge the object. The zoom out is just opposite to the action of zoom in. Here we need to bring the fingers closer from a distance. These zoom in and out can also be done with mouse scrolls.

The medical images contain lots of slices that can be processed and visualized in a 3Dimensional volumetric model [20]. The medical visualization applications accept to change the portion of the image from multiple directions. For changing the image slice, use a hand up and down movement by swiping on the screen. This gesture is valid only in 2Dimensional medical imaging.

11.3.1 Overview

Medical imaging is the technique of representing the interior of the body in 2D space. The 2D image will give a good classification of anatomical structure, but the tumor which might have the same contrast like the neighbor region is not distinctive in 2D images, thus certain pre-processing methodologies are adopted to enhance the image followed by extracting the tumor for further analysis and visualization as shown in Fig. 11.2.

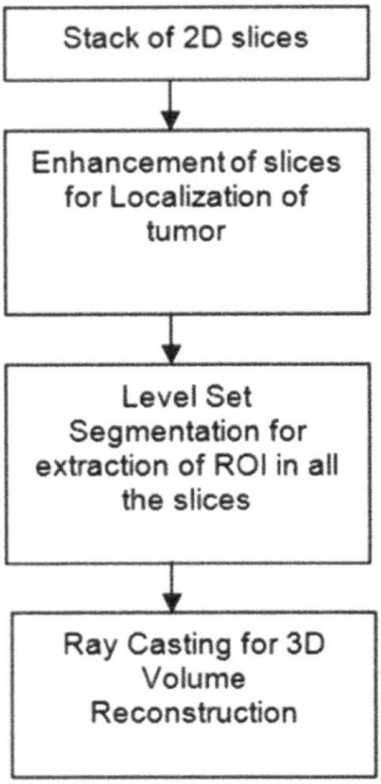

Fig. 11.2 Visualization

11.3.2 Image Enhancement

The purpose of enhancements to image was to get better interpretation and understanding about information. Several publications agitate the improvement of frames from scrutiny videos to boost the video's visual quality; which underlies information, that the individual shelves' pixel, aren't only analyzed however also changed. At the same time, alternative analysis approaches delineated within the approaching sections solely attempt to dig up information with no changes to the content [19–22]. During the context, many image process procedures are applied. It concentrates on methods as well as the analysis that addresses the domain of endoscopy. Further, side notably necessary during this context is time period capability as a optimized result ought to instantaneously visible on-screen throughout the procedure [23]. Though, image improvement and pre-processing don't seem to be interesting among real-time applications. Still, it may also have importance as a preparation step to extent the automatic process. Earlier works embraces automatic adjustment of contrast with the assistance of cluster and bar chart modification; removal of temporal noise, i.e., removing the tiny flying particles or else fast-moving smoke to show a brief moment at a position, employing a temporal median filter of color values. Color standardization uses an affine transformation to urge obviate a reddish tinge caused by the blood throughout therapeutic interventions and acquire a lot of natural colors [24, 25].

11.3.2.1 Anisotropic Diffusion

The extracted anisotropic scattering false preprocessing technique is the transformation that allows changes in the distance and that the image was made. Frequency and high margins algorithm maintain and improves the image elements of low-frequency diffusion by applying the law (Fig. 11.3).

By an equation,

$$\partial I/\partial \tau = \delta\iota\varpi(\chi(\xi, \psi, \tau)\ \nabla I) = \nabla\chi.\nabla I + \chi(\xi, \psi, \tau)\ \Delta I \qquad (11.1)$$

In Eq. 11.1 Where Δ is Laplace's slope, div is the divergence operator and C (x, y, t) is the coefficient of diffusion. C (x, y, t) controls the diffusion coefficient and is generally chosen according to the image's slope to maintain the image's edges.

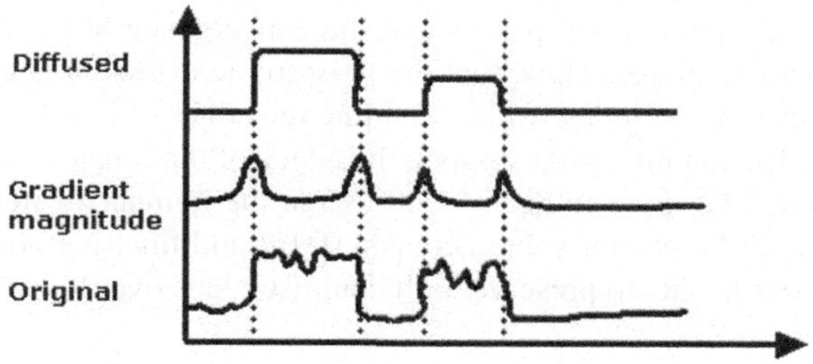

Fig. 11.3 Anisotropic diffusion

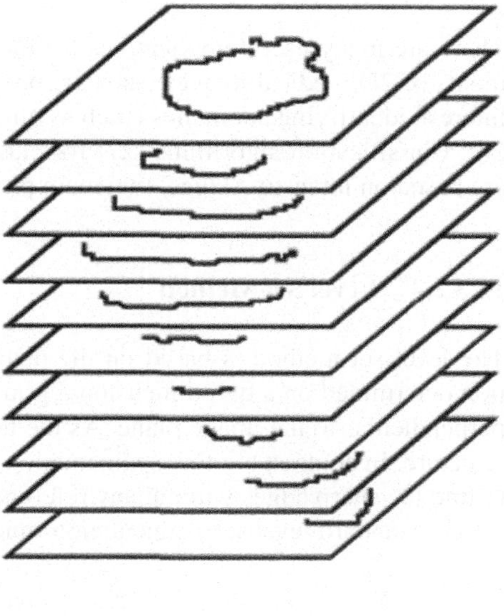

Fig. 11.4 Reconstruction of the 3D dataset by a series of 2D slices

11.3.2.2 Description of Algorithm

For Anisotropic diffusion, description is as follows. Digital images get suffered from noisiness rarely. But we require the perfect noiseless images. This work utilizes diffusion equations, especially anisotropic diffusion, to cut off the image's noise level. Applying these kinds of methods is a trade-off between retaining information and the noise level. Diffusion equations may reduce the noise level, but they also may blur the edges and thus information is lost. We discuss the mathematics and theoretical results behind the diffusion equations. We start with continuous equations and build towards discrete equations as digital images are fully discrete.

The main focus is on iterative method, that is, we diffuse the image step by step. As it occurs, we need certain assumptions for these equations to produce good results, one of which is a time step restriction and the other is a correct choice of a diffusivity function. We construct an anisotropic diffusion algorithm to denoise images and compare it to other diffusion equations. We discuss the edge-enhancing property, the noise removal properties and the convergence of the anisotropic diffusion. Results on test images show that the anisotropic diffusion is capable of reducing the noise level of the image while retaining the edges of image and as mentioned, anisotropic diffusion may even sharpen the edges of the image. The steps area follows: Initially read the input image second assign the number of iterations, third set the integration of constant value between 0–1/7 and finally gradient modules and conduction coefficients to preserve high contrast edges over low contrast.

11.3.2.3 Image Segmentation

There are many useful applications for medical professionals to differentiate fragments of 2D medical images, such as: predicting sounds of interest and objects of interest, identifying anomalies (such as tumors, polyps, etc.), of tissue Quantity [14, 26]. Classification algorithms [27] for classification, other objects and boundaries are based on intensity values' two main properties: continuity and homogeneity.

11.3.2.4 Level Set Method

The level set method is based on the determination of the initial level C(t) function determined on a two-dimensional grid (x, y). The zero level function is moved perpendicular to the image plane. As the iteration increases the size will define the structure. In contrast to other segmentation algorithms, the Level set method is used to find the sharp edges without any reference template.

The standard level set segmentation function is given by Eq. 11.2.

$$F = 1 - \varepsilon\kappa + \beta(\nabla\varphi \cdot \nabla\nabla I) \tag{11.2}$$

Here "1" represents the outline inside the object. "εκ" is a viscous term that reduces the curvature of the outline. The last term is an edge attraction term that outlines the edge.

11.3.2.5 Volume Rendering

Volume rendering (Fig. 11.5.) of the medical images provide quantitative information about the properties of anatomic tissues and their coordination with the surrounding. Volume is the cumulative representation of the 2D slices as shown in Fig. 11.4. The volume of 2D sampled data can be rendered either by surface or volume rendering methods. Surface rendering just gives the surface representation of the volume by removing the hidden part, thus lag in the classification of internal objects. So, Volume

Fig. 11.5 Volume rendering

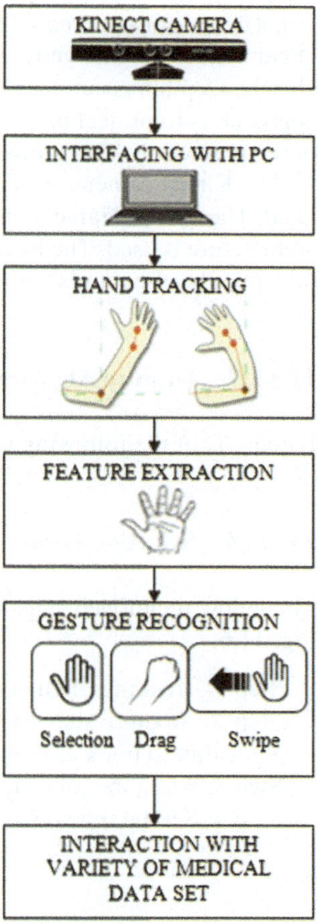

Rendering based on ray casting was used to reconstruct the 3D from slices efficiently. Volume rendering provides both surface and opacity of the volume.

11.3.2.6 Interaction Using Kinect

Kinect is capable of capturing the depth of each pixel in the scene by using infrared emitter and camera. The data gives the geometric information about the scene. The resolution of the sensor is 640 $\times$ 480 pixels in 30 Hz [15]. The user's skeleton image is obtained from the depth data, which is used to define the gestures. The common gestures used for interacting with the medical images are select, drag, swipe, rotate, and zoom. The gesture analysis in Kinect is achieved by three major steps like tracking, recognition, and user interface. The system's field of view is 58° horizontally, 45° vertically, and 70° diagonally, with a working radius of 0.8 m (2.6 feet) to 3.5 m (11 feet). depth. An IR laser emitter projects a well-known bitmap [28, 29]. These points are recorded by an IR camera and compared with a known model. Disturbances are known to be superficial changes and can be detected more or less closely. Depth measurements are performed using structured light technology. This approach is to project an image of pixels into scene and capture the transformation of the projection. This allows you to calculate the distance from the pixel (depth).

The Kinect camera, located in front of the screen, captures a series of images by hand. The current frame number represents the time information [30, 31]. A two-tier architecture is used. The lower level provides tracking, recognition functionality and the upper level controls the user interface.

11.3.2.7 Gesture Algorithm

It consists of the following steps.

11.3.2.8 Selection Gesture

The below mentioned steps explain the procedure of selection gesture as shown in Fig. 11.6.

Step 1: Tracking of cursor path to define the mouse movement
Step 2: Acquire the shape of hand by executing Contour and Convexity hull algorithm to track each node point of hand
Step 3: Align the joints to recognize the gesture
Step 4: Set the time delay to hold a position for clicking the image.

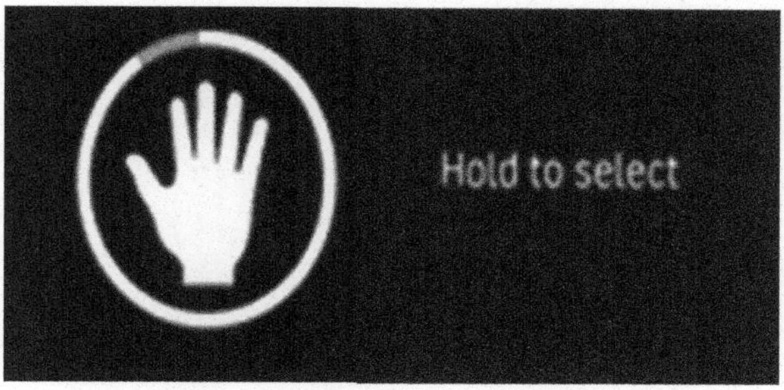

Fig. 11.6 Selection gesture

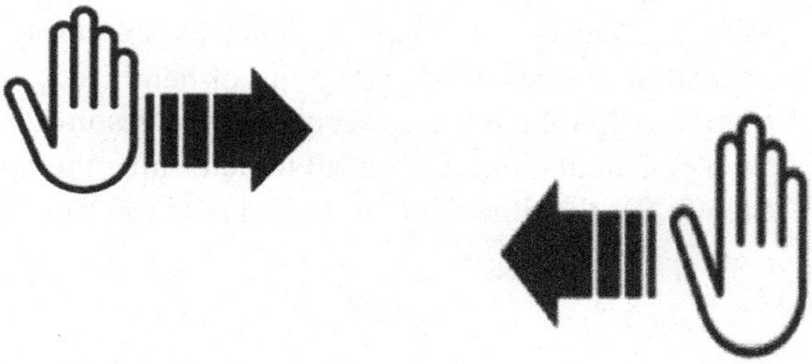

Fig. 11.7 Swipe gesture

11.3.2.9 Swipe Gesture

In the swipe gesture (Fig. 11.7), the hand remains above the elbow and moves periodically from left to right. The below mentioned steps explain the procedure.

Step 1: Tracking of cursor path to define the mouse movement
Step 2: Acquire the shape of hand by executing Contour and Convexity hull algorithm to track each node point of hand
Step 3: Create a recognizer function to recognize the gesture for running the slideshow
Step 4: Assign swipe right leads to the next slide and swipe left will go to the previous slide
Step 5: Load the set of medical data with a common path and assign index value to follow the sequence
Step 6: Create a function to display previous, current and next image for sliding when swiping occurs.

11.3.2.10 Fist Gesture

The gesture is activated based on the distance measure from the centroid of the palm and the fingers. Initialize the header function to interface the Kinect with the selection gesture. The below mentioned steps explain the procedure of fist gesture (Fig. 11.8).

Step 1: Tracking of cursor path to define the mouse movement

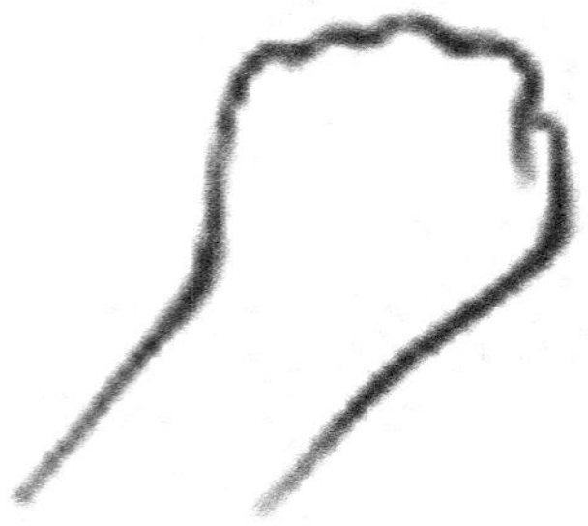

Fig. 11.8 Fist gesture

Step 2: Acquire the shape of hand by executing Contour and Convexity hull algorithm to track each node point of hand
Step 3: Align the joints to recognize the gesture
Step 4: Calculation of centroid to determine the opening and closing of the fist.
Step 5: Set the time delay to hold a position for clicking the image.

11.4 Results and Discussion

A frequent drawback is we have a tendency to use to face throughout low-level visualization consists of eliminating noise and small-scales from a picture at the same time, maintain or perhaps enhance the edge structure. Anisotropic diffusion filtering use Non-linear equations could one among the various solutions to accumulate the goals uses a single image to boost image resolution using interpolation and forward-and-backward non-linear diffusion post-processing that suppresses ringing (Fig. 11.9).

The process is incredibly productive in distinctive those medical pictures that provide similar pictures for two or more dangerous diseases. The approach respects the boundaries between the edges.

The level set segmentation was performed on all slices. Then the volume was rendered using a volume rendering technique as shown in Fig. 11.10.

The process experimented with two unique users (Fig. 11.11): the primary one that has recorded (U1) and another one without abundant sports background (U2). The score was calculated using the two movement comparison algorithms: the joint rotation (A1) and the angle between joints (A2). We are able to notice that the scores are much lower as the complexity of the experiment rises. The Kinect sensor's capture wasn't good to enhance skeletal animation. However, there was a pair of common observations to require under consideration.

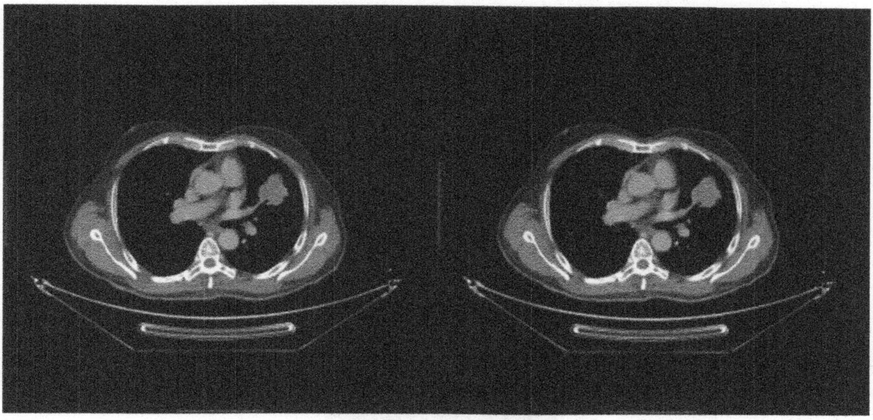

(a) (b)

Fig. 11.9 Image enhancement by anisotropic diffusion. **a** Initial stage image, **b** Final stage image

11.4.1 Selection Gesture

The selection gesture concentrates on (1) how to choose a suitable set of gestures with an adequate level of discrimination power, and (2) comparing invariant moments as well geometric properties while recognizing hand gestures (Fig. 11.12).

Two-dimensional structures, specifically cluster property and features matrices, are utilized for gesture selection and for evaluation of different gesture characteristics. For classification, method uses Moment invariants, Zernike moments, and geometric features. Correspondingly compared recognition rates as well as comparative results make sure the best performance of geometric features.

11.4.2 Swipe Gesture

A **swipe gesture** occurs when the user moves one or more fingers across the screen in a specific horizontal or vertical direction. Use the UISwipeGestureRecognizer class to detect **swipe gestures** as shown in Fig. 11.13.

11.4.3 Drag Gesture

If we rotate then offset, then the offset is applied based on our view's rotated axis. For example, if we move something 100 pixels to its left then rotate 90°, we would end up with it being 100 pixels to the left and rotated 90°. But if we rotated 90° then moved

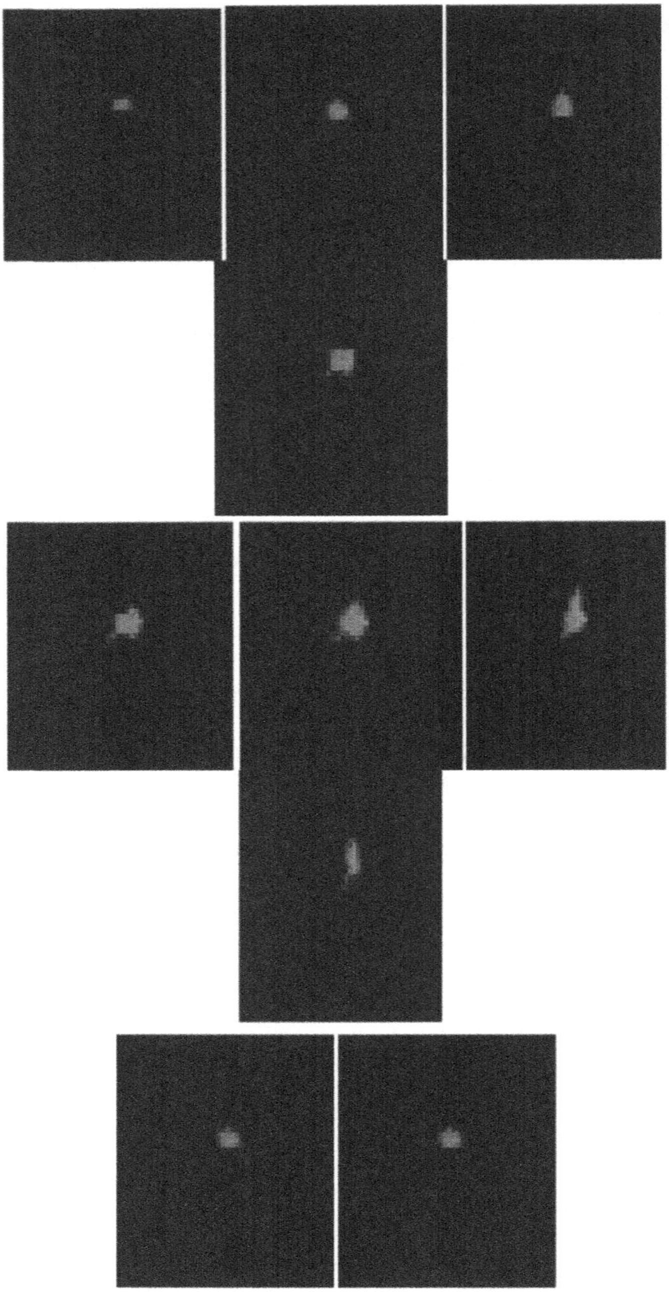

Fig. 11.10 Segmented tumor from the stack of slices

Exercise	Score A1		Score A2	
	U1	U2	U1	U2
Arm stretches	95	81	98	94
Lateral Stretch	80	77	97	91
Quadriceps Stretch	86	69	93	90
Lateral Lunge	79	70	91	90
Squats	80	61	87	75
Hip Extension	75	52	80	65

Fig. 11.11 Performance analysis

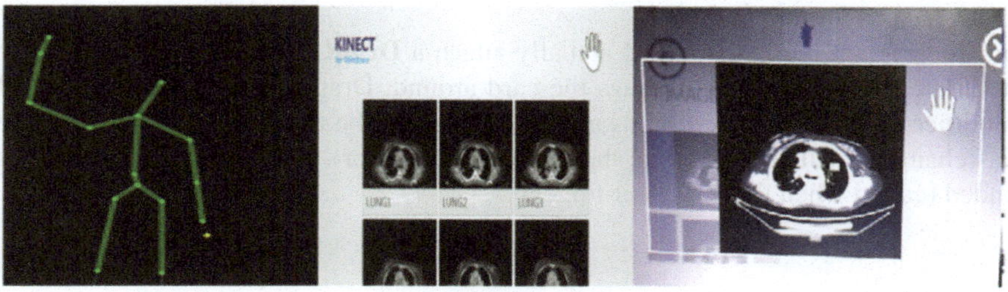

(a) (b) (c)

Fig. 11.12 **a** Tracked skeletal image **b** 2D slices loaded in program **c** Opening of image using gesture

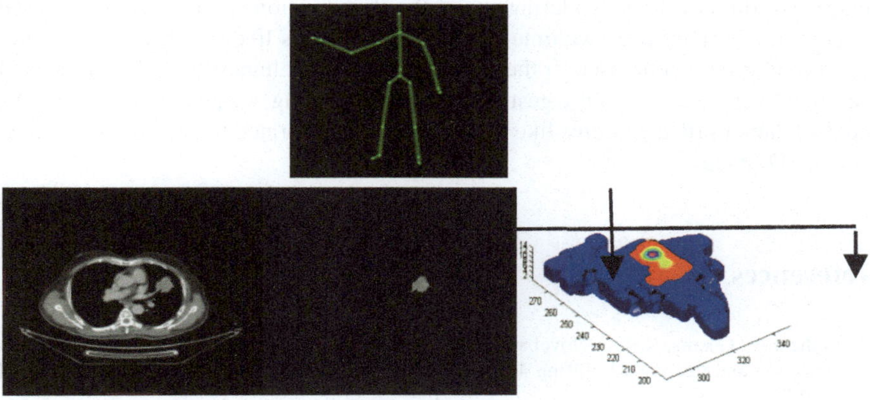

Fig. 11.13 Track skeleton and swipe set of medical data

it 100 pixels to its left, we would end up with something rotated 90° and moved 100 pixels directly down, because its concept of "left" got rotated (Fig. 11.14).

So, we have created a property to store the drag amount, and added three modifiers that use the drag amount to change the way the view is rendered. What remains is the

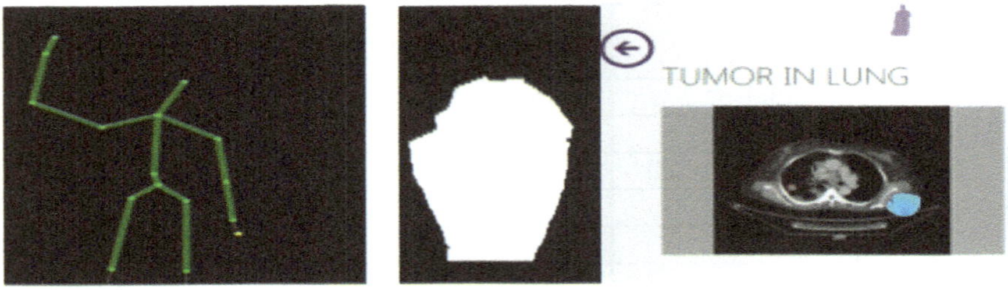

(a) (b) (c)

Fig. 11.14 **a** tracked skeletal image, **b** depth image of fist, **c** drag image using gesture

most important part: we need to actually attach a **DragGesture** to our card so that it updates **offset** as the user drags the card around. Drag gestures have two useful modifiers of their own, letting us attach functions to be triggered when the gesture has changed (called every time they move their finger), and when the gesture has ended (called when they lift their finger).

11.5 Conclusion

The diagnosis of lung tumors based on severity and depth has been achieved. The lung tumor was localized by improving the contrast and homogeneity of the input image. The direct volume rendering attains the classification of internal objects based on contrast. Further direct volume rendering techniques like splatting and texture-based rendering can be used in the case of 3D space volumetric rendering. Kinect was effectively used to acquire gestures for selection, drag, swipe to interact with the medical data. Further gestures like rotate can be incorporated to control the medical data in 3D space.

References

1. Judice, A., Geetha, K.P.: A Novel assessment of various bio-imaging methods for lung tumor detection and treatment by using 4-d and 2-d ct images. Int. J. Biomed. Sci.: IJBS **9**(2), 54 (2013)
2. Al-Tarawneh, M.S.: Lung cancer detection using image processing techniques. Leonardo Electron. J. Pract. Technol. **11**(21), 147–158 (2012)
3. Wason, J.V., Nagarajan, A.: Image processing techniques for analyzing CT scan images towards the early detection of lung cancer. Bioinformation **15**(8), 596 (2019)
4. Siegel, R.L., Miller, K.D., Goding Sauer, A., Fedewa, S.A., Butterly, L.F., Anderson, J.C., Cercek, A., Smith, R.A., Jemal, A.: Colorectal cancer statistics, 2020. A Cancer journal for clinicians, CA (2020)

5. Chaudhary, A., Singh, S.S.: Lung cancer detection on CT images by using image processing. In: 2012 International Conference on Computing Sciences, pp. 142–146. IEEE (2012)
6. Makaju, S., Prasad, P.W.C., Alsadoon, A., Singh, A.K., Elchouemi, A.: Lung cancer detection using CT scan images. Procedia Comput. Sci. **125**, 107–114 (2018)
7. Senthil Kumar, K., Venkatalakshmi, K., Karthikeyan, K.: Lung cancer detection using image segmentation by means of various evolutionary algorithms. Comput. Math. Methods Med. (2019)
8. Kasturi, M.M., Sutha, P., Jayanthi, V.E.: Efficient edge detection method for diagnosis of 2D and 3D lung and liver images. In: 2017 International Conference on Inventive Systems and Control (ICISC), pp. 1–5. IEEE (2017)
9. Alabbasi, H., Gradinaru, A., Moldoveanu, F., Moldoveanu, A.: Human motion tracking & evaluation using Kinect V2 sensor. In: 2015 E-Health and Bioengineering Conference (EHB), pp. 1–4) IEEE (2015)
10. Vijh, S., Gaur, D., Kumar, S.: An intelligent lung tumor diagnosis system using whale optimization algorithm and support vector machine. Int. J. Syst. Assu. Eng. Manag., 1–11 (2019)
11. Kumar, S., Scholar, M.T., Kumar, A.: Lung Segmentation Using Region Growing Algorithm (2014)
12. Prabin, A., Veerappan, J.: Automatic segmentation of lung ct images by CC based region growing. J. Theor. Appl. Inform. Technol. **68**, 63–69 (2014)
13. Cruz, L., Lucio, D., Velho, L.: Kinect and RGBD Images: Challenges and Applications (2012). https://doi.org/10.1109/sibgrapi-t.2012.13
14. Kaur, A.R.: Feature extraction and principal component analysis for lung cancer detection in CT scan images. Int. J. Adv. Res. Comput. Sci. Softw. Eng. **3**(3) (2013)
15. Molina, Javier., Escudero-Viñolo, Marcos., Signoriello, Alessandro., Pardàs, Montse., Ferrán, Christian., Bescós, Jesús., Marqués, Ferran, Martínez, José M.: Real-time user independent hand gesture recognition from time-of-flight camera video using static and dynamic models. Mach. Vis. Appl. **24**(1), 187–204 (2013)
16. Chourmouzios, T., Maria, P.: On the choice of the parameters for anisotropic diffusion in image processing. Pattern Recogn. **46**(5), 1369–1381 (2013)
17. Gallo, L., Placitelli, A.P., Ciampi, M.: Controller-free exploration of medical image data: experiencing the Kinect. In: 2011 24th International Symposium On Computer-Based Medical Systems (CBMS), pp. 1–6. IEEE (2011)
18. Pedro, L.M., de Paula Caurin, G.A.: Kinect evaluation for human body movement analysis. In: 2012 4th IEEE RAS & EMBS International Conference on Biomedical Robotics and Biomechatronics (BioRob), pp. 1856–1861. IEEE (2012)
19. Staub, C., Lucio, D., Velho, L.: Human—computer Interfaces for Interaction with surgical tools in robotic surgery. IEEE RAS/EMBS International Conference on Biomedical Robotics and Bio-mechatronics (2013)
20. Granum, E., Kufaisal bin Mohd Sidik, M., Shahrizal bin Sunar, M., bin Ismail, I.: A novel gesture-based interface e for a VR simulation. Workshop on Digital Media and Digital Content Management (2012)
21. Fabian, J., Can, S., Jensen, B.: Integrating the Microsoft Kinect with Simulink: real time object tracking example. IEEE/ASME Trans. Mechatron. (2014)
22. Mohd Sidik, M.K., Sunar, M.S., Ismail, I., Mokhtar, M.K.: A Study on natural interaction for human body motion using depth image data. In: Digital Media and Digital Content Management, Workshop on, pp. 97–102. IEEE Computer Society (2011)
23. Jeena Jacob, I., Srinivasagan, K.G., Ebby Darney, P., Jayapriya, K.: Deep learned inter-channel colored texture pattern: a new Chromati-texture descriptor. Pattern Anal. Appl., Springer, Vol. 23, 239–251 (2020)
24. Apirajitha, P.S., Gopala Krishnan, C., Aravind Swaminathan, G., Manohar, E.: Enhanced secure user data on cloud using cloud data centre computing and decoy technique. Int. J. Innov. Technol. Expl. Eng. https://doi.org/10.35940/ijitee.i7777.078919 (IJITEE) ISSN: 2278–3075, Volume-8 Issue-9, July 2019

25. Münzer, B., Schoeffmann, K., Böszörmenyi, L.: Content-based processing and analysis of endoscopic images and videos: a survey. Multimed Tools Appl. **77**, 1323–1362 (2018)
26. Khehrah, N., Farid, M.S., Bilal, S., Khan, M.H.: Lung nodule detection in CT images using statistical and shape-based features. J. Imaging **6**(2), 6 (2020)
27. Prasannavenkatesan, T.: Probable forecasting of epidemic COVID-19 in using COCUDE model, EAI Endorsed Transactions on Pervasive Health and Technology, Online First, https://doi.org/10.4108/eai.3-2-2021.168601 (2021)
28. Theerthagiri, P., Jeena Jacob, I., Usha Ruby, A. et al.: Prediction of COVID-19 Possibilities using KNN Classification Algorithm, 03 November 2020, PREPRINT (Version 2) available at Research Square
29. Antony Judice, A., Parimala Geetha, K.: A Novel assessment of various bio-imaging methods for lung tumor detection and treatment by using 4-D and 2-D CT images. Int. J. Biomed. Sci. **9**(2), 54–60 (2013)
30. Sen, S., Garg, A., Gealy, D.V., McKinley, S., Jen, Y., Goldberg, Y.: Automating multi-throw multilateral surgical suturing with a mechanical needle guide and sequential convex optimization. In: 2016 IEEE International Conference on Robotics and Automation (ICRA), pp. 4178–4185. IEEE (2016)
31. Prasannavenkatesan, T.: Forecasting hyponatremia in hospitalized patients using multilayer perceptron and multivariate linear regression techniques. Concurrency and Computation: Practice and Experience. Springer, e6248 (2021)

Part III
Advanced Machine Learning Paradigms for Cancer Diagnosis

Chapter 12
Deep MammoNet: Early Diagnosis of Breast Cancer Using Multi-layer Hierarchical Features of Deep Transfer Learned Convolutional Neural Network

K. O Mohamed Aarif, P. Sivakumar, Caffiyar Mohamed Yousuff, and B. A. Mohammed Hashim

Abstract Deep Convolutional Neural Network (CNN) comprises of multiple convolutional layers which learn feature form input image with different levels of abstraction; In this work, we address the issue to improvise the recognition accuracy of CNN for classification of breast cancer from mammogram images. To achieve optimize classification we propose a multilayer hierarchical convolutional feature integration in deep transfer learned CNN. In Deep CNN the last layer learns significant features that are highly invariant but their spatial resolutions are too stiff to exactly confine the target. In contrast, features from earlier layers offer more exact localization and hold more fine-grained spatial subtleties for exact confinement but are less invariant. This observation recommends that reasoning with multiple layers of CNN features for breast cancer detection from mammogram images is of great importance. In this work, we proposed to integrate the features extracted from the earlier layer and the last layer of deep CNN to train and improvise the classification accuracy of breast cancer detection in the mammogram image. We also discussed that consistent improvement in accuracy is obtained by using mammogram augmentation and different weight learning factors across different layers.

Keywords Deep learning · Breast cancer detection · Mammogram · Herirchical convolutional feature · Convolutional neural network

---

K. O. Mohamed Aarif (✉) · C. Mohamed Yousuff · B. A. Mohammed Hashim
C.Abdul Hakeem College of Engineering and Technology, Melvisharam, Tamil Nadu, India
e-mail: aarifko.ece@cahcet.edu.in

C. Mohamed Yousuff
e-mail: yousuff.ece@cahcet.edu.in

B. A. Mohammed Hashim
e-mail: hashimba.ece@cahcet.edu.in

P. Sivakumar
Dr. N.G.P. Institute of Technology, Coimbatore, Tamil Nadu, India

J. Nayak et al. (eds.), *Advanced Machine Learning Approaches in Cancer Prognosis*, Intelligent Systems Reference Library 204,
https://doi.org/10.1007/978-3-030-71975-3_12

12.1 Introductions

Cancer is a genetic disorder that results from the uncontrolled division of abnormal cells and destroys the body tissue [1]. Generally, a flaw in cell separation during the progression course results in genetic alterations, and it may be gained or caused a twisting of DNA because of specific revelations. Scientifically three basic kinds of nucleic acid add to malignancy development, they are malignant growth drivers (to be specific DNA repair gene), tumor silencer gene, and proto-oncogenes [2]. Proto-oncogenes are nothing but the genes allowing cells to develop and isolate when they shouldn't do as such, tumor silencer is the permitting cells to run wild in their division procedure and DNA repair gene is the one leaving the dented DNA without a real fixing. Malignant growth may extent to another part of the body from tissues or an organ, in such cases, the malignant growth type is called metastatic cancer [3]. Malignant growth fluctuates in the area they are framed at, and the level of their seriousness of disease will generally vary with time.

There are more than 100 chronicled sorts of cancer, which are given names taking into account the organ or tissue they are formed at [2]. Understanding the procedure of the malignant growth process, the organ it is created in, and the reasons for its expansion has aid treatment revelation. Despite the ongoing advances in medicine and the medication industry, an ideal remedy for the disease is yet to be found and assessed. Malignancy influences all classes of individuals, young and old, yet it is discovered more in senior individuals than youth. There are various intuitions for the types of cancer which are based on positions and gender. Among the regular disease types in females are breast cancer [4].

Breast cancer starts and develops in the breast tissue and occurs due to abnormal cell division which develops a mass in the breast called a tumor. Breast cancer influence gender independently, but it is more common in women and the second leading cause of death. According to the WHO report, breast cancer is the most prevalent and widespread in women with over 2 million cases in 2018 and 15% of cancer death in 2019. An indication of breast cancer is any new hard mass or lump in breast tissue. However, not all hard masses are cancerous. Medically breast cancer is classified as benign (non-cancerous) and malignant (cancerous) as shown in Fig. 12.1.

The following changes in the breast denote the breast cancer proliferation:

1. A lump or pain in the breast
2. Pain in the nipple area
3. Itching or Irritation of breast skin
4. The structural change in the breast
5. Leakage of nipple including blood.

Therefore, early diagnosis and medication of breast cancer are crucial for a patient's health and to improve a higher endurance rate. In the last decade, 15% of women were diagnosed with the most advanced stage survival rate, and 90% diagnosed at earlier

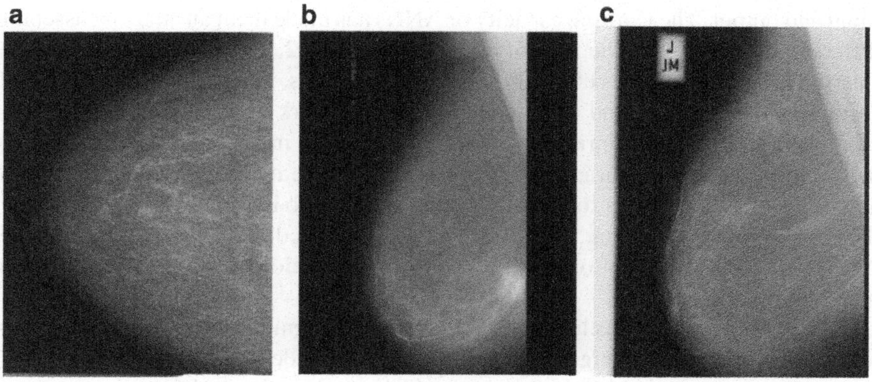

Fig. 12.1 **a** A normal breast **b** Benign mass and **c** malignant mass

stages [5]. The most universally used practices for diagnosis are self-examination, clinical examination, and screening tools like mammography, MRI, histopathology, and fine-needle aspiration cytology (FNAC) [6].

Of these, mammography is the most prevalent screening technique which helps in achieving quick, stable, and reliable diagnosis [7]. Mammography is the noninvasive screening method that involves the use of low-energy X-rays to detect the mass [8] and also a crucial factor in decreasing breast malignant growth mortality. The standard methodology of mammography coordinates tapping the breast inside a unit joint to the mammogram. When the breast is set up, steady weight is applied on the breast to have an even thickness, which improves the overall picture quality and facilitates the covering of the breast structure in the final image [9]. Usually, the mammographic pictures are taken in two views to the breast; Cranio-Caudal (CC) imaged from top and Medio-Lateral Oblique (MLO) from left to right [10].

Mammography is practiced using advanced hardware that gives significant level differentiation and contiguous goals required for dependable results. This is because mammography can give breast malignancy screening hypothesis much before any unmistakable indications. With extraordinary acuteness to calcification, mammographic assessment is extremely superior at identifying micro-calcifications and calcification clusters, which are significant delineations of breast cancer [11]. Mechanized screening of mammograms or PC supported the analysis of breast malignant growth is an immense field of exploration.

An exact and dependable prognosis can give data on the sort of required helpful mediation. This will spare numerous patients from experiencing needless agonizing and costly treatment. The most challenging part includes the characterizing of cancer tumors as benign or malignant. Studies have shown the adequacy of CAD frameworks; among the different methodologies in the field of clinical finding, Artificial Neural Network (ANN) is one of the computing techniques, which has pulled in the consideration of numerous analysts for clinical choice support. The ANNs are adaptable numerical structures that can distinguish complex connections among input and output. The learning capacity of ANNs has made them an amazing asset for different applications in the field of computer vision [12, 13]. A Standard Machine Learning (ML) procedures utilized for CAD frameworks, incorporate a hand-crafted feature extraction stage and an efficient learning network for classification. Numerous machine learning algorithms have been presented in the literature. Regarding the performance and accuracy of various classes where it focuses on segmentation as a crucial part and didn't follow any viable measures to improve the reparability of the classes before preparing their ML model [8]. Proceeding onward from old-style AI later exertion has been outfitted towards the utilization of Deep Learning (DL) methods.

Deep learning strategies have achieved enormous significance in the field of clinical image analysis and huge endeavors have been made in CAD frameworks. As opposed to conventional ML techniques, which require a manual feature extraction stage, which in turn depends on domain-specific information. Deep learning strategies adaptively gain proficiency with the fitting component extraction process from the information concerning the objective yield. This removes the dreary procedure of building and examining the ability of features while encouraging the reproducibility of the systems. With the evolution of deep learning, massive research works in breast cancer detection have been presented exploiting various CNN architecture. Deep learning analyze suspected lesions especially & precisely through quantitative investigation [14].

12.2 Literature Study

Several investigations have been reported for breast cancer using a mammogram and have applied various ways to deal with the related issues and achieve high classification exactness. Here we will be looking at the exploration done using deep learning for mammogram based breast cancer detection in the past four years. We categorized the literature study into three subsections. (Literature study in Reviews & survey; In Machine learning: In Deep learning).

12.2.1 In Reviews & Surveys

A systematic review & future scope of breast cancer modalities using deep learning radiomics is presented in [15] with the present research to make the deep learning-based radiomics accountable and narrow down the attention on the analytic estimation of deep learning-based CAD frameworks to give recommendations and to lessen the outstanding burden of radiologists. Similarly in Ref. [16], a review has been presented on the current status of high-density breast cancer detection. Here the authors discussed shifting breast densities over the globe, the gust of breast thickness data identified with imaging supported determination, and how the diagnosis has seen a sensational move in new screening proposals in mammography and physical assessment. The authors conclude that for patients with suspected/ known breast neoplasia, the breast thickness is also a prime risk factor. In Ref. [17] the author surveys the components impacting mammographic density (MD), the accessible strategies for MD evaluation, its impact on breast malignancy, and discussed the supplemental screening strategies for ladies with thick breast tissue. The study on deep learning in breast cancer has been presented in [18], where the authors discoursed the most normal breast malignancy imaging modalities and breast disease databases that are mostly referred in the recent research articles. Then the authors audited the application regions of deep learning in clinical image examination and finally listed the exploration gap for advanced research.

12.2.2 In Machine Learning

A Multi-million Mammography Image Dataset—the Cohort of Screen-Aged Women is presented in [19] where they have developed a dataset from the women's summoned to screening examinations between 2008 and 2015, about 2 million mammography images have presently been collected. In Ref. [20] the authors have constructed a mammogram dataset with masses by selecting the 106 best mammography images form INbreast [21] dataset and performed augmentation to generate around 7000 images. In Ref. [22] a breast Cancer detection utilizing Anthropometric and Clinical Features has been presented where the authors find the most pertinent biomarkers of breast disease, which can be accomplished from customary blood investigation and anthropometric estimations to improve the exhibition of current CAD arrangement of early breast malignant growth recognition. This examination used an ongoing informational collection containing nine anthropometric and clinical qualities. The SVM model with radial basic function (RBF) part gave off an impression of being the best classifier by using six features. Similarly in [23] varying parameters of machine learning are utilized for prediction of breast cancer by taking six supervised machine learning algorithms with radial basis function kernel.

12.2.3 In Deep Learning

A deep learning architecture is presented in [24] with semantic segmentation for breast cancer classification which eliminates the noise and artifacts from the mammogram after the dense muscles area is removed. In Ref. [25] the authors presented a CAD-based diagnosis of breast cancer embracing You-Only-Look-Once (YOLO) for classification and full-resolution convolutional network (FrCN). They took three different deep CNN models and independently analyzed using the INbreast dataset.

In Ref. [26] a breast density based tumor detection and classification have been presented, the authors have applied the Seeded Region Growing (SRG) technique for segmentation of tumors from the mammogram and performed experimentation on three freely accessible datasets; RIDER Breast MR Pictures, Mammographic Image Analysis Society (MIAS), and Digital Database for Screening Mammography (DDSM) and attained an averaged accuracy of 91.4%. A fast and compact MobileNet based architecture for breast cancer detection has been presented in [27], here the author has experimented with 2 above mentioned standard datasets. The proposed network is faster and consumes less memory but not won the race in recognition accuracy which is around 86%.

The author in this study [28] has given a diagram of the fundamental ideas and improvements in the field of AI for breast malignant growth recognition in advanced mammography and computerized breast tomosynthesis. Capacities that ought to be utilized in the clinical domain has been evaluated.

A comparative analysis of different CNN models on various publicly available dataset has been presented in [29, 30]. Here the authors have compared the performance of seven models experimented on four benchmark datasets and highlighted the pros and cons of these models. In [31] a lightweight deep CNN model has been showcased vigorously which identifies, portion, and characterizes the mammogram image irregularities and assesses the possibilities of transfer learning procedures by reusing pre-prepared models to encourage training and evade the datasets hazards. The outcomes show that the framework associates well with the ground truth explanations and can distinguish 85% of the majority at three false positives.

Hybrid network, CNN–Linear classifier [32] & CNN–Multiple Linear classifiers [33] based breast cancer detection has been presented, in which CNN is used as a feature extractor, and the linear classifiers are used for classification. They experimented with their hybrid network on two datasets; (1) the DDSM and (2) the Curated Breast Imaging Subset of DDSM (CBIS-DDSM) and have achieved 94% and 85% recognition accuracy respectively. Ting et al. [34] prepared a network from scratch for breast masses classification. Their system involves 28 convolutional and completely associated layers and it is taken care of by proposition ROIs recognized by a one-shot indicator. They led their examinations in the MIAS database.

Yeman et al. [35] introduced a deep CNN model to learn balanced reflective highlights from dual-sided perspectives on mammograms. The CAD framework was dependent on three consecutive advances. To extricate breast lesions, both right and left mammograms were overturned to place the two pictures in a similar direction. Features extracted are concatenated finally to serve the neural system (NN) classifier. By this methodology, they accomplished an exceptional precision of 93.33% in terms of AUC. Rampun et al. [36] utilized a group of an ensemble altered rendition of AlexNet pre-prepared and adjusted on CBIS-DDSM. At the inference, they picked the three best performing models and combined their potentials.

Over the most recent couple of years, deep learning models including AlexNet, VGG16, GoogleNet, DenseNet, Inception, and ResNet have been effectively proposed accomplishing a superior order execution contrasted with the shallower ones. In Ref. [37], the author introduced a correlation for breast lesions determination utilizing three deep CNN pre-trained models in which completely associated layers were utilized as the final layer for classification and accomplished acceptable recognition accuracies of 95.0%.

Lan et al. [38] examined different information mining and deep learning techniques in bioinformatics. The authors gave an actual comprehensive discussion on how deep learning impacts the clinical image investigation enormously. The authors also gave a synopsis on different improved neural systems in deep realizing which extraordinarily affected the exploration work. Mohsin Jadoon et al. [39], got an exactness of 83.74% by utilizing the CNN curvelet strategy in the MIAS database.

In Ref. [40] Three primary viewpoints are being engaged by the analysts to improve the presentation perspective of deep learning models, which shows the huge number of concealed layers go on better than the smaller systems. The self-governing execution of each layer is likewise conceivable with the bigger systems and the outcome is acquired by consolidating all the feedback from each layer.

From the literature, we identified that the CNN based classifiers outflanked the conventional classifiers with the most noteworthy accomplished precision. We also observe that the current CNN based breast cancer detection using trained models ends up in inadequate classification due to the following reasons.

12.2.4 Problem Statement

(i) In Mammogram screening: The Primary issue largely implicates the classification of breast cancer tumors as benign or malignant using a mammogram. But accurate classification using the current CNN models is difficult due to the following reasons.

(a) Concealing of prominent features due to poor brightness and contrast
(b) Integument of masses
(c) Hard to distinct thick tissues
(d) Inconsistent tissue circumstance.

And mostly all the classifier models extract significant features from the last layer of CNN for classification which are invariant and their spatial resolutions are too stiff to exactly confine the target. In contrast, features from earlier layers offer more exact localization but are less invariant [41].

(ii) Resource scarcity in Deep learning. The outstanding success of DL significantly depends on the training of CNN with the large and diverse labeled dataset, whereas in mammograms we have little datasets openly accessible. Deep CNN when trained with such a small dataset leads to convergence issues and influence in drastic performance reduction.

12.2.5 *Contribution*

The chief contributions of this work are (i). Exploiting integration of multi-layer hierarchical features of deep transfer learned network which integrates the features from earlier layers that offer more exact localization of masses but are less invariant and the significant features from the last layer of CNN for classification.

(ii). Mammogram image augmentation using GAN to generate batches of augmented images that improvise the training efficiency and classification accuracy.

(iii). The proposed network accomplishes a high classification accuracy, beating current methodologies in literature mainly concerning breast cancer detection using a mammogram.

12.3 Proposed Method

In this work, we propose the integration of multi-layer hierarchical features from pre-trained CNN for breast cancer detection based on the observation that the features of deeper layers of CNN are more significant and are invariant in all aspects. Whereas features at early layers hold all the more fine-grained spatial subtleties and are helpful for exact confinement. Figure 12.2 shows the framework of our proposed work.

Initially, the mammogram images are pre-processed with the regular deep network-oriented methods. Then we utilized Generative Adversarial Network (GAN) network to augment the dataset for generating augmented batches on mammogram images. This dataset is then used to train six powerful deep transfer learning models (AlexNet, SqueezeNet, GoogleNet, MobileNetV2, ResNet18, and DarkNet19) individually. From the trained network we extract the feature map from the first convolution layer and the last layer. These feature maps are fed to the feature concatenation function

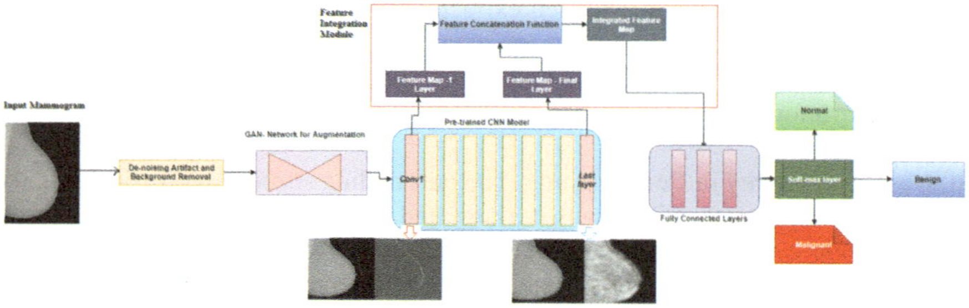

Fig. 12.2 Complete framework of the proposed method for breast cancer detection using mammograms. The pre-trained network represents the 6 CNN transfer learned models through adopting fine-tuning for some of the last convolutional blocks

unit which provides an integrated feature map. The integrated feature map is a robust and more significant feature vector which is passed on to the fully connected layers followed by a soft-max layer. The softmax layer assigns normalized positive values to each class so that they can be interpreted as probabilities. In our case, the Normal, Benign, and Malignant are the three probabilities of output class.

12.3.1 Hierarchical Features

The behavior of distinctive CNN layers for object recognition can be found in [42]. In this work, we propose to utilize the features from the various leveled layers of CNNs as opposed to as it were the last layer to confine to target.

Our methodology is based on the perception that although the last layers of pre-prepared CNNs are more compelling to catch semantics, on the other hand, they are lacking to encode the fine-grained spatial subtleties, for example, (Integument of masses and thick tissues) in the mammogram. The prior layers, on the other hand, are exact in restriction however don't catch semantics as delineated in Figs. 12.3 and 12.4. This perception proposes that the different layers of CNN highlights for mammogram screening is critical as semantics are stiff to contrast and brightness variations and spatial subtleties are successful for exact confinement of masses.

As can be seen from Figs. 12.3 and 12.4 feature activation of Conv1 has fine details of masses structure and integument of massed in both strongest and weakest activation. In contrast feature activation of the fc8 layer has consolidated details of masses and thick tissues but lags in fine-grained spatial subtleties. So in our proposed network we extract and integrate the features of each mammogram image from the final as these layer extract features which are progressive details of the masses and from the initial convolutional as these layers have specific structural details of the masses in the mammogram image.

12.3.2 Mammogram Augmentation

There are numerous approaches to address difficulties related to constrained resources in deep learning. Image Augmentation is one valuable procedure in building convolutional neural systems that can expand the size of the preparation set without obtaining new images. The thought is straightforward; replicate pictures with verities so the model can gain from more samples. By augmentation we can increase the picture in such a way that it protects the key highlights to making expectations, yet revises the pixels enough that it includes some commotion. Data Augmentations come from simple to basic changes, for example, even flipping, shading space enlargements, and irregular editing. For radiography images, the most widely used augmentation procedure is of Generative Adversarial Network (GAN) [43].

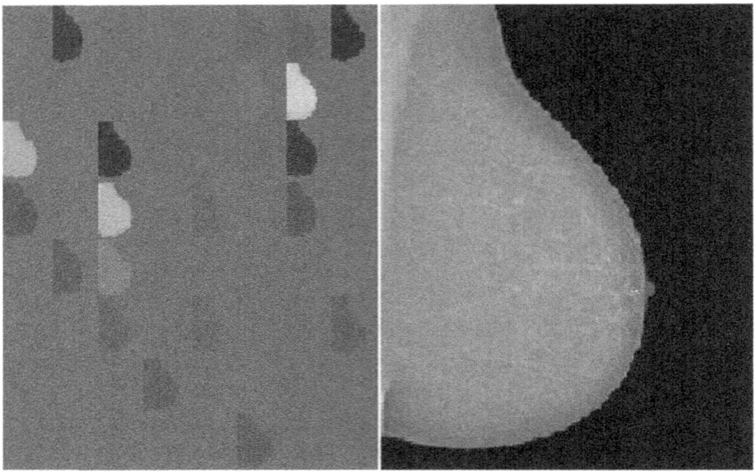

(a)

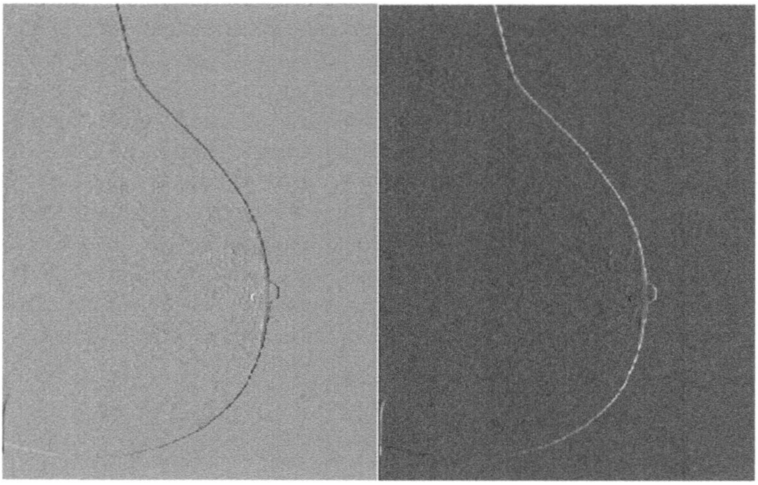

(b)

Fig. 12.3 Feature visualization of AlexNet form different layers. **a** Conv1 features activation, **b** Strongest weakest activation in conv1

Generative Adversarial Network (GAN) is a class of deep learning models that has two principle systems, called the generative system and discriminative system. The principal neural system is the generator arranges, liable for producing new replicate information cases that resemble the training information. The discriminator attempts to recognize genuine data and fake data produced by the generator network. Figure 12.5 shows the Generic GAN Model. There are several variants of GAN presented in the literature, but just for the augmentation of a mammogram, the traditional

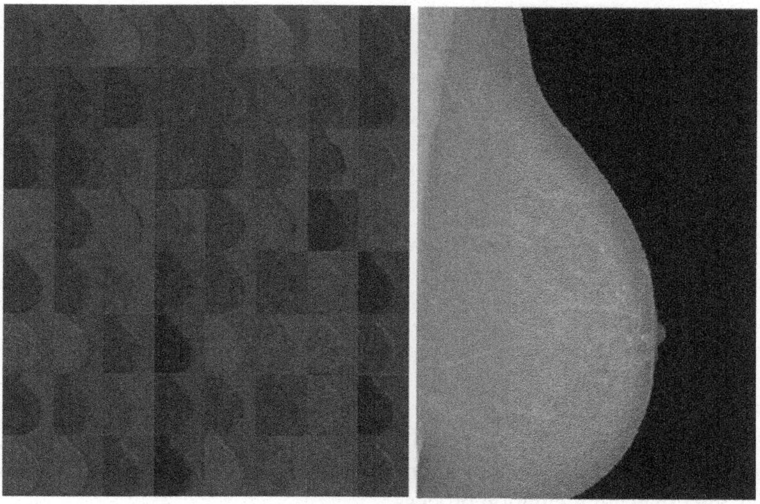

(a)

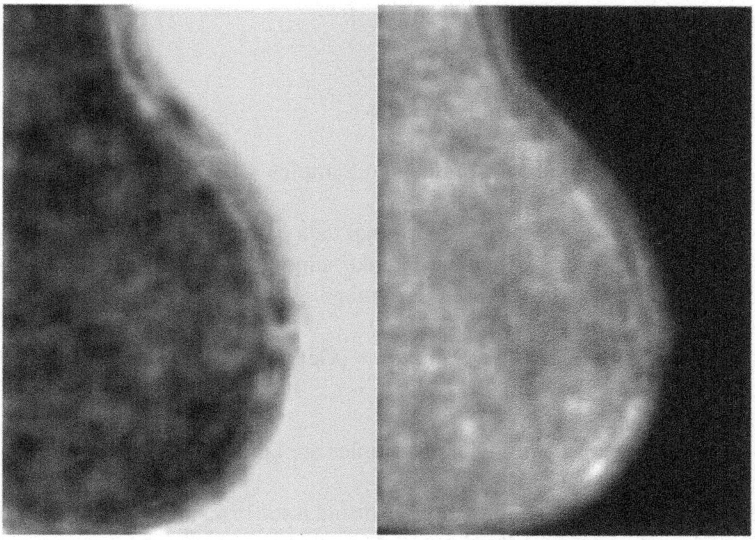

(b)

Fig. 12.4 Feature visualization of AlexNet form different layers. **a** fc8 (last layer) features activation, **b** Strongest & weakest activation in fc8

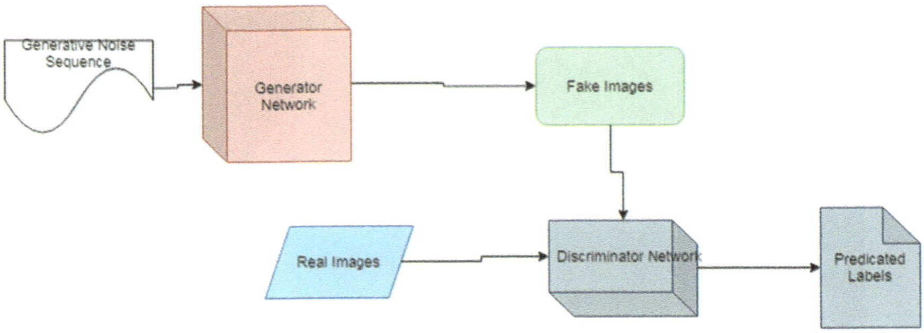

Fig. 12.5 GAN–Model for Mammogram augmentation

GAN is sufficient. Our GAN network is similar to [43] which investigates GAN for augmentation of available mammogram datasets. Our Algorithm mentioned below explains the GAN augmentation process.

Algorithm: Generative Adversarial Network

Input: Mammogram Datasets
Output: Augmented Mammogram Images

Step 1: Input to the generator—Augmented Samples = {Generative Noise Sequence + Dataset};
Step 2: Train the Discriminator with original data
Step 3: Discriminator—discriminate the fake samples with from the real dataset
–Assign labels: 0–Fake image & 1–Real Image
–Generate Feedback to Generator
Step 4 : Generator—Augmented Samples = {Generative Noise Sequence + Dataset + Feedback};
Generate new samples
Step 5: Go to step 3 until Augmented Samples are approved

The GAN aided in overcoming the overfitting issue brought about by the predetermined number of pictures in the dataset. Also, it expanded the dataset pictures to be multiple 20 times higher than the first dataset. The dataset images in the wake of utilizing the GAN arrange for 3 classes Normal, benign, and malignant. This will help in accomplishing surprising testing precision and execution lattices. The accomplished results will be pondered in detail in the experimental results segment. Figure 12.6 presents tests of the yield of the GAN network for the mammogram cases.

Mammograms can't be considered as a basic image ordering task, because there is a runoff in small regions inside a whole picture. For example, a mammogram with 2000×3600 pixels size incorporates just about 150×150 (pixels) of deformities.

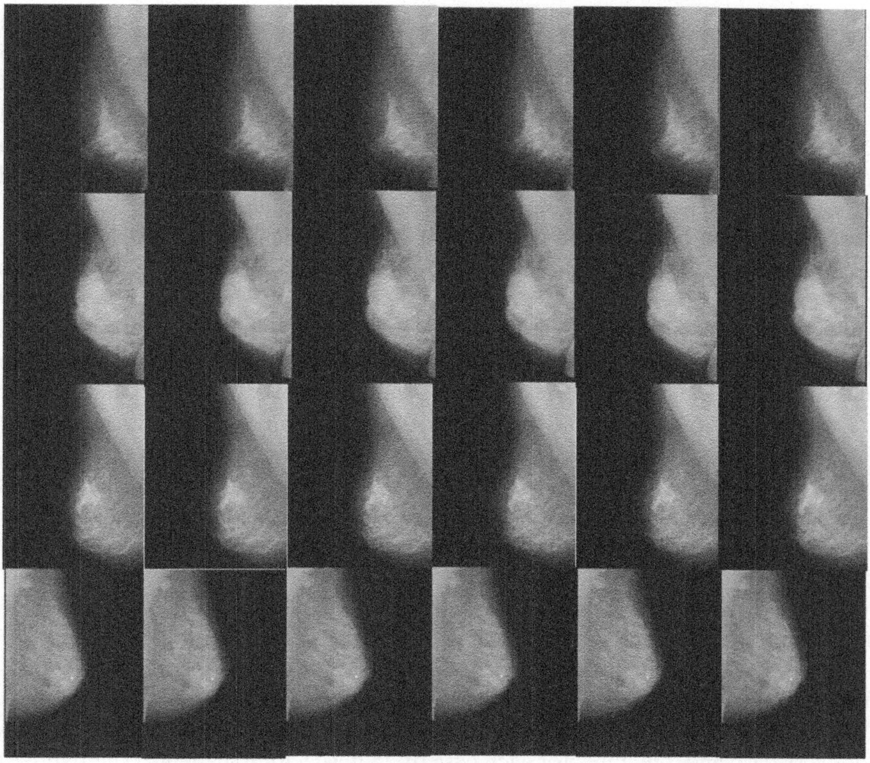

Fig. 12.6 Samples of images generated using the proposed GAN structure

To utilize a pre-prepared deep model for transfer learning, it is important to resize and standardize the contribution to a similar configuration that the system was at first prepared.

12.4 Experimental Analysis and Discussion

12.4.1 Corpus

In this study five publically available datasets, DDSM [44], CBIS-DDSM [45], MIAS [46] INbreast [21], and BCDR [47] are used to evaluate our proposed method.

DDSM Dataset: The Digital Database for Screening Mammography (DDSM) is the biggest online accessible dataset gathered by South Florida University for research in the breast malignant growth recognition and characterization frameworks. It is gathered to characterize actual breast information which is arranged as indicated by the level of seriousness of the discoveries, related ground truth, and other data of 2600 cases. The database includes about 2,500 preliminaries and ordered into 43 volumes, each one of which incorporates two perspectives for each breast, Cranial Caudal (CC) view took from the top of the breast, and the other is Medium Lateral Diagonal (MLO) took from the side point at 45°. Benign and malignant masses in all mammograms are perceived and clarified by master radiologists. So we utilized a batch of 1200 cases comprising an aggregate of 5000 pictures.

CBIS DDSM: Curated Breast Imaging Subset of DDSM (CBISDDSM) is a revised and normalized variant of the (DDSM). In CBIS-DDSM dataset comprises 6775 examinations and specialists trimmed the abnormality ROIs and removed 339 faulty mass cases physically. The pictures have been decompressed and changed over to DICOM design. Restored ROI division and bounding boxes, and pathologic analysis for training information are additionally included.

MIAS: The Mammographic Image Analysis Society (MIAS) is an association of UK research groups on breast cancer detection. The dataset comprises 322 pictures of 161 patients and all pictures are MLO view mammograms. Besides, the pictures were in PGM format and 1024 × 1024 pixels with 8-bit depth. The pictures in the database comprise left and right breast images of the fatty-glandular, thick and fatty breast. The mammogram pictures are grouped into three significant classes: normal, benign, and malignant. Of the database, 207 mammograms are normal, 63 are benign and 52 are malignant.

INbreast: The INbreast database is a mammographic database, with pictures obtained at a University (Hospital de São João, Breast Center, Porto, Portugal). INbreast has a sum of 115 cases with 410 pictures. The mammogram has 4 pictures for every case and 2 pictures for each case of 25 mastectomy patients. The INbreast database presents a wide fluctuation of cases which incorporates a few sorts of lesions (masses, calcifications, asymmetries, and twists) are incorporated. An XML sheet is also provided with the radiologist review on contours. INbreast doesn't exist freely on the web yet it tends to be obtained by request and agreement [21]. We were keen on the benign and malignant cases, so we collected a batch of 40 cases comprising a sum of 150 pictures.

BCDR: The Breast Cancer Digital Repository (BCDR) is a gathering of breast cancer anonymized patients cases clarified by master radiologists containing clinical information like distinguished inconsistencies, breast depth, BIRADS order, etc. The dataset consists of film mammography formed by 736 images of 344 patients with lesions, and picture-based highlights processed from CC and MLO mammography picture views which are accessible along with the directions of the outline of the lesion. BCDR-FM is a subdivided dataset made out of benign and malignant discoveries. We collected a batch of 400 images of 250 patients. The MLO and CC images are grey-level digitized mammograms with a resolution of 720 × 1168 and an 8-bit depth TIFF format.

12.4.2 Preprocessing

The acquired mammograms may contain noises and artifacts like labels and marks, which unfavorably influence the classification result. These are expelled by using the median filtering & global thresholding. The median filter is a non-linear filter popularly used to remove noise, labels, and identification marks in a mammogram and it also preserves the sharpness of the image's edges. The key advantage of median filters is that expanding the size of the window in the channel prompt better productivity in noise expulsion. Figure 12.7a shows the Original mammogram picture, Fig. 12.7b shows a mammogram after filtering through the median filter. Table 12.1 shows the filtered output image correlations in terms of PSNR and MSE. Thresholding the mammogram is to separate the background and the breast tissue using the histogram. So we have employed Otsu's thresholding method, as proven to the best in the literature for background separation in radiology images. Otsu's is a non-parametric unsupervised automatic threshold selection method with high sensitivity and specificity. It uses the cumulative initial order moments of the histogram to separate the background from the breast tissue establishing the optimal threshold by tuning inter-class variance. Figure 12.7c shows a mammogram after pectoral muscle removal (mass tissue which supports the breast body).

The background separation is required in a few datasets as normal just 60% of the zone is canvassed by breast area in the whole mammogram. The mammogram artifacts removal and background separation are shown in Figs. 12.8 and 12.9 respectively. The extraction of ROIs from the mammograms was performed by trimming a window of fixed size for all lesions, based on the mass. The picture size was chosen as such in request to be adequate for all the majority in the dataset. Along these lines, resize-prompted bending is kept away, while the adequate neighboring tissue is incorporated for learning features on a larger scale.

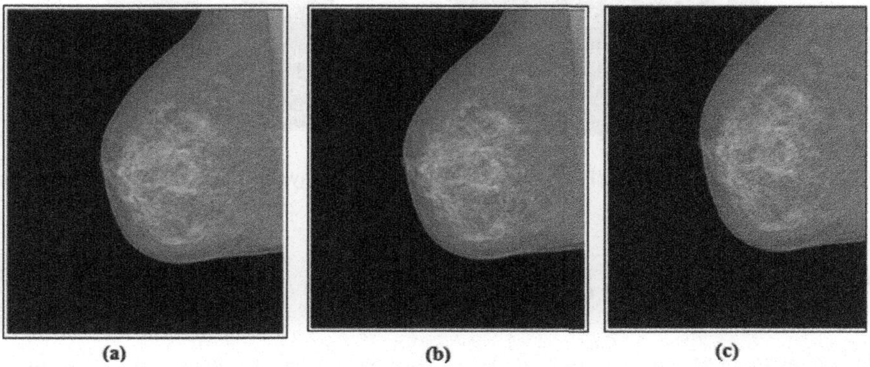

Fig. 12.7 **a** A mammogram form INbreast 2nodulos mama direita + micros, **b** Filtered version of (**a**) and **c** After removal of the pectoral muscle

Table 12.1 PSNR and MSE values of Sample Mammogram from each datasets

Sample image no	MSE	PSNR
MIAS—mdb322	0.2968	50.21
DDSM: 1-1	6.99E+03	45.70
CRDB;09c17b23-7deb-43b8-81a9—967501d7af3c_454_overlay	0.7176	44.88
CBIS-DDSM	5.89E+03	49.78
INBreast	5.5477E+03	50.02

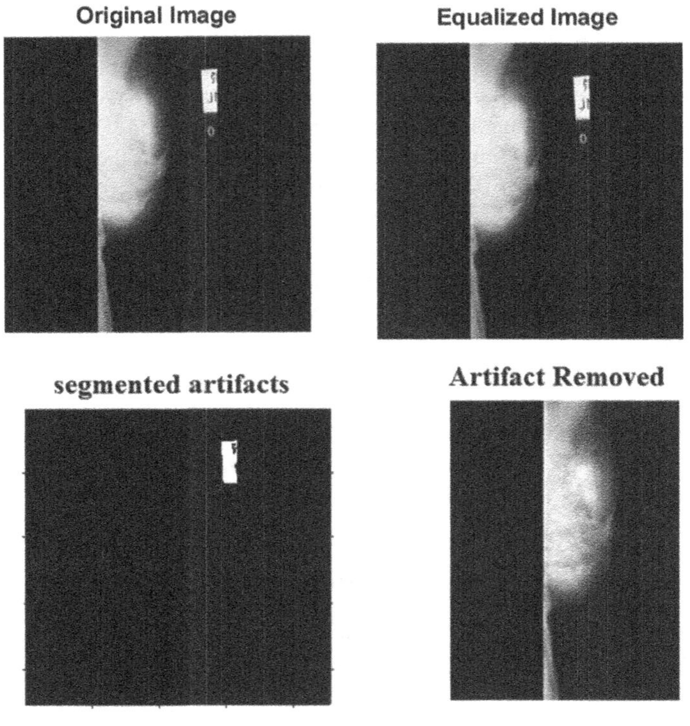

Fig. 12.8 MIAS–dataset alone has few visible artifacts which have been removed by segmentation

12.4.3 Analysis and Discussion

We experimented our proposed method using the six most powerful CNN Models (AlexNet, SqueezeNet, GoogleNet, MobileNetV2, ResNet18, and DarkNet19). We evaluated the individual model performance in two-mode (i). Random initialization (RI) mode and (ii) Pre-trained mode or transfer learning modes (TF). Experimen-

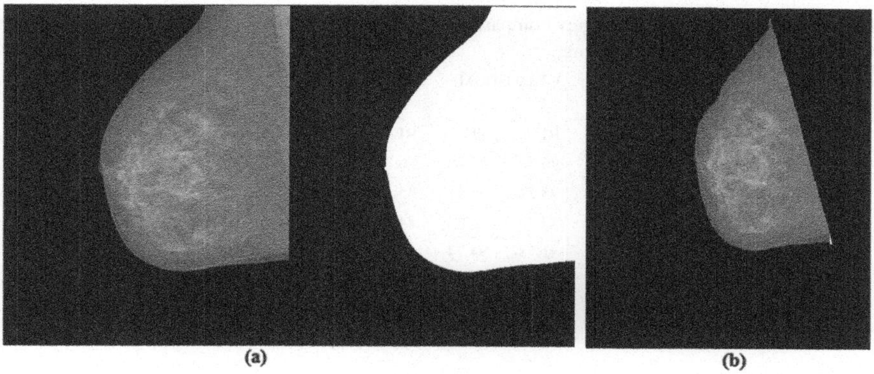

Fig. 12.9 **a** Mammogram with the background **b** Isolated breast without background

tal results show the outcomes from the correlation between the two unique modes prepared on all our five selected datasets. All through this investigation, a NVIDIA–1060 graphics Zotak (CUDA v10.0) was utilized for the fast response. Each dataset is divided into multiple ratios for training, testing and validation, for the ratio 8:1:1 we achieved the maximum recognition accuracy. For all the CNN models we preserved the initial learning to 0.9 and for every fold we gradually reduce the learning rate for every iterations.

(i) Random initialization (RT) Mode. Random initialization assigns random values to the weight which trials each weight from norm dissemination with a little deviance. The thought is to choose weight esteems arbitrary after a conveyance which would support the streamlining procedure to merge to a significant arrangement. The systems loads were instated to a little arbitrary number produced from a normal appropriation. The low deviance permits inclination to the system towards a straightforward 0 arrangement.
(ii) Pre-trained Initialization or TF Mode. In the Pre-trained Initialization mode, we transfer learn CNN models acquired by training on ImageNet, as initialization for our systems loads. The calibrating methodology here is the feature extraction component which is the fundamental method of performing transfer learning. We first expel the characterization part of the network (for example the completely associated layers) which was liable for giving the probabilities of a picture as being from every one of the trained class. At that point, we utilize the remaining structure of the models as a stable feature extractor that processes the CNN codes of each picture from our datasets. We at last utilize a Softmax classifier to prepare the acquired high-dimensional CNN codes. Table 12.2 shows the performance comparison of CNN models in random initialization versus Pre-trained transfer learning. Table 12.3 shows that the proposed method steadily performs superior compared to the other three individual CNN layers feature models on the dataset.

Figure 12.10 show the classification accuracy comparison of six CNN models with different weight learning factor in all the five datasets. From Fig. 12.10 we also

Table 12.2 Classification accuracy comparison of different CNN models in random initialization versus Pre-trained transfer learning

CNN models or Dataset	DDSM		CBIS-DDSM		MIAS		INbreast		BCDR	
Mode	RI	TF	RI	TF	RI	TF	RI	TF	RI	TF
AlexNet	87.24	96.7	86.84	97.12	86.84	96.89	85.74	97.24	86.74	96.44
SqueezeNet	86.84	96.5	95.74	95.17	85.23	95.17	82.74	96.14	85.77	95.3
Google Net	87.45	94.7	82.23	93.33	84.56	94.37	79.65	95.63	80.59	95.22
MobileNetV2	88.32	96.21	81.78	94.74	80.23	92.81	72.28	95.77	80.54	95.19
ResNet18	82.75	95.74	79.25	95.21	79.54	94.29	76.98	95.21	80.10	95.09
DarkNet19	84.78	94.11	79.84	92.14	76.11	94.78	71.45	95.18	79.48	95.23

Table 12.3 Performance comparison of the proposed method to other individual CNN layers feature on the dataset

CNN models or Dataset	DDSM			CBIS-DDSM			MIAS			INbreast			BCDR		
Layers	1st	Final	INTG	1st	Final	INTG	1st	Final	INTG	1st	Final	INTG	1st	Final	INTG
AlexNet	88.23	92.74	96.7	86.97	92.55	97.1	79.25	90.74	96.89	88.41	90.74	97.24	72.21	90.77	96.44
SqueezeNet	85.25	90.85	96.5	85.47	92.87	95.17	77.21	90.45	95.17	87.21	88.27	96.14	66.85	90.21	95.3
Google Net	86.78	89.74	94.7	86.21	91.57	93.33	76.21	91.33	94.37	84.96	87.64	95.63	69.45	90.38	95.22
MobileNetV2	82.14	88.33	96.21	83.74	93.74	94.74	74.23	90.27	92.81	83.55	88.21	95.77	69.74	90.85	95.19
ResNet18	81.66	88.57	95.74	81.27	90.12	95.21	79.22	91.45	94.29	84.85	88.23	95.21	66.87	90.36	95.09
DarkNet19	79.87	84.45	94.11	80.88	89.64	92.14	75.21	89.94	94.78	82.11	88.74	95.18	66.17	90.14	95.23

observe and confirm that the weight learning factor has a quite moderate influence on the classification accuracy. We even evaluate the assessment for the region based classification accuracy (RCA) and the overall classification accuracy (OCA). As appeared in Fig. 12.11, CNNs prepared under the transfer learn accomplished better execution contrasted than the ones prepared without any pre-learning. This affirms the tendency in cutting edge efforts to show an inclination to the fine-tuning situation. This distinction in execution is credited to the way that the inspected systems are planned and advanced for datasets a several order bigger than the accessible mammographic ones. Still, when the system is prepared, the learned highlights can address an assortment of issues distinctive in nature after the fine-tuning stage. From Tables 12.2 and 12.3, it is also witnessed that compare to all the models AlexNet performs outstandingly well in all the datasets. The possible reason for AlexNet outperforming other networks could the simplest structure of it.

Table 12.4 shows that our proposed method performs comparably well with a consistent averaged accuracy of about 97% in detection and classification against the latest works. The above observation and evidence confirm that electing features from a single layer of CNN that ensembles all datasets at hand with an individual transfer learning network are hard to differentiate the thick tissues and masses in the mammogram. From the above correlations, we conclude that the utilization of multiple layers of hierarchical integrated features that are robust and more significant enables higher accuracy gain in the classification of breast cancer in mammograms.

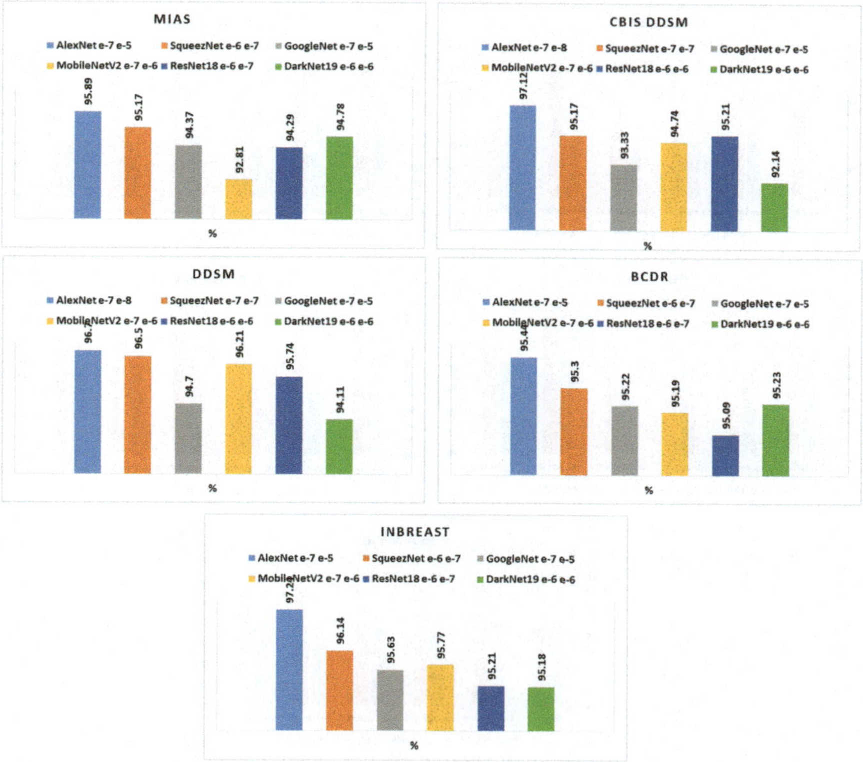

Fig. 12.10 Classification accuracy comparison of CNN models concerning various weight learning factors in all the datasets

Table 12.4 Classification comparison of proposed work against the latest work

Reference	Datasets	Classification accuracy (%)
Lizhen Shen et al. [48]	MIAS	91.5
Ansar et al. [27]	CBIS-DDSM	V1-74.5, V2-73.0
Mugahed et al. [40]	INbreast	97.2
Moreira et al. [21]	INbreast	95.0
Shrivastava and Bharti [26]	MIAS, DDSM	94.0, 95.3
Jiang et al. [49]	BCDR-F03	83.0
Proposed method	DDSM, CBIS-DDSM, MIAS, INbreast, BCDR	96.7, 97.12, 96.89, 97.24, 96.44

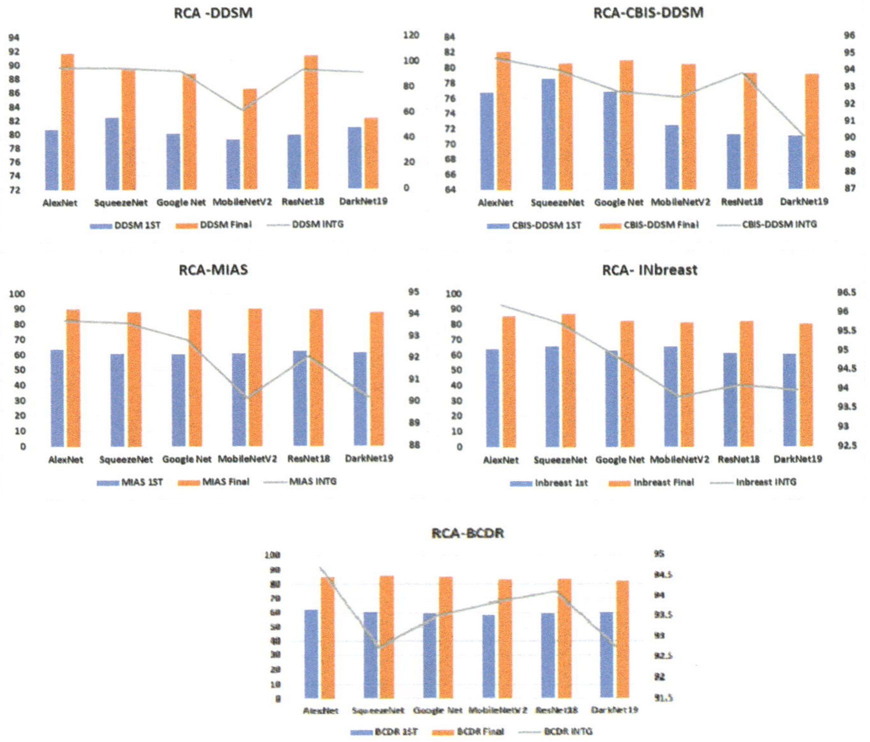

Fig. 12.11 Performance comparison of CNN models with ROI–classification accuracy in all the datasets

12.5 Conclusion and Future Scope

To reduce the mortality rate of breast malignant growth in women, legitimate treatment must be given which is trailed by early identification of cancer. Mammogram screening with deep transfer learning is the most reliable method for early diagnosis of breast cancer. But the current deep learning-based breast cancer detection using pre-trained models ends up in inadequate classification due to dependency of the utilization of the features extracted from the last layer of the network which conceals the prominent feature of mammograms for accurate classification. So In this chapter, an Early Diagnosis of Breast Cancer Using Multi-Layer Hierarchical Features of Deep Transfer Learned Convolutional Neural Network is presented. Our proposed method exploits the integration of multi-layer hierarchical features of deep transfer learned network which incorporates the features from earlier layers that offer more exact localization but are less invariant and the significant features from the last layer of CNN for classification. Our method is supported by the GAN network mammogram image augmentation to generate batches of augmented images that improvise the training efficiency and classification accuracy. We experimented our proposed method on five standard publicly available mammogram datasets on six benchmarks deep learn models. The experimental results show that for all the dataset our proposed method achieved 97% averaged accuracy which outperforms all other recent models in this class. The integration of hierarchical features and handcrafted features to further improve the classification performance is our future consideration. The proposed system mainly goes in the direction of developing an ideal most reliable early detection of breast cancer.

References

1. Chakraborty, S., Rahman, T.: The difficulties in cancer treatment. E-cancer medical science. 6, ed16 (2012). https://doi.org/10.3332/ecancer.2012.ed16. (14 Nov 2012)
2. Ekicia, S., Jawzal, H.: Breast cancer diagnosis using thermography and convolutional neural networks. Med. Hypotheses **137** (2020). https://doi.org/10.1016/j.mehy.2019.109542
3. Memorial Sloan Kettering Cancer Center, What Is Metastatic Cancer? Answers to Six Common Questions, about-cancer/causes-of-cancer/age-and-cancer (2019). https://www.mskcc.org/blog/what-metastatic-canceranswers-six-common-questions
4. American Cancer Society, How Common Is Breast Cancer? (2019). https://www.cancer.org/cancer/breast-cancer/about/how-common-is-breast-cancer.html
5. Howlader, N., Noone, A.M., Krapcho, M., Garshell, J., Miller, D., Altekruse, S.F., Kosary, C.L., Yu, M., Ruhl, J., Tatalovich, Z.: SEER cancer statistics review, 1975–2012, Bethesda. MD Natl, Cancer Inst (2015)
6. Jalalian, A., Mashohor, S., Mahmud, R., Karasfi, B., Saripan, M.I., Ramli, A.R.: Review article: foundation and methodologies in computer-aided diagnosis systems for breast cancer detection. EXCLI J **16**, 113–137 (2017)
7. Raghavendra, U., et al.: Application of Gabor wavelet and locality sensitive discriminant analysis for automated identifcation of breast cancer using digitized mammogram images. Appl Soft Comput J (2016). https://doi.org/10.1016/j.asoc.2016.04.036
8. Saxena, S., Gyanchandani, M.: Machine learning methods for computer-aided breast cancer diagnosis using histopathology: a narrative review. J. Med. Imaging Radiat. Sci. **51**(1), 182–193 (2019). https://doi.org/10.1016/j.jmir.2019.11.001. (PMID: 31884065)
9. Radiological Society of North America, Breast Cancer Screening (2019). https://www.radiologyinfo.org/en/info.cfm?pg=screening-breast. Accessed 26 Sept 2019
10. Agarwal, R., Díaz, O., Yap, M.H., Lladó, X., Martí, R.: Deep learning for mass detection in Full Field Digital Mammograms. Comput. Biol. Med. **121** (2020)
11. Horsch, K., Giger, M.L., Vyborny, C.J., Lan, L., Mendelson, E.B., Hendrick, R.E.: Classification of breast lesions with multimodality computer-aided diagnosis: Observer study results on an independent clinical data set. Radiology **240**(2), 357–368 (2006). https://doi.org/10.1148/radiol.2401050208
12. Ahmadizar, F., Soltanian, K., AkhlaghianTab, F., Tsoulos, I.: Artificial neural network development by means of a novel combination of grammatical evolution and genetic algorithm. Eng Appl Artif Intell **39**, 1–13 (2015)
13. Sadoughi, F., Kazemy, Z., Hamedan, F., Owji, L., Rahmanikatigari, M., Talebi, A.T.: Artificial intelligence methods for the diagnosis of breast cancer by image processing: a review. Breast Cancer (Dove Med Press) **10**, 219–230 (2018). https://doi.org/10.2147/BCTT.S175311
14. Holst, H., Ohlsson, M., Peterson, C., Edenbrandt, L.: Intelligent computer reporting 'lack of experience': a confidence measure for decision support systems. Clin. Physiol. **18**, 139–147 (1998)

15. Pang, T., Wong, J.H.D., Ng, W.L., Chan, C.S.: Deep learning radiomics in breast cancer with different modalities: overview and future. Expert Syst. Appl. **158** (2020). https://doi.org/10.1016/j.eswa.2020.1135010957-4174/2020. (Elsevier Ltd.)
16. Ghieh, D, Saade, C., Najem, E., El Zeghondi, R., Rawashdeh, M.A., Berjawi, G.: Staying abreast of imaging e Current status of breast cancer detection in high density breast. Radiography 28. In Press. Corrected Proof (2020). https://doi.org/10.1016/j.radi.2020.06.003. (June)
17. Lian, J., Li, K.: A review of breast density implications and breast cancer screening. Clin. Breast Cancer (2020). https://doi.org/10.1016/j.clbc.2020.03.004
18. Debelee, T.G., Schwenker, F., Ibenthal, A., et al.: Survey of deep learning in breast cancer image analysis. Evol. Syst. **11**, 143–163 (2020). https://doi.org/10.1007/s12530-019-09297-2
19. Dembrower, K., Lindholm, P., Strand, F.: A multi-million mammography image dataset and population-based screening cohort for the training and evaluation of deep neural networks-the cohort of screen-aged women (CSAW). J. Digit. Imaging **33**, 408–413 (2020). https://doi.org/10.1007/s10278-019-00278-0
20. Huang, M.-L., Lin, T.-Y.: Dataset of breast mammography images with masses. Data in Brief, vol. 31, pp. 105928 (2020). https://doi.org/10.1016/j.dib.2020.1059282352-3409/. (© 2020 Published by Elsevier Inc.)
21. Moreira, I.C., Amaral, I., Domingues, I., Cardoso, A., Cardoso, M.J., Cardoso, J.S.: INbreast: toward a full-field digital mammographic database. Acad. Radiol. **19**(2), 236–248 (2012)
22. Rahman, M.M., et al.: Machine learning based computer aided diagnosis of breast cancer utilizing anthropometric and clinical features. IRBM (2020). https://doi.org/10.1016/j.irbm.2020.05.005
23. Guptaa, P., Garg, S.: Breast cancer prediction using varying parameters of machine learning models. Proc. Comput. Sci. **171**, 593–601, 1877–0509 (2020). https://doi.org/10.1016/j.procs.2020.04.064. (© 2020)
24. Ahmed, L., Iqbal, M.M., Aldabbas, H., et al.: Images data practices for semantic segmentation of breast cancer using deep neural network. J. Ambient Intell. Human. Comput. (2020). https://doi.org/10.1007/s12652-020-01680-1
25. Al-antari M.A., Al-masni M.A., Kim, T.S.: Deep learning computer-aided diagnosis for breast lesion in digital mammogram. In: Lee, G., Fujita, H. (eds.) Deep Learning in Medical Image Analysis. Advances in Experimental Medicine and Biology, vol. 1213. Springer, Cham (2020). https://doi.org/10.1007/978-3-030-33128-3_4
26. Shrivastava, N., Bharti, J.: Breast tumor detection and classification based on density. Multimedia Tools and Applications (IF 2.313). https://doi.org/10.1007/s11042-020-09220-x. (Pub Date : 2020-07-16)
27. Ansar, W., Shahid, A.R., Raza, B., Dar, A.H.: Breast cancer detection and localization using mobilenet based transfer learning for mammograms. In: Brito-Loeza, C., Espinosa-Romero, A., Martin-Gonzalez, A., Safi A. (eds.) Intelligent Computing Systems. ISICS 2020. Communications in Computer and Information Science, vol. 1187. Springer, Cham (2020). https://doi.org/10.1007/978-3-030-43364-2_2
28. Sechopoulos, I., Teuwen, J., Mann, R.: Artificial intelligence for breast cancer detection in mammography and digital breast tomosynthesis: state of the art. Semin. Cancer Biol. (2020). https://doi.org/10.1016/j.semcancer.2020.06.002
29. Hamed, G., Marey, M.A.E.R., Amin, S.E.S., Tolba, M.F.: Deep learning in breast cancer detection and classification. In: Hassanien, A.E., Azar, A., Gaber, T., Oliva, D., Tolba, F. (eds.) Proceedings of the International Conference on Artificial Intelligence and Computer Vision (AICV2020). AICV 2020. Advances in Intelligent Systems and Computing, vol. 1153. Springer, Cham (2020). https://doi.org/10.1007/978-3-030-44289-7_30
30. Tsochatzidis, L., Costaridou, L., Pratikakis, I.: Deep learning for breast cancer diagnosis from mammograms-a comparative study. J. Imaging **5**, 37 (2019)
31. Oliveira, H.S., Teixeira, J.F., Oliveira, H.P.: Lightweight deep learning pipeline for detection, segmentation and classification of breast cancer anomalies. In: Ricci, E., Rota Bulò, S., Snoek, C., Lanz, O., Messelodi, S., Sebe, N. (eds.) Image Analysis and Processing - ICIAP 2019. ICIAP 2019. Lecture Notes in Computer Science, vol. 11752. Springer, Cham (2019). https://doi.org/10.1007/978-3-030-30645-8_64

32. Ragab, D.A., Sharkas, M., Marshall, S., Ren, J.: Breast cancer detection using deep convolutional neural networks and support vector machines. Peer J. **7** (2019). https://doi.org/10.7717/peerj.6201
33. Agrawal, S., Rangnekar, R., Gala, D., Paul, S., Kalbande, D.: Detection of breast cancer from mammograms using a hybrid approach of deep learning and linear classification. In: 2018 International Conference on Smart City and Emerging Technology (ICSCET), Mumbai, pp. 1–6 (2018). https://doi.org/10.1109/ICSCET.2018.8537250
34. Ting, F.F., Tan, Y.J., Sim, K.S.: Convolutional neural network improvement for breast cancer classification. Expert Syst. Appl. **120**, 103–115 (2019)
35. Hagos, Y.B., Mérida, A.G., Teuwen, J.: Improving breast cancer detection using symmetry information with deep learning. In: Image Analysis for Moving Organ, Breast, and Thoracic Images, pp. 90–97. Springer (2018)
36. Rampun, A., Scotney, B.W., Morrow, P.J., Wang, H.: Breast mass classification in mammograms using ensemble convolutional neural networks. In: Proceedings of the 20th International Conference on e-Health Networking, Applications and Services (Healthcom), Ostrava, Czech Republic, 17–20 September 2018, pp. 1–6. IEEE, Piscataway, NJ, USA (2018)
37. Chougrad, H., Zouaki, H., Alheyane, O.: Deep convolutional neural networks for breast cancer screening. Comput. Methods Programs Biomed. **157**, 19–30 (2018). Apr
38. Lan, K., Wang, D.T., Fong, S., Liu, L.S., Wong, K.K., Dey, N.: A survey of data mining and deep learning in bioinformatics. J. Med. Syst. **42**(8), 139 (2018)
39. Jadoon, M.M., Zhang, Q., Haq, I.U., Butt, S., Jadoon, A.: Three-Class mammogram classification based on descriptive CNN features. BioMed Res. Int. (2017)
40. Mugahed, A., Al-antari, P.D., Kim, T.S.: Evaluation of deep learning detection and classification towards computer-aided diagnosis of breast lesions in digital X-ray mammograms. Comput. Methods Programs Biomed. (2020). https://doi.org/10.1016/j.cmpb.2020.105584
41. Ma, C., Huang, J.-B., Yang, X., Yang, M.-H.: Robust visual tracking via hierarchical convolutional features. IEEE Trans. Pattern Anal. Mach. Intell. (2017). https://doi.org/10.1109/TPAMI.2018.2865311
42. Guo, Y., Liu, Y., Oerlemans, A., Lao, S., Wu, S., Lew, M.S.: Deep learning for visual understanding: a review. Neurocomputing **187**, 27–48 (2016)
43. Madani, A., Moradi, M., Karargyris,A., Syeda-Mahmood, T.: Chest x-ray generation and data augmentation for cardiovascular abnormality classification. In: Proceedings SPIE 10574, Medical Imaging 2018: Image Processing, 105741M (2018). https://doi.org/10.1117/12.2293971. (2 March 2018)
44. Heath, M., Bowyer, K., Kopans, D., Moore, R., Kegelmeyer, W.P.: The digital database for screening mammography. In: Proceedings 5th International Workshop Digital Mammography, Medical Physics Publishing, pp. 212–218 (2000)
45. Lee, R.S., Gimenez, F., Hoogi, A., Rubin, D.: Curated breast imaging subset of DDSM. Cancer Imaging Arch. (2016). https://doi.org/10.7937/K9/TCIA.2016.7O02S9CY
46. Suckling, J., et al.: The mammographic image analysis society digital mammogram database exerpta medica. In: International Congress Series, vol. 1069, pp. 375–378 (1994)
47. Lopez, M.G., Posada, N.G., Moura, D.C., Pollán, R.R., Valiente, J.M.F., Ortega, C.S., Solar, M., Diaz-Herrero, G., Ramos, I., Loureiro, J.: BCDR: a breast cancer digital repository. In: Proceedings of the 15th International Conference on Experimental Mechanics (2012)
48. Shen, L., He, M., Shen, N., Yousefi, N., Wang, C., Liu, G.: Optimal breast tumor using discrete wavelet transform and deep belief network based on improved sunflower optimization method. Biomed. Signal Process. Control **60** (2020). https://doi.org/10.1016/j.bspc.2020.101953
49. Jiang, F., Liu, H., Yu, S., Xie, Y.: Breast mass lesion classification in mammograms by transfer learning. In: Proceedings of the 5th International Conference on Bioinformatics and Computational Biology, pp. 59–62. ACM (2017)

Chapter 13
Study on Gene Alterations in Cervical Cancer Using Computational Genomics Tools

B. Sai Lalitha, M. Malini, M. Venkateswara Rao, E. Satya Mounika Sravani, and M. A. Mandira

Abstract Cervical cancer is one of the leading causes of cancer-related deaths in women. Genomics deals with genome structure, function, development, and mapping. It is known that the expression of genes changes in cancer cells. Computational surveys are one of the most significant means of biological discovery due to the present abundance of huge biological datasets. Contributions of computational genomics research to biology include proposing cell signalling human genes using comparative genomics techniques and statistical assessment with multiple mammalian and vertebrate species. In our study, we aimed to identify the alterations of genes involved in cervical cancer. Using tools of computational genomics, a data set on cervical cancer as from NCBI-GEO and the Series Matrix and Platform files and sorted the information to prepare a gene expression table. The Gene expression table was then uploaded on Network Analyst for protein-protein interaction and Gene expression analysis. In N/A genes are mapped for transcription factor and protein-protein interactions of different pathways are identified from molecular interaction databases (KEGG, Reactome, GO_BP, GO_MF). The pathway is studied in GeneMANIA and gene cards. Two genes CDC6 and CDKN2A are identified and are studied for alterations in cervical cancer. In cervical squamous cell carcinoma, CDC6 is amplified by 0.4% and no mutation and deletion of genes is found. CDKN2A gene showed mutation by 1.99% and deep deleted by 0.4% but no amplification was found. In our study, the analysis is done on 607 cases in which, in cervical adenocarcinoma CDC6 gene is amplified by 2.17% with deep deleted by 2.17% gene and no mutation is found in CDKN2A whereas no amplification, deep deletion and mutation are seen. Our finding would help the researchers to conduct future studies on CDC6 and CDKN2A genes for better treatments.

Keywords Cervical cancer · Computational genomics · Gene expression · Cancer signalling pathways

B. Sai Lalitha (✉) · M. Malini · M. Venkateswara Rao · E. Satya Mounika Sravani
Department of Biomedical Engineering, University College of Engineering, Osmania University, Hyderabad, India

M. A. Mandira
Department of Biotechnology, SRM Institute of Science and Technology, Chennai, India

J. Nayak et al. (eds.), *Advanced Machine Learning Approaches in Cancer Prognosis*, Intelligent Systems Reference Library 204,
https://doi.org/10.1007/978-3-030-71975-3_13

13.1 Introduction

Genes are in every cell DNA in the body and regulate cell growth, division, and protein production in cells. Every protein has a specific role, and it serves as messengers of the cell. A Mutated gene produces the malfunctioned protein or prevents the synthesis of protein. Mutation can lead to an uncontrollable proliferation of cells known as cancer. Among women worldwide, cervical cancer is 2nd most life-threatening cancer. Cervical cancer develops in women's cervix, which is the entrance to the womb from the vagina (Fig. 13.1). Mutated Cervix cells are known as dysplasia. The uncontrolled growth of cancer cells leads to the formation of primary tumor and spreads to other parts of the body forming secondary tumors.

Clinically there are three main types of cervical cancer: squamous cell carcinoma, adenocarcinoma, adeno-squamous carcinoma. Squamous cell carcinoma develop from cells in the exocervix, which is the outer part of the cervix and can typically be triggered by the cervical epithelium. The squamous cell type constitutes 90% of all cervix carcinomas. Adenocarcinoma is a type of glandular cell cancer. Adenocarcinoma in the cervix grows from endocervix mucus-producing gland cells. Adeno-squamous cell carcinoma develops from both Squamous cells and glandular cells. Compared to squamous cell carcinoma, adeno and adeno-squamous carcinoma are less common. Cervical cancer is usually caused by smoking, long-term use of oral contraceptives, chlamydia infection, human papillomavirus (HPV) etc., Long-term infection of the Human Papilloma Viruses triggers most cervical cancers (HPVs). There are over 100 HPV types and mostly 16 and 18 types are associated with to cervical cancer.

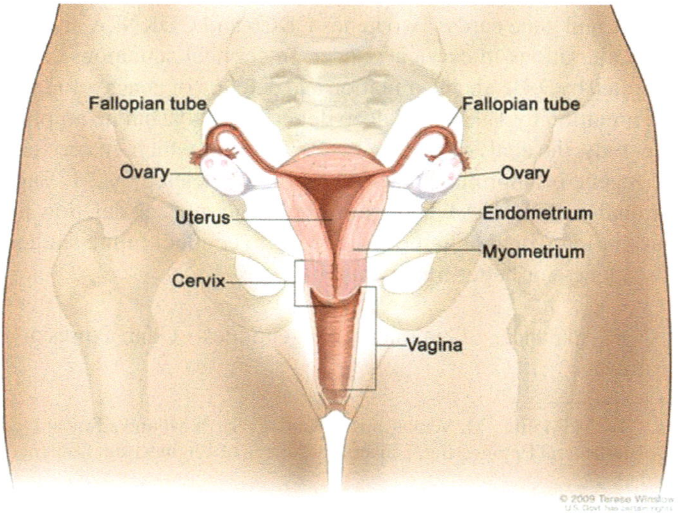

Fig. 13.1 Cervix [National Cancer Institute dictionary]

Computational genomics uses statistical and numerical analysis to translate biological information of biomolecules such as DNA and RNA. Computational genomics is a division of computational biology and bioinformatics which concentrates on an entire set of genomes instead of a specific gene. Computational studies have been one of the most effective ways for biological research to understand the concept of DNA regulation at the molecular level which is beyond the current abundance of large biological data sets. With the help of computational genomics, researchers can analyze the enormous data, build a model biological phenomenon, and make predictions to understand the mechanism of genome. It can also determine potential links between tissue-specific gene expression and the regulation of a gene in different pathways. Networks represent the interactions and the interdependency of the genes or proteins present. In biology, networks give us a holistic approach where biological systems are often represented graphically. Network Interactions are usually represented as physical interactions, genetic interactions, and co-expressions of one gene or multiple genes which help to analyze various connections present between the entities. The protocol for computational genomics for studying the gene network, identifying gene of interest, and studying the gene using online tools. Computational genomics is widely used in single cell RNA- sequencing experiments where tools like FASTQC, Kraken, and RNA-SeQC are used for the mapping the genome [1]. Not only for studying human genomes it can also be widely used in the study of plants. Tools like Ensembl Plants, Gramene, PLAZA, PoGs etc. provide databases and platforms for sequencing, BLAST and gene function studies [2]. GeneMania is GO annotation database and widely used in gene function studies. clusDCA is used for analysing gene [3]. In the paper NCBIGEO, Network Analyst, GeneMANIA, Genecards and CBioPortal computational tools are discussed.

13.1.1 Gene Expression Omnibus (GEO)

GEO is a public functional genomics data repository, supporting MIAME-compliant data submissions, arrays, and sequence-based data. Gene expression profiles can be downloaded from NCBI GEO [4]. The gene expression omnibus stores the functional genomic data in the versatile database. It offers procedures of annotated data in a simple and easy format, mechanisms to search, preview, and download data of interest[1] (Fig. 13.2).

The records available on Geo are published data submitted by various researchers. The data is available in three types. They are as follows:

i. **Platforms**—The platform consists of a summary and description of the array or sequencer. For identification they are assigned with specific GEO accession number. GPL represents the platform files with a four-digit number, which can act as a reference for various samples. GEO consists of the title of the research, the sample organism, submitter, link for series, sample, file, and data [4].

[1] https://www.ncbi.nlm.nih.gov/geo/.

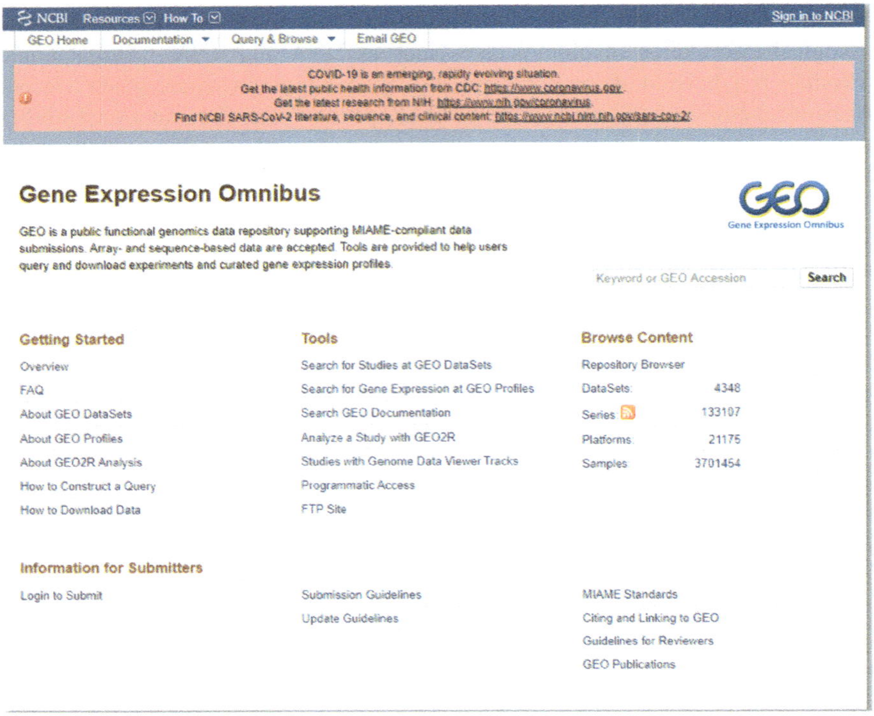

Fig. 13.2 NCBI GEO [4]

ii. **Sample**—Microarray Data is represented as GSE with a unique GEO accession number and of the sample. Represented as GSM [4].

iii. **Series**—The series file consists of gene expression of each sample. They are given an accession number of their own for identification and representational purpose. It is represented by GSE followed by the number assigned [4]. NCBI also provides information through datasets and profiles. Datasets consists of transfomed biological data that can be easily studied statisticaly. Profiles determine the expression of genes across datasets. They can be viewed using the GEO profile interface [4].

13.1.2 NetworkAnalyst

NetworkAnalyst enables the user to visualize and interpret the data and is first released in 2014 [5]. One of the significant functions of NetworkAnalyst is the protein-protein interactions (PPI) used to understand protein and gene pathways. Most graphs are visualized with nodes as proteins and edges as interactions. Data visualization follows steps: identification of gene proteins, retrieval of identified gene proteins, and analysis.

Once the data is uploaded, annotate, specify the normalization and network type, the network is further created according to the database. Different nodes can be selected and studied individually. Functional enrichment analysis can be performed with varying databases like KEGG, GO, or REACTOME. Remove or delete specific nodes as per convenience or study upregulated or downregulated genes. Apart from this, there are other graphs like heatmaps, enrichment networks, Venn diagrams, and chord diagrams. Using Network Analyst we can perform gene-expression meta-analysis and profiling of 17 different species. The networks can be viewed in 2D, 3D, and virtual reality space. In addition, meta-analysis is another feature offered by NetworkAnalyst [5–7].

The work flow followed in NetworkAnalyst—(Fig. 13.3).

i. The various databases used by NetworkAnalyst.

   (a) KEGG (Kyoto Encyclopedia of Genes and Genomes)
   (b) REACTOME
   (c) GO:BP (Gene Ontology: Biological Process), GO: CC (Gene Ontology: Cellular Component) andGO:MF (Gene Ontology: Molecular Function)
   (d) PANTHER:BP (PANTHER: Biological Process), PANTHER: MF (PANTHER: Molecular Function) and panther: CC (PANTHER: Cellular Component)
   (e) MOTIF

ii. The various interaction networks handled by Network Analyst.

   (a) Protein-protein interactions (PPI)—To understand the various biological processes that affect the body's basic functioning, including cell-cell interactions, metabolic process, and so on [8, 9].
   (b) Gene regulatory networks—It governs the transcription of mRNA of the genes with an assortment of DNA segments that interact with other segments or parts of segments [10].
   (c) Gene co-expression network—It shows networks of various genes with different roles in different biological processes.
   (d) Disease-gene—The genes are responsible for the occurrence of genetic diseases or diseases that are inherited. They are mainly caused by mutation or inheritance and many times due to external factors.
   (e) Chemical-gene—The biochemistry of gene functioning and how different genes are affected by the chemical processes carried or how they could be causing chemical changes [8–10].

The visualization tools play an essential role in understanding and interpreting data. They can be broadly divided into the following:

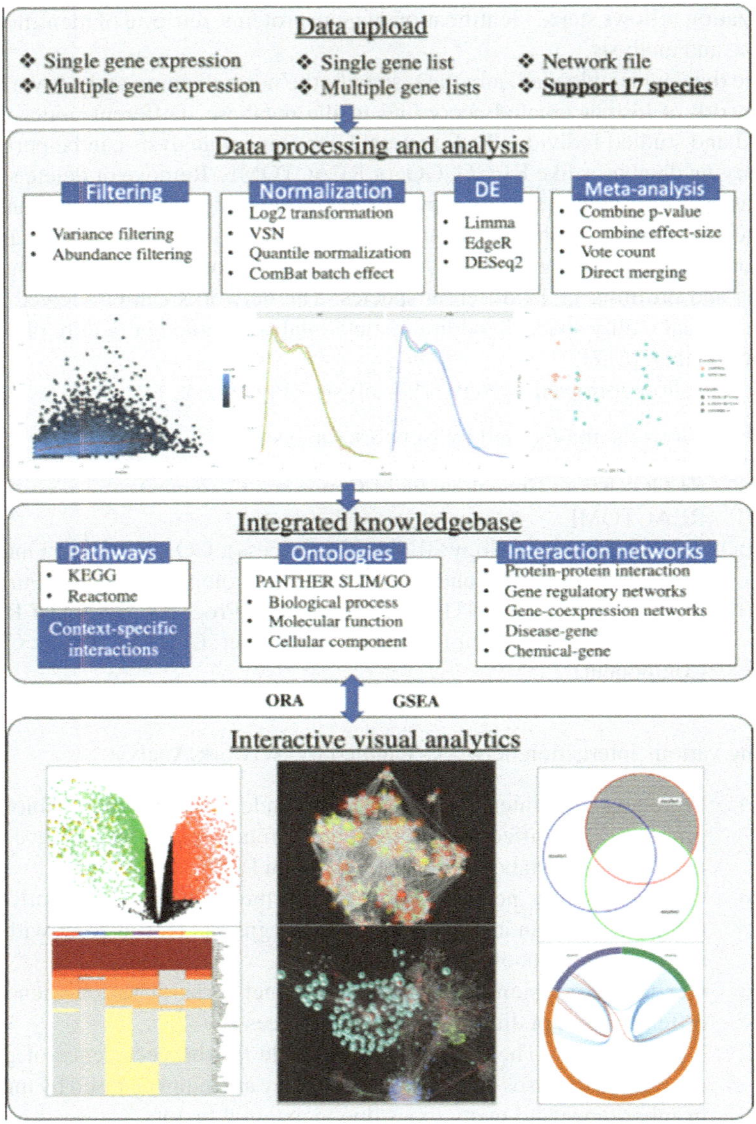

Fig. 13.3 Workflow of NetworkAnalyst [9]

i. **Over Representation Analysis (ORA)**

In ORA, genes could be sorted under the specific lists according to their functions, certain criteria like SNPs or insertion or deletions, etc. It determines the significant enrichment and the differentially expressed genes that are part of a specific pathway

[11, 12]. The hypergeometric tests are used to determine the repeated genes in the given gene list and annotated gene list. A necessary cutoff like fold change is provided to get the required overlapping data [13]. The significant genes are determined and then can be used to understand the biological mechanism [12].

ii. **Gene Set Enrichment Analysis (GSEA)**

GSEA is an analytical tool that focuses on gene sets (i.e., genes with common functions, regulation, etc.) and interprets gene expression data of functionally related genes [14–16]. It forms a connection between various biological processes and co-expressions. The data is taken from multiple individual studies and enables us to study and understand how they interact and get influenced by different states of health and diseases [13].

The following are some of the interactive visual analytics that is present in the NetworkAnalyst platform:

(a) **Volcano plot**

A volcano plot is a scatterplot that shows the data in the form of a graph between the statistical differences and magnitude of change, i.e., P-value and fold change. This helps us view the upregulated, downregulated genes, and the insignificant genes according to the specified information. The upregulated genes are towards the right and the left side consists of downregulated genes with the significant genes towards the top, as shown in (Fig. 13.4) [17, 18]. It is used for proteomics, genomics, transcriptomics, and metabolomics studies to understand the significant changes between the two points in the plot [19].

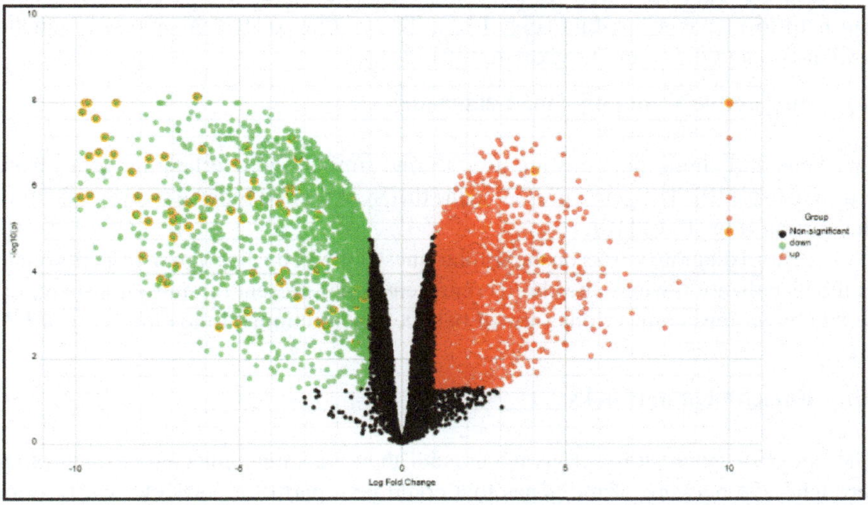

Fig. 13.4 Volcano plot with the upregulated and downregulated genes [10]

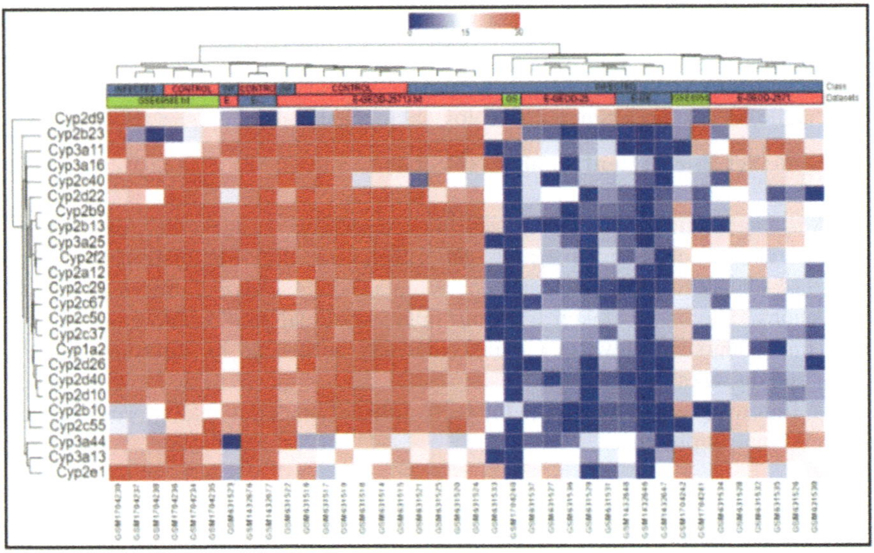

Fig. 13.5 Heatmap [10]

(b) Heatmap

Heatmap is used to visualize the biological data by comparing multiple lists [10]. The genes and the samples are represented by the rows and the columns respectively in a particular colour scheme mostly grouped based on the gene expression data [20]. Colour codes represent specific data, and the understanding of the colour coding can help to interpret the data (Fig. 13.5). The colour codes can represent genetic similarities and the level of expression [21, 22].

(c) Interactive Venn and chord diagrams

The Venn and chord diagrams are used to find similar and overlapping genes from multiple lists [10]. The genes present in the different sections can be seen by selecting the portion (Fig. 13.6) [10].

The chord diagram works on the similar lines of the Venn diagram with a difference in the visualization where the chords represent genes present in multiple lists represented by various connections formed between the sections of the circle (Fig. 13.7) [10].

(d) Enrichment networks

The enriched genes are seen as nodes, and they are interconnected to each other through edge network of the genes that could be a part of a particular pathway or several pathways. It groups similar gene sets and helps to visualize them. The nodes are presented as meta-nodes that open into various other nodes of the gene set. By

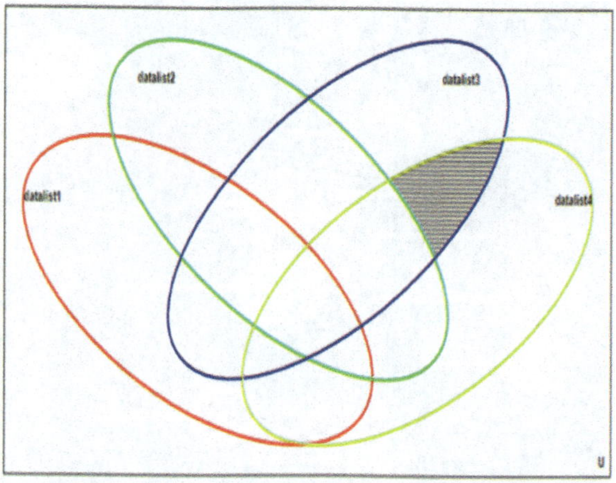

Fig. 13.6 Venn diagram with genes [10]

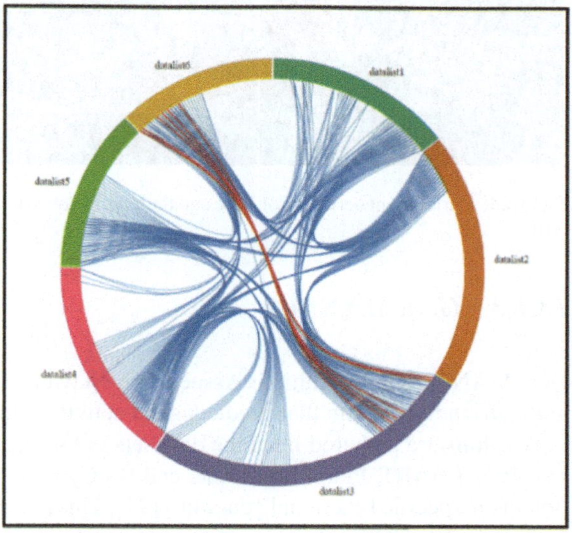

Fig. 13.7 Chord diagram with genes [10]

analyzing various nodes, we can derive the gene or gene-sets of our interest and study them separately [10] (Fig. 13.8).

For further information (www.networkanalyst.ca) official site can be visited. All the information has been provided in the form of tutorials and FAQs.

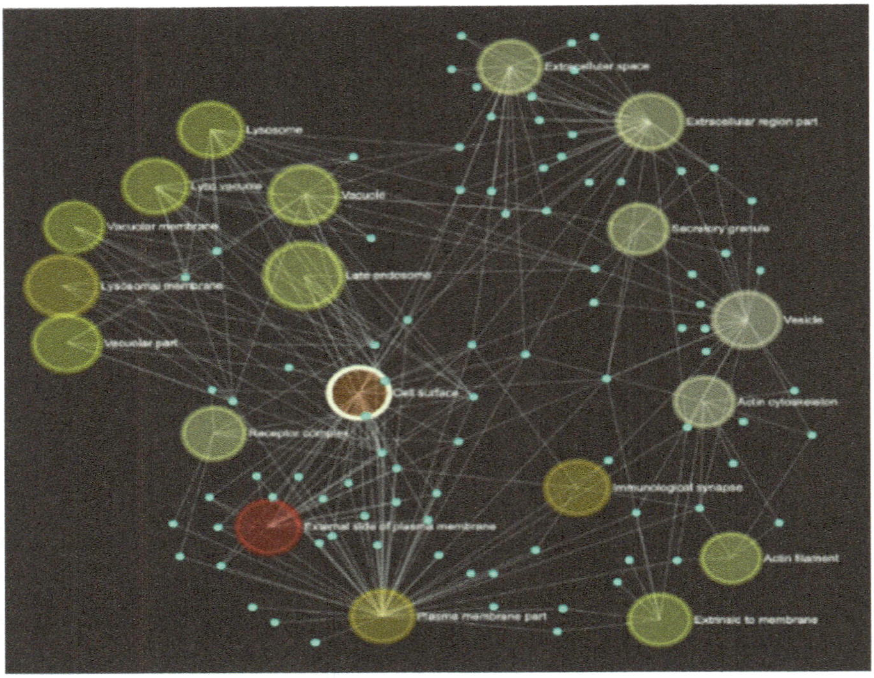

Fig. 13.8 Enrichment networks of gene and their pathways with the different nodes and meta-nodes [10]

13.1.3 GeneMANIA

GeneMANIA (Gene Multiple Association Network Integration Algorithm) [20] is a user-friendly website that predicts gene activity. Many data sets and thousands of interactions are gathered from the data sets of GEO, BioGRID, IRefIndex and I2D, InterPro, SMART, Pfam, Reactome, and BioCyc, via Pathway Commons as well as organism-specific functional genomics [24]. This portal offers a resilient interface for analyzing data about genomic, proteomic, and gene function. It also provides single-gene queries, multiple gene queries, and network searches. By selecting different data sets or by uploading own data sets, the search can be customorised.

Using a vast collection of functional association data, the genes linked to the query gene can be found. And this functional association data includes Protein and Genetic Interactions, Co-expression, Co-localization, Pathway, and Protein Domain Similarity and Physical Interactions.

Protein and Gene interaction data are represented with two genes linked functionally, depicting if the effects of perturbation of a gene were altered by disturbance of the second gene. Co-expression of the gene can be determined by the study of gene expression where two genes are related when their rates of expression. Co-localization is estimated by genes in the same tissue or proteins on the same site. Two genes are related when both are expressed in the same tissue or when both of their gene products are found in the same cell site. The pathway is formulated when two gene products are related and are involved in the same pathway reaction. Protein Domain Similarity is evaluated on genes having the same protein domain and gene products are linked. Physical Interactions are described when they are found to interact in an analysis of protein-protein interaction showing the two gene products are related together [25].

Upon entering a specific gene, within the chosen datasets, GeneMANIA will identify associated genes. When a gene list is entered within the selected datasets, GeneMANIA gives the relations between the genes. The interconnection of the attributes like physical interactions, co-expression, prediction, co-localization, pathway, Genetic Interactions, and shared protein domain of a particular gene (Fig. 13.9).

Open GeneMANIA https://GeneMANIA.org and Homo sapiens is selected for human subjects and particular genes of interest are entered in the text box.

The interactions required for the study can be selected by clicking on the three-point icon next to the search box. This reveals all the sources of interaction and enables to choose by checking their attributes like co-expression, co-localization, genetic interactions, pathways, physical interactions, shared protein domains, and others. To create network visualization, click on the magnifying glass icon is selected and the final network will appear on the main screen.

Different types of interactions are characterized by various coloured connector paths. Select three horizontal line icon on the right side of the screen to see a colour legend and choose the particular interactions of interest. Select a specific gene. It provides data and offers options to delete this from the network and repeat a network

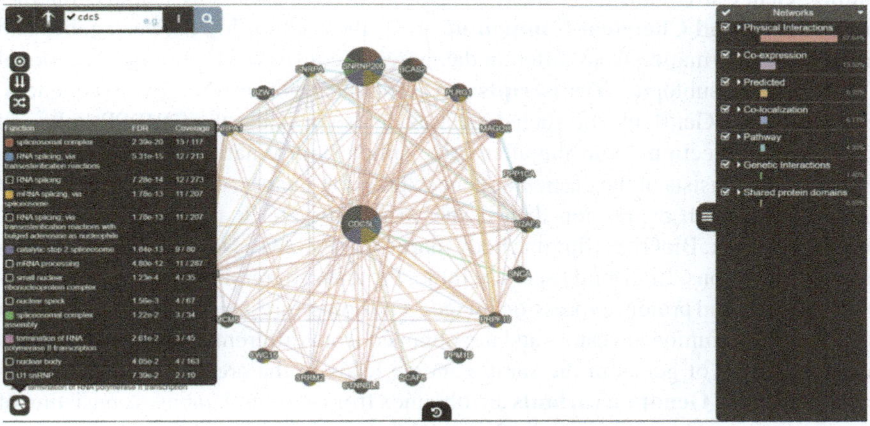

Fig. 13.9 Features of GeneMANIA

study solely on that gene. Select the data icon on the left of the screen, displays simple network data, such as gene interactions. Select the data icon again to delete from the screen. The pie chart icon at the bottom left of the screen displays a set of genes classified with that function in the genome.

13.1.4 GeneCards

GeneCards is a human genome database created by the Department of Molecular Genetics at the Weizman Institute of Science in Israel in 1977 [23]. It is an automated database that mines through data to find all the information of the gene. It retrieves the data from various datasets like NCBI, HGNC, ENSEMBL, and UniProtKB. Genecards also consists of genomic, proteomic, and transcriptomic data, as well as their functions with respect to the disease [26, 27].

GeneCards provides data in sections as **Aliases or number of RNA transcript sources** obtained from different databases. **Summaries** obtained from different databases talk about the function, localization, etc. **Genomics** display the genomic structure and its chromosomal location. **GeneHancer regulatory elements** is about the regulatory elements acquired from the GeneHancer database. **Proteins** provide the information of the proteins encoded by the genes from the UniProtKB database. **Domains** is about the protein domains with data taken from various databases. **Function** gives information about various functions of the gene consisting of GWAS catalog and Human Phenotypic Ontology (HPO). **Localization** provides the gene localization according to various databases. It consists of Subcellular locations from COMPARTMENTS and Subcellular locations from the Human Proteins Atlas (HPA). **Pathways and Interactions** provides the links of multiple pathways to which the gene belongs that is taken from various databases. It consists of SuperPaths: unified GeneCards Pathways, Interacting proteins, and SIGNOR Curated Interactions. **Drugs and Chemical Compounds** gives the relationship between genes and drugs with information from different databases. It consists of Drugs and Additional Compounds as subtopics. **Transcripts** consist of the cDNA, mRNA, exon sequences, etc. taken from GenBank and such databases. It also provides the CRISPR links and contains a subsection about the alternative splicing information taken from ASD. **Expression** consists of the particular gene expression images, data on overexpressed tissues, table with expression data tissue specificity, etc. It has various subparts, including GTEx, BioGPS, Illumina body map, CGAP: SAGE Normal, mRNA Differential Expressions, LifeMapDiscoveryTable, Protein differential expression, expression partners, and protein expression images. **Orthologs** are genes present in different species with common ancestors and are obtained from different databases. **Paralogs** are duplication of genes in the same genome leads to the creation of gene copies called paralogs. **Genomic variants** are obtained from various databases consisting of sequence variations, additional dbSNP identifiers, structural variation table, generic variance classification, and scores and GDI or Gene damage index. **Disorders and diseases** are the diseases and disorders in which the gene is involved. **Publication** shows the name, publication year, and links to articles. **Products** include the products that are using or contains the query gene [26].

13.1.5 cBioPortal

cBioPortal (https://www.cbioportal.org) [28] is a web-based tool used for research, visualization, and evaluation of multidisciplinary cancer genomics results. The database provides details on molecular profiling in cancer tissues and cell lines to conveniently accessible genomic, epigenetic, gene expression, and proteomic occurrences. The portal provides graphic summaries of multi-platform gene data, network visualization and analysis, survival analysis, Patient-centric requests, and programmatic software access.

The portal's interactive user application allows detailed cancer genomics profiles available to researchers and clinicians without the need for bioinformatics knowledge, thereby promoting biological observations. It also provides a complete approach to the analysis and visualization of the features of the cBioPortal for Cancer Genomics [29].

cBioPortal uses data from large consortium like TCGA and ICGC and publications from Pubmed. These data sources support a range of omics data, which are DNA methylation, RNA based data levels, protein levels, mutations, fusions. It provides a wide range of features and analysis tools. Visualizing the distribution of genomic alterations in multiple genes across many data samples, calculating mutual exclusivity of genomic events, visualizing the distribution of mutations within a gene, and copying the number and expression for a gene. Performing analysis, identifying mutated genes present in the same set of samples as per the particular gene of interest (Fig. 13.10). Depicts the query interface of all lists of the studies organized by the tissue of origin and sorted by the particular tissue of origin and provides the option to quickly select tissue data samples. It provides the data of the number of samples, and one can view the clinical and genomic data of the particular study by selecting the info and pie- chart icons which are beside the sample studies.

A query window appears on selecting a particular tissue from the study and querying it by the gene. Both boxes are checked (Mutation, copy number of alterations, and type of particular gene of interest) in the section and query of the gene is submitted.

After submitting the query, results like Oncoprint, Cancer type summary, Mutations, Comparison/Survival, CN Segments, Pathways, Expression are displayed. Mutations, copy number of alterations, deletions through colour codes in different patients [28, 29].

Oncoprints (Fig. 13.11) are visualizing medium of genomic data in the form of heat maps [28, 30, 31]. They show the various genomic alterations. They can show data of somatic mutations, copy number alterations, and mRNA changes in different cases. The rows show the genes, and the columns show the individual patient. It is a very simple and straightforward way of representation [28, 29].

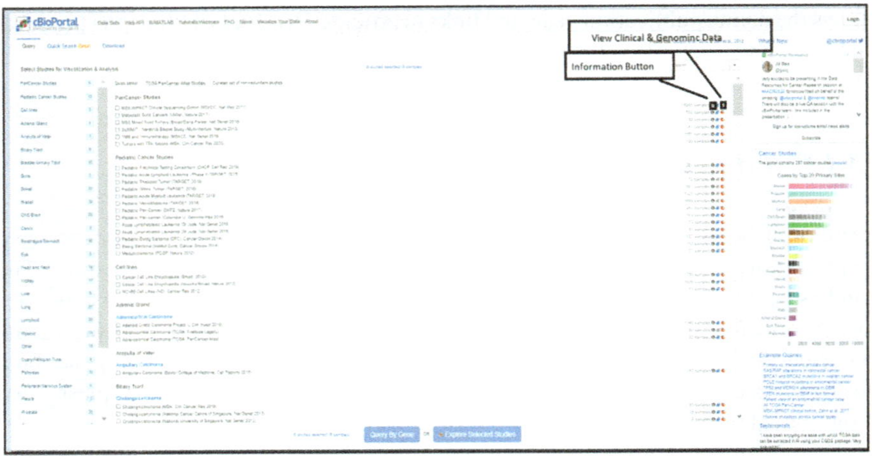

Fig. 13.10 Features of cBioPortal

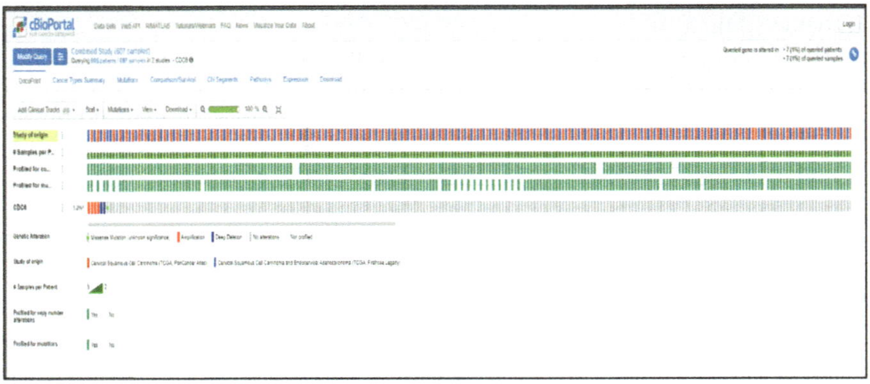

Fig. 13.11 Oncoprint

Data for different cell types are shown as bar graphs (Fig. 13.12). The option can be changed accordingly to get the alteration frequency or absolute count of different cell types. The bar graph is obtained for all the genes together or individual genes separately. The data also shows whether it is for mutation or CNA (circulating nucleic acids) etc.

The whole genome or specific genes can be selected. The structure of the genome is shown, and selecting a specific site on the genome highlights the CNA of that site. CNA or circulating nucleic acids act as biomarkers in the identification of cancers. They can be very beneficial in carrying out studies. The red lines indicate amplification and the blue one deletion. The RefSeq and amino gene sequence can be observed by zooming in, the amino gene sequence (Fig. 13.13).

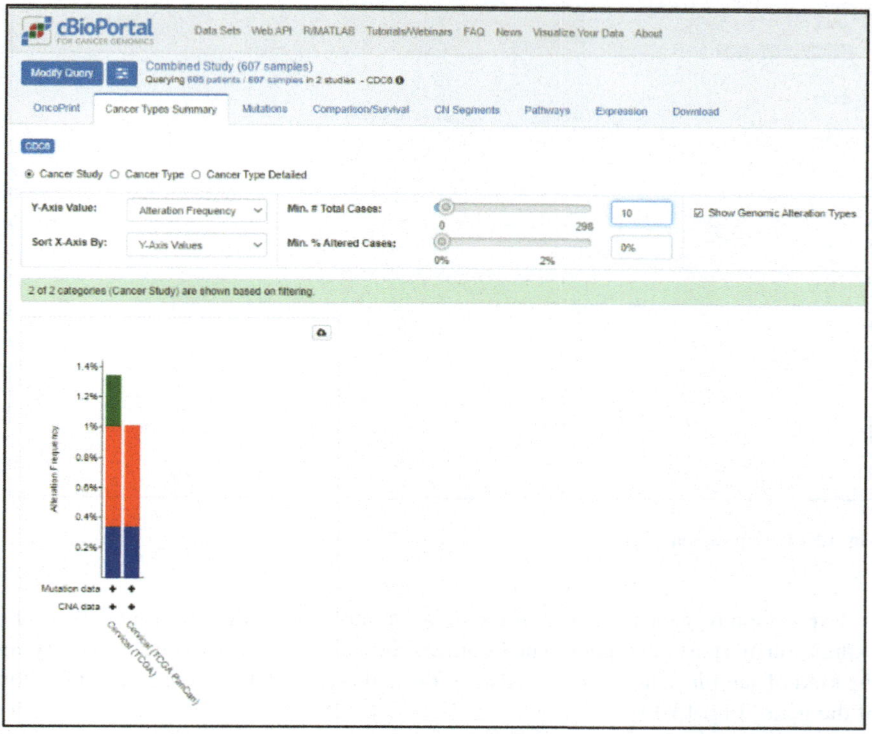

Fig. 13.12 Cancer type summary

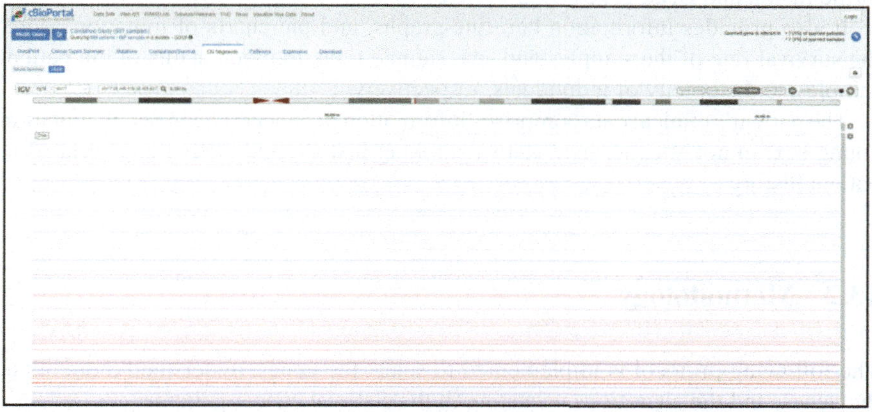

Fig. 13.13 CN segments

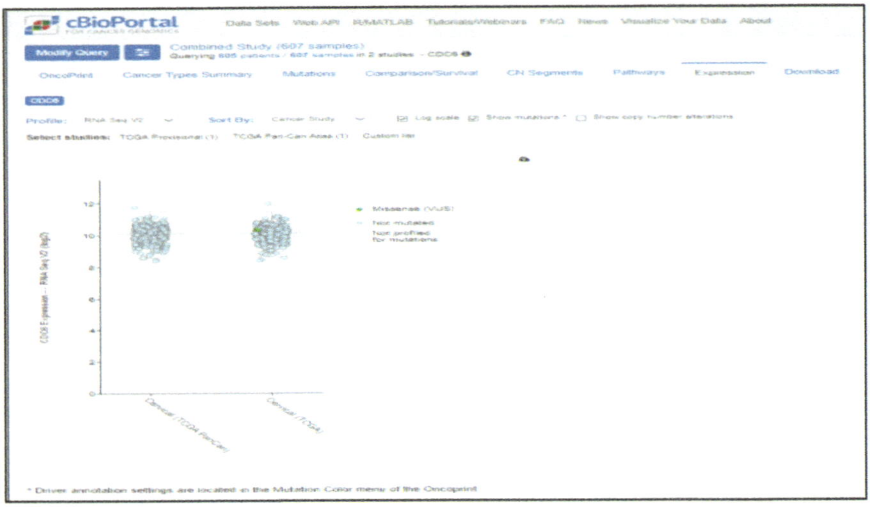

Fig. 13.14 Expression of genes

Expression of genes consists of the data for variation of the different cells to the expression of a particular gene. The sample is shown as color-coded circles specifying the kind of sample. The x-axis consists of the cell type and the y-axis, the expression of the gene (Fig. 13.14).

The summary window provides information on cancer type with the number of samples, genomic profile sample count, mRNA data, and the frequency percentage of the fusion and CNA genes (Fig. 13.15).

It also provides information bar, line graphs, and pie charts of mutation count, the survival rate of the samples and sex, sample type, the vital status of the patient samples, and ethnicity of individuals, respectively.

The patient's clinical data comprises information of cancer type in detail, mutation count, sex, tumor site, survival status, smoking history, and other things related to patient history.

13.2 Methodology

The following protocol is implemented to select the genes, understand more about the genes, and the alterations occurring in the cervical cancer genome.

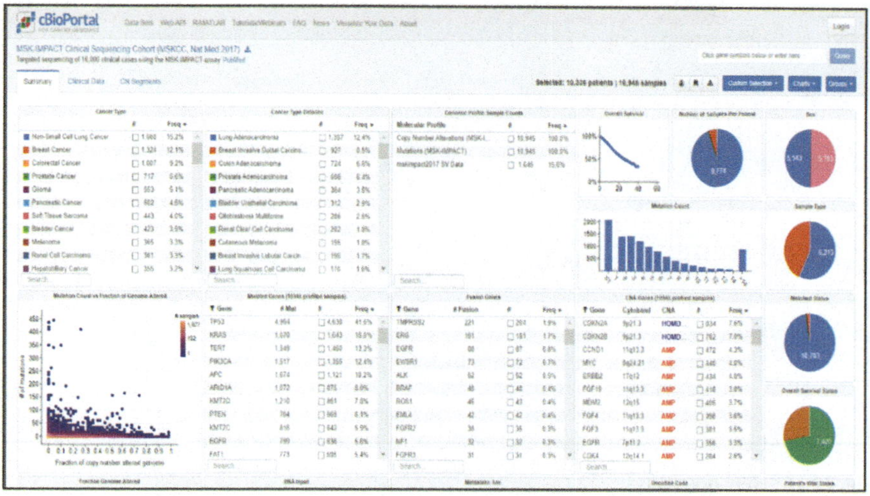

Fig. 13.15 Summary of the samples

13.2.1 NCBI Geo

In NCBI GEO portal,[2] the dataset on cervical cancer is opened using accession number (i.e. GSE63514), and GEO2R file is downloaded. The 'normal' and 'cancer' sample groups are defined and a table of TOP 250 genes is downloaded by selecting TOP 250. The data is pasted in an excel sheet using 'paste special option' (i.e. unicode). As we require only gene related tabular data, other introductory part is deleted in the series matrix file. For gene ID, platform files are downloaded in notepad format and symbol is transferred to another excel file sheet. The gene symbol and gene ID are copied from the platform file to the series matrix file corresponding to the gene. The #class data is added to the second row by comparing it with the headings, which are normal and cancer, as arranged in GEO 2R in the original dataset. As Network analyst accepts only tab delimilited format the edited file is saved in the 'tab delimited' format.

13.2.2 Data Analysis in NetworkAnalyst

As discussed in the introduction section from NetworkAnalyst (13.1.2), we obtain the converted data used for analysis. NetworkAnalyst has seven steps. They are as follows:

[2] www.ncbi.nlm.nih.gov.

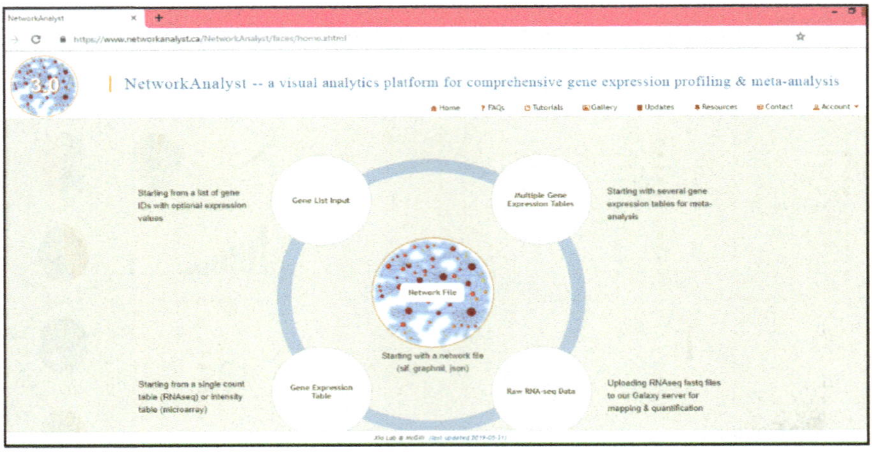

Fig. 13.16 NetworkAnalyst

i. The front page of NetworkAnalyst has options, as shown in (Fig. 13.16). According to our uploading file, we select the required option. In our study, we used 'Gene Expression Table'. The gene expression profiling and functional analytics support 17 common organisms. Homo sapien (human) organism is specified. A datatype is selected as microarray data, and ID type organism is chosen as the official gene symbol. The gene expression table is uploaded. The file size limit is 50mb. (Fig. 13.17).
ii. After this gets uploaded, proceed with the 'Quality check'. Quality check does a review of the data provided like data type, matched and unmatched gene number, etc. The review of our dataset is shown in (Fig. 13.18). The group names (i.e., cancer and normal) are denoted as C and N. After checking the data's accuracy, proceed with data filling and normalization.
iii. Filtering is used to delete data which is either not useful or is actually incorrect. Normalization is critical for accurately identifying transcriptional variations and ensuring that each sample's expression distributions are identical throughout the experiment. No log normalization is performed with a variance filter of 15, as seen in (Fig. 13.19). The genes were filtered with annotation preserved for further analysis.
iv. For differential gene expression analysis, the LIMMA3, EDGE, and DESEQ 2 can be selected. The analysis of differential expression involves using standardized read count data and statistical analysis to distinguish differences in expression between experimental groups (i.e., C and N). The statistical method LIMMA (Linear modelling with empirical Bayes Moderation) is selected. The differential analysis was performed successfully by comparing a comparison of interest (C vs. N), as shown in (Fig. 13.20).

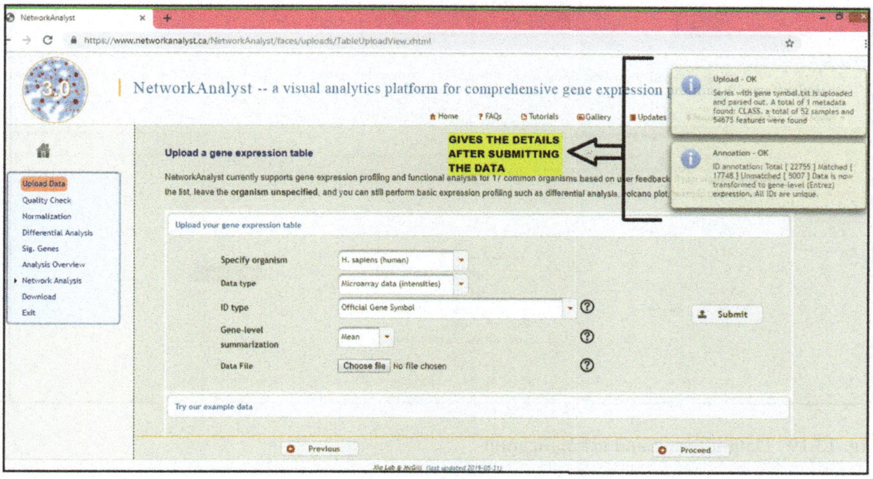

Fig. 13.17 Upload data

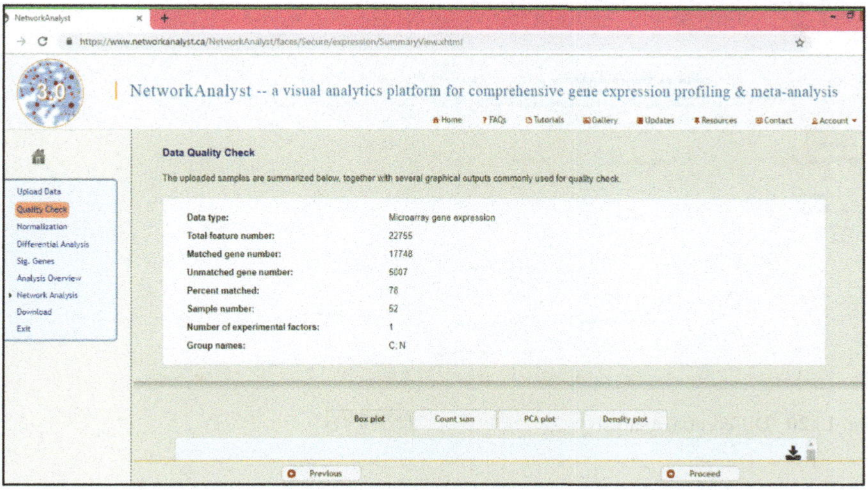

Fig. 13.18 Quality check

v. A threshold of p-value and log 2 fold change are specified to identify significant genes. In our study, the p-value of 0.05 and log 2 fold change is 1.0. The total significant genes were identified and listed (i.e., 1974 genes) as in (Fig. 13.21).

vi. Analysis overview in visual analytics is a human perceptual system to uncover the hidden hands in big data. It integrates visualization with statistical analysis in understanding the complex omics data. After analysis, visualization of the network is performed (Figs. 13.22 and 13.23).

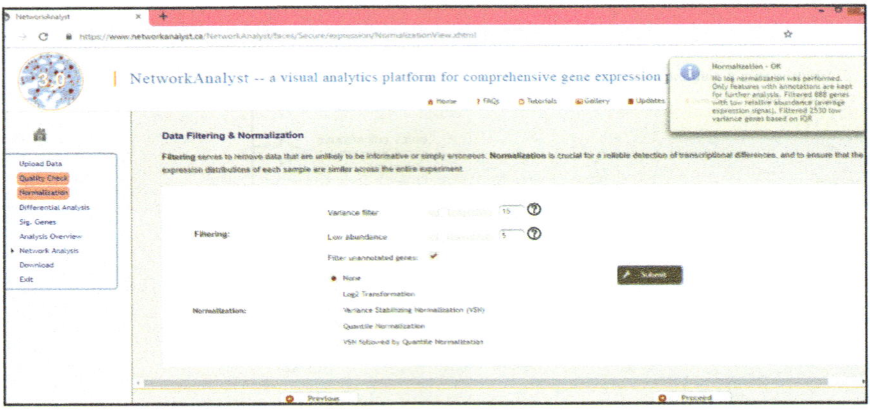

Fig. 13.19 Data filtering and normalization

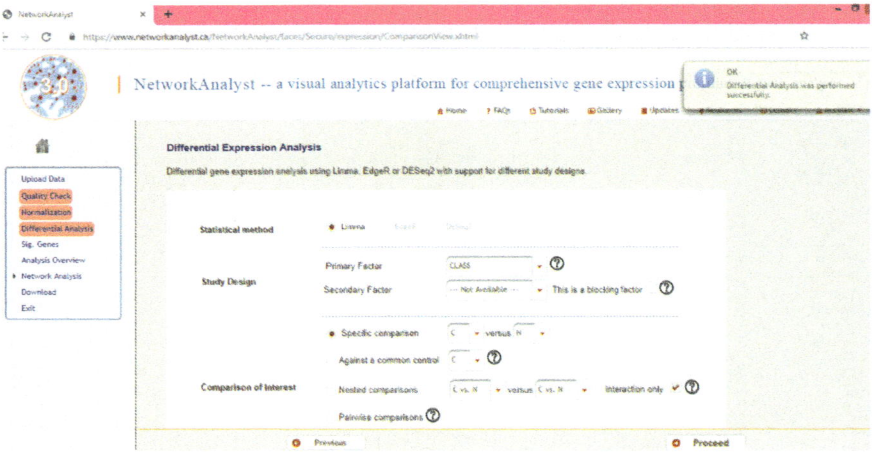

Fig. 13.20 Differential analysis

vii. On proceeding a graphical representation of the data is obtained. Here it is an ORA enrichment network that has been discussed in the introduction. Here changes to the network can be made accordingly, find the various genes involved, and see the data in various forms like 3D and VR. The nodes can be zoomed into, and on clicking on a specific one, they split into different genes involved in the pathway (Fig. 13.24).

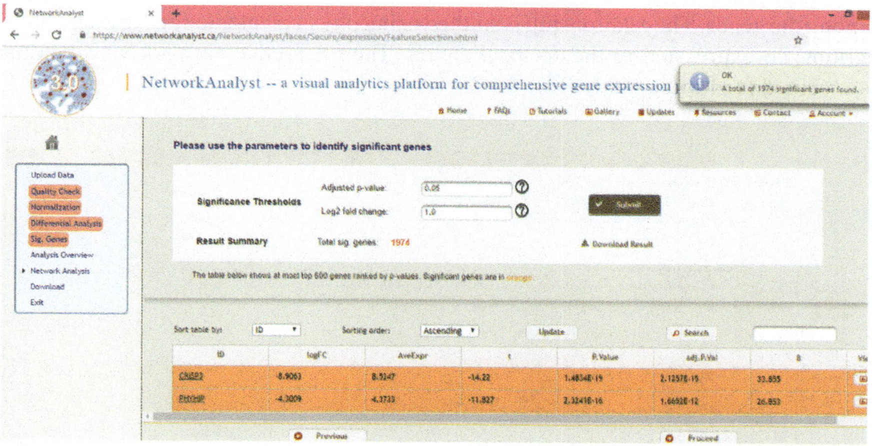

Fig. 13.21 Significant genes

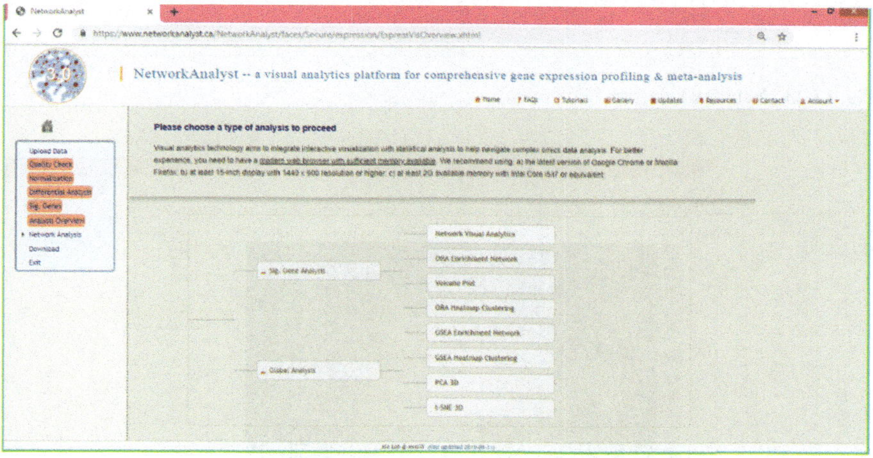

Fig. 13.22 Analysis overview

13.2.3 *Identifying Co-expressed Genes Using GeneMANIA*

As discussed in the introduction (refer Sect. 13.1.3) GeneMANIA is used for analyzing a particular gene list to acquire biological relationships among the cellular components. We can obtain physical interactions, genetic interactions, co-expression or the co-localization of molecules. Open GeneMANIA (https://GeneMANIA.org) the gene pathway selected from NetworkAnalyst, i.e., cell cycle pathway TTK, CDKN2A, CDK1, DBF4, CDC25B, CCNB1, DC45, CDC6, CDC7, PKMYT1, and MCM2 genes are analysed to construct a gene network and explore the relationships among the genes. The relationship is studied using physical interactions, genetic interactions, co-expression or the co-localization. The interactive network visualization is obtained for further study (Fig. 13.25).

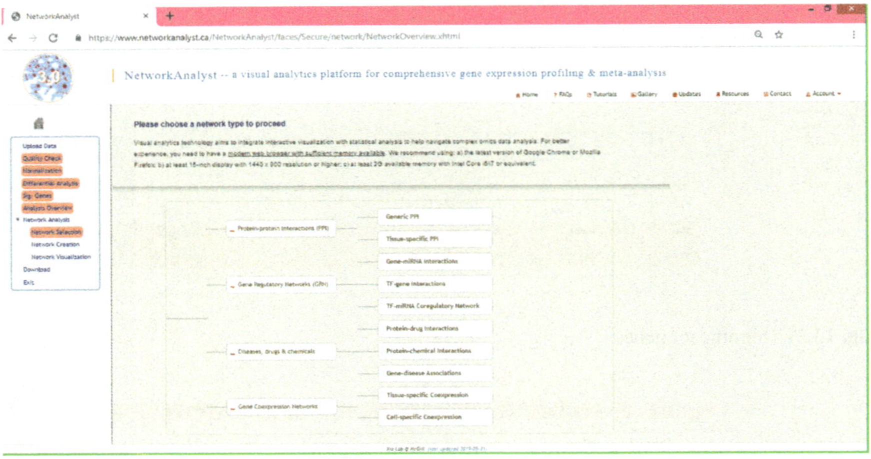

Fig. 13.23 Network selection

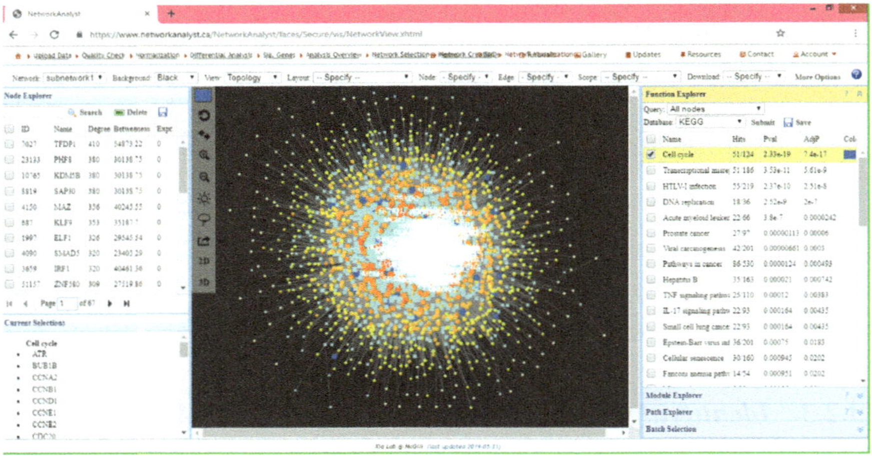

Fig. 13.24 Enrichment network of genes

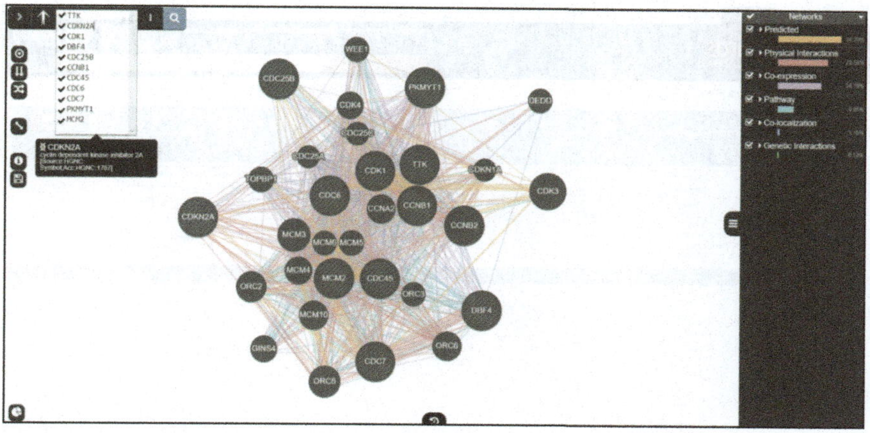

Fig. 13.25 Network visualization on GeneMANIA

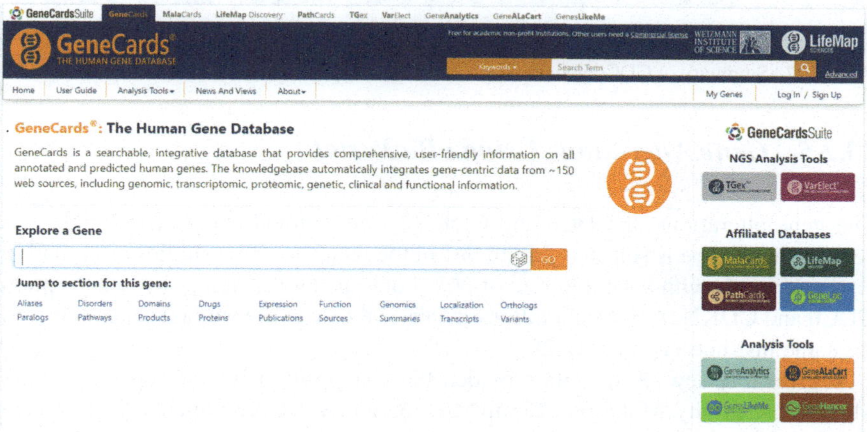

Fig. 13.26 GeneCards portal

13.2.4 *Summary of Genes Using GeneCards*

i. Once the gene of interest is identified from NetworkAnalyst and GeneMANIA, the detailed information of genes are studied in GeneCards. We open GeneCards using the link (Fig. 13.26).[3]
ii. The gene is given in the search box (i.e., CDC6 and CDKN2A). A detailed summary of the genes CDC6 and CDKN2A are studied. The details like expression, previous publications are considered from the data (Fig. 13.27).

[3]https://www.genecards.org/.

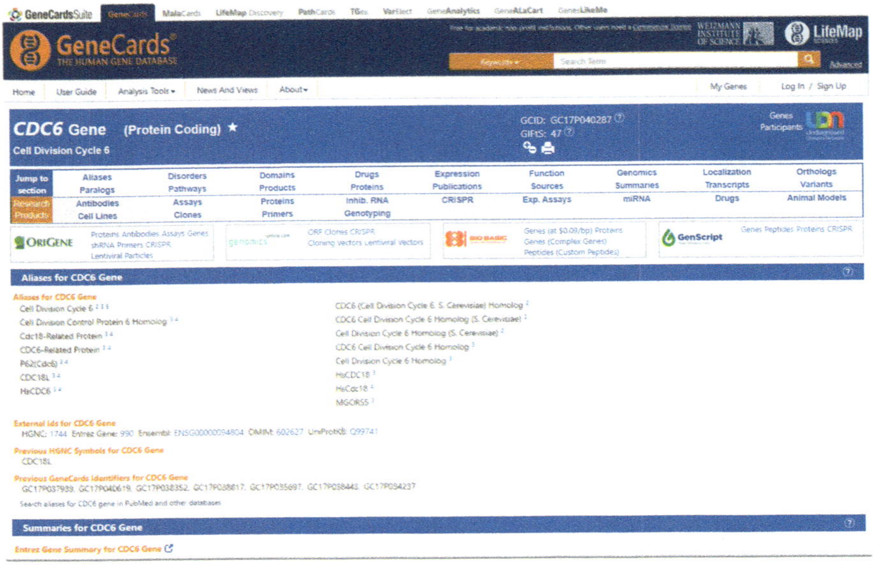

Fig. 13.27 Summary of CDC6 genes

13.2.5 Gene Alterations Using cBioPortal

The gene alterations of CDC6 and CDKN2A are studied using cBioPortal.[4] The cervix cancer type is selected for studies in the database. Two studies are found on cervical cancer with a sample size of 607. Later, using the 'query by gene' option, CDC6 and CDKN2A gene alterations in cervical cancer are studied separately with the same instructions (Fig. 13.28).

It gives a review of the data provided like Oncoprint, Clinical Types Summary, Mutual Exclusivity, Mutations, Comparison & Survival, CN Segments, Pathway, and Expression of the gene.

13.3 Results

The results of each step in the protocol are obtained and analyzed. NCBI GEO is used to download the series matrix and platform files for the samples (normal and cancer). All the genes are listed with respect to their p-values. After sorting with gene symbols, the excel file is converted to notepad (i.e. tab delimited), as shown in (Fig. 13.29).

[4]https://www.cbioportal.org.

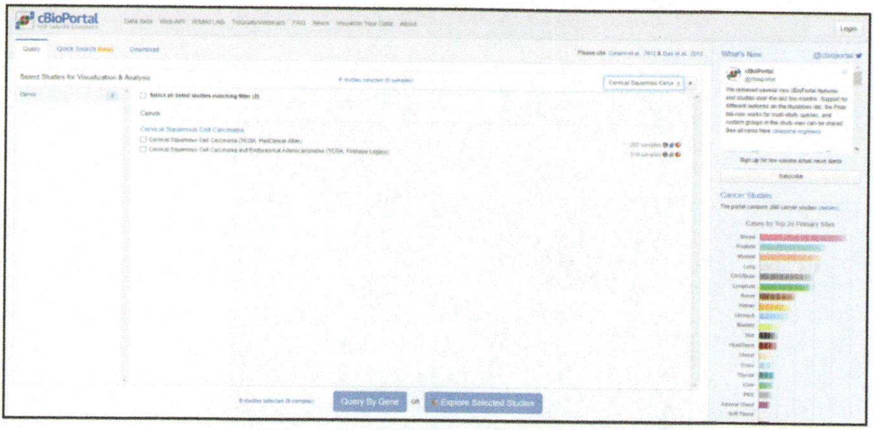

Fig. 13.28 cBioPortal webpage

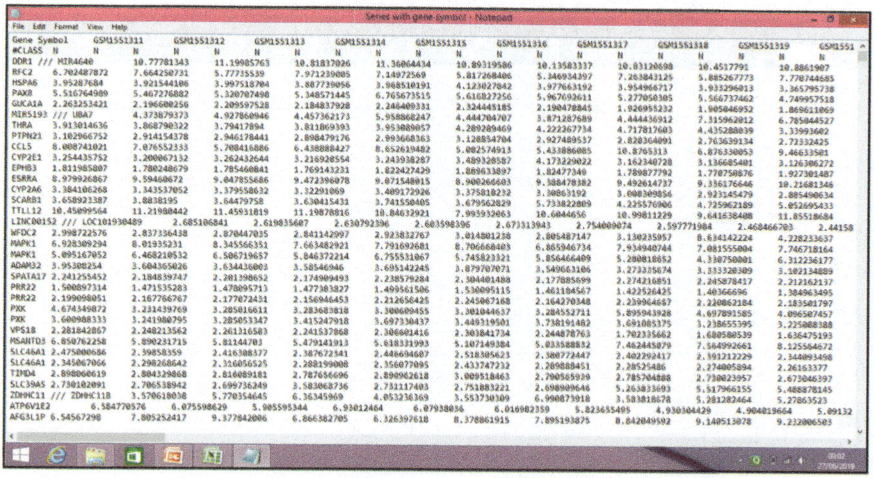

Gene Symbol	GSM1551311	GSM1551312	GSM1551313	GSM1551314	GSM1551315	GSM1551316	GSM1551317	GSM1551318	GSM1551319	GSM1551
#CLASS	N	N	N	N	N	N	N	N	N	N
DDR1 /// MIR4640	10.77781343	11.19985763	10.81837026	11.36064434	10.89319586	10.13583337	10.83120698	10.4517791	10.8861907	
RFC2	6.702487872	7.664250731	5.77735539	7.971239005	7.14972569	5.817268406	5.346934397	7.263843125	5.885267773	7.770744685
HSPA6	3.95287684	3.921544106	3.997518704	3.887739056	3.968510191	4.123027842	3.977663192	3.954966717	3.933296013	3.365795738
PAX8	5.516764989	5.467276882	5.320707498	5.348571445	6.765673515	5.616827256	5.967692611	5.277050305	5.566737462	4.749957518
GUCA1A	2.263253421	2.196600256	2.209597528	2.184837928	2.246409331	2.324445185	2.190478845	1.926955232	1.905046952	1.869611069
MIR5193 /// UBA7	4.373879373	4.927860946	4.457362173	5.958868247	4.444704707	3.871287689	4.444436912	7.315962012	6.785044527	
THRA	3.913014636	3.868790322	3.79417894	3.811869393	3.953089057	4.289289469	4.222267734	4.717817603	4.435288039	3.33993602
PTPN21	3.102966752	2.914154378	2.946178441	2.898479176	2.993668363	3.128854704	2.927489537	2.828364091	2.763639134	2.72332425
CCL5	8.008741021	7.076552333	5.708416886	6.438888427	8.652619482	5.082574913	5.433886085	10.8765313	6.876330053	9.46633501
CYP2E1	3.254435752	3.200067132	3.262432644	3.216928554	3.243938287	3.489328587	4.173229022	3.162340728	3.136685401	3.126306272
EPHB3	1.811985807	1.780248679	1.785460841	1.769143231	1.822427429	1.889633897	1.82477349	1.789877792	1.770750876	1.927301487
ESRRA	8.979926867	9.59460672	9.047855686	9.472396078	9.071548015	8.900266603	9.388478382	9.492614737	9.336176646	10.21681346
CYP2A6	3.384106268	3.343537052	3.379558632	3.32291069	3.409172926	3.375818232	3.30863192	3.008309856	2.923145479	2.885490634
SCARB1	3.658923387	3.8838195	3.64479758	3.630415431	3.741550405	3.679562829	5.733822809	4.225576906	4.725962189	5.052695433
TTLL12	10.45099564	11.21980442	11.45931819	11.19878816	10.84632921	7.993932063	10.6044656	10.99811229	9.641638408	11.85518684
LINC00152 /// LOC101930489	2.685106841	2.619835607	2.630792396	2.603598396	2.673313943	2.754009074	2.597771984	2.468466703	2.44158	
WFDC2	2.998722576	2.837336438	2.870447035	2.841142997	2.923832767	3.014801238	2.805487147	3.130235957	8.634142224	4.228233637
MAPK1	6.928309294	8.01935231	8.345566351	7.663482921	7.791692681	8.706668403	6.865946734	7.934940744	7.081555004	7.746718164
MAPK1	5.095167052	6.468210532	6.506719657	5.846372214	6.755531067	5.745823321	5.856466409	5.280818652	4.330750001	6.312236177
ADAM32	3.95308254	3.604365026	3.634436003	3.58546946	3.695142245	3.879707071	3.549663106	3.273335674	3.333320309	3.102134889
SPATA17	2.241255452	2.184839747	2.201398652	2.174909493	2.238579284	2.304401488	2.177885699	2.274216851	2.245878417	2.212162137
PRR22	1.500897314	1.471535283	1.478095713	1.477383827	1.499561506	1.530095115	1.461184567	1.422526425	1.40366696	1.384963495
PRR22	2.199098051	2.167766767	2.177072431	2.156946453	2.212656425	2.245067168	2.164270348	2.239964657	2.220862184	2.183501797
PXK	4.674349872	3.231439769	3.285016611	3.283683818	3.300609455	3.301044637	3.284552711	5.895943928	4.697891585	4.096507457
PXK	3.600988333	3.241980795	3.285053347	3.415247918	3.697330437	3.449319501	3.738191482	3.691085375	3.238655395	3.225088388
VPS18	2.281842867	2.248213562	2.261316583	2.241537868	2.306601416	2.303841734	2.244878763	1.702335662	1.680580539	1.636475193
MSANTD3	6.850762258	5.890231715	5.81144703	5.479141913	5.618331993	5.107149384	5.033588832	7.462445079	7.564992661	8.125564672
SLC46A1	2.475000686	2.39858359	2.416308377	2.387672341	2.446694607	2.518305623	2.380772447	2.402292417	2.391212229	2.344093498
SLC46A1	2.345067066	2.298268642	2.316056525	2.288199008	2.356077095	2.433747232	2.289888451	2.28525486	2.274005894	2.26163377
TIMD4	2.898060619	2.804329868	2.816089181	2.787656696	2.890962618	3.009518463	2.790565939	2.785704888	2.730023957	2.673046397
SLC39A5	2.730102091	2.706538942	2.699736249	3.583068736	2.731117403	2.751883221	2.698909646	5.263833693	5.517966155	5.488878145
ZDHHC11 /// ZDHHC11B	3.570618038	5.770354645	6.36345969	4.053236369	3.553730309	6.990873918	3.583818678	5.281282464	5.27863523	
ATP6V1E2	6.584770576	6.075598629	5.905595344	6.93012464	6.07938036	6.016982359	5.823655495	4.930304429	4.904019664	5.09132
AFG3L1P	6.54567298	7.805252417	9.377842006	6.866382705	6.326397618	8.378861915	7.895193875	8.842049592	9.140513078	9.232006503

Fig. 13.29 Series matrix

The result obtained from NCBI GEO is uploaded to the NetworkAnalyst, and further steps were carried out as mentioned in Sect. 13.2.2. A gene enrichment plot with various genes involved in different pathways is obtained. The meta-node gene pathways from different databases: KEGG, REACTOME, GO–BP, GO–MF, are copied separately into an excel sheet. All the pathways are studied, and the cell cycle pathway from the KEGG database is selected for the study (Figs. 13.30 and 13.31).

The gene pathway obtained from NetworkAnalyst is further studied using GeneMANIA to identify associated genes with a set of input genes at the genetic level. The underlying similar co-expressed genes are obtained in gene-gene interactions.

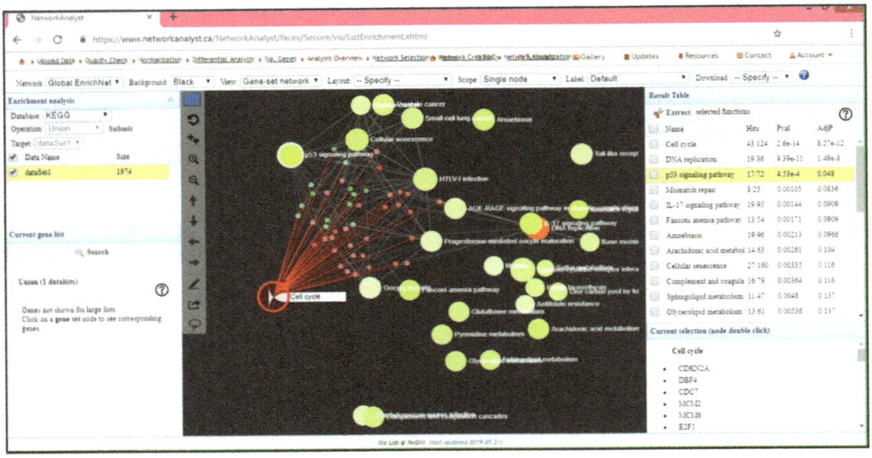

Fig. 13.30 Genes involved in cell cycle pathway

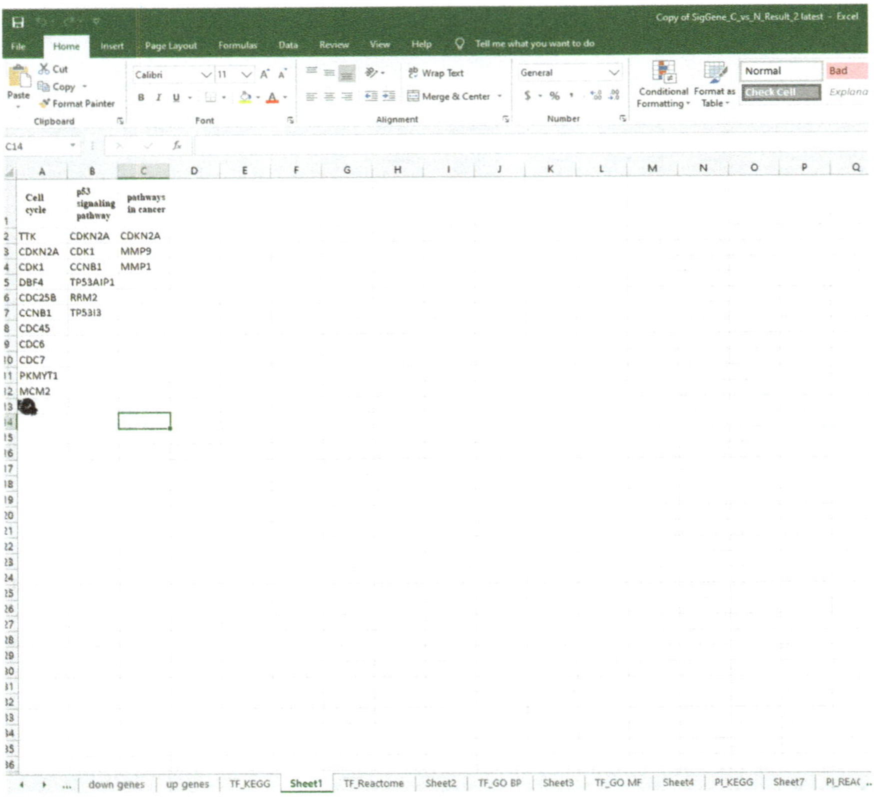

Fig. 13.31 Cell cycle pathways

GeneMANIA shows gene interactions using physical interaction, co-expression, co-localization from the source databases. CDKN2A is co-expressed with PKMYT1, CDC45, TTK, CDC25C, CCNB1, CDC25A, MCM6 genes as shown in (Fig. 13.32) CDC6 is co-expressed with CDC25C, ORC3, ORC6, PKMYT1, WEEE1, CDC25B, CDC25A,TTK, CDK1, CCNA2,CCNB1, MCM6, CCNB2, MCM4 genes as shown in (Fig. 13.33). Furthermore, the co-localization, co-expression of CDKN2A and CDC6 were determined.

The particular genes obtained from the GeneMANIA are studied further in GeneCards. GeneCards provides the complete data and summary of the query genes CDC6 and CDK2NA. The data fields of GeneCards are discussed in Sect. 13.1.4. In our study, the data field focused was the past research publications on the genes. From the latest publications, CDC6 gene was studied in 257 publications and CDKN2A in 4154 publications, as shown in (Figs. 13.34 and 13.35). This data is used as literature survey.

In cBioPortal, after all the studies on cervical cancer are obtained, the interpretation of data to identify different events in the gene is done. The total studies found in cervical cancer are studies with 607 samples. The cancer type data showed that CDC6 had been altered in 4.35% of 46 cases. It is deep deleted by 2.17% in one case and amplified by 2.17% in one case with no mutation in Cervical Adenocarcinoma, whereas in Cervical Squamous Cell Carcinoma, CDC6 is altered by 0.4% in 251 cases, amplified by 0.4% in one case with no deep deletion and mutation. The red, blue, and green show the amplification, deep deletion, and mutation data, respectively (Fig. 13.36).

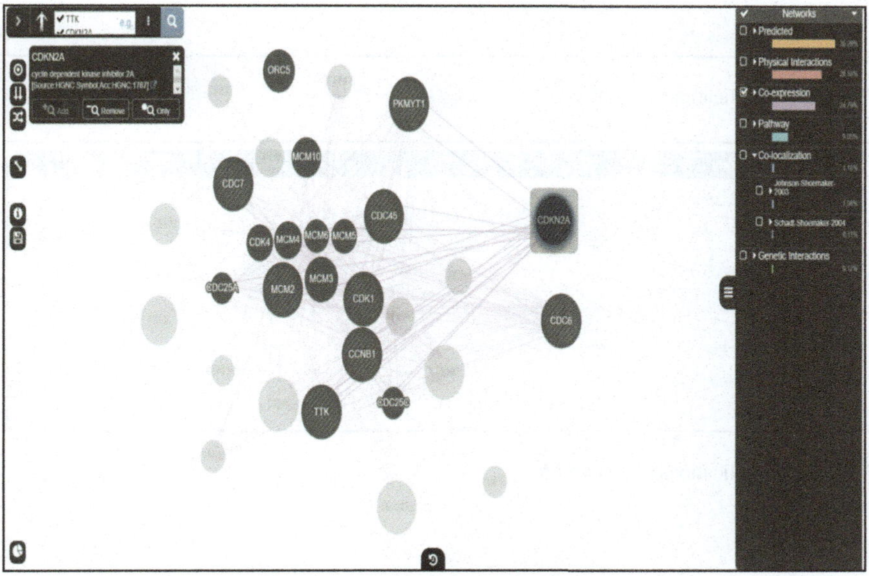

Fig. 13.32 Network Visualization for CDKN2A

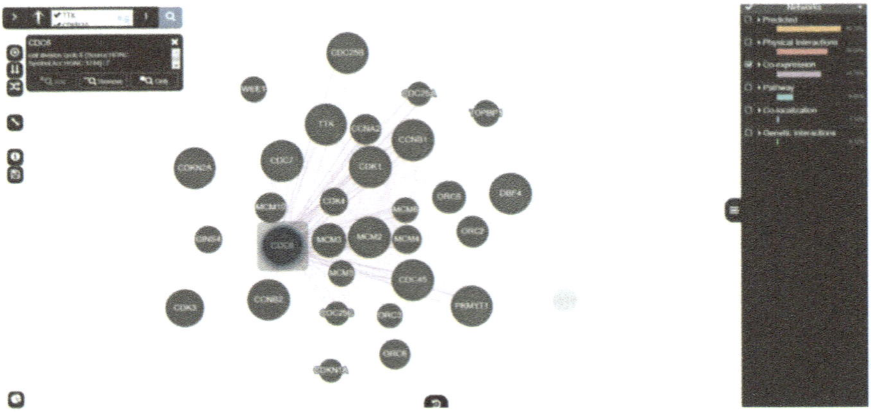

Fig. 13.33 Network visualization for CDC6

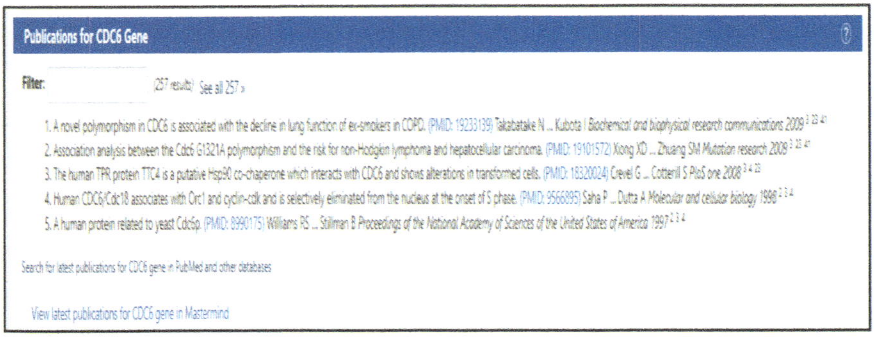

Publications for CDC6 Gene

Filter: (257 results) See all 257 »

1. A novel polymorphism in CDC6 is associated with the decline in lung function of ex-smokers in COPD. (PMID: 19233139) Takabatake N ... Kubota I *Biochemical and biophysical research communications* 2009 [3 23 41]
2. Association analysis between the Cdc6 G1321A polymorphism and the risk for non-Hodgkin lymphoma and hepatocellular carcinoma. (PMID: 19101572) Xiong XD ... Zhuang SM *Mutation research* 2009 [3 23 41]
3. The human TPR protein TTC4 is a putative Hsp90 co-chaperone which interacts with CDC6 and shows alterations in transformed cells. (PMID: 18320024) Crevel G ... Cotterill S *PloS one* 2008 [3 4 23]
4. Human CDC6/Cdc18 associates with Orc1 and cyclin-cdk and is selectively eliminated from the nucleus at the onset of S phase. (PMID: 9566895) Saha P ... Dutta A *Molecular and cellular biology* 1998 [2 3 4]
5. A human protein related to yeast Cdc6p. (PMID: 8990175) Williams RS ... Stillman B *Proceedings of the National Academy of Sciences of the United States of America* 1997 [2 3 4]

Search for latest publications for CDC6 gene in PubMed and other databases

View latest publications for CDC6 gene in Mastermind

Fig. 13.34 Publications of CDC6

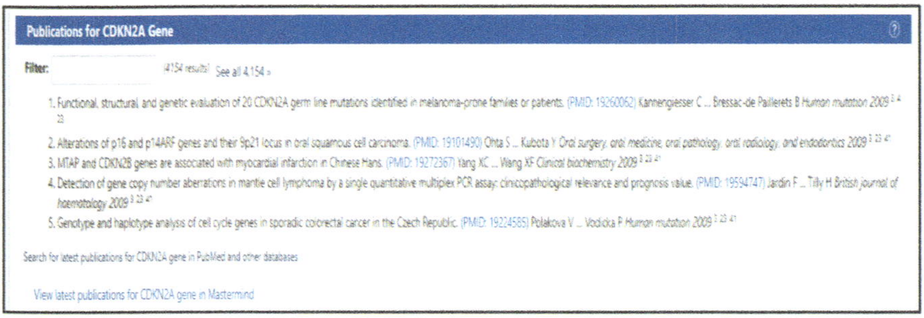

Publications for CDKN2A Gene

Filter: (4154 results) See all 4,154 »

1. Functional, structural, and genetic evaluation of 20 CDKN2A germ line mutations identified in melanoma-prone families or patients. (PMID: 19260062) Kannengiesser C ... Bressac-de Paillerets B *Human mutation* 2009 [3 4 23]
2. Alterations of p16 and p14ARF genes and their 9p21 locus in oral squamous cell carcinoma. (PMID: 19101490) Ohta S ... Kubota Y *Oral surgery, oral medicine, oral pathology, oral radiology, and endodontics* 2009 [3 23 41]
3. MTAP and CDKN2B genes are associated with myocardial infarction in Chinese Hans. (PMID: 19272367) Yang XC ... Wang XF *Clinical biochemistry* 2009 [3 23 41]
4. Detection of gene copy number aberrations in mantle cell lymphoma by a single quantitative multiplex PCR assay: clinicopathological relevance and prognosis value. (PMID: 19594747) Jardin F ... Tilly H *British journal of haematology* 2009 [3 23 41]
5. Genotype and haplotype analysis of cell cycle genes in sporadic colorectal cancer in the Czech Republic. (PMID: 19224585) Polakova V ... Vodicka P *Human mutation* 2009 [3 23 41]

Search for latest publications for CDKN2A gene in PubMed and other databases

View latest publications for CDKN2A gene in Mastermind

Fig. 13.35 Publications of CDKN2A

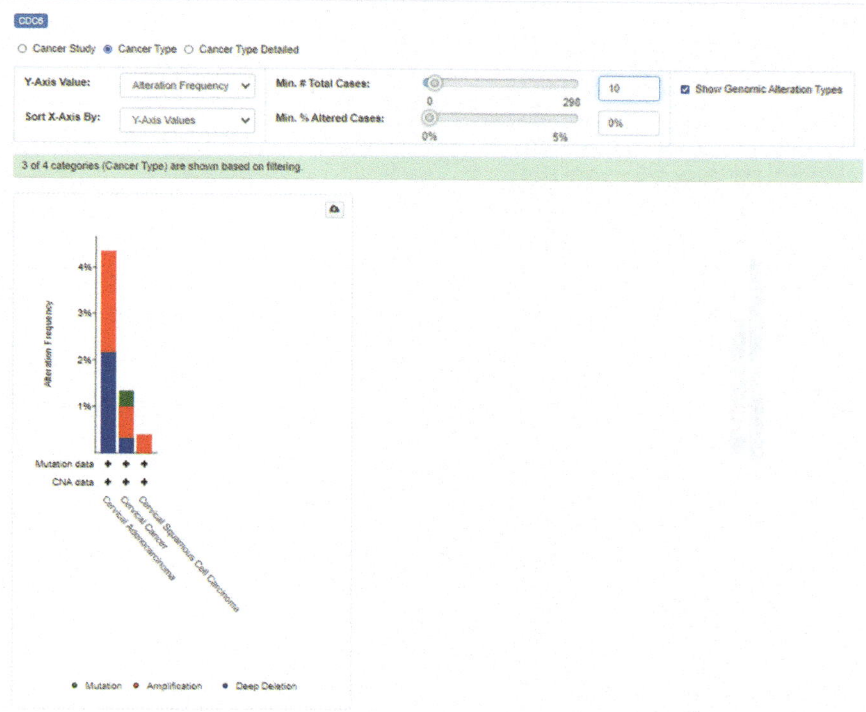

Fig. 13.36 Cancer type summary for CDC6

In 607 samples, CDKN2Agene is altered in 2.39% of 251 cases, mutated by 1.99% in 5 cases and deep deleted by 0.4% in one case and no amplification in cervical squamous carcinoma, whereas no alterations were found in Cervical Adenocarcinoma (Fig. 13.37).

This study is helpful in understanding alterations in the cervical genes and expression studies through genetic pathways. The paper also gives a framed protocol to study any type o cancer through computational genomics tools.

The methodology and NCBI GEO, Omics datasets NetworkAnalyst, GeneMANIA, Genecards, cBioPortal tools for identifying and studying the genes were supported with similar studies from literature. Differentially expressed genes (DEGs) in cancer patients from datasets GSE12251, GSE16879, and GSE23597 were integrated using NetworkAnalyst. The proportion of immune cell types was estimated via CIBERSORT. While NetworkAnalyst provided gene expression profiles and data, CIBERSORT provided the immune cell types and the cellular content [32]. The lncRNA immune prognostic signature (LIPS) (used for predicting survivability) was predicted and validated using different datasets. The study was conducted at mRNA level of cervical cancer [33] CIBERSORT was used to analyze the immune-related genes (IRGs) to find the immune checkpoint inhibitors. The research group conducted functional enrichment plots from the protein–protein interaction network to find

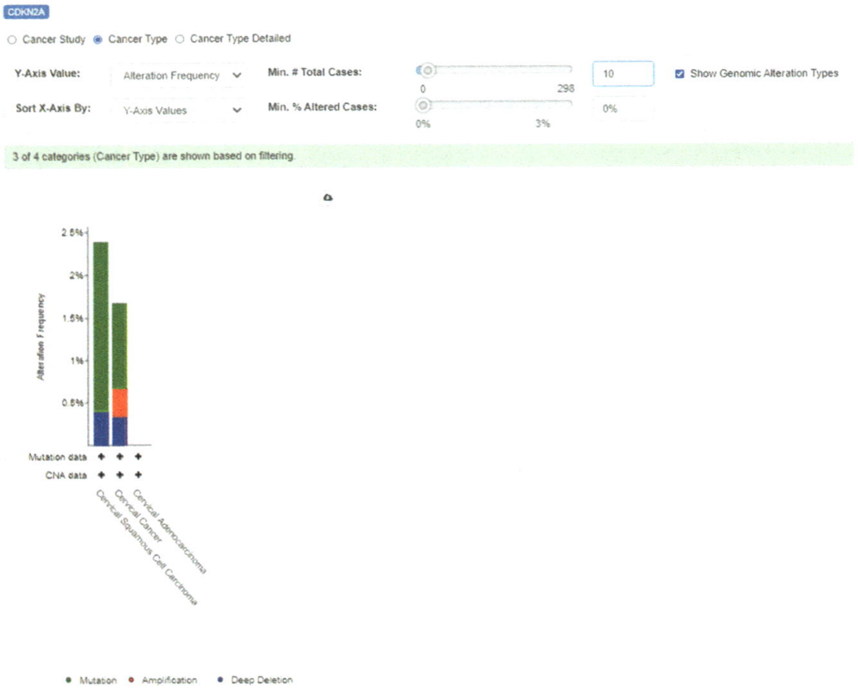

Fig. 13.37 Cancer type summary for CDKN2A

upregulated and downregulated genes [34] Shibo Yu et al., studied mRNA levels of the prognostic gene GINS2 in patients was studied using GeneMANIA, cBioPortal, TIMER, The Human Protein Atlas, GEPIA, Oncomine etc. [35]. Salma Begum Bhyan et al., used ECGene, OCGene, G2SBC and CCDB tools to determine the genes in breast, ovarian, endometrial and cervical cancer and studied for mutations in cBioPortal [36]. Cava, C., Bertoli studied driver genes in regulating the pathways in cancer using Gene Ontology, Reactome, KEGG, Biocarta databases. The functional pathways were obtained from GeneMANIA for further study on driver genes [37]. Darya V Telegina et al., used GeneMANIA to construct interaction networks for differentially expressed (DE) apoptosis-related genes at ages 20 days, 3 and 18 months [38]. Chen, M., Wang constructed Gene network in Genemania. CCND2, CDKN2A, CADM1, CCL2, CTNNB1, ERBB2, PHGDH, TP53BP1, TP63, TGFBR2, EGFR, PRKCB, SH3KBP1, KDELR1, NFATC1, PPP2R5D, HSPA6, PIKFYVE, RABEP1, PRKCI, PTGS2, STK11, FOXO1, TP53, PIK3CA, MYC, IMP3 and MAPK1 were explored in cervical intraepithelial neoplasia patients. The significant genes at the core of the network were selected, and the signaling pathways associated with these genes were studied using KEGG database [39].

Overall, our paper demonstrated the working of tools in computational genomics to identify, visualize, analyse, and understand the complex biological interaction network of the genes.

13.4 Conclusion

Analyzing the biological network is essential in gaining an understanding of the complex biological processes. Omics datasets are becoming increasingly common, but they can be hard to access, analyze, and visualize, especially without a computational skillset. The various computational genomics tools offer much easier integration of more extensive data and data visualization without having to go through advanced graphical representation. The protocol of computational analysis has many steps. Foremost from NCBI GEO, the experimental data is acquired. The dataset is submitted to NetworkAnalyst to visualize the meta-node network of genes based on functional enrichment analysis using various gene interaction pathways from databases (KEGG, REACTOME, GO). The visualization as a network makes it easy to analyze and understand. The gene pathway of interest is submitted in GeneMANIA where the Co-expression of similar genes is obtained. In our study, CDC6 and CDKN2A are selected for the study of alterations in cervical cancer. GeneCards provides is a human genome database and genomic, proteomic, and transcriptomic data of the gene. The literature for CDC6 and CDKN2A are reviewed using 257 publications for CDC6 and 4154 publications for CDKN2A. It can be hard to interpret the data and identify different events (Mutations/amplification/deletion) from large datasets. cBioPortal is an exclusive cancer study portal with the data collected from a wide range of databases. The alterations in the genes CDC6 and CDKN2A are analyzed and found to alter in cervical cancer. More cases need to be studied for a better understanding of the mechanism of genes. The tools used and step by step process of studying the data through these analytical platforms are provided with results. In our study, the pre-researched data from computational genomics tools is used.

Acknowledgements We would like to acknowledge Dr. Ayyavu Mahesh, Centre for Stem Cell and Cancer Genomics, AMI BioScience, Coimbatore, Tamil Nadu, India, for his constant guidance and support throughout the study.

References

1. Bacher, R., Kendziorski, C.: Design and computational analysis of single-cell RNA-sequencing experiments. Genome Biol. **17**, 63 (2016). https://doi.org/10.1186/s13059-016-0927-y
2. Martinez, M.: Computational tools for genomic studies in plants. Curr. Genomics **17**(6), 509–514 (2016). https://doi.org/10.2174/1389202917666160520103447

3. Wang, S., Cho, H., Zhai, C., Berger, B., Peng, J.: Exploiting ontology graph for predicting sparsely annotated gene function. Bioinformatics **31**(12), i357–364 (2015). https://doi.org/10.1093/bioinformatics/btv260
4. Barrett, T., Wilhite, S.E., Ledoux, P., Evangelista, C., Kim, I.F., Tomashevsky, M., Marshall, K.A., Phillippy, K.H., Sherman, P.M., Holko, M., Yefanov, A., Lee, H., Zhang, N., Robertson, C.L., Serova, N., Davis, S., Soboleva, A.: NCBI GEO: archive for functional genomics data sets–update. Nucleic Acids Res. **41**(Database issue), D991-5. https://doi.org/10.1093/nar/gks1193
5. Ijaz, M., Mahmood-ur-Rahman Ansari, Iqbal, M.: Introductory chapter: protein-protein interactions and assays, protein-protein interaction assays. https://doi.org/10.5772/intechopen.77337
6. Rao, V.S., Srinivas, K., Sujini, G.N., Sunand Kumar, G.N.: Protein-protein interaction detection: methods and analysis (2014). https://doi.org/10.1155/2014/147648
7. Wang, Y.: Gene regulatory networks. In: Dubitzky, W., Wolkenhauer, O., Cho, K.H., Yokota, H. (eds.) Encyclopedia of Systems Biology. Springer, New York (2013). https://doi.org/10.1007/978-1-4419-9863-7
8. Xia, J., Benner, M.J., Hancock, R.E.: NetworkAnalyst–integrative approaches for protein-protein interaction network analysis and visual exploration. Nucleic acids Res. **42**(Web Server issue), W167–W174 (2014). https://doi.org/10.1093/nar/gku443
9. Zhou, G., Soufan, O., Ewald, J., Hancock, R.E.W., Basu, N., Xia, J.: NetworkAnalyst 3.0: a visual analytics platform for comprehensive gene expression profiling and meta-analysis. Nucleic Acids Res **47**(W1), W234–W241. https://doi.org/10.1093/nar/gkz240. (02 July 2019)
10. Xia, J., Lyle, N.H., Mayer, M., Pena, O.M., Hancock, R.E.W.: INVEX-a web-based tool for integrative visualization of expression data. Bioinformatics **29**(24), 3232–3234. (gene expression data analysis)
11. Pathway Analysis in Bioinformatics: Mapping Data to Information. https://www.kolabtree.com/blog/pathway-analysis-in-bioinformatics-mapping-data-to-information/
12. Tsuyuzaki, K., Morota, G., Ishii, M., et al.: MeSH ORA framework: R/Bioconductor packages to support MeSH over-representation analysis. BMC Bioinform. **16**, 45 (2015). https://doi.org/10.1186/s12859-015-0453-z
13. Liu, L., Ruan, J.: Network-based pathway enrichment analysis. In: Proceedings. IEEE International Conference on Bioinformatics and Biomedicine, pp. 218–221 (2013). https://doi.org/10.1109/BIBM.2013.6732493
14. Subramanian, A., et.al.: Gene set enrichment analysis: a knowledge-based approach for interpreting genome-wide expression profiles. In: Proceedings of the National Academy of Sciences. https://doi.org/10.1073/pnas.0506580102
15. Mootha, V., Lindgren, C., Eriksson, K., et al.: PGC-1α-responsive genes involved in oxidative phosphorylation are coordinately downregulated in human diabetes. Nat. Genet. **34**, 267–273 (2003). https://doi.org/10.1038/ng1180
16. Huang, D.W., Sherman, B.T., Lempicki, R.A.: Bioinformatics enrichment tools: paths toward the comprehensive functional analysis of large gene lists. Nucleic Acids Res. **37**(1), 1–13. https://doi.org/10.1093/nar/gkn923. (1 January 2009)
17. Li, W., et al.: Using volcano plots and regularized-chi statistics in genetic association studies. Comput. Biol. Chem. **48**, 77–83 (2014). https://doi.org/10.1016/j.compbiolchem.2013.02.003
18. Doyle, M.: Visualization of RNA-Seq results with Volcano Plot (Galaxy Training Materials) (2019). https://galaxyproject.github.io/training-material/topics/transcriptomics/tutorials/rna-seq-viz-with-volcanoplot/tutorial.html. (Batut et al.: Community-driven data analysis training for biology cell systems (2018). https://doi.org/10.1016/j.cels.2018.05.012)
19. Volcano plot service. https://www.creative-proteomics.com/services/volcano-plot-service.htm
20. Biological interpretation of gene expression data. https://www.ebi.ac.uk/training/online/course/functional-genomics-ii-common-technologies-and-data-analysis-methods/biological-0#:~:text=In%20heat%20maps%20the%20data,absolute%20values)%20of%20gene%20expression

21. Institute of canine biology. https://www.instituteofcaninebiology.org/heat_map.html. Accessed 5 Jan 2021
22. Zhao, S., Guo, Y., Sheng, Q., Shyr, Y.: Advanced heat map and clustering analysis using heatmap3, vol. 2014, Article ID 986048, pp. 6 (2014). http://dx.doi.org/10.1155/2014/986048
23. Mostafavi, S., Ray, D., Warde-Farley, D., Grouios, C., Morris, Q.: GeneMANIA: a real-time multiple association network integration algorithm for predicting gene function. Genome Biol. **9**(Suppl 1), S4 (2008). https://doi.org/10.1186/gb-2008-9-s1-s4
24. Franz, M., Rodriguez, H., Lopes, C., Zuberi, K., Montojo, J., Bader, G.D., Morris, Q.: GeneMANIA update 2018. Nucleic Acids Res. **46**(W1), W60–W64 (2018). https://doi.org/10.1093/nar/gky311
25. Warde-Farley, D., et.al.: The GeneMANIA prediction server: biological network integration for gene prioritization and predicting gene function. Nucleic Acids Res. **38**(suppl_2), W214–W220 (2010). https://doi.org/10.1093/nar/gkq537. (1 July 2010)
26. Stelzer, G., et al.: The GeneCards suite: from gene data mining to disease genome sequence analysis. Current Protoc. Bioinform. **54**, 1.30.1–1.30.33 (2016). https://doi.org/10.1002/cpbi.5
27. Safran, M., et al.: GeneCards Version 3: the human gene integrator. Database J. Biol. Databases Curation. baq020 (2010). https://doi.org/10.1093/database/baq020
28. Cerami, E., Gao, J., Dogrusoz, U.: The cBio cancer genomics portal: an open platform for exploring multidimensional cancer genomics data. https://doi.org/10.1158/2159-8290.cd-12-0095
29. Gao, J., Aksoy, B.A., Dogrusoz, U.: Integrative analysis of complex cancer genomics and clinical profiles using the cBioPortal. https://doi.org/10.1126/scisignal.2004088
30. Gu, Z.: Oncoprint (2015-10-14). https://bioconductor.riken.jp/packages/3.2/bioc/vignettes/ComplexHeatmap/inst/doc/s8.oncoprint.html
31. Cisowski, J., Bergo, M.O.: What makes oncogenes mutually exclusive?. Small GTPases, **8**(3), 187–192 (2017). https://doi.org/10.1080/21541248.2016.1212689
32. Liu, Y., Duan, Y., Li, Y.: Integrated gene expression profiling analysis reveals probable molecular mechanism and candidate biomarker in Anti-TNFα Non-response IBD patients. J. Inflamm. Res. 13, 81–95 (2020 Feb 12). https://doi.org/10.2147/jir.s236262. (PMID: 32104045; PMCID: PMC7024800)
33. Chen, Q., Hu, L., Huang, D., Chen, K., et al.: Six-lncRNA immune prognostic signature for cervical cancer. Front. Genet. **11**, (2020). https://doi.org/10.3389/fgene.2020.533628
34. Yang, S., Wu, Y., Deng, Y., et al.: Identification of a prognostic immune signature for cervical cancer to predict survival and response to immune checkpoint inhibitors. Oncoimmunology **8**(12):e1659094 (2019). https://doi.org/10.1080/2162402x.2019.1659094. (2019 Oct 3, PMID: 31741756; PMCID: PMC6844304)
35. Yu, S., Zhu, L., Xie, P., Jiang, S., et al.: Mining the prognostic significance of the GINS2 gene in human breast cancer using bioinformatics analysis. Oncol. Lett. **20**, 1300–1310 (2020)
36. Bhyan, S.B., Wee, Y., Liu, Y., Cummins, S., Zhao, M.: Integrative analysis of common genes and driver mutations implicated in hormone stimulation for four cancers in women. Peer J. **7**, e6872 (2019). https://doi.org/10.7717/peerj.6872. (Published 2019 Jun 6)
37. Cava, C., Bertoli, G., Colaprico, A., et al.: Integration of multiple networks and pathways identifies cancer driver genes in pan-cancer analysis. BMC Genom. **19**, 25 (2018). https://doi.org/10.1186/s12864-017-4423-x
38. Telegina, D.V., Korbolina, E.E., Ershov, N.I., et al.: Identification of functional networks associated with cell death in the retina of OXYS rats during the development of retinopathy. Cell Cycle **14**(22), 3544–3556 (2015). https://doi.org/10.1080/15384101.2015.1080399
39. Chen, M., Wang, H., Liang, Y., et al.: Establishment of multifactor predictive models for the occurrence and progression of cervical intraepithelial neoplasia. BMC Cancer **20**, 926 (2020). https://doi.org/10.1186/s12885-020-07265-7

Chapter 14
Prostate Cancer: Cancer Detection and Classification Using Deep Learning

Sampurna Mandal, Debanik Roy, and Sunanda Das

Abstract Cancer has already taken the second leading position as the cause of death making the global burden world wide. There is an estimate of 9.6 million deaths in 2018 as per the survey of US cancer statistics. Prostate cancer is an abnormal, malignant growth of cells in the prostate gland uncontrollably. This disease mainly affects either middle-aged or older thousands of men each year. Cancer till now is a major issue that is continuously creating a burden to the individuals as well as health systems. Therefore, it is a big concern in front of health systems demanding a strong system which can detect early and help for treatment. Here, we have applied some deep learning models to study the classification for the detection of clinically significant prostate cancer from the large-scale cancer image data for each patient. This paper investigates the effect of deep learning architecture like VGG16, EfficientNet, Dense Net121, ResNext50 in the large-scale cancer image data classification setting. Our main contribution is to focus on the high-level accuracy because these deep learning algorithms have the capability of transfer learning with image instant segmentation.

Keywords Prostate cancer · Deep learning network · Medical imaging · Statistical analysis · Image data classification

14.1 Introduction

Prostate cancer is a common cancer mostly found in men. In Europe, approximately 417,000 cases are found having prostate cancer and 92,000 deaths are recorded in each year [1]. As per survey [2], the statistics say that prostate cancer is commonly occurring cancer type in men. Nowadays, one out of seven men of middle age is

S. Mandal · D. Roy
Department of Robotics Engineering, The Neotia University, South 24 Pargana 743368, WB, India

S. Das (✉)
Department of Computer Science and Engineering, SVCET, RVS Nagar, Chittoor 517127, AP, India

J. Nayak et al. (eds.), *Advanced Machine Learning Approaches in Cancer Prognosis*, Intelligent Systems Reference Library 204,
https://doi.org/10.1007/978-3-030-71975-3_14

having prostate cancer in Europe. More than 2 million men in Europe are currently living with prostate cancer. Prostate cancer is nothing but a malignant tumour present in the prostate. These tumour will grow very slowly and have no symptoms at the starting. The chance of prostate cancer mainly is at higherage. In most of the cases, urinating related issues can be the cause of Benign Prostatic Enlargement (BPE). BPE is nothing but a non-cancerous growth of the prostate. If prostate cancer causes any symptoms, then there is a high possibility that it is at critical stage. The symptoms at this level include: pain in the hips, back, chest, or rapid onset of local symptoms or legs from cancer which has spread to the bones and blood in the semen.

Around 95% among prostate cancers are of type adenocarcinomas. Approximately 4% prostate cancer cell grow this generally found in transitional epithelium of the urethra or from ducts. Primary carcinoid tumours of the sarcomas, prostate, and primary small cell carcinomas are rare kind of the prostate cancer. With the time, any other organ's tumour may spread into the prostate cancer. In many researches for prostate cancer classification, generally texture features are carried out for tissue pattern classification. Paper [3] shows how texture features are used to classify tissue patterns. The history of biological structure recognition for prostate cancer mainly depends on individual cells of the body. Prostate cancer tumor cells are different from other tumour cells. The study of immune histochemistry for the antigens helps to distinguish these different tumors. The Gleason grading system [4] is a multidisciplinary approach for prostate adenocarcinoma. This grading is to find Gleason patterns (3, 4, or 5) and classify cancer. At first the biopsy sample is considered as Gleason score, then this score is assigned into an ISUP grade of scale 1–5. Actually, this grading score is very important biomarkers used to measure the progress of a disease for prostate cancer; while ISUP grade is significant for making decision for treatment for a patient. Sometimes over grading can result to wrong diagnosis and unnecessary treatment. A segmentation-based approach is presented in paper [5] where automated detection and segmentation of prostate gland regions is found by utilizing low-level image features.

14.2 Dataset

The dataset used here is taken from Kaggle Prostate Cancer Grade Assessment [6] contributed by the Medical Centre of Radboud University. These images are labelled with several scanner's maximum microscope resolutions. For training and testing of model, 75 and 25% of data are used. In the training dataset, the severity of the cancer is on 0–5 scale. Approximately 1,000 images are taken as hidden test set. Different procedures are applied on the images of test data and the training data. On few images of training data, stray pen marks are used, while test dataset images are kept free of pen marks. Segmentation masks represents the ISUP grade of the image. Some training images may have false positives or may have false negatives in the label masks. These masks are actually essential for selecting the important subsamples from the images. These mask values generally depend on the data provider:

Table 14.1 Determination of isup_grade score based on Gleason-score

ISUP grade score	Gleason-score	Risk_group
0	0	Very low
1	<=6	Low
2	7 (3 + 4)	Intermediate favourable
3	7 (4 + 3)	Intermediate unfavourable
4	8	High
5	09-Oct	Very high

Radboud: Here, prostate glands are independently labelled having several values as below:

0: background (non-tissue) or unknown
1: stroma (connective tissue, non-epithelium tissue)
2: healthy (benign) epithelium
3: cancerous epithelium (Gleason 3)
4: cancerous epithelium (Gleason 4)
5: cancerous epithelium (Gleason 5).

The ISUP grade scores are classified into risk_group from very low to very high based on the gleason-score of the dataset shown in Table 14.1.

The characteristics and distributions of the dataset from two different sources are shown in Fig. 14.1. Figure 14.2 is showing that (i) Majority of data samples in train set have ISUP grade values 0 or 1 (total >50%). (ii) Rest of the data samples have associated ISUP grades from 2 to 5 with all ranging in the 11–12% each. Figure 14.3 shows that (i) From above graph, it is clear that Gleason score distribution is not uniform. (ii) Few Gleason score like (3 + 3) and (0 + 0) are more frequent while others like (3 + 5) and (5 + 3) are very rare in this dataset. Figure 14.4 shows that (i) All exams with ISUP grade = 0 have Gleason score 0 + 0 or negative. (ii) All exams

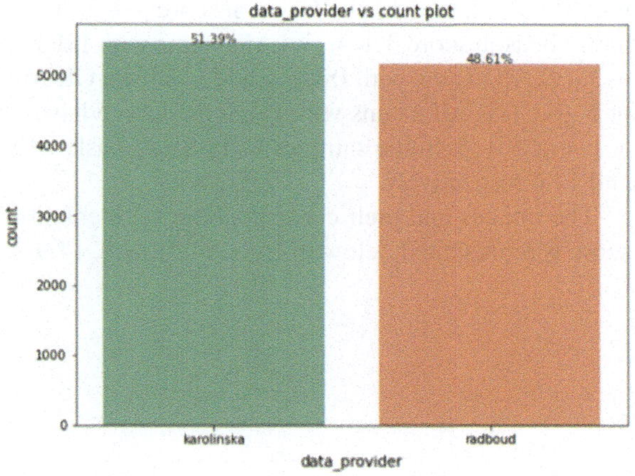

Fig. 14.1 Source distribution

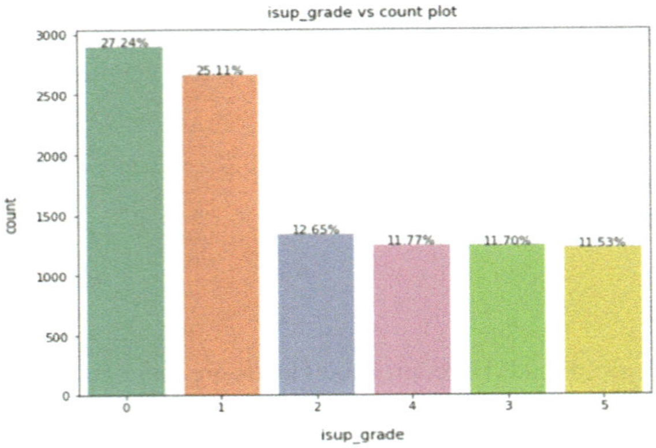

Fig. 14.2 ISUP grade distribution

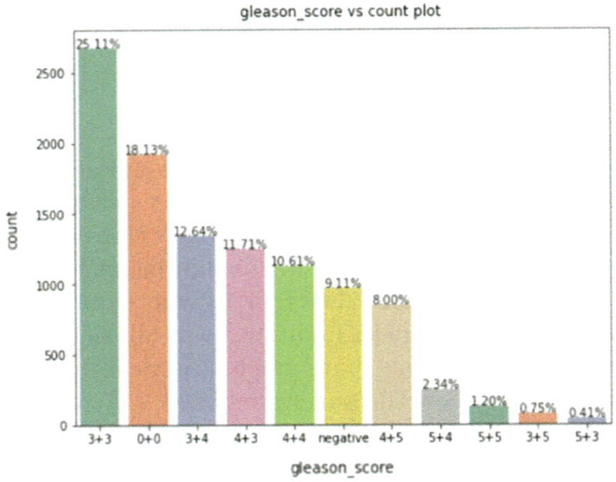

Fig. 14.3 Gleasonscore distribution

with ISUP grade = 1 have Gleason score 3 + 3. (iii) All exams with ISUP grade = 2 have Gleason score 3 + 4. (iv) All exams with ISUP grade = 3 have Gleason score 4 + 3. (v) All exams with ISUP grade = 4 have Gleason score 4 + 4 (majority), 3 + 5 or 5 + 3. (vi) All exams with ISUP grade = 5 have Gleason score 4 + 5 (majority), 5 + 4 or 5 + 5. Some samples and image-masks of images are shown in Figs. 14.5 and 14.6 respectively.

The images and their corresponding segmentation mask for various ISUP grade score is represented below in Figs. 14.7, 14.8, 14.9, 14.10, 14.11 and 14.12.

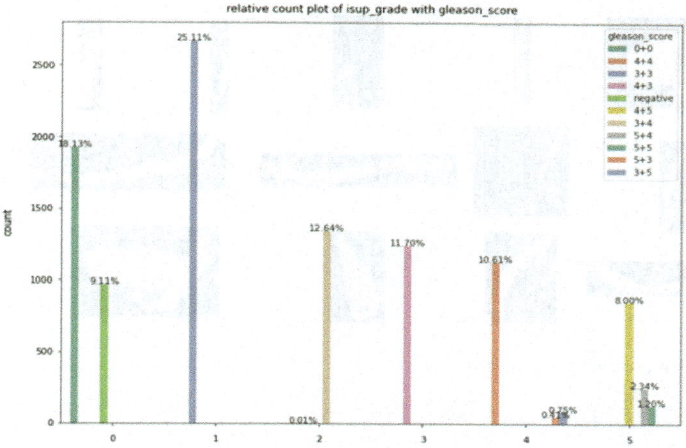

Fig. 14.4 Relative distribution

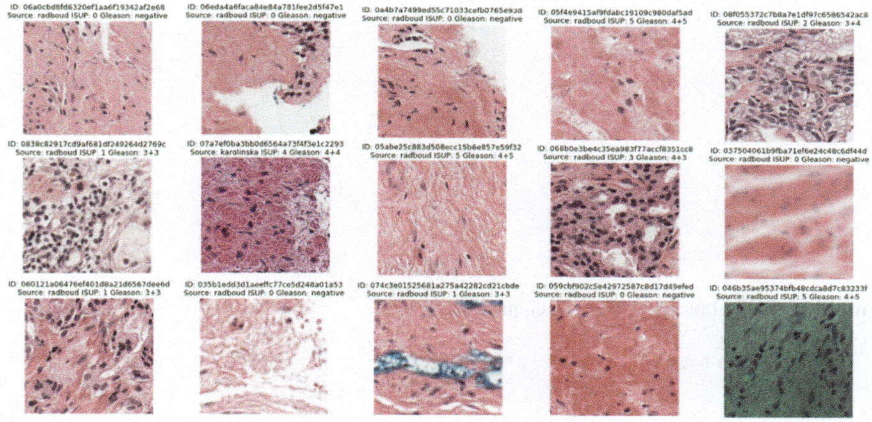

Fig. 14.5 Samples of images

14.3 Methodology

Several Deep Learning (DL) models like VGG16, EfficientNet, ResNeXT50 are used here to train the dataset.

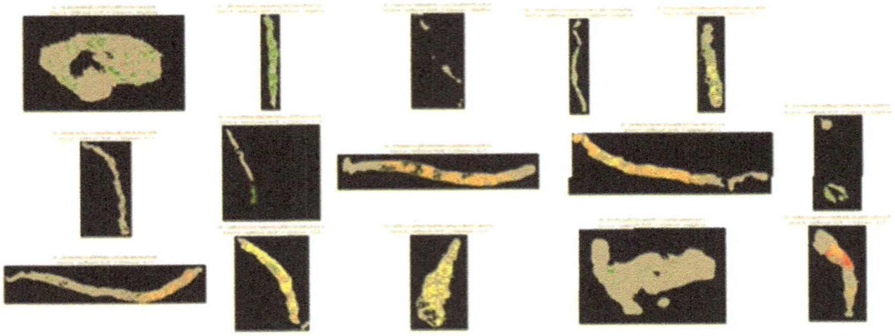

Fig. 14.6 Samples of image-masks

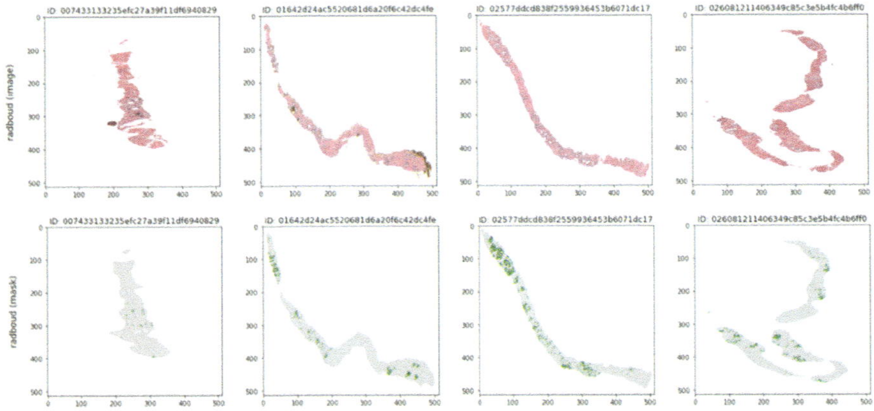

Fig. 14.7 ISUP grade score 0 for Radboud dataset

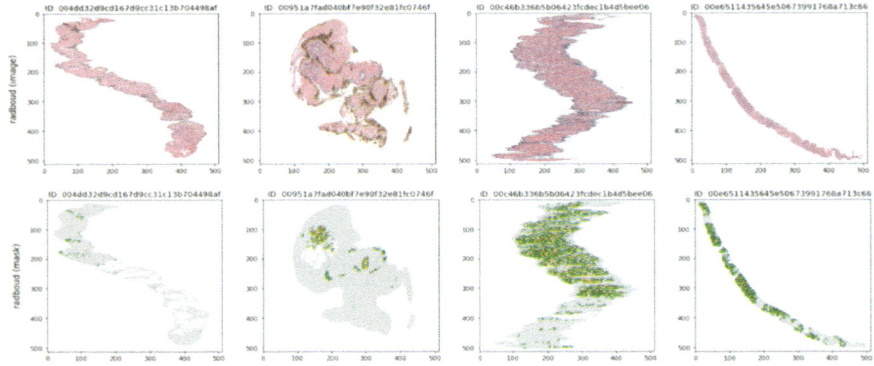

Fig. 14.8 ISUP grade score 1 for Radboud dataset

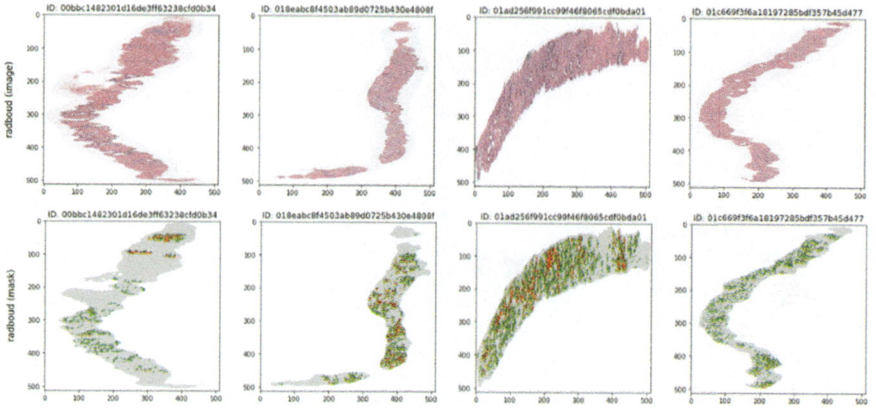

Fig. 14.9 ISUP grade score 2 for Radboud dataset

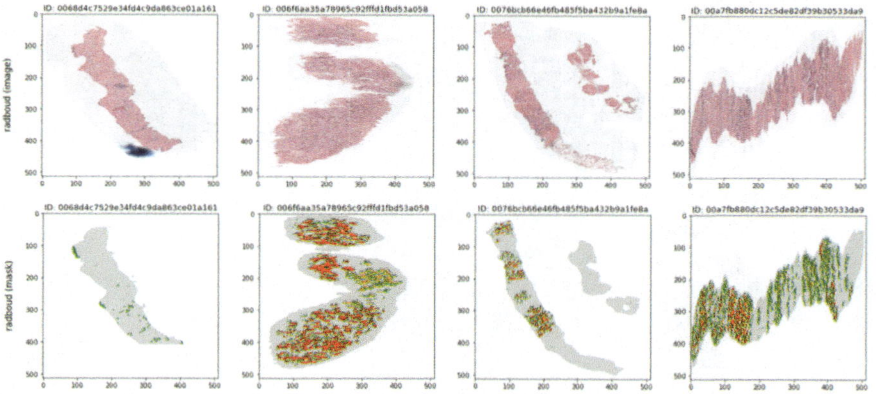

Fig. 14.10 ISUP grade score 3 for Radboud dataset

14.3.1 Data Pre-processing

To optimize the training process, the input images are pre-processed utilizing various pre-processing techniques [7]. The main reason for pre-processing the images is to enhance the visual quality of the input image by increasing contrast, by deleting low or high frequencies in the image and by reducing the noise from the original images. Image resizing and image normalization pre-processing techniques are used for enhancing the quality of image.

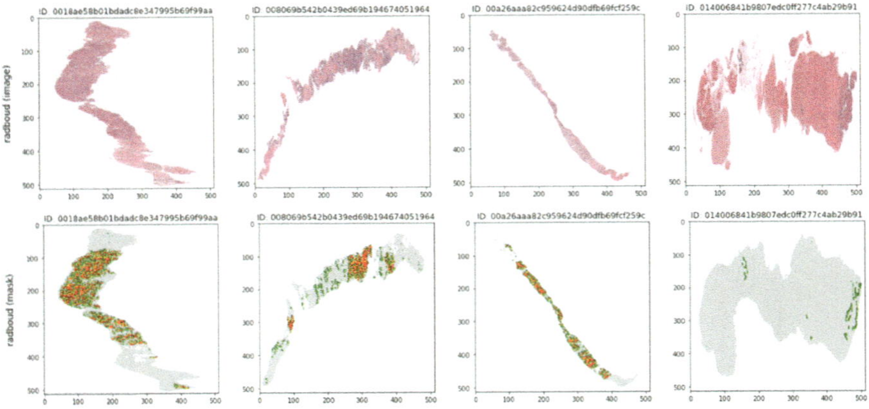

Fig. 14.11 ISUP grade score 4 for Radboud dataset

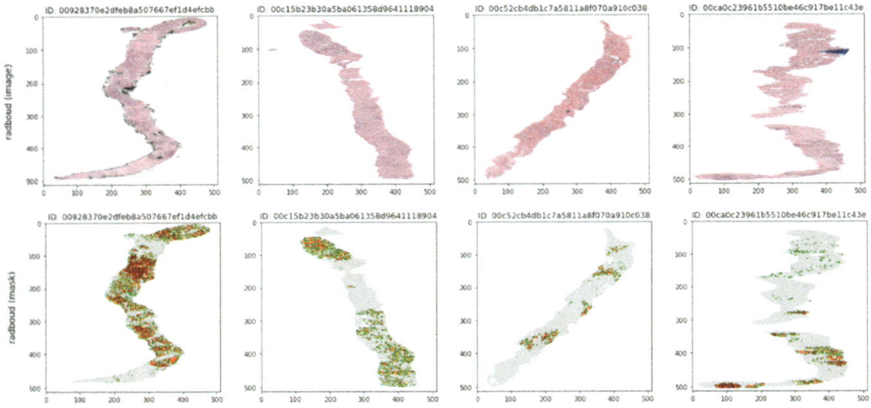

Fig. 14.12 ISUP grade score 5 for Radboud dataset

14.3.1.1 Image Resizing

The dimensions of the images used in this proposed method, are of different ranges. Therefore, to achieve fixed dimensions of all images, the original images are re-scaled to 224 × 224. Further, these images were re-scaled to size of 224 × 224 pixels to fit to the size of the input image in VGG16, EfficientNet, DenseNet121 and ResNeXt50 pretrained models.

14.3.1.2 Image Normalization

In this paper, intensity normalization as pre-processing technique is applied which is widely used in image processing applications. The intensity values (from 0 to 255) are normalized to a standard normal distribution [8] with the help of min-max normalization as shown in Eq. 14.1. As this technique removes bias and achieves uniform distribution, it assists in accelerating the convergence of the model.

$$x_{norm} = \frac{x - x_{min}}{x_{max} - x_{min}} \tag{14.1}$$

where, 'x' represents the pixel intensity and the x_{min} and x_{max} signifies the minimum and maximum intensity values of input images respectively. The objective of this function is to enhance the convergence of the model to get a uniform distribution throughout the dataset.

14.3.1.3 Data Augmentation

Data augmentation [9] is a technique to artificially expand the size of a training dataset by modifying the images in the dataset. Cropping, horizontal flipping and padding belong to the data augmentation. Deep learning neural network generates efficient results on more data. Augmentation techniques can improve the efficiency of deep learning neural network models. Data augmentation can significantly increase the diversity of data to train. This feature of augmentation helps the deep learning models to improve the performance on image recognition tasks.

14.3.2 Deep Learning (DL) Models

This section describes the working of deep learning models used in this study.

14.3.2.1 Vgg16 Architecture

The model VGG16 [10] belongs to convolutional neural network architecture. This network is carrying total 16 layers. Convolutional layers, Activation layers, Max Pooling layers and Fully connected layers are the part of this network. It is excelled to AlexNet network where filter size is increased in the first and second convolution layers having small filters of size 3×3. Therefore, VGG16 is the modified version of AlexNet. This network is too large with having 138 million parameters. For forward propagation only 96 MB memory is required for each image. The overall block diagram of VGG-16 architecture is mentioned in Fig. 14.13.

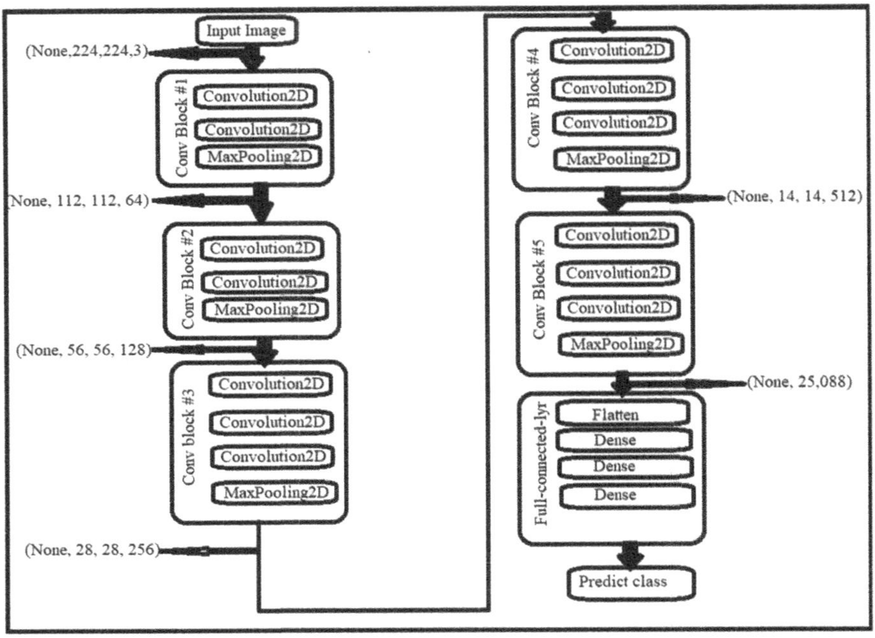

Fig. 14.13 Block diagram of VGG16

14.3.2.2 EfficientNet

Convolutional Neural Networks (CNN) has three scaling dimensions: depth, width and resolution. Number of CNN layers are depth, where, CNN each layer wide is width and number of channels are resolution. EfficientNet [11] is rethinking model scaling for CNN. Better accuracy can be achieved by simply scaling each of width/depth/resolution with constant ratio. The width, depth, and resolution of the network are uniformly scaled with fixed coefficients for scaling as shown in Eqs. 14.2–14.4

$$dept : d = \propto^{\phi} \tag{14.2}$$

$$width : w = \beta^{\phi} \tag{14.3}$$

$$resolution : r = \gamma^{\phi} \tag{14.4}$$

where, $\alpha \,.\, \beta^2 \,.\, \gamma^2 \approx 2$ and $\alpha \geq 1, \beta \geq 1, \gamma \geq 1$, ϕ is a coefficient that controls availability of resources and α, β, γ are assigned depth, width and resolution in the Eqs. 14.2–14.4 respectively.

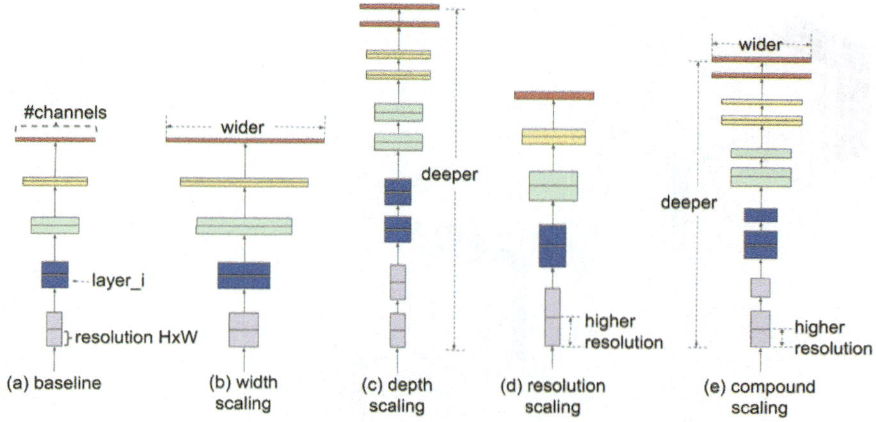

Fig. 14.14 EfficientNetincluding base, width, depth, resolution and compound scaling

Table 14.2 EfficientNet-B0 baseline network architecture

Stage	Operator	Resolution	Channels	Layers
1	Conv 3 × 3	224 × 224	32	1
2	MBConv1, K3 × 3	112 × 112	16	1
3	MBConv6, K3 × 3	112 × 112	24	2
4	MBConv6, K5 × 5	56 × 56	40	2
5	MBConv6, K3 × 3	28 × 28	80	3
6	MBConv6, K5 × 5	14 × 14	112	3
7	MBConv6, K5 × 5	14 × 14	192	4
8	MBConv6, K3 × 3	7 × 7	320	1
9	Conv 1 × 1 & Pooling & FC	7 × 7	1280	1

In Fig. 14.14, the diagram of EfficientNet is shown. Here, layer operation is not changed by scaling. It is a multi-objective search for Neural Architecture search (NAS) that optimizes not only accuracy but also floating-point operations (FLOPS). Its architecture is same as of M-NASNET. The network blocks/layers are as shows below in Table 14.2.

14.3.2.3 DenseNet

Dense Convolutional Network (DenseNet) [12] works substantially deeper and more accurate. Here, each layer is connected to each of other layer through feed-forward way as shown in Fig. 14.15.

In traditional feed-forward neural networks, the output of one layer is connected to the next layer with applying some composite functions. The multiple inputs of

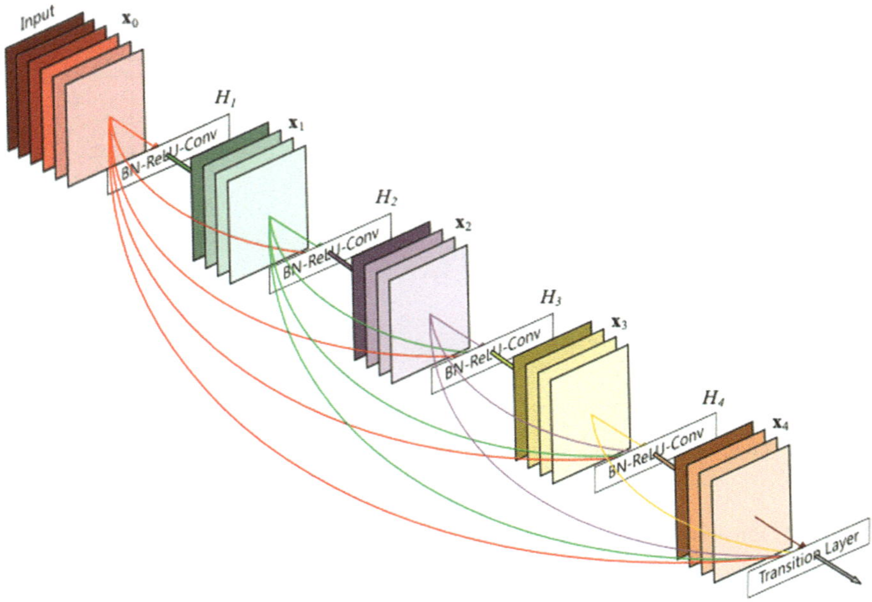

Fig. 14.15 Block diagram of DenseNet

$H\ell(\cdot)$ is concatenated into a single tensor as mentioned in Eq. 14.5.

$$x_l = H_l(x_0, x_1, \ldots, x_{l-1}) \tag{14.5}$$

where, $x_0, x_1, \ldots, x_{l-1}$ represents the series of the feature-maps which are generated in layers 0, . . ., $\ell-1$. The network blocks/layers are as shows below in Fig. 14.16.

14.3.2.4 ResNeXt50

ResNeXt-50 is a highly modularized network architecture for image classification. It is advanced versions of ResNet model [13] with increase in convolution layer, MaxPool and average pool layer. 3.8 × 10^9 Floating points operations are carried out here. All parameters of this network are mentioned in Table 14.3. The block diagram of ResNeXt-50 is mentioned in Fig. 14.17.

In artificial neural network, weighted sum is measured by fully-connected and convolutional layers. It is nothing but the form of aggregating transformation shown in Eq. 14.6.

$$\sum_{i=1}^{D} w_i x_i \tag{14.6}$$

Layers	Output Size	DenseNet-121	DenseNet-169	DenseNet-201	DenseNet-264
Convolution	112 × 112	7 × 7 conv, stride 2			
Pooling	56 × 56	3 × 3 max pool, stride 2			
Dense Block (1)	56 × 56	$\begin{bmatrix}1\times1 \text{ conv}\\3\times3 \text{ conv}\end{bmatrix}\times 6$	$\begin{bmatrix}1\times1 \text{ conv}\\3\times3 \text{ conv}\end{bmatrix}\times 6$	$\begin{bmatrix}1\times1 \text{ conv}\\3\times3 \text{ conv}\end{bmatrix}\times 6$	$\begin{bmatrix}1\times1 \text{ conv}\\3\times3 \text{ conv}\end{bmatrix}\times 6$
Transition Layer (1)	56 × 56	1 × 1 conv			
	28 × 28	2 × 2 average pool, stride 2			
Dense Block (2)	28 × 28	$\begin{bmatrix}1\times1 \text{ conv}\\3\times3 \text{ conv}\end{bmatrix}\times 12$	$\begin{bmatrix}1\times1 \text{ conv}\\3\times3 \text{ conv}\end{bmatrix}\times 12$	$\begin{bmatrix}1\times1 \text{ conv}\\3\times3 \text{ conv}\end{bmatrix}\times 12$	$\begin{bmatrix}1\times1 \text{ conv}\\3\times3 \text{ conv}\end{bmatrix}\times 12$
Transition Layer (2)	28 × 28	1 × 1 conv			
	14 × 14	2 × 2 average pool, stride 2			
Dense Block (3)	14 × 14	$\begin{bmatrix}1\times1 \text{ conv}\\3\times3 \text{ conv}\end{bmatrix}\times 24$	$\begin{bmatrix}1\times1 \text{ conv}\\3\times3 \text{ conv}\end{bmatrix}\times 32$	$\begin{bmatrix}1\times1 \text{ conv}\\3\times3 \text{ conv}\end{bmatrix}\times 48$	$\begin{bmatrix}1\times1 \text{ conv}\\3\times3 \text{ conv}\end{bmatrix}\times 64$
Transition Layer (3)	14 × 14	1 × 1 conv			
	7 × 7	2 × 2 average pool, stride 2			
Dense Block (4)	7 × 7	$\begin{bmatrix}1\times1 \text{ conv}\\3\times3 \text{ conv}\end{bmatrix}\times 16$	$\begin{bmatrix}1\times1 \text{ conv}\\3\times3 \text{ conv}\end{bmatrix}\times 32$	$\begin{bmatrix}1\times1 \text{ conv}\\3\times3 \text{ conv}\end{bmatrix}\times 32$	$\begin{bmatrix}1\times1 \text{ conv}\\3\times3 \text{ conv}\end{bmatrix}\times 48$
Classification Layer	1 × 1	7 × 7 global average pool			
		1000D fully-connected, softmax			

Fig. 14.16 Network layers of DenseNet architecture

Table 14.3 ResNeXt-50(32 × 4d) architecture

Stage	Output	ResNeXt-50 (32 × 4d)
Conv1	112 × 112	7 × 7, 64, stride 2
Pool1		3 × 3 max pool, stride2
Conv2	56 × 56	[(1 × 1, 128), (3 × 3, 128, C = 32), (1 × 1, 256)] × 3
Conv3	28 × 28	[(1 × 1, 256), (3 × 3, 256, C = 32), (1 × 1, 512)] × 4
Conv4	14 × 14	[(1 × 1, 512), (3 × 3, 512, C = 32), (1 × 1, 1024)] × 6
Conv5	7 × 7	[(1 × 1, 1024), (3 × 3, 1024, C = 32), (1 × 1, 2048)] × 3
Pool2		Global avg pool 100-d fc, sofmax
# params		25.0 × 10^6
FLOPS		4.2 × 10^9

where, $x = [x_1, x_2, \ldots, x_D]$ is input vector of neurons in D channel and w_i represents filter weights of ith channel. The transformations are aggregated by $\sum_{i=1}^{D} w_i x_i$ are mentioned in Eqs. 14.7 and 14.8.

$$\mathcal{F}(x) = \sum_{i}^{C} \tau_i(x) \tag{14.7}$$

$$y = x + \sum_{i}^{C} \tau_i(x) \tag{14.8}$$

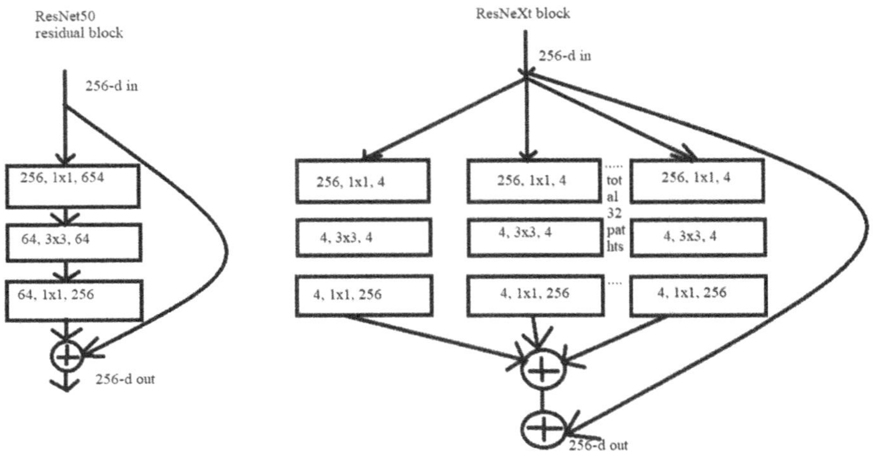

Fig. 14.17 Building blocks of ResNeXt-50

where, $\tau_i(x)$ is an arbitrary function. C is the size of the set of transformations to be aggregated.

14.3.3 Evaluation Metrics

This section describes the evaluation metrics used in evaluating the performance of the model.

14.3.3.1 Statistical Analysis

Classification accuracy represents the total number of correct predictions divided by the total number of predictions made for a dataset. For the performance measurement, accuracy is important term for classification problems. Recall, Precision, F-score, Specificity, Confusion Matrix, Mean and Standard Deviation are the base case levels for the statistical analysis. Confusion Matrix is a performance measurement for machine learning classification problem where output can be two or more classes. Confusion matrix is based on counts from predicted and actual values. For the proposed method, confusion matrix is generated as shown in result section. The calculation equations of Recall, Fall_out, Specificity and F1-score are mentioned in Eqs. 14.9–14.12 respectively.

$$Recall = \frac{TP}{P} = \frac{TP}{TP + FN} \tag{14.9}$$

$$Fall\_out = \frac{FP}{N} = \frac{FP}{FP + TN} \tag{14.10}$$

$$Specificity = \frac{TN}{N} = \frac{TN}{FP + TN} = 1 - Fall\_out \tag{14.11}$$

$$F1\_score = \frac{2 \times TP}{2 \times TP + FP + FN} \tag{14.12}$$

where, *TP* = True Positive, *FP* = False Positive, *TN* = True Negative, *FN* = False Negative of data set.

14.3.3.2 Quadratic Weighted Kappa (QWK) Score

The Quadratic Weighted Kappa (QWK) [14] is a popular metric for classification tasks where the classes are hierarchical. The metric usually ranges from 0 (random agreement) to 1 for complete agreement. The QWF is calculated as shown below.

At first, a histogram matrix *O* of size *N* x *N* is generated, where, O_{ij} represents the number of its ISUP grade score where *i* is actual value and *j* is a value which is predicted. *w* is a weighted matrix of size $N \times N$. It generates differences between actual and predicted values mentioned in Eq. 14.13.

$$w_{i,j} = \frac{(i - j)^2}{(N - 1)^2} \tag{14.13}$$

E, a *N* x *N* histogram matrix is the outer product generated from the actual histogram vector of outcomes and the predicted histogram vector. The normalization is done in such a way that *E* and *O* have the same sum value. Finally, taking the value of O_{ij}, *w* and *E*, the quadratic weighted kappa is evaluated as in Eq. 14.14.

$$k = \frac{\sum_{i.j} w_{i,j} O_{i,j}}{\sum_{i.j} w_{i,j} E_{i,j}} \tag{14.14}$$

14.4 Results and Discussions

The evaluation of Deep Learning (DL) models is done by Quadratic Weighted Kappa (QWK) score. Table 14.4 depicts the QWK scores for various DL models. Among all these methods, EfficientNet model is showing the highest QWK score as 0.913.

A confusion matrix based on Radboud dataset [6] is generated using Eqs. 14.9–14.12 respectively which is shown in Table 14.5. In VGG16 net, for 0 category, the

Table 14.4 Evaluation of DL models based on QWK score

Model name	QWK score
VGG16	0.631
EfficientNet	0.913
DenseNet121	0.712
resNext50	0.795

Table 14.5 Confusion matrix of several Deep Learning (DL) models

Serial no	Model name	Category	0	1	2	3	4	5
1	VGG16	0	181	250	16	57	15	67
		1	155	244	17	44	19	54
		2	90	96	8	27	15	28
		3	64	114	10	25	12	17
		4	77	108	8	25	8	35
		5	65	102	11	27	8	25
2	EfficientNet	0	304	82	21	9	21	13
		1	162	119	35	9	31	27
		2	101	42	28	3	20	24
		3	77	31	16	23	13	34
		4	83	29	8	4	33	28
		5	73	15	4	4	9	65
3	DenseNet121	0	161	192	1	94	0	2
		1	84	259	1	39	0	0
		2	34	146	6	32	0	0
		3	14	103	0	67	0	10
		4	26	86	1	68	0	4
			15	74	0	48	0	33
4	ResNeXt50	0	2000	697	123	40	23	9
		1	527	1605	428	69	31	6
		2	76	525	515	105	102	20
		3	24	158	273	223	370	194
		4	34	125	152	136	356	446
		5	22	50	76	70	270	736

number of correctly classified samples are 181 and 250, 16, 57, 15, 67 are the incorrectly classified samples for category 1, 2, 3, 4 and 5 respectively. Similarly, for other categories of VGG16 net, the all correctly classified and incorrectly classified sample numbers are mentioned in this table. In this way, confusion matrix for EfficientNet, DenseNet121 and ResNeXt50 is represented in Table 14.5.

In Table 14.6, precision, recall, f1-score and support values for VGG16, EfficientNet, DenseNet121 and ResNeXt50 are represented.

Figure 14.18 shows the heat map for confusion matrix of VGG16, EfficientNet, DenseNet121 and ResNeXt50.

Table 14.6 Classification Report of DL models showing their precision, recall, f1-score, support

Serial no	Model name	Category	Precision	Recall	F1-score
1	VGG16	0	0.29	0.31	0.30
		1	0.27	0.46	0.34
		2	0.11	0.03	0.05
		3	0.12	0.10	0.11
		4	0.10	0.03	0.05
		5	0.11	0.11	0.11
		Macro avg	0.17	0.17	0.16
		Weighted avg	0.20	0.23	0.20
2	EfficientNet	0	0.38	0.68	0.49
		1	0.37	0.31	0.34
		2	0.25	0.13	0.17
		3	0.44	0.12	0.19
		4	0.26	0.18	0.21
		5	0.34	0.38	0.36
		Macro avg	0.34	0.30	0.29
		Weighted avg	0.35	0.36	0.33
3	DenseNet121	0	0.48	0.36	0.41
		1	0.30	0.68	0.42
		2	0.67	0.03	0.05
		3	0.19	0.35	0.25
		4	0.00	0.00	0.00
		5	0.67	0.19	0.30
		Macro avg	0.39	0.27	0.24
		Weighted avg	0.39	0.33	0.28
4	ResNeXt50	0	0.75	0.69	0.72
		1	0.51	0.60	0.55
		2	0.33	0.38	0.35
		3	0.35	0.18	0.24
		4	0.31	0.29	0.30
		5	0.52	0.60	0.56
		Macro avg	0.46	0.46	0.45
		Weighted avg	0.51	0.51	0.51

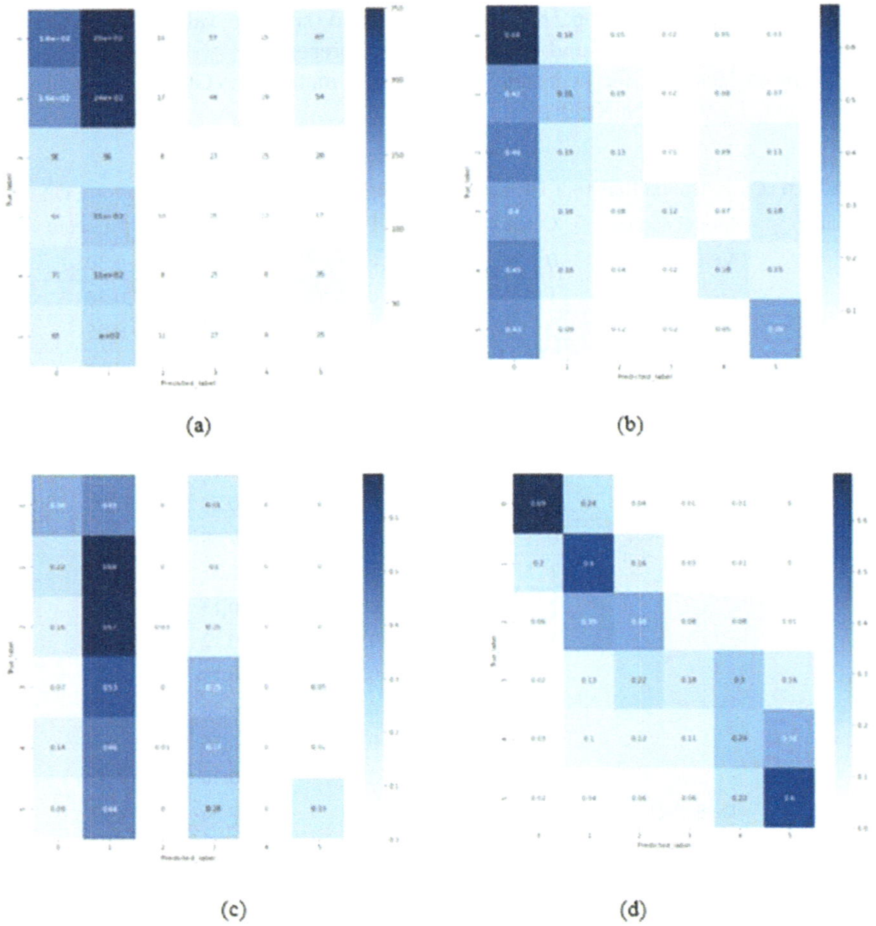

Fig. 14.18 Heat map of confusion matrix for **a** VGG16 **b** EfficientNet **c** Densenet121 **d** ResNeXt50

Here Table 14.7 shows the comparative result among several methods. Among all other methods, the proposed method is having always above the 93% accuracy value which proves the efficiency of the proposed method.

Table 14.7 Comparative study among several methods with proposed method

Method	Approach used	Merits	Performance metrics (%)
CNN	Image classification	High accuracy, best classification	Accuracy: 86.3
SVM	Image classification	Good classification accuracy	Accuracy: 87
KNN	Image classification	Good classification accuracy	Accuracy: 76
Proposed method	VGG16, EfficientNet, Resnext 50, Dense Net 12 based convolution with deep network	Very High classification best detection	Accuracy: 93.28

14.5 Conclusion

In maximum cases, it is observed that conventional methods for the analysis of cancer samples to the normal samples is usually not significant. This paper shows the efficient results using Deep Learning (DL) approaches for prostate cancer data classification. The score of Quadratic Weighted Kappa (QWK) signifies the EfficientNet as the best net for classification of the cancer data among other DL nets. As per result of confusion matrix based on precision, recall, f1-score, support, ResNeXt50 net shows best accuracy results in comparative to other models.

References

1. Ferlay, J., et al.: Cancer incidence and mortality patterns in Europe: estimates for 40 countries. Eur. J. Cancer 49, **201**, 1374–403 (2012)
2. U.S. Cancer Statistics Working Group, United States Cancer Statistics: 1999–2005 Incidence and Mortality Web-based Report, Atlanta: U.S. Department of Health and Human Services, Centers for Disease Control and Prevention and National Cancer Institute (2009). www.cdc.gov/uscs. Accessed 5 May 2020
3. Diamond, J., Anderson, N., Bartels, P., Montironi, R., Hamilton, P.: The use of morphological characteristics and texture analysis in the identification of tissue composition in prostatic neoplasia. Hum. Pathol. **35**, 1121–1131 (2004)
4. Suhail, Z., Mahmood, A., Wang, L., Malcolm, P.N., Zwiggelaar, R.: A voting-based encoding technique for the classification of gleason score for prostate cancers. In: Nixon, M., Mahmoodi, S., Zwiggelaar, R. (eds.), Medical Image Understanding and Analysis. MIUA 2018. Communications in Computer and Information Science, vol. 894. Springer, Cham (2018). https://doi.org/10.1007/978-3-319-95921-4_9
5. Naik, S., Doyle, S., Madabhushi, A.: Gland segmentation and computerized gleason grading of prostate histology by integrating low-high-level and domain specific information, MIAAB Workshop (2007)
6. https://www.kaggle.com/c/prostate-cancer-grade-assessment/data. Accessed 10 May 2020
7. Sonka, M., Hlavac, V., Boyle, R.: Image pre-processing. In: Image Processing, Analysis and Machine Vision. Springer, Boston, MA (1993). https://doi.org/10.1007/978-1-4899-3216-7_4

8. Lemaitre, G., Mojdeh, R., Joan, M, Joan, V., Paul, W. et al.: Normalization of T2W-MRI Prostate Images using Rician a priori. SPIE Medical Imaging, Feb 2016, San Diego, United States. ffhal-01265774f
9. Zhu, Q., Du, B., Turkbey, B., Choyke, P.L., Yan, P.: Deeply-supervised CNN for prostate segmentation. In: Proceedings of the 2017 International Joint Conference on Neural Networks (IJCNN), San Francisco, CA, USA, 4–9 Feb 2017, pp. 178–184 (2017)
10. Guan, Q., Wang, Y., Ping, B., Li, D., Du, J., Qin, Y., Lu, H., Wan, X., Xiang, J.: Deep convolutional neural network VGG-16 model for differential diagnosing of papillary thyroid carcinomas in cytological images: a pilot study. J. Cancer **10**(20), 4876–4882 (2019). https://doi.org/10.7150/jca.28769
11. Mingxing, T, Quoc, V.L: EfficientNet: rethinking model scaling for convolutional neural networks. In: Proceedings of the 36 th International Conference on Machine Learning, Long Beach, California, PMLR 97, (2019)
12. Huang, G., Liu, Z, Maaten, L., Weinberger, K.: Densely connected convolutional networks. In: IEEE conference Computer Vision and Pattern Recognition (CVPR), pp. 4700–4708 (2017)
13. He, K., Zhang, X., Ren, S., Sun, J.: Deep residual learning for image recognition. In: Computer Vision and Pattern Recognition (CVPR), pp. 770–778 (2016)
14. Brenner, H., Kliebsch, U.: Dependence of weighted kappa coefficients on the number of categories. Epidemiology **7**(2), 199–202 (1996). https://doi.org/10.1097/00001648-199603000-00016

Chapter 15
A Deep Learning Prediction Model for Detection of Cancerous Lesions from Dermatoscopic Images

Ankita Pramanik and Rivu Chakraborty

Abstract Skin cancer is a major issue regarding public health and mostly affects the Caucasians every year. It is the leading form of cancer affecting the people of USA. The mortality rate of skin cancer can be reduced to 2% if detected early. Dermatoscopy is a very popular tool in the diagnosis of benign as well as cancerous pigmented skin lesions. Dermatoscopy images are also suitable for automated diagnosis of pigmented skin lesions using deep learning techniques. This espouses the need of building an easily accessible, portable, faster and cheaper diagnostic system. The existing works mainly use pretrained network and huge processing resource. In this work, a 16-layer deep convolutional neural network is developed from the scratch. The network consists of 9 convolutional layers, 4 maxpool layers and 3 fully connected layers. The validation of the proposed architecture is done on the dermatoscopic images of the Kaggle dataset archive without augmentation. The proposed work offers an accuracy value of 87.58% which is much better than the existing works on the Kaggle dataset without augmentation. skin cancer, Dermatoscopic Images, convolutional neural network, Kaggle.

Keywords Skin cancer · Dermatoscopic images · Convolutional neural network · Kaggle

15.1 Introduction

The cells in the body are expected to divide in an orderly fashion to give rise to new cells. However, when the cells grow abnormally they give rise to cancer. The cancerous cells gives rise to new cancerous cells and throttle the normal cells, thus spreading the disease [1]. The cancer can spread from the region of origin to other

A. Pramanik (✉) · R. Chakraborty
Indian Institute of Engineering Science and Technology, Shibpur, Howrah, India
e-mail: ankita@telecom.iiests.ac.in

R. Chakraborty
e-mail: rivuchakraborty17@gmail.com

J. Nayak et al. (eds.), *Advanced Machine Learning Approaches in Cancer Prognosis*,
Intelligent Systems Reference Library 204,
https://doi.org/10.1007/978-3-030-71975-3_15

organs. This is called metastasis [2]. In the case of metastasis, the cancer though has spread to other organs will still bear the name of the organ it originated from. For example, the cancer that originated in the liver will be called liver cancer. If the cancerous cells from the liver spread to pancreas, the cancer in the pancreas will have the characteristics of liver cancer and will be called liver cancer. In other words, the characteristics of the cancer that has spread to the pancreas from other organs is markedly different from pancreas cancer and so the cancer that originated in the pancreas will be the only one to be called pancreas cancer. The most common cancer types are [3] the cancers originating in bladder, breast, colon and rectal region, endometrial lining, kidney, liver, lung, pancreas, prost ate, skin and thyroid gland. Apart from these, Leukemia and Non-Hodgkin Lymphoma are also widely occurring cancer types.

Skin cancer is a common cancer affecting people globally. It is the most commonly occurring form of cancer in the USA where 5 million plus cases are diagnosed every year [4]. The situation is so grim in USA that 20% of the American population is feared to be affected by skin cancer by the time they reach the age 70 [5]. Globally too the figure of non melanoma skin cancer is very grim with a fatality rate more than 5,400 people per month [6]. The fatality can be reduced if detected in the earlier stages. The 5-year survival rate for melanoma is 99% if detected at an early stage of the cancer [4].

The various types of skin cancers are shown in Fig. 15.1 [7]. Skin cancers are classified into the following two broad categories:

- Melanoma and
- Non melanoma.

Non melanoma is further classified into:

- basal cell carcinoma (BCC) and
- squamous cell carcinoma (SCC).

Apart from these two, few rarely occurring cancerous forms, namely skin adnexal tumors, Kaposi sarcoma, cutaneous (skin) lymphomas, and sarcomas, also fall under the category of non-melanoma skin cancers. Melanoma and non melanoma skin cancers are shown in Fig. 15.2.

The appearance and severity of the three types of cancer are summarised in Table 15.1.

The non-melanoma type of skin cancer is the more prevalent variety. If treated early, this cancer is unlikely to spread to other regions of the body. However, the malignant variety of melanoma spreads rapidly to other body parts and turns fatal in the event of lack of early treatment. Some not so common varieties of skin cancer are dermato fibro sarcoma protruberans and Merkel cell tumors. The later type of cancer is a very aggressive cancer usually affecting hormone-producing cells lying under skin and in follicles of hair. It is usually found in the neck and head region. It is also known as neuroendocrine carcinoma of the skin. The possible reasons of getting affected from skin cancer are as follows:

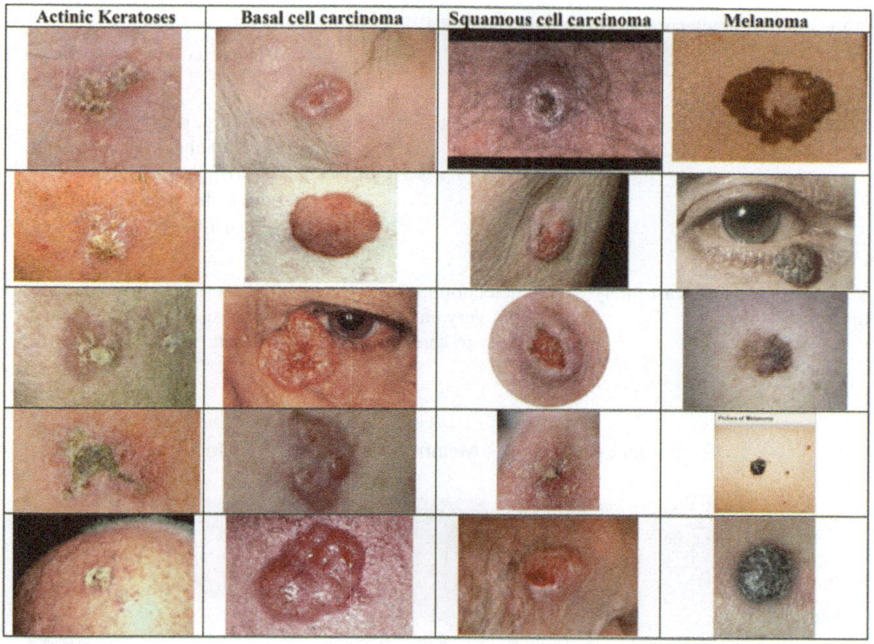

Fig. 15.1 Types of skin cancer [7]

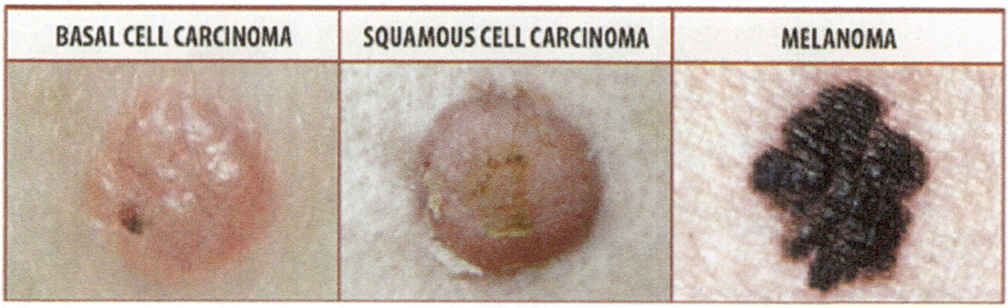

Fig. 15.2 Types of skin cancer

- Over exposure to ultraviolet light
- Tanning booths
- Immunosuppression
- Exposure to radiation
- Exposure to carcinogens.

Skin cancers are malignant skin lesions. Not all lesions are cancerous. Figure 15.3 gives a pictorial representation of all the different varieties of skin lesions. Malignant skin lesions are classified into stages 0 to 4 based on the level of the spread of the cancer. The lower the number of the cancer stage, lesser the spread of cancer in the

Table 15.1 Characteristics of typical skin cancers

BCC	SCC	Melanoma
Appearance		
Pearly/ waxy bump or flat brown lesion	Firm red pimple/ nodule or scaly patch	Bleeding, itching or colour/ shape changes of an already occurring mole; large brownish patch; smaller spot with white/ red/ black speckles
Severity		
Very easily treated; least likely to spread	Early detection makes treatment very easy; probability to spread more than BCC	Most serious form; late diagnosis makes treatment difficult; spreads very rapidly

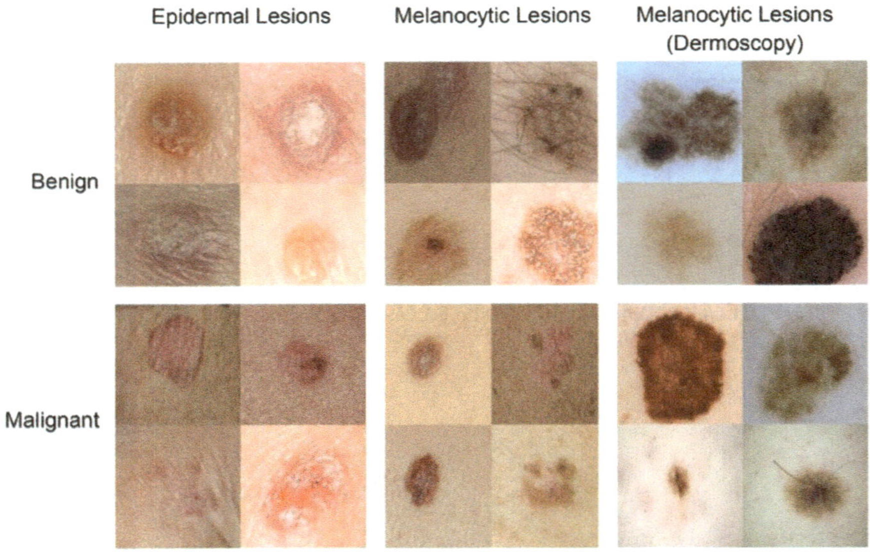

Fig. 15.3 Types of skin lesions

body. Stage 0 indicates that abnormal cells have been formed. However the cells have not metastasized. The cancer is in most advanced form in stage 4 where it has spread to other regions of the body. The lower the stage of the cancer, the better is the chance of survival. A plot of survival probability to the survival years is given in Fig. 15.4 [8].

The survival probability of stage 0 cancer patients are fairly high, approximately 100% hence not much detailed study of the survival probability of overall skin cancer patients in stage 0 has been undertaken. So, the Fig. 15.4 does not give the survival probability of such patients. However, detailed study into the various stages

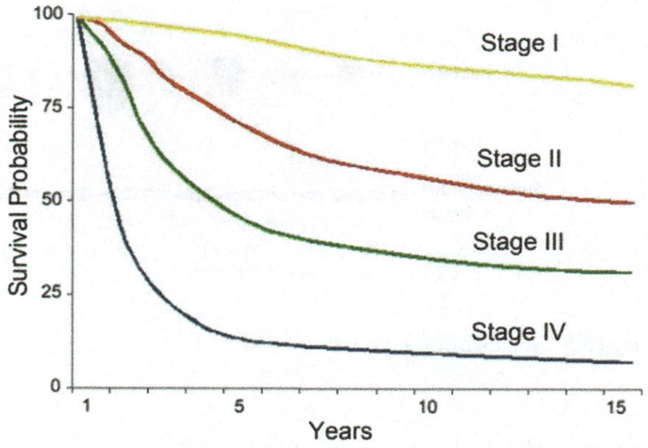

Fig. 15.4 Survival years versus survival probability

Table 15.2 5-year survival probability of melanoma

Stage	Probability (%)
0	99.9
1/2	89–95
2	45–79
3	24–70
4	7–19

Table 15.3 Stages of skin non Melanoma

Stage	Size of tumor
0	Upper layer of skin
1	≤ 2 cm
2	Between 2 and 4 cm
3	More than 4 cm
4	Any size

of melanoma right from Stage 0 has been done. The work in [9] gives 5-year survival probability of melanoma based on stage and is reproduced below in Table 15.2.

The stages of the spread of non melanoma cancer are given in the following Table 15.3, [10]. The stages of spread of melanoma cancer are not as straight forward as in Table 15.3. It depends on the size of the skin lesion, stage of ulceration (break of skin) and the spread area. In stage 0, the melanoma affects the outermost skin layer and does not affect the nearby regions. In stage 4, the cancer spreads to organs like bone, brain, lungs, etc. The changes in the various stages of melanoma are shown in Fig. 15.5. The stages are further broken down into substages. The various substages of melanoma are as follows:

- **Stage 0**: in outermost layer of skin
- **Stage 1A**: <1 mm tumor, may or may not be ulcerated

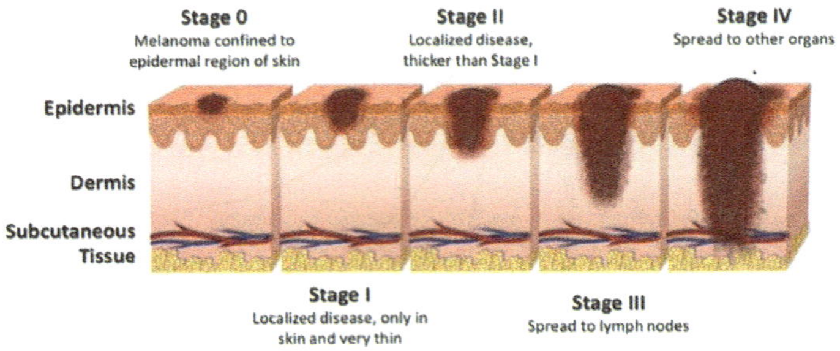

Fig. 15.5 Stages of Melanoma

- **Stage 1B**: 1–2 mm tumor, no ulceration
- **Stage 2A**: 1–2 mm if ulcerated, or 2–4 mm if not ulcerated.
- **Stage 2B**: 2–4 mm tumor if ulcerated, >4 mm if not ulcerated
- **Stage 2C**: >4 mm and ulcerated
- **Stage 3A**: <1 mm if ulcerated, or 1–2 mm if not ulcerated. Cancer develops in 1–3 sentinel lymph nodes.
- **Stage 3B**: ≤2 mm if ulcerated, or 2–4 mm if no ulceration, plus cancer in one of 1–3 lymph nodes or microsatellite tumors very close to primary tumor or satellite tumors ≤2 cm of primary tumor or in-transit metastases
- **Stage 3C**: ≤4 mm if ulcerated, or >4 mm if no ulceration, plus cancer in one 2–3 lymph nodes, ≥1 nodes, plus microsatellite tumors, satellite tumors, or in-transit metastases or ≥4 nodes or any number of fused nodes
- **Stage 3D**: ≥4 mm and ulcerated and cancer in any of these ≥4 lymph nodes or numerous fused nodes or ≥2 nodes or multiple fused nodes, plus microsatellite tumors, satellite tumors, or in-transit metastases
- **Stage 4**: has spread to far away body parts.

Surgery, immunotherapy, cryotherapy, radiation therapy, photodynamic therapy, chemotherapy etc. are certain varieties of treatment of skin cancer. The treatment type depends on the type and spread of the cancer. The treatment is started immediately after the diagnosis. The diagnosis is made by trained health experts by identifying the skin changes. The health expert usually after visual diagnosis prescribes further tests to confirm the findings. Skin biopsy is the most common diagnostic procedure for cancer. The procedure is painful as the suspicious skin needs to be removed for testing. Imaging or removal of lymph cells for detailed diagnosis are also popular. Use of dermascopy can improve the diagnostic accuracy by 30% [11] as compared to the naked eye. For general practitioners the accuracy of correct diagnosis is 62–63% [12]. Thus it is evident that the accuracy of diagnosis of skin cancer is very much dependant on human judgement. So it can be safely concluded that missing a fine detail from the skin lesion can prove fatal for the patient. Thus to remove such uncertainties, artificial intelligence (AI) is being used for skin cancer detection in recent times. The distinct boundaries and color of the lesions gives AI the best edge to detect skin cancer features. AI has been used to detect skin cancer from Raman spectra [13].

Preprocessing to remove the shortcomings of image acquisition and artifacts like hair removal is done in the first step of medical image diagnosis. However some databases offer clean images so this step can be skipped. As the field of medical diagnosis using image processing is quite mature, there are numerous works on skin cancer detection by image processing. Some works like [14, 15] have used genetic algorithm for classification. But the later works using CNN have shown improved results. The work in [16] uses support vector machine (SVM) for skin cancer detection. Apart from SVM, transform techniques have also been used for feature extraction [17, 18]. The later works use a combination of SVM and convolutional neural network (CNN) for the task [19]. For feature extraction, gray level co-occurrence matrix (GLCM) has also been used [14, 20]. Few works like have used the pretrained networks, namely AlexNet [14, 21, 22], ResNet [21, 22], VGGNet19 [21, 22] etc. for the task of skin cancer classification. The main problem of using a pretrained network is that the network size is huge and it is difficult to fine tune the parameters. So to mitigate these problems, the present work develops a CNN model to classify benign and malignant skin lesions, from scratch. The model has just 16 layers and can be tuned as the need be.

The main contributions of this study can be summarized below:

- understanding skin cancer
- Understanding deep learning (DL) in image processing
- Propose a novel 16-layer deep CNN model to extract skin cancer fetures
- Perform binary classification to detect if the skin lesion is cancerous or non cancerous.

The rest of the paper is organized as follows: Sect. 15.2 discusses briefly the various existing works on skin caner detection. The survey is not restricted to the works using CNN only. Thus it gives a good flavour of the state of the art in skin cancer detection through image processing. Section 15.3 of this chapter presents a brief introduction to the various tools and techniques used in this work. A brief introduction to CNN and the other tools commonly used in DL like Adam optimizer, categorical cross entropy and softmax is also discussed in the section. The various dataset available for skin images are discussed briefly in Sect. 15.4. The dataset used in this particular work is also discussed in this section. The proposed methodology is discussed in Sect. 15.5. The overall methodology, the proposed network architecture and the various parameters are discussed in this section. The obtained results, analysis and comparison with existing works are given in Sect. 15.6. Finally the paper is concluded in Sect. 15.7 with a discussion on the results obtained, limitations and possible scope of future works.

15.2 Literature Study

In this section, the existing works on skin cancer detection using AI is discussed briefly.

In the work [22], comparative study on different DL architecture; like: ResNet50, VGGNet19, AlexNet and Xception in skin cancer detection is done. The study concludes that best performance is obtained by using ResNet50 with data augmentation steps. One experiment is also conducted by the authors to enhance the speed of training and deployment process by using Graphics Processing Unit (GPU). From the comparative study it is observed that robustness of the skin image analysis can be mutilated because of presence of noise, shadows or artefacts on the image. Thus to improve the image quality different pre-processing steps are introduced by the authors. Along with this, class skewness problem is minimized by proposing data augmentation methods like: horizontal and vertical flipping techniques in the work.

An automated computer-aided model to detect skin cancer is proposed in [19]. The algorithm proposed incorporates an enhanced segmentation phase to identify the infected lesion of the skin. Authors also use CNN to extract features from the image dataset. Using multiclass linear SVM, a classifier model is developed. Total 337 images are captured from three different dataset, like: Dermatology Information System, DermQuest, DermNet Skin Disease Atlas website in three different stages. The proposed model is able to obtain accuracy of 93.75%.

In the paper [23] a novel segmentation neural network, *skin-segnn* to obtain high lesion boundary detection accuracy is proposed. Another model *skin-segnn* is developed utilizing CNN architecture GoogleNet Inception v3. Dataset comprises of 13,000 images collected by combining open-access dermatology repositories, namely the ISIC Dermoscopic Archive [24] and the Edinburgh Dermofit Library [25]. Though the exact accuracy level is not mentioned in the paper but high prediction accuracy is achieved from the proposed system.

Authors in the paper [20] collected dermoscopic images of total 50 cases from Internet and hospitals for classification. In the first step, filtering, segmentation and feature extraction were done on the images. Dull Razor software was used for hair removal and then Fast Median Filtering was used to filter the images. For segmentation purpose maximum entropy threshold segmentation was used. Finally, IMAGEJ and MATLAB software was used for feature extraction based on GLCM technique. Log Sigmoid activation function was used. The function gives 0 to indicate non-cancerous condition and 1 for cancerous condition. Accuracy of 88% was achieved by this technique.

In the work [18], the authors proposed a model for early detection of cancer of skin using artificial neural network (ANN) with the aim of classifying malignant melanoma and other skin diseases. Combination of digital image processing and ANN is used for classification purpose. Total 21 cases of dermoscopic images were used. Pre-processing and post-processing was done to eliminate noise and preserve edges of the images respectively. Segmentation was done to isolate cancerous skin from healthy skin. Finally, two dimensional wavelet transform is used for extracting unique features of cancer from the images. Extracted features ere fed to feed forward multiplier network for classification in this proposed system. For training purpose back propagation algorithm was used. The authors claimed to achieve satisfactory accuracy by their algorithm. However the exact accuracy has not been given in the paper.

In [26] a unique human and AI combination is presented by the authors. Altogether 11,444 dermatoscopic images were considered for experimentation. The images were segregated into 5 diagnostic categories. A single CNN was trained by novel DL techniques. Classification of total 300 biopsy-verified skin lesions into five predetermined categories were done by 112 dermatologists of thirteen University Hospitals of German along with trained CNN. Study was done based on two distinguished stages. First end point confirms the classification of the images into 5 different stages. Second end point of the study was about the classification of benign or malignant of the skin disease. This classification was done using binary numbers. The combining classification technique based on human and AI achieved accuracy of 82.95%, higher than 1.36% if done individually.

Simple classification model is proposed in [14]. Digital format dermoscopic images were considered for image processing. Images were processed in two stages. In pre-processing stage hair removal and filtering was done using Dull razor and filtering software. In post processing stage image enhancement and contrast adjusting was done. In the next stage, Otsu colour threshold segmentation was done using IMAGEJ software. Next, contrast, correlation, homogeneity and energy features were extracted using GLCM. In the last stage a hybrid classifier using genetic algorithm with ANN instead of the conventional classifier, is used. It was trained by 30 known values. Overall 88% accuracy was achieved by the proposed model.

The work in [15] used 1300 images from the dermoscopic image database, Dermofit [25] with an aim to classify skin lesions into benign and malignant. The algorithm involves multiple steps including pre-processing, post-processing, feature extraction and classification. Genetic algorithm is employed as the classifier. The result shows 92% accuracy in case of benign and 84% accuracy in malignant cases.

Computer-aided diagnosis is used to detect lesion borders in [27]. Analysis of dimension of symmetry of the lesion pigmentation of skin is done here. Epiluminescence microscopy (ELM) is used for making the outer layer of skin translucent as the preliminary process. Then image segmentation process is performed to detect the lesion. Once the lesion is detected it is used for extracting features and classification purpose.

In the work, [16] 199 skin lesion images were considered to develop classification model using image processing and SVM. Proposed model achieved specificity of 72%, and sensitivity 86%.

The paper in [17] introduced DL architecture based on convolutional auto-encoder for classification of histopathology images for BCC diagnosis. Dataset of 1417 images collected from 308 regions of interest of slides of skin histopathology were used. Evaluation and comparison were done on different image representation strategies like: bag of features or transforms like discrete cosine transform or Haar wavelet and proposed learned-from-data representations. The system was able to achieve accuracy of 91.4% and F-measure of 89.4%.

Three different tasks, namely segmentation of lesion, dermoscopic feature extraction from the lesion and classification of lesion, using two DL methods were performed in [28]. 2000 skin lesion images were considered by the publicly available dataset [29]. Segmentation result and coarse classification result were simultaneously obtained by the proposed DL framework. The proposed frame work consists of two fully convolutional residual network. Coarse classification result is refined with the calculation of distance heat-map done by lesion index calculation unit. Feature extraction is done by the proposed CNN. 75.3, 84.8 and 91.2% accuracy level is acquired for task 1, task 2 and task 3 respectively from the proposed system.

For skin cancer detection 3551 patients were chosen for 5846 clinical images with pigmented skin lesions that includes both malignant tumours and benign tumors in [30]. Randomly 666 patients were selected for training and faster, region based CNN was developed and its performance was also presented. Accuracy offered by the proposed algorithm was 86.2%.

In [31] transfer learning tecnique is used along with pre-trained deep neural network to increase the classification rate in automatic skin lesion classification system. Transfer learning was then applied to Alex-net framework. This application is done in three different ways, like: weights of the architecture is finely tuned, replacement of classification layer by softmax layer and augmenting dataset by various rotation angles which maybe fixed or random. Images are taken from three datasets, MED-NODE, Derm (IS & Quest) [32] and ISIC [24]. The accuracy achieved with the three datasets are 96.86, 97.70 and 95.91%, respectively.

In the paper [33], the authors combined DL with machine learning to build a method for segmentation of skin lesions and also to identify the detected area and surrounding tissues. Largest available dataset [29] at that time was considered. The dataset contained 900 training and 379 testing images. The proposed system achieved 75% accuracy and 59% specificity with 82% sensitivity.

Authors in [21] use CNN models to study the effect of external factors like: ruler, hair present on the skin. The authors also study the effect of the quality of the image in classification of melanoma. Dataset given in [34] was used. ResNet50, DenseNet121, VGG16 and AlexNet: these four common CNN models were used. Among them DenseNet121 had given the best accuracy. 6 different test set was considered. DenseNet has given accuracy of 89.22% with hair set, 86% with ruler set and 88.81% with none-set.

15.3 Preliminaries, Tools and Techniques

In this section the different aspects of CNN with special focus on application in image processing is discussed briefly.

15.3.1 Convolutional Neural Network (CNN)

ANNs are designed by imitating the structures and working principles of the human nervous system. A single-layered neural network is the simplest neural network to be designed. It is called the 'perception'. The mathematical model is represented in the Fig. 15.6. By concatenating numerous single-layered structures, a fully-connected neural network is developed as shown in Fig. 15.7.

In image analysis by a fully connected network every raw pixel of the image is considered. Every pixel is used for training the neural network in fully connected network. The entire numbers of trainable parameters of the neural network is increased in a large number. This leads to a huge computational complexity in the neural network. For example, the present work uses Kaggle dataset [35] for testing and validation purpose. The dataset consists of RGB images of size 224×224. So, the number of weights in the first layer is $224 \times 224 \times 3 = 150528$.

The use of a large number of weights can give rise to over-fitting of the network. For this reason, the total process could become very much time consuming and the system could occupy huge storage. So for image classification fully connected layers in ANN are not suitable. To solve this issue a different kind of neural network architecture is applied. It is popularly known as CNN. CNN is designed mainly for working on the different types of images. The Kaggle image can be converted to $1 \times 1 \times 10 = 10$ in the first layer itself.

DL is a sub-domain of the machine learning. It is a brain-inspired machine learning approach. In the DL approach, computer intelligence learns from the data presented to it. From that, it will make predictions on the same or related data. The DL can overcome the drawbacks present in the traditional approaches. For this reason, DL has rapidly found usage in diverse fields like bioinformatics, medical image analysis,

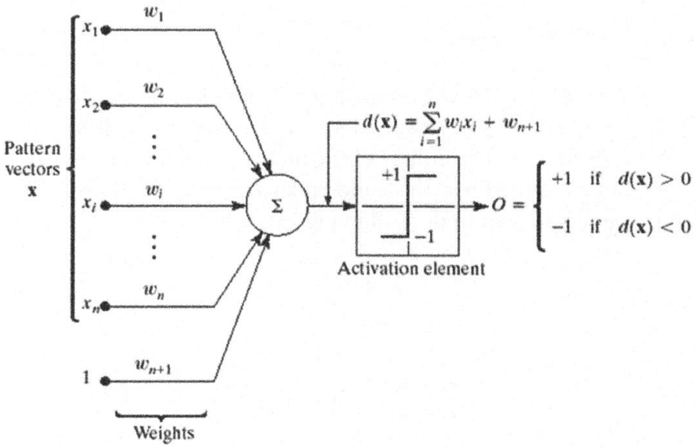

Fig. 15.6 A mathematical model of a perceptron

health industries, finance, agriculture, and many different fields [36]. CNN is one of these types of efficient application of DL models. It is based on the existing theories of traditional ANN.

CNN is a type of ANN. The working principal of CNN imitates the visual cortex of the human brain. The visual cortex receives the information relayed from the different layers from the retina. In this process, the cells respond only to the visual stimuli at a certain orientation. One of the important advantages of CNN is unlike ANN, it scales the image during the training process itself. Unlike fully connected ANN, a layer of CNN is connected with a smaller number of neurons of the next layer determined by the need of the network. The scaling down of the images also reduces computational complexity. CNN takes the close proximity of the pixels under consideration thus requiring a smaller number of parameters for training. Thus, the training process is easier than fully connected ANN. There are mainly 5 layers of CNN. The various layers of CNN are as follows:

1. Input
2. Convolution
3. Activation
4. Pooling
5. Fully Connected.

15.3.1.1 Input Layer

In this layer, the image is fed to the input. This layer analyses the pixel values and introduces the values to the next layer. The functionality of this layer is similar to the layers of ANN in general.

15.3.1.2 Convolution Layer

This layer makes use of convolutional filters. These filters detect patterns of the images, i.e. edges, geometric shapes, and so on. The size of each filter is termed as F_k and is a $F_k \times F_k$ matrix. The values of the matrix are random values. This is also known as the features of the filter, these are updated during the training process. The convolution process is shown in the following Eqs. 15.1 and 15.2

$$G = H * F \tag{15.1}$$

$$G[i, j] = \sum_{s=-k}^{k} \sum_{t=-k}^{k} H[s, t] F[i - s, j - t] \tag{15.2}$$

The convolutional operation is done by each filter with the image matrix. After pass through each filter, a reduction of the number of image pixels is achieved. So

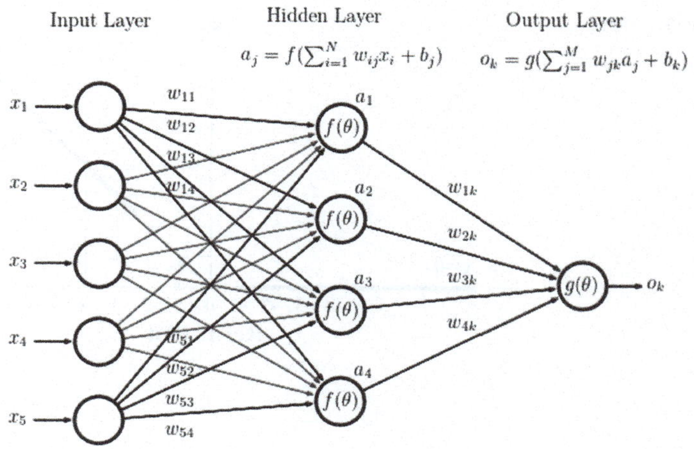

Fig. 15.7 A mathematical model of a fully-connected neural network (*Source* [38])

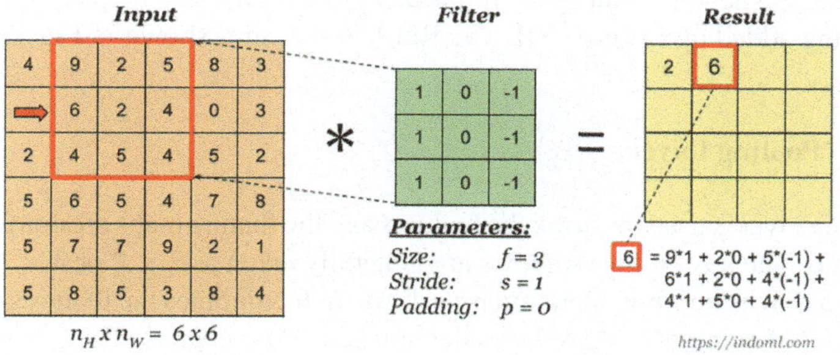

Fig. 15.8 An example of convolution operation (*Source* [37])

that the size of the image is reduced. This pixel reduction is done without losing the relationship with the nearby pixels. For example, as be scan be seen in Fig. 15.8, the convolution operation is applied on an image of size 6×6, and the filter size is taken to be 3×3. The stride size is 1×1. The output obtained is of size 4×4. Without padding the image size gets reduced and the complexity is reduced by 55.5%.

15.3.1.3 Activation Layer

The output of the convolution layer is passed on to this layer. The output is passed through an activation function. Here a rectified linear unit (ReLU) is used. The activation functions enable the neuron if its input is a positive value. A linear relationship with the input variable is present in those cases. If the input of the activation is negative zero output is obtained. The mathematical expression of the ReLU is given in Eq. 15.3.

Fig. 15.9 ReLU plot

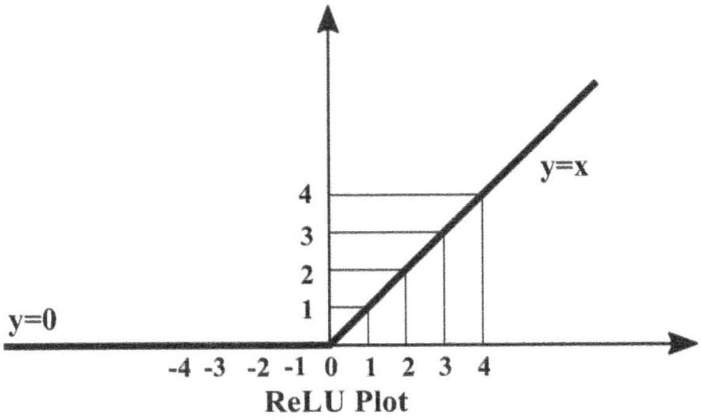

$$f(x) = \max(0, x) \tag{15.3}$$

In this layer, the negative values are replaced by zero. This step helps to avoid all the values being added up to zero [39]. The ReLU function is shown in Fig. 15.9.

15.3.1.4 Pooling Layer

The pooling layer is used to shrink the features and the feature maps are converted into smaller size. The size of the windows are generally taken as 2×2 or 3×3 sizes. In this layer, a downsampling operation is performed. It combines the features of nearby related pixel. It automatically reduces the number of parameters. The computational load on the next layer is reduced in this way. It results in a faster training. Let the dimension of the feature map be $mp_h \times mp_w \times mp_c$. The output of the pooling layer is shown in the Eq. 15.4. An example case of maxpooling operation is shown in Fig. 15.10.

$$mp'_h \times mp'_w \times mp'_c = \frac{mp_h - f + 1}{s} \times \frac{mp_w - f + 1}{s} \times mp_c \tag{15.4}$$

Here mp_h, mp_w, mp_c denotes the original dimension of the image. After pooling operations, the dimensions become mp'_h, mp'_w, mp'_c. f is the filter size and s is the length of the stride.

15.3.1.5 Fully Connected Layer

Like every ANN the fully connected layers in CNN takes the output of the convolution layer or the max-pooling layer as the input. Then it flattens the input images and classifies the images according to a label. The filtered images received from the previous layers are put in a list or vector. The neurons present in this layer follow

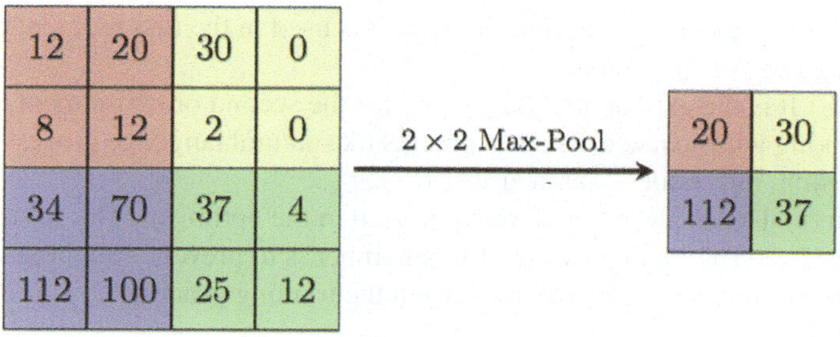

Fig. 15.10 An example of max-pooling operation by 2 × 2 (*Source* [40])

a back-propagation process for optimization. It optimizes the accurate weights for the neurons. The weights are defined in such a way that the difference or the error between the actual output and the desired output is reduced as much as possible. The weights are then allotted on a priority basis. Then the neuron 'vote' among them and the winner is the decision of that classification. For the improvement of the performance, ReLU or Softmax activation function is used [41].

15.3.2 Adams Optimizer

Optimizers are used to tune the characteristics of a neural network i.e. learning rates and weights to reduce the losses in the training process. The choice of the optimizers are vital in determining the network performance. Various optimizers like gradient descent and it variants, momentum, Nesterov accelerated gradient etc. have been used in neural network. In recent times, adaptive moment estimation (Adam) optimizer is becoming highly popular. It is the first optimizer to work with first and second order moments, m(t) and v(t) respectively, in place of the classical stochastic gradient descent procedure [42].

The main objective behind Adam is not to proceed instantly although there is a chance to jump on the minimum. The speed of the operation of Adam is decreased little for better searching of the attributes. The motivation of this application was to update neural network weights iteratively and is dependent on the training data. It also stores few average squared gradients like m(t), v(t) etc. v(t) is the uncentered variance of the gradient.

15.3.2.1 Parameters of Adam

- **Alpha** (α) It is the learning rate or step size. If the value of α is less (e.g. 0.01, 2.0E-4), that means the system training rate is slow. If the initial value is large then the training process is faster before the increase of the rate.

- **Beta** (β_1) It is the exponential decay rate. It is used in the first moment estimates. Typical value is kept around 0.9.
- **Beta** (β_2) It is the exponential decay rate for the second order moment estimates. For working with sparse gradient problems like natural language processing, computer vision, this value is set near to 1.0.
- **Epsilon** (ϵ) This is a very small number used in the optimizer. The value is nearly 10^{-7} to 10^{-9}. The main purpose of this number is to prevent obtaining undefined numbers in division operations by zero in the training process.

$$\hat{m}_t = \frac{m_t}{1-\beta_1^t}\hat{v}_t = \frac{v_t}{1-\beta_2^t} \tag{15.5}$$

Here, mean of the variables m(t) and v(t) is calculated, where E[m(t)] evaluates to E[g(t)] and E[f(x)] is the representation of the expected value of f(x). The parameter is update as follows:

$$\theta_{t+1} = \theta_t - \frac{\eta}{\sqrt{\hat{v}_t} + \epsilon}\hat{m}_t \tag{15.6}$$

Adams weight decay upgradation rule is as follows [42],

$$w_t = w_{t-1} - \eta\left(\frac{\hat{m}}{\sqrt{\hat{v}_t} + \epsilon} + \lambda w_{t-1}\right) \tag{15.7}$$

here λ is the weight decay function.

Although Adams optimizer is computationally intensive it offers the following advantages:

- This optimizer performs rapidly.
- The convergence speed of this optimizer is also very high.
- Another advantage of this algorithm is it can correct and disappear the rate of learning, it provides a high variance.

15.3.3 Categorical Cross Entropy

Categorical cross entropy is a loss function implemented in multi-class classification tasks. This function calculates the total entropy between the distributions and gives a very good measure of how they are different from each other. It is also called log loss. The loss is calculated as

$$Loss = -\Sigma_{i=1}^{outputsize} l_i.log(\hat{l_i}) \tag{15.8}$$

where $\hat{l}_i$ is the i-th scalar value in the output of the model, l_i is the target value corresponding to it, and *output size* is the total number of scalar values in the output of the model. It is recommended to use softmax activation function with this loss function.

15.3.4 Softmax

The softmax function is very popularly used in the last step of a neural network. Some vector components in the network may take values below 0 or greater than 1 or may not add to 1, which is undesirable. After application of the softmax function, all the vector components take distribution in the range (0,1) and add to 1. The softmax function is calculated as

$$\sigma(x_j) = \frac{e^{x_j}}{\Sigma_i x_i} \tag{15.9}$$

where x_i are the elements of the input vector and can take any values.

15.4 Dataset

Researchers require standard dataset to compare their work with other published works. Not just for bench marking but datset is needed for carrying our preliminary tests. Some commonly available datasets are described below.

15.4.1 ISBI Challenge Dataset

Since 2016–2019 till now, ISBI has released dataset for their public ISBI Challenge [29, 43–45]. The ISBI Challenge 2016 Dataset contained melanoma images. Gradually over the years, images for other pathologies like nevi, actinic keratosis, vascular lesions and Bowen's disease etc. were added over the years.

15.4.2 PH2 Dataset

The PH2 [46] database contains 200 dermoscopic images of melanoma and non melanoma sourced from the Pedro Hispano Clinic, Portugal Dermatology Service. Thus earning the name PH2.

Table 15.4 Datasets [45]

Data set	No. of dermascopic images	Melanoma images
2016 ISBI Challenge [44]	900	273
2017 ISBI Challenge [29]	2000	374
2018 ISBI Challenge [43]	10000	1113
2019 ISBI Challenge [45]	25333	4522
PH2 [46]	200	40
ISIC Archive [24]	23906	21659

15.4.3 ISIC Challenge

The ISIC [24, 47] has run challenges in 2018 and 2019 for classification of skin diseases. The dermatoscopy images have been sourced from various datasets and clinics all over the world. The dataset contained more than 23,000 dermoscopic images of seven different diseases including melanoma.

15.4.4 Kaggle

This dataset contains about 2600 benign and malignant images of skin moles [35]. Unlike other image repositories discussed above, this dataset does not distinguish between the types of malignant or benign images.

A brief comparison of the datasets are given in Table 15.4.

Apart from these dataset other datasets like DermIS [32], and Dermofit Image Library [25] are also popular.

15.5 Proposed Methodology

The present work proposes a CNN model developed from the scratch to classify dermascopic images into two groups, benign and malignant. A block diagram representation of the proposed model is shown in Fig. 15.11. The proposed model works in two stages. In the first stage of the algorithm, training is done and in the second stage, testing is done. The two stages are described briefly in Sects. 15.5.1 and 15.5.2, respectively.

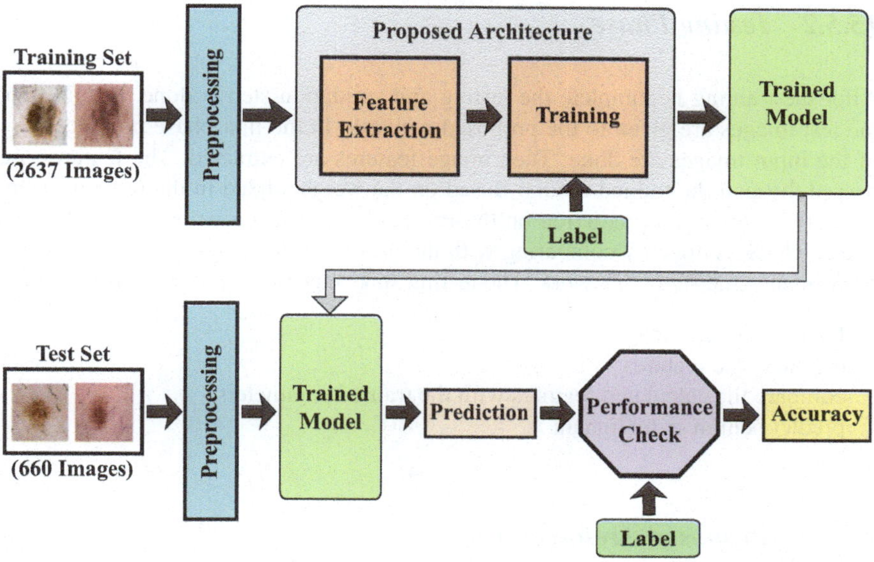

Fig. 15.11 Proposed training and testing model

15.5.1 Training Phase

This is the first phase of implementing any neural network. In the training phase, the features are extracted and are used to train the model. The broad steps of the training stage of the proposed model are summarized below:

1. feed the training images
2. preprocess data
3. feed the preprocessed data to the propose CNN network
4. train the network
5. save the model.

In the first step of this stage, preprocessing is done on the input image. This helps in improving the image quality and minimising the unwanted features. Then the preprocessed image is passed on to the proposed architecture. The proposed network extracts features from the images and passes on the features for training the network. The information from the ground truth is also passed. The network learns the characteristics of the two classification levels from the ground truth and the extracted features. The training model is thus developed. The vital parameters of the model like layer position, filter size, stride length etc. needs to be saved for reproducing during the testing phase and during actual field deployment.

15.5.2 Testing Phase

After the training is complete the testing and validation step is done. In this step, the test images are given to the proposed network. In the first phase preprocessing of the input images are done. Then image features are extracted. The features are passed through the trained model. Based on the weights fixed in the previous step, the network makes a prediction on the images being cancerous or benign. Performance check is done by comparing with the ground truth. Accuracy is chosen as a performance metric in this work. The testing stage can be summarized as follows:

1. feed the testing images
2. calculate the features
3. compare the calculated features with the trained parameters
4. predict benign or malignant.

15.5.3 Proposed Architecture

The proposed method aims to automatically classify photographs of skin lesions into two groups—cancerous and non-cancerous skin lesions. To solve this problem a novel 16-layer DCNN is proposed which is fully trained by the training set of images given in the dataset [35]. The proposed architecture is built from scratch. There are 9 convolutional layers, 4 maxpool layers and 3 fully-connected layers present in the architecture. The architecture is graphically described in the Fig. 15.12.

The input layer is followed by two convolutional layers with ReLU activation function. The convolution layers extract the special features from an image. The activation function as uses the ReLU approach, discards the negative value of the images. The resultant feature maps are passed to the maxpool layers, which decrease the dimension size, and hence complexity of the images. In the proposed algorithm, the two convolutional layers are followed by a maxpool layer. The unit of two convolutional layers with ReLU and one maxpool layer are repeated for three more stages. In the subsequent stage, three fully connected layers are present. The fully collected layers compile the data of the previous layers to form the final output. The last fully connected layer has only two outputs, benign or malignant. The last fully connected layer uses the softmax function. The composition of the proposed network is summarised in Table 15.5.

The layers of the network and their associated features are as follows:

1. Conv: n = 32, f = 3
2. Conv: n = 64, f = 3
3. Maxpool: f = 4
4. Conv: n = 64, f = 5
5. Conv: n = 64, f = 5
6. Maxpool: f = 2

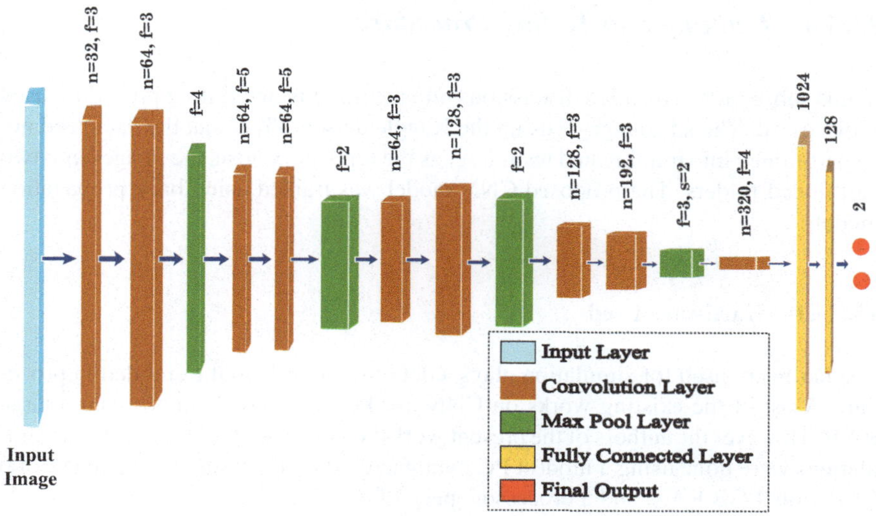

Fig. 15.12 Proposed methodology

Table 15.5 Number of layers

Name of the layer	Number
Convolutional	9
Maxpool	4
Fully-connected	3

7. Conv: n = 64, f = 3
8. Conv: n = 128, f = 3
9. Maxpool: f = 2
10. Conv: n = 128, f = 3
11. Conv: n = 192, f = 3
12. Maxpool: f = 3, s = 2
13. Conv: n = 320, f = 4
14. Fully connected: 1024
15. Fully connected: 128
16. Fully connected: 2.

where Conv stands for convolutional layer, Maxpool for maxpool layer, n for number of filters, f for filter size and s for stride.

15.5.4 Training and Testing Procedure

In this subsection, a detailed discussions into the training and testing procedure used is discussed. The advantage of using the Kaggle datset [35] is that the data need not be partitioned into training and testing set as the repository hosts the images into two partitioned folders. The proposed CNN model was trained using back propagation model.

15.5.4.1 Hardware Used

The hardware used for simulation plays a determining role in the simulation procedure. Most of the existing works on CNN use PCs with GPU support and a large RAM. However the authors of the present work did not have a GPU support. The simulations were done using a modest PC manufactured by HP with Intel Core i5-8500 CPU with 4 GB RAM and a processor speed of 3.0 GHz.

15.5.4.2 Dataset Used

Most of the recent works make use of the ISBI dataset [43] or ISIC dataset [24]. The authors of this work had a modest PC as discussed in Sect. 15.5.4.3. The PC is inadequate to handle the above mentioned datasets. So the authors chose the Kaggle dataset [35]. These images in the Kaggle repository are selected and processed from ISIC archive [29, 34, 47] which contains eight categories of cancerous and non-cancerous skin lesions. The chosen dataset [35] is already partitioned into two sets - Training and Testing. The dataset contains 1440 benign images and 1197 malignant images for training purpose and 360 benign images and 300 malignant images for testing purpose. All the images are color images with 224 × 224 sizes.

15.5.4.3 Training Parameters

As previously mentioned, back propagation is used to train the CNN model. The loss is calculated using categorical cross entropy over a bath size of 32 for 25 epochs. The proposed work implements binary classification. Categorical cross entropy, described briefly in Sect. 15.3.3 is one of the losses which is used for binary and multiclass classification. The softmax activation function described briefly in Sct. 15.3.4 is used in the final layer of the proposed architecture. So the loss calculation using categorical cross-entropy becomes much easier and faster when softmax is present in the last layer [48]. So this loss is widely applied for binary and multiclass classification in the field of computer vision [49]. It is to be noted that as only binary classification is done in this work, the term binary cross entropy should be used instead of categorical cross entropy. However as the inbuilt python function uses the term categorical cross

Table 15.6 Adam optimizer parameters

Name of the parameter	Value
α	0.001
β_1	0.9
β_2	0.999
ϵ	10^{-8}

Table 15.7 Model hyperparameters

Name of the parameter	Value
Optimizer	Adam
Loss	Categorical cross entropy
Epoch	25
Batch	32

entropy even for binary classification so the present work uses the term categorical cross entropy for the employed loss function.

The errors were calculated in the forward pass. Based on these values, the weights were adjusted in the backward pass. For optimization of the network Adam optimizer was used. The parameters chosen for the optimizer are learning rate $\alpha = 0.001$, first moment of exponential decay rate $\beta_1 = 0.9$, second moment of exponential decay rate $\beta_2 = 0.999$ and the small number epsilon $\epsilon = 10^{-8}$. The parameters for Adams learning are summarized in Table 15.6.

The proposed network is built from the scratch in Python using TFLearn with TensorFlow as backend. The same parameters are used for training and testing purpose too. The model was tested by varying the hyperparameters. The hyperparameters offering the best results are chosen for the proposed network. The chosen hyperparameters are summarized in Table 15.7.

15.6 Results

The proposed algorithm is a two part classification algorithm. The images are classified as either benign (Class 0) or malignant (Class 1). To quantify the performance the parameter accuracy is chosen.

15.6.1 Accuracy

To understand accuracy, the following four attributes needs to be discussed first:

1. True Positive (TP): Cancerous lesion is present and is detected correctly.
2. True Negative (TN): Cancerous lesion is absent and that is detected correctly.

Table 15.8 Performance on test data

TP	TN	FP	FN
249	329	31	51

3. False Positive (FP): Cancerous lesion is present but is not detected.
4. False Negative (FN): Cancerous lesion is absent but is detected in the image incorrectly.

Accuracy is calculated as

$$Accuracy = \frac{TP + TN}{TP + TN + FP + FN} \tag{15.10}$$

Accuracy is a measure of actual classification. The proposed work is tested on Kaggle dataset [35]. It has 660 test images. For the testing purpose malignant images are considered as the positive class. The test results obtained are TP = 249, TN = 329, FP = 31, FN = 51. The test results are presented in Table 15.8.

$$Accuracy = \frac{249 + 329}{249 + 329 + 31 + 51} \tag{15.11}$$

By applying (15.10) to the parameters of Table 15.8 the accuracy of the present algorithm can be calculated as per (15.11). So, from (15.11) it can be seen that the proposed algorithm offers an accuracy of 87.58%. The confusion matrix is shown in Fig. 15.13.

15.6.2 Comparison with Existing Works

To establish the efficacy of the proposed network built from scratch, a comparison with existing works is essential. For a fair comparison, the most recent works (published in 2020) working on the Kaggle dataset [35] or using DCNN for classification are chosen. It is to be noted that there are other works on DL based skin cancer detection but they use other datasets or other approaches but not DCNN. It is to be noted that the accuracy of an algorithm is highly dependent on the dataset size. The larger the repository size better the training and testing performance.

The work in [50] proposed a two stage algorithm. In the first step preprocessing was done to remove clutter and hair. In the second stage two DL models, namely Inception-v3 and MobileNet were used separately. The simulation results demonstrated that the Inception-v3 network achieved better validation accuracy and thus was used for validation of test data. The final accuracy with Inception-v3 network was 81% when trained on original images but improved to 86% on using images after refinement or processing.

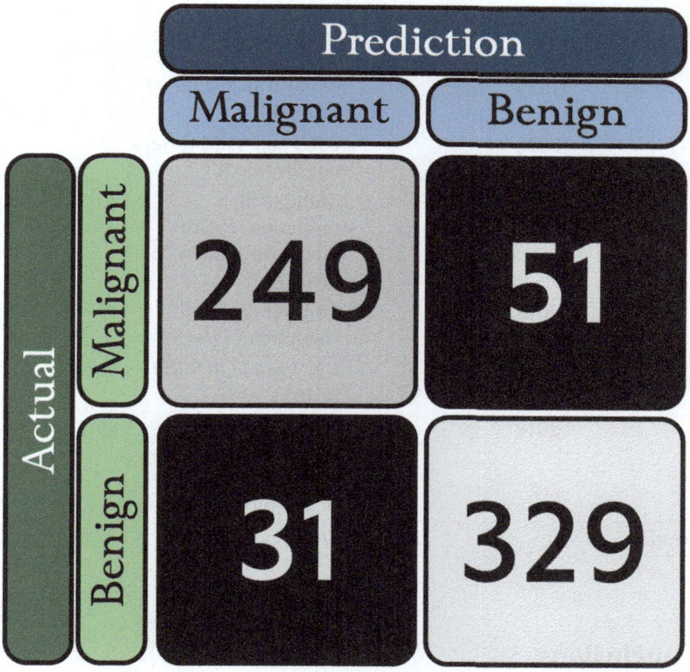

Fig. 15.13 Confusion matrix

The work in [51] did a comparative study of skin cancer by using CNN and SVM. The simulation studies proved that the former approach offered a better accuracy and the accuracy value obtained was 83%.

A CNN with attention mechanism, to preserve edge details had been proposed in [52]. The work gives an accuracy of 80.5% on the PH2 [46] database.

The work in [53] on the PH2 [46] database and a fusion of CNN and full convolutional residual network (FCRN) gives and accuracy of 86.81%.

An accuracy of 86.5% is obtained in the work [28]. It also proves its algorithm using the PH2 [46] database. The work [28] uses dual DCNN which learns mutually from each other.

DCNN and optimization of coloured features of the segmented lesion has been applied in [54]. The work on the ISIC challenge dataset [43] offers an accuracy of 85.1%. A comparison of the proposed work with the most recent work are given in Table 15.9.

From Table 15.9 it is clearly visible that the proposed algorithm offers better accuracy than the existing works. Also the proposed work has distinctive advantage over the other works as it offers smaller customised network.

Table 15.9 Comparison with existing works

Work	Year of publication	Approach used	Accuracy (%)
[50]	2020	48-layer Inception-v3 network	81% (original images), 86 (refined images)
[51]	2020	CNN and SVM (layers not specified)	83
[52]	2020	Multiple high resolution feature blocks (minimum 20 layers)	80.5
[53]	2018	18-layer deep full resolution CNN	86.81
[28]	2018	CNN and FCRN (50 & 101)	86.5
[54]	2018	Aggregated deep convolutional features (Multiple ResNet 50 or 101 blocks)	85.1
Proposed work		16-layer DCNN	87.58

15.7 Conclusions

This work proposes a 16-layer CNN architecture for classifying skin lesion. The network in the present work is developed from scratch and does not use any pre-trained networks. The developed model offers an accuracy of 87.58% with the Kaggle dataset [35] which is a much better than the state of the art works on the same dataset. The use of a smaller network gives the distinctive advantage of smaller computational time and lower hardware cost.

It is to be noted that the performance of any CNN is highly dependent on the size of the dataset. The larger the dataset, more efficient the training of the network. In the future the team expects to upgrade the hardware and test the proposed algorithm on large datasets like ISBI [43] or ISIC [24].

The present algorithm does a two part classification of the skin lesions. The algorithm can be modified for multi part classification like actinic keratosis, BCC, SCC, melanoma, to name a few.

The existing works on skin cancer detection from images does not make use of vital data like gender, race, age etc. The authors conjecture that the segmentation process of the lesions can be improved by incorporating these features. So, the authors propose to incorporate these features in their future work.

Acknowledgements The authors would like to thank Avik Kumar Das for his immense help during the manuscript preparation stage.

References

1. Society, A.C.: What Is Cancer? (2020). https://www.cancer.org/content/dam/cancer-org/research/cancer-facts-and-statistics/annual-cancer-facts-and-figures/2020/cancer-facts-and-figures-2020.pdf. Accessed 2 Oct 2020
2. WebMD: Skin Cancer (2020). https://www.webmd.com/melanoma-skin-cancer/melanoma-guide/skin-cancer#1. Accessed 2 Oct 2020
3. Cokkinides, V., Albano, J., Samuels, A., Ward, M., Thum, J.: American cancer society: cancer facts and figures. Am Cancer Soci Atlanta (2005)
4. Society, A.C.: Cancer Facts and Figures 2020 (2020). https://www.cancer.org/content/dam/cancer-org/research/cancer-facts-and-statistics/annual-cancer-facts-and-figures/2020/cancer-facts-and-figures-2020.pdf. Accessed 2 Oct 2020
5. Stern, R.S.: Prevalence of a history of skin cancer in 2007: results of an incidence-based model. Arch. Dermatol. **146**(3), 279–282 (2010)
6. Fitzmaurice, C., Akinyemiju, T.F., Al Lami, F.H., Alam, T., Alizadeh-Navaei, R., Allen, C., Alsharif, U., Alvis-Guzman, N., Amini, E., Anderson, B.O., et al.: Global, regional, and national cancer incidence, mortality, years of life lost, years lived with disability, and disability-adjusted life-years for 29 cancer groups, 1990 to 2016: a systematic analysis for the global burden of disease study. JAMA Oncol. **4**(11), 1553–1568 (2018)
7. Dorj, U.O., Lee, K.K., Choi, J.Y., Lee, M.: The skin cancer classification using deep convolutional neural network. Multimed. Tools Appl. **77**(8), 9909–9924 (2018)
8. Esteva, A., Kuprel, B., Novoa, R.A., Ko, J., Swetter, S.M., Blau, H.M., Thrun, S.: Dermatologist-level classification of skin cancer with deep neural networks. Nature **542**(7639), 115–118 (2017)
9. Bauman, C.A., Emary, P., Damen, T., Dixon, H.: Melanoma in situ: a case report from the patient's perspective. J. Can. Chiropr. Assoc. **62**(1), 56 (2018)
10. Healthline: Skin Cancer Stages: What Do They Mean? (2020). https://www.healthline.com/health/stages-of-skin-cancer#melanoma. Accessed 2 Oct 2020
11. Mayer, J.: Systematic review of the diagnostic accuracy of dermatoscopy in detecting malignant melanoma. Med J. Australia **167**(4), 206–210 (1997)
12. Masood, A., Ali Al-Jumaily, A.: Computer aided diagnostic support system for skin cancer: a review of techniques and algorithms. Int. J. Biomed. Imaging **2013** (2013)
13. Sigurdsson, S., Philipsen, P.A., Hansen, L.K., Larsen, J., Gniadecka, M., Wulf, H.C.: Detection of skin cancer by classification of Raman spectra. IEEE Trans. Biomed. Eng. **51**(10), 1784–1793 (2004)
14. Aswin, R., Jaleel, J.A., Salim, S.: Hybrid genetic algorithm-artificial neural network classifier for skin cancer detection. In: 2014 International Conference on Control, Instrumentation, Communication and Computational Technologies (ICCICCT), pp. 1304–1309. IEEE (2014)
15. Tong, S.T., Sopory, P.: Does integral affect influence intentions to use artificial intelligence for skin cancer screening? A test of the affect heuristic. Psychol. Health **34**(7), 828–849 (2019)
16. Gilmore, S., Hofmann-Wellenhof, R., Soyer, H.P.: A support vector machine for decision support in melanoma recognition. Exp. Dermatol. **19**(9), 830–835 (2010)
17. Cruz-Roa, A.A., Ovalle, J.E.A., Madabhushi, A., Osorio, F.A.G.: A deep learning architecture for image representation, visual interpretability and automated basal-cell carcinoma cancer detection. In: International Conference on Medical Image Computing and Computer-Assisted Intervention, pp. 403–410. Springer (2013)
18. Jaleel, J.A., Salim, S., Aswin, R.: Artificial neural network based detection of skin cancer. Int. J. Adv. Res. Electr. Electron. Instrum. Eng. **1**(3) (2012)
19. Shoieb, D.A., Youssef, S.M., Aly, W.M.: Computer-aided model for skin diagnosis using deep learning. J. Image Graph. **4**(2), 122–129 (2016)
20. Jaleel, J.A., Salim, S., Aswin, R.: Computer aided detection of skin cancer. In: 2013 International Conference on Circuits, Power and Computing Technologies (ICCPCT), pp. 1137–1142. IEEE (2013)

21. Akkoca-Gazioğlu, B.S., Kamasak, M.: Effects of objects and image quality on melanoma classification using deep neural networks (2020)
22. Kassani, S.H., Kassani, P.H.: A comparative study of deep learning architectures on melanoma detection. Tissue Cell **58**, 76–83 (2019)
23. Chang, H.: Skin cancer reorganization and classification with deep neural network (2017). arXiv:1703.00534
24. Collaboration, I.S.I.: ISIC 2019 (2019). https://challenge2019.isic-archive.com. Accessed 1 Apr 2020
25. Ballerini, L., Fisher, R.B., Aldridge, B., Rees, J.: A color and texture based hierarchical k-nn approach to the classification of non-melanoma skin lesions. In: Color Medical Image Analysis, pp. 63–86. Springer (2013)
26. Hekler, A., Utikal, J.S., Enk, A.H., Hauschild, A., Weichenthal, M., Maron, R.C., Berking, C., Haferkamp, S., Klode, J., Schadendorf, D., et al.: Superior skin cancer classification by the combination of human and artificial intelligence. Eur. J. Cancer **120**, 114–121 (2019)
27. Schmid, P.: Segmentation of digitized dermatoscopic images by two-dimensional color clustering. IEEE Trans. Med. Imaging **18**(2), 164–171 (1999)
28. Li, Y., Shen, L.: Skin lesion analysis towards melanoma detection using deep learning network. Sensors **18**(2), 556 (2018)
29. Codella, N.C., Gutman, D., Celebi, M.E., Helba, B., Marchetti, M.A., Dusza, S.W., Kalloo, A., Liopyris, K., Mishra, N., Kittler, H., et al.: Skin lesion analysis toward melanoma detection: A challenge at the 2017 international symposium on biomedical imaging (ISBI), hosted by the international skin imaging collaboration (ISIC). In: 2018 IEEE 15th International Symposium on Biomedical Imaging (ISBI 2018), pp. 168–172. IEEE (2018)
30. Jinnai, S., Yamazaki, N., Hirano, Y., Sugawara, Y., Ohe, Y., Hamamoto, R.: The development of a skin cancer classification system for pigmented skin lesions using deep learning. Biomolecules **10**(8), 1123 (2020)
31. Hosny, K.M., Kassem, M.A., Foaud, M.M.: Classification of skin lesions using transfer learning and augmentation with alex-net. PloS One **14**(5) (2019)
32. DermIS Dermatology Information System|Home (2019). https://www.dermis.net. Accessed 30 Nov 2019
33. He, K., Zhang, X., Ren, S., Sun, J.: Deep residual learning for image recognition. In: Proceedings of the IEEE Conference on Computer Vision and Pattern Recognition, pp. 770–778 (2016)
34. Combalia, M., Codella, N.C., Rotemberg, V., Helba, B., Vilaplana, V., Reiter, O., Carrera, C., Barreiro, A., Halpern, A.C., Puig, S., et al.: Bcn20000: dermoscopic lesions in the wild (2019). arXiv:1908.02288
35. Fanconi, C.: Kaggle Skin Cancer: Malignant versus Benign dataset—Processed Skin Cancer pictures of the ISIC Archive (2019). https://www.kaggle.com/fanconic/skin-cancer-malignant-vs-benign. Accessed 7 May 2020
36. Seetha, J., Raja, S.S.: Brain tumor classification using convolutional neural networks. Biomed. Pharmacol. J. **11**(3), 1457 (2018)
37. Indonesia, B.P.M.: Convolutional neural networks (CNN) introduction (2018). https://indoml.com/2018/03/07/student-notes-convolutional-neural-networks-cnn-introduction/. Accesed 03 Oct 2020
38. Ivezić, Ž., Connolly, A.J., VanderPlas, J.T., Gray, A.: Statistics, Data Mining, and Machine Learning in Astronomy: A Practical Python Guide for the Analysis of Survey Data. Princeton University Press (2019)
39. Pavan, M.S., Jagadeesh, P.: Brain tumor segmentation using covolutional neural network in MRI images. Int. J. Pure Appl. Math. **119**, 1585–1592 (2018)
40. https://i.stack.imgur.com/6WbWu.png: Imgur.com. Accessed: 03 Oct 2020
41. O'Shea, K., Nash, R.: An introduction to convolutional neural networks (2015). arXiv:1511.08458
42. Kingma, D.P., Ba, J.: Adam: A Method for Stochastic Optimization (2014). arXiv:1412.6980

43. Codella, N., Rotemberg, V., Tschandl, P., Celebi, M.E., Dusza, S., Gutman, D., Helba, B., Kalloo, A., Liopyris, K., Marchetti, M., et al.: Skin lesion analysis toward melanoma detection 2018: a challenge hosted by the international skin imaging collaboration (ISIC) (2019). arXiv:1902.03368
44. Gutman, D., Codella, N.C., Celebi, E., Helba, B., Marchetti, M., Mishra, N., Halpern, A.: Skin lesion analysis toward melanoma detection: a challenge at the international symposium on biomedical imaging (ISBI) 2016, hosted by the international skin imaging collaboration (ISIC) (2016). arXiv:1605.01397
45. Naeem, A., Farooq, M.S., Khelifi, A., Abid, A.: Malignant melanoma classification using deep learning: datasets, performance measurements, challenges and opportunities. IEEE Access **8**, 110575–110597 (2020)
46. Mendonça, T., Ferreira, P.M., Marques, J.S., Marcal, A.R., Rozeira, J.: Ph 2-a dermoscopic image database for research and benchmarking. In: 2013 35th Annual International Conference of the IEEE Engineering in Medicine and Biology Society (EMBC), pp. 5437–5440. IEEE (2013)
47. Tschandl, P., Rosendahl, C., Kittler, H.: The ham10000 dataset, a large collection of multi-source dermatoscopic images of common pigmented skin lesions. Sci Data **5** (2018)
48. Hinton, G., Vinyals, O., Dean, J.: Distilling the knowledge in a neural network (2015). arXiv:1503.02531
49. Murugan, P.: Implementation of deep convolutional neural network in multi-class categorical image classification (2018). arXiv:1801.01397
50. Farooq, M.A., Khatoon, A., Varkarakis, V., Corcoran, P.: Advanced deep learning methodologies for skin cancer classification in prodromal stages (2020). arXiv:2003.06356
51. Brindha, P.G., Rajalaxmi, R., Kabhilan, S., Sangitkumar, C., Sanjeevan, L.: Comparative study of SVM and CNN in identifying the types of skin cancer. J. Crit. Rev. **7**(11), 640–643 (2020)
52. Xie, F., Yang, J., Liu, J., Jiang, Z., Zheng, Y., Wang, Y.: Skin lesion segmentation using high-resolution convolutional neural network. Comput. Methods Programs Biomed. **186** (2020)
53. Al-Masni, M.A., Al-Antari, M.A., Choi, M.T., Han, S.M., Kim, T.S.: Skin lesion segmentation in dermoscopy images via deep full resolution convolutional networks. Comput. Methods Prog. Biomed. **162**, 221–231 (2018)
54. Yu, Z., Jiang, X., Zhou, F., Qin, J., Ni, D., Chen, S., Lei, B., Wang, T.: Melanoma recognition in dermoscopy images via aggregated deep convolutional features. IEEE Trans. Biomed. Eng. **66**(4), 1006–1016 (2018)

Chapter 16
Deep Learning Based Classification of Brain Tumor Types from MRI Scans

Jyotishka Das, Suvadeep Ghosh, Rivu Chakraborty, and Ankita Pramanik

Abstract Patients suffering from brain tumors have significant rate of mortality. The diagnosis of brain tumors, if carried out erroneously, may result in incorrect medical intervention and hence may reduce the chance of survival of the patient. Since the risk of developing brain tumors increases with age and as there has been an increase in the aging population in the world, an urgent need is felt to develop simple and low cost analytical tools for its early diagnosis. Usually, MRI scans are used to image a patient's brain. In recent times, machine learning and its subdomain, deep learning has reduced the need for human judgment in the diagnosis of diseases. Deep learning models are increasingly being adopted in lieu of traditional supervised learning algorithms due to their inherent advantages owing to their ability to gather requisite details from the images automatically. One of the most difficult bio-medical imaging problems is to detect whether a patient has developed brain tumor. Despite having literatures dedicated to detect or classify various types of brain tumors through deep learning approaches, they lack high accuracy. Here, a solution for the classification of two types of brain tumors, namely Meningioma and Glioma is presented. A novel 13-layer deep convolutional neural network (CNN) architecture is used, that is built from scratch. The proposed system after performing 10-fold cross-validation gives an average validation accuracy of 100%. It is the highest attainable accuracy among existing works performed on axial MRIs, and on the same dataset.

Keywords CNN · Deep learning · Brain tumor · MRI

J. Das · S. Ghosh · R. Chakraborty · A. Pramanik (✉)
IIEST Shibpur, Howrah, India
e-mail: ankita@telecom.iiests.ac.in

S. Ghosh
e-mail: suvadeep.ug2016@telecom.iiests.ac.in

J. Nayak et al. (eds.), *Advanced Machine Learning Approaches in Cancer Prognosis*, Intelligent Systems Reference Library 204,
https://doi.org/10.1007/978-3-030-71975-3_16

16.1 Introduction

Brain tumor is an abnormal cell mass, growing at an uncontrollable pace inside the human brain. Asia has the highest fatality rate of people suffering from brain tumor [13, 30]. Unlike any other tumors in our body, brain tumors have a limited space for growth due to the presence of cranium. This in turn means, that a growing brain tumor can squeeze vital parts of the brain causing major injuries and health problems by affecting the endocrine system. Hence, it is essential to detect brain tumors correctly at the nascent stage to provide necessary treatment.

Brain tumors can be classified based on their region of inception, characteristics, behaviour and growth rate. They can be differentiated into different types based on various parameters [52, 55]:

- **Characteristics and Behaviour**: Based on their characteristics and behaviour, brain tumors can be either benign or malignant.
  - ***Benign Brain Tumor***: They are non-progressive and have distinguished boundaries. Their rate of progression is slow. Since benign brain tumors do not spread beyond the region of its origin, it is considered to be less feisty than malignant ones. The abnormal mass of cells may press upon a region of the brain as they grow. After correct diagnosis, this can be easily removed in time by surgery.
  - ***Malignant Brain Tumor***: Malignant brain tumor cells, on the other hand have fuzzy borders and rapid rate of progression. Since malignant brain tumors have undefined boundaries, they can invade and spread to other healthy cells of the body parts [33].
- **Growth Rate**: Based on the growth rate, malignant tumors can be of the following types:
  - ***Grade I***: Least malignant
  - ***Grade II***: Less malignant
  - ***Grade III***: More malignant
  - ***Grade IV***: Most malignant
- **Region of Inception**: Based on the region of inception, brain tumors can be classified into two types - primary and secondary brain tumor.
  - ***Primary Brain Tumor***: These tumors arise from the tissues in the brain. These can either be benign or malignant. According to the WHO, primary brain tumors can also be classified in more than 100 ways based on their types, the most common being Gliomas and Meningiomas. Different types of primary brain tumor are discussed below:

    Gliomas: Gliomas, either low-grade (LGG Grades I-II) or high-grade (HGG Grades III-IV) are malignant tumors which are intrinsic to the cerebral cavity and may affect the central nervous system causing tumor-infiltrative edema [53]. On the basis of their grades and characteristics, Gliomas can have

varying degrees of vascularity, some which can even disrupt the blood-brain barrier. These characteristics can potentially allow their differentiation [7]. The prognosis of subjects with Gliomas are low ($\leq$15 months). Astrocytomas, Oligodendrogliomas and Ependymomas are examples of different types of Gliomas.
Meningiomas: Meningiomas are mostly benign, extrinsic cerebral tumors in the meninges (the membrane that seperates the brain from the spinal cord). Mengingiomas may disrupt the blood-brain barrier, and form vasogenic edema in the peritumoral tissue. However, edema may not always be present, in both Gliomas and Meningiomas [39].
Pituitary tumors: These tumors originate from the region of the pituitary gland that sits at the base of the brain. Most of them are benign, but some can develop to be malignant. These tumors can interfere with the normal hormone levels, thus affecting the whole body. Some common types of pituitary tumors are Craniopharyngiomas, Adenomas and Rathke's cleft cysts.
Schwannomas: These tumors arise from Schwann cells, which produce the protective membrane called myelin sheet, in our nerve cells. These are usually benign and mostly affect adult females.
Pineal region tumors: Developing in and around the pineal gland, these tumors cannot be removed because the pineal gland is hard to be accessed.

- ***Secondary or Metastatic Brain Tumor***: These tumors can spread inside the brain from other parts the body. Tumors such as lung cancer, breast cancer and skin cancer can metastasize to brain.

The growth of brain tumor has external symptoms like:

- Headaches, that might worsen in the morning
- Nausea and drowsiness
- Vision problems
- Speech problems
- Hearing problems
- Seizures
- Fatigue
- Dizziness and stumbling
- Increased intracranial pressure
- Confusion and sluggishness in everyday activity
- Depression and personality changes.

The symptoms that manifest are typical to the type of brain tumor the patient has and also on the location of the tumor. If the doctor suspects a patient with brain tumor, the patient is usually advised to undergo either some medical imaging techniques (like magnetic resonance imaging (MRI), computer tomography (CT), cerebral angiogram, etc.) or some other tests (like audiometry, visual field acuity measure or endocrine evaluation) according to the standard operating procedure. Based on the final test results, the doctor performs a final diagnoses and treats the patient accordingly. MRI is a preferred technique over others due to its non-ionising and non-invasive properties, as well as due to its good spatial and temporal resolution. MRI is used to image the soft tissues of the brain using a magnetic field and radio frequency waves. For conducting MRI scans, a particular orientation and coverage area needs to be decided to better visualize the tumor affected area [18]. To increase the contrast of the resulting MRI scans for the purpose of better visualization of the brain tumors, a dye or a contrast material, such as gadolinium is injected into the bloodstream. Normally, T-weighted MRI images are employed to classify primary (such as Meningioma, Glioma, Pituitary tumor, Schwannomas, Pineal region tumors), and secondary (Metastates) brain tumors. After performing suitable MRI scan, if brain tumor is detected, a doctor is consulted for confirming the type and class of it. Keeping track of the progression of brain tumor is a herculean task, hindered by the necessity to make careful observations about a plethora of features that may change with time. Some of these features like heterogeneity, iso/hypo-intense properties, and perilesional edema have to be carefully monitored to classify brain tumors manually [43]. To expedite the process of brain tumor classification, relevant features must be extracted from the MRI scans of the brain.

To detect a brain tumor in its nascent stage, the experience of the radiologist matters a lot. Since, the diagnosis of the tumor and evaluating its type, is the primary task at hand before suggesting any further medication, a biopsy ought to be performed. A definitive brain surgery is essential to perform biopsy of the brain tumor, unlike other body parts. To prevent the potential subjectivity of biopsy, it is necessary to develop an efficacious tool which can help in accurate diagnosis by segmenting and classifying tumors from MRI images. Research and development of robust machine learning technologies has opened a new frontier in medical imaging and diagnostics [3]. Initially, conventional brain tumor classification algorithms based on manual expertise were used for this process. Conventional brain tumor classification algorithms rely heavily on region-based tumor segmentation rather than extracting relevant number of features from the MRI scans to aid the classification process. These days, the growing adaptation of deep learning (DL) techniques has brought a paradigm shift in the classification process. Recent studies have shown promising results by the application of AI in detecting the presence and also the type of brain tumor directly from the medical images, thus reducing human intervention and delay. Therefore, manual expertise, which is subject to error and time consumption, can be avoided.

Machine Learning (ML) is a discipline of computer science for solving complex problems that have no proper model or equation. It trains the computers to learn from examples and experiences using a data-driven approach. It is an approach to achieve Artificial Intelligence (AI) [6]. A Venn-diagram representing the relationship between different approaches in AI methodologies is shown in Fig. 16.1. Many ML computation approaches are inspired by how the human brain learns and solves problems. A biological neuron or nerve-cell is the basic unit of the human nervous system. It is also the basic computational element of our brain. The mathematical equivalent of a biological neuron is known as an *artificial neuron* or *perceptron*, as shown in Fig. 16.2. A complex connected network of neurons, called ANN is designed in such a way that it mimics the sensory network of the human nervous system. It is

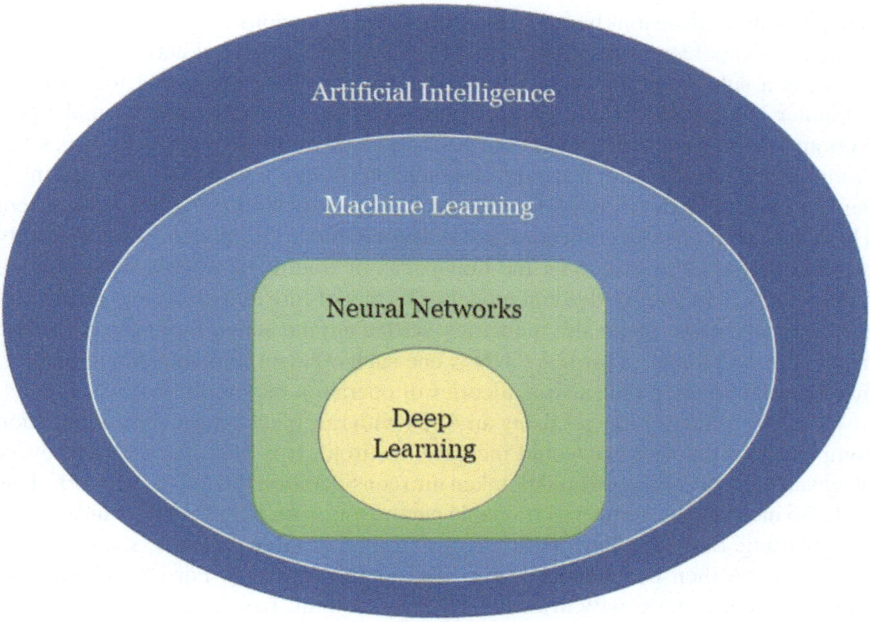

Fig. 16.1 Venn diagram representing the relationship between Artificial Intelligence, Machine Learning and Deep Learning

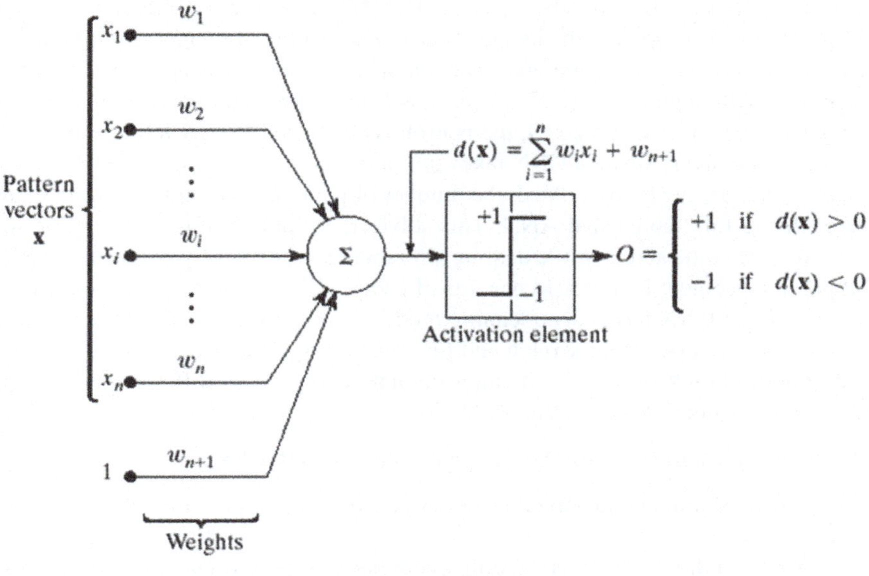

Fig. 16.2 A mathematical model of a Perceptron (*Source* [16])

capable to make decisions based on the gathered informations. As shown in Fig. 16.5, multi-layered perceptrons (MLP) forms a *fully-connected* neural network.

DL is a subdomain of brain-inspired ML approaches, attempting to make the computer intelligent to learn representations on data, and subsequently make predictions on the same. A recent boom in computational intelligence techniques has promoted extensive research and development on DL approaches. DL is increasingly being adopted in a diversity of domains including medical imaging practises, where a high degree of classification accuracy is desired. Since DL models have inherently better capabilities to overcome the drawbacks of traditional approaches, they are radically efficient over traditional models. DL models are quickly being adapted by professionals across the health industries, setting a trend across bio-informatics and medical image analytics [46]. A CNN is one such efficient implementation of a DL model, building upon the existing theories of operation of a traditional ANN.

If we try to classify images using an ANN with raw pixel values, the computation complexity of the network would increase manifold. It is because, each and every pixel values of the images would be taken into consideration to train the network. This will also increase the number of trainable parameters, which may in turn quickly lead to overfitting. Since the network has to optimize all of these parameters, the training process could then become very time and storage intensive. For classification of images, the full connectivity in an ANN is thus wasteful. To solve this computational problem, a diferent kind of network architecture is popularly used, specially designed for working with images. CNN is a special kind of ANN motivated by the working of the visual cortex of our brains, which receives and processes information relayed from the retinas. These cells respond only to the visual stimuli at a certain orientation. CNN has an advantage of scaling the images over ANN. Scaling of images is important as scaling down reduces the computational complexity and processing time of training the model. Although in an ANN, a neuron is fully-connected to every neurons in a previous layer, in case of a CNN, the neuron is connected to only a few neurons in the preceding layer. Since, a CNN takes into account that pixels in close proximity to each other are generally related, the number of parameters required to train it are lesser than a fully-connected ANN. This solves the problem of overfitting that we so frequently come across while dealing with images using a fully-connected ANN. Taking into account the inherant benefits of using a CNN for a classification task, a novel 13-layer CNN based deep leaning model was deployed for the current study, which was developed from scratch and fine-tuned to give an accurate result for the brain tumor classification task. It can accurately classify two different varieties of brain tumor, namely Meningioma and Glioma.

The main contributions of this study can be summarized below:

- To provide a simple understanding about the working of a DL model in an image processing task.
- To provide a thorough understanding about how the performance analysis of different DL based classification algorithms are conducted.
- Propose a novel 13-layer deep CNN based DL model which is capable of extracting relevant features from brain MRI images.

- Use those relevant features to perform a binary classification task, i.e., the model would be able to distinguish two different varieties of brain tumor (i.e., Meningioma and Glioma).
- To compare the performance of the proposed model with various other DL models that performs a binary or a ternary classification task on the same Figshare dataset.

Section 16.2 of this book offers a brief literature study conducted on various ML and DL methodologies adopted in brain tumor prognosis. Section 16.3 explains the methodology used in the current discussion. It offers a brief description of the functionalities of the various types of layers of a typical CNN model. It also discusses various performance metrics used to assess the accomplishment of a classification mechanism. This is followed by Sect. 16.4, which explains the proposed method offered by this manuscript regarding the classification task. Section 16.5 discusses the experimental setup of the current work. It also explains the details about the preparation of the dataset and the data pre-processing technique adopted. It also explains how the model was trained and tested, along with the optimal values of the hyperparameters used. Sect. 16.6 presents the analysis of the results, and offers a comparison of the current work with other existing works conducted on the same dataset. This chapter is concluded in Sect. 16.7, with a discussion on the limitations of the current architecture, possible improvement(s) and future scope(s) of work.

16.2 Literature Study

Brain tumor modeling process is usually performed on the basis of MRI images. To treat a brain tumor, it is important to extract essential information from the MRI scans of the patient's brain as it is considered to be more reliable for the detection of anomalies than more traditional diagnostic procedures like ultrasound imaging or CT scan. For decades, data mining techniques have been used to extract relevant pieces of information from a large dataset. Classification of images or parts of them, is one of the main tasks in medical image analysis. Many methods such as support vector machine (SVM), decision tree, random forest, fuzzy c-means (FCM), Bayesian classifier and ANN have been used to classify or detect brain tumor from MRI scans [11, 31, 47, 48, 54]. In [54], the authors used a colour based segmentation technique using K-means clustering to do semantic segmentation of tumor regions from MRI images. By combining colour translation, histogram and K-means clustering, the efficiency of the algorithm was improved. The past decade has also seen an increased adoption of SVM for detecting, or classifying brain tumors [51]. For a similar kind of segmentation task, FCM was used in [48]. After the features were extracted by grey level run through matrix, SVM was used for the classification task. The work had obtained an accuracy of 91.66% and a sensitivity of 83.33% using linear kernel function.

In recent years, DL algorithm models are adopted in lieu of traditional ML models since DL models does not need a large number of nodes compared to traditional architectures like SVM or K-nearest neighbor [32]. Damodharan and Raghavan [12] presented a brain tumor detection algorithm, which utilises a feature based segmentation technique. MRI images of the brain (10 images with brain tumor, and 10 images without brain tumor) were segmented according to the tissue types. Each of these tissue segmented images were divided into a number of blocks. Features such as entropy, mean, variance and energy were calculated for each of the blocks, and were aggregated to evaluate the feature vector. This feature vector, when passed through a neural network classifier, gave the performance metrics of the model. The authors had claimed a highest classification accuracy of 80%.

Rao et al. [41] proposed a stacked prediction framework based CNN model to segment brain tumor affected areas from MRI scans. BRATS-2015 dataset [15] was used for training purpose. Multimodal representation of each pixel was obtained by combining its neighbourhood based learnt deep representations in each modalities. The segmentation was done by aggregating the classification results of each pixels in the image. An accuracy of 67% was obtained for the segmentation task.

Seetha and Raja [46] presented a simple CNN based classification model to detect brain tumors. The dataset was created from Radiopaedia [40] and BRATS 2015 testing dataset [15]. In the training phase, the images were divided into two categories by their label names (tumor or no-tumor). After pre-processing, the features extracted were passed through a CNN to compute the loss function. Using gradient descent algorithm, the value of the loss function was reduced so that the accuracy can be improved. In the testing phase, the features extracted from the test image was passed through the trained CNN model to get the performance metrics. An accuracy of 97.5% was obtained.

Ozyurt et al. [35] had proposed a neuroscopy and CNN (NS-CNN) based algorithm to segment and then classify brain MRI images as benign and malignant. 500 samples taken from TCGA-GBM dataset [45] was used for training. The NS-EMFSE + CNN + SVM model gave the best performance metrics with an accuracy of 95.62%, and sensitivity of 96.25%.

Numerous literature are available attempting to classify brain tumor based on their types. The authors in [1, 2, 5, 9, 21, 22, 24, 25, 36, 37, 43, 44, 50] used T1-weighted MRI images obtained from "brain tumor dataset", built by Cheng et al. [8] to classify brain tumors into Meningioma or Glioma or Pituitary tumor. Cheng et al. [9], besides building the public Figshare repository, also compared the performance of various feature extracting methods for the extraction of the region of interests (ROI) and their subsequent classification. The tumor regions were first augmented, and then divided into many subregions. It was shown that the feature extracting techniques such as intensity histogram, bag-of-words (BoW), and gray-level co-occurrence matrix gives better accuracies using augmented ROI than non-augmented ROI. If ring-form partition was used along with augmentation, the accuracies obtained were further improved. The highest accuracy of 91.28% was obtained for the BoW model, with augmented ROI and ring-form partition.

Abiwinanda et al. [1] built a CNN model to classify brain tumors. Data augmentation techniques were not employed. The CNN based architecture consists of one each of convolution, maxpool, flattening, hidden, and fully connected layers. The simple CNN model gave the highest validation accuracy of 84.19%.

Afshar et al. [2] employed a CapsNet architecture which takes into account the brain tumor MRI images along with the course boundaries of the tumors as extra inputs, to classify them into Meningioma or Glioma or Pituitary tumor. The proposed method was claimed to have an accuracy of 90.89%, better as compared to CNNs or normal CapsNet architectures. The increase in the classification accuracy was claimed to be primarily due to the elimination of the requirement for exact annotation of the tumor region, and the novelty of the algorithm which aids the CapsNet to focus only on the main region of interest.

Paul et al. [37] employed a CNN model to classify brain tumor MRI images. Data augmentation was performed on the original images to prevent overfitting. A six-layed deep CNN was modelled. After a five-fold cross validation process, the highest classification accuracy was obtained as 91.43%.

Pashaei et al. [36] proposed a CNN based architecture to extract hidden features from MRI images by applying the convolution and max-pooling operations. These extracted features were fed to a kernel extreme learning machine (KELM) to classify the MRI images into either Meningioma, Glioma or Pituitary tumor. The KE-CNN model gives an improved accuracy of 93.68%, over other different classifiers like SVM and radial base function.

Ismael et al. [22] employed a modified ResNet50 architecture [17] to classify brain tumor types from MRI images. 3064 T1-weighted MRI images were used for training, giving an overall accuracy of 99% with data augmentation, and 95% without augmentation for a three-class classification problem (Meningioma or Glioma or Pituitory tumor).

Rehman et al. [43] performed a comparative analysis of three popular CNN networks, namely AlexNet, VGGNet and GoogleNet to classify brain tumors types. Transfer learning techniques and data augmentation were employed on the training dataset resulting in the highest classification accuracy of 98.69% on the VGG16 architecture.

Kaplan et al. [25] employed a modified local binary pattern (nLBP) feature extracting method to design the classification task using a KNN model. The highest accuracy obtained was 95.56%.

Bhanothu et al. [5] proposed using a faster R-CNN DL algorithm to mark the region of the occurrence of the tumor using Region Proposal Network (RPN). Both the RPN and the classifier network used a VGG-16 based architecture as backbone. Using [8] as the training dataset, the model obtained a precision of 75.18% (against Glioma), 89.45% (against Meningioma) and 68.18% (against Pituitary tumor). The mean average precision was obtained as 77.60%.

In [21, 44, 50], the authors of each of the respective studies employed various statistical models for the evaluation of the classification task. Abdel-Qader et al. [21] gathered statistical features from MRI images using 2D Discrete Wavelet Transformation (DWT) combined with 2D Gabor filter techniques. These features were used for training a neural network. A classification accuracy of 91.9% was obtained. Tahir et al. [50] compared the performance of various popular preprocessing methods employed in improving the classification accuracy of statistical models. They reported the highest obtained accuracy as 86%, benchmarked against a SVM classifier. Sarhan et al. [44] proposed using wavelet decomposition on the brain MRI images as obtained from [8], before passing it to a CNN classifier. The proposed method was shown to significantly reduce the complexities of the CNN classifier. An overall accuracy of 99.3% was obtained for the three class classification.

Kaldera et al. [24] employed a DL model to segment and classify brain tumors into two classes, namely Glioma and Meningioma. A CNN was used for the classification task and a Faster Region based CNN was used for the segmentation task. 218 T1-weighted MRI images from the public "brain tumor dataset" built by Cheng was used as the training set [8, 9]. The model gave an accuracy of 100% for Meningioma and an accuracy of 87.5% for Glioma classifications. Also, a confidence level of 94.6% was obtained when Meningioma tissues were segmented.

A review on recent studies on the detection of brain tumors using MRI scans is shown in Table 16.1.

16.3 Methodology Used

In this section, an overview of the methodology used in the current study is presented. The principles involved in the functioning of a CNN used in the classification task is presented in Sect. 16.3.1. The metrics used to quantify the classification results are discussed in Sect. 16.3.2.

16.3.1 Convolutional Neural Network (CNN)

In recent years, CNN has become the most popular deep-learning based architecture because it is able to compute complex operations using convolution filters. It is a series of feed-forward layers which implements convolutional and pooling operations. The 2D feature maps obtained after the last pooling layer is converted into an 1D vector, by adopting several fully-connected layers. This 1D vector is used for the actual classification task.

The details regarding the various types of layers in the CNN architecture is discussed below:

- **Input Layer**: The image is taken as the input. The input layer of a CNN introduces the pixel values to its next layer, just like any other form of ANN.
- **Convolution Layer**: This layer contains filters which can detect patterns like edges, geometric shapes etc. Each filter has to have a specified with a filter size F_k. The filter is an $F_k \times F_k$ matrix filled with random values, also known as features

Table 16.1 A review on recent studies on detection of brain tumors using MRI scans

Author	Year	Dataset Used	Purpose	Technique	Highest Performance	Remarks
Bhanothu et al. [5]	2020	Cheng's figshare repository- "brain tumor dataset"	Classification : Meningioma / Glioma / Pituitary Tumor	Faster R-CNN	Prec. : 77.60%	VGG network is used as backbone
Kaplan et al. [25]	2020			KNN	Acc. : 95.56%	Modified nLBP feature extracting method used
Rehman et al. [43]	2020			VGG16	Acc. : 98.69%	VGG16 gives better classification accuracy than AlexNet and GoogleNet
Sarhan et al. [44]	2020			WCNN	Acc. : 99.30 %	Wavelet decomposition feature extracting technique used
Tahir et al. [50]	2019			SVM	Acc. : 86.00%	Data preprocessing improved accuracy
Ismael et al. [22]	2019			ResNet50	Accuracy : 99.00% Precision : 99.00% Recall : 99.00% F1- Score : 99.00%	Data augmentation improved accuracy
N. Abhiwinanda et al. [1]	2018			CNN	Acc. : 90.89%	Simplest network used, consisting of only 5 layers
Parian Afshar et al. [2]	2018			Capsnets	Acc. : 90.89%	High classification accuracy obtained because CapsNet only focuses on the region of interest
Abdel-Quader et al. [21]	2018			ANN	Acc. : 91.90%	Statistical features obtained by 2D DWT and 2D Gabor filtering techniques
A. Pashaei et al. [36]	2018			KELM+CNN	Acc. : 93.68%	KELM+CNN gives improved classification accuracy over SVM and Radial base function
J. Paul et al. [37]	2017			CNN	Acc. : 91.43%	Six layer deep architecture used, along with data augmentation
Cheng et al. [9]	2015			SVM SRC KNN ROI	Acc. : 91.28% (SVM [BoW])	Using ring-form partition along with augmented region of interest increased classification accuracy
Kaldera et al. [24]	2019		Classification: Meningioma / Glioma Segmentation : Meningioma	CNN	Acc. (Glioma) : 87.50% Acc. (Meningioma) : 94.00% Acc. (Net) : 94.60%	For the segmentation of Meningioma, affected tumor region also obtained
Ozyurt et al. [35]	2019	TCGA-GBM dataset	Classification : Benign / Malignant Segmentation : Tumor region	NS-CNN	Acc. : 95.62%	Expert maximum fuzzy-sure entropy (NS-EMFSE) along with CNN and SVM classifier gave highest accuracy
Seetha and Raja [46]	2018	Radiopaedia and BRATS-2015 dataset	Classification : Tumor / No tumor	CNN	Acc. : 97.50%	Pre-trained network used
Rao et al. [41]	2015	BRATS-2015 dataset	Segmentation : Tumor regin	CNN	Acc. : 67.00%	Stacked prediction framework used
Damodharan and Raghavan [12]	2015	Dataset not mentioned	Classification : Tumor / No tumor	Neural Network	Acc. : 80.00%	Neural network gave better accuracy than SVM or Bayesian classification
Singh et. al. [48]	2015	Dataset not publicly available	Segmentation : Tumor region	SVM + Fuzzy c means	Acc. : 100.00%	GLRLM feature extraction technique is used

of the filter. These features are updated in back propagation when the model is trained. The convolution operation is given by Eqs. (16.1, 16.2), as follows:

$$G = H * F \tag{16.1}$$

$$G[i, j] = \sum_{u=-k}^{k} \sum_{v=-k}^{k} H[u, v]\, F[i-u, j-v] \tag{16.2}$$

There is a convolution operation on each filter with the image matrix. It filters the image with a smaller pixel value filter, reducing the image size without compromising on losing the relationship between the adjacent pixels. For example, in Fig. 16.3, when we apply convolution operation on a 6×6 image using a 3×3 filter with 1×1 stride, we obtain a 4×4 output if no padding is applied (55.5% decrease in complexity).

- **Activation Layer**: After the convolution operation is performed, the output is usually passed through an activation function. The activation layer also can be placed after fully-connected layer, which is explained later. One of the mostly used activation function is Rectified Linear Unit (ReLU). It fires a neuron if the input contains positive values, with the activation function having a linear relationship with the input variable. If the input is negative, the output is zero. The ReLU activation function is expressed by Eq. (16.3), as follows:

$$f(x) = max(0, x) \tag{16.3}$$

In the ReLU activation layer, the negative values from the filtered image are replaced with zeros. This prevents the negative values being summed up to zero in the next convolutional layer [38].

- **Pooling Layer**: This layer is used to shrink the feature maps into smaller sizes. A window size of usually 2×2 or 3×3 is considered. The pooling layer performs a downsampling operation on the image stacks, i.e., combines spatially closer features which in turn reduces the number of parameters required. The redundancy obtained makes the image representation more compact which reduces the computation load for the next stages, thus resulting in faster training. A max-pooling operation is demonstrated in Fig. 16.4. For a feature map having dimensions $n_h \times n_w \times n_c$, the dimensions of output obtained after a pooling layer is given by Eq. (16.4), as follows:

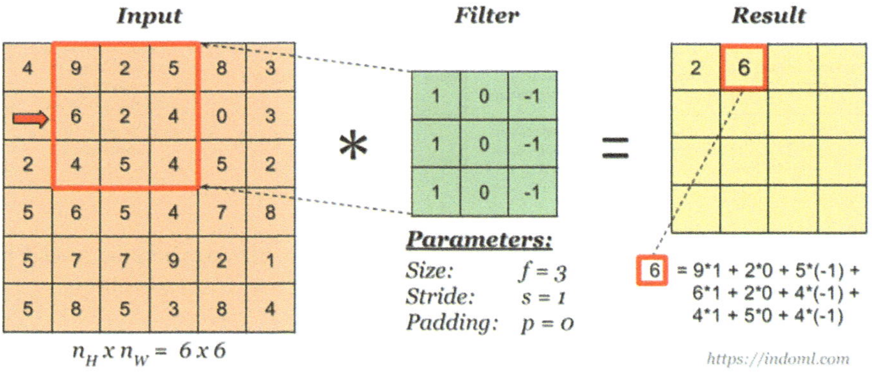

Fig. 16.3 An example of convolution operation (*Source* [20])

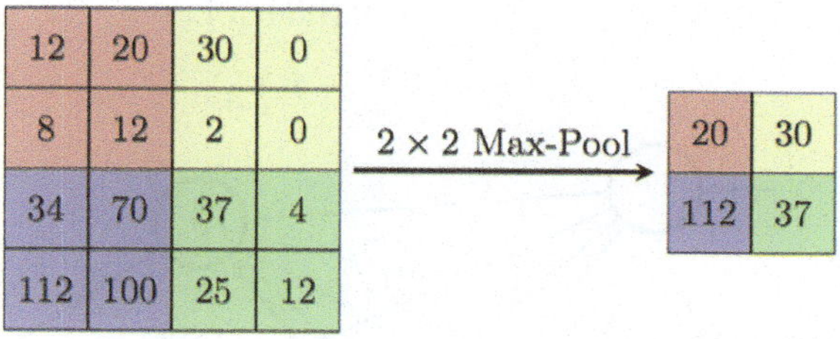

Fig. 16.4 An example of max-pooling operation by 2 × 2 (*Source* [19])

$$n'_h \times n'_w \times n'_c = \frac{n_h - f + 1}{s} \times \frac{n_w - f + 1}{s} \times n_c \tag{16.4}$$

where n_h, n_w, n_c are the original dimensions (height, width and number of channels) of the feature maps before the pooling operation is performed, n'_h, n'_w, n'_c are their new dimensions after the pooling operation is performed, f is the filter size, and s is the stride length.

- **Fully Connected Layer**: Similar to multi-layered perceptrons of a fully-connected ANN as described in Fig. 16.5, the fully connected layers in a CNN receive the results of the convolution or pooling layer as inputs, flattens them and classifies the image into a label.
  The filtered images obtained from the convolution/maxpool operations, are put in a single list/vector. The single vector represents a probability of labelling a certain feature in the image. The neurons in a fully-connected layers goes through a *backpropagation* process. This process is used to optimize the most accurate weights that are assigned to the neurons. The weights are determined in such a way that the error between the actual output and the desired output is minimized. The weights that are being allocated to each of the neurons are used to prioritize the most appropriate label. The neurons then "vote" on each of the labels, the winner of that vote being the decision of the classification task. ReLU or Softmax activation function may be used between these layers to improve performance [34]. Overfitting can be reduced by using regularization and dropout processes.

16.3.2 Evaluating the Performance of a Classification Model

To quantify the performance of any testing algorithm, various performance metrics have been developed. Knowledge of these metrics is essential while designing any test system. These system parameters are convenient to validate the usefulness of a classification model. Most commonly used among them are system accuracy, sensitivity, specificity and F1 score. These system parameters can be measured on the basis of TP, FP, TN, and FN values, obtained from the confusion matrix at the end of testing phase of a model. A confusion matrix showing the calculation of performance metrics of a model from TP, FP, TN and FN results is shown in Fig. 16.6. For the

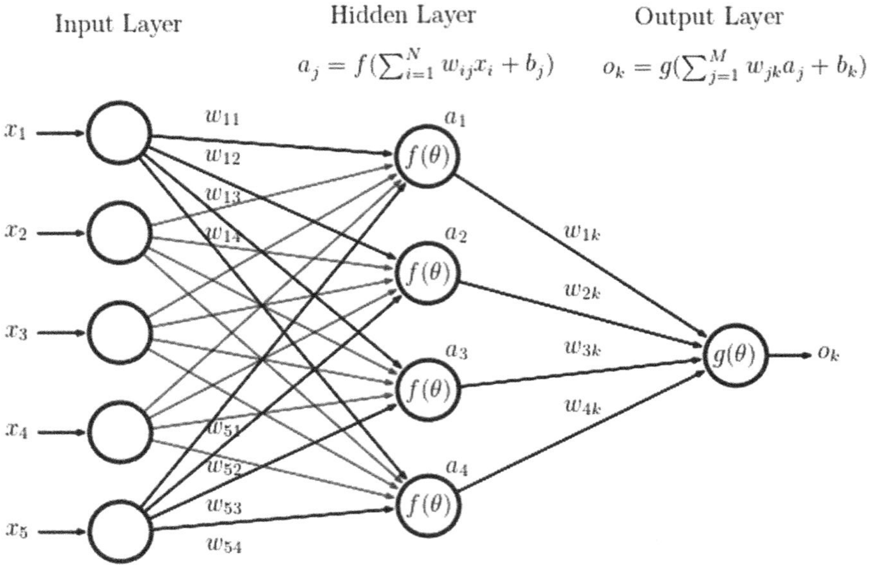

Fig. 16.5 A mathematical model of a *fully-connected* neural network (*Source* [23])

		Predicted Class		
		Positive	**Negative**	
Actual Class	**Positive**	True Positive (TP)	False Negative (FN) Type II Error	**Sensitivity** $\frac{TP}{(TP+FN)}$
	Negative	False Positive (FP) Type I Error	True Negative (TN)	**Specificity** $\frac{TN}{(TN+FP)}$
		Precision $\frac{TP}{(TP+FP)}$	**Negative Predictive Value** $\frac{TN}{(TN+FN)}$	**Accuracy** $\frac{TP+TN}{(TP+TN+FP+FN)}$

Fig. 16.6 A confusion matrix showing the calculation of performance metrics of a model (*Source* [49])

evaluation of these system parameters, the following four attributes are used in the measurement :

1. True Positive (TP): Cases with the abnormality, that are correctly predicted.
2. True Negative (TN): Cases without the abnormality, that are correctly predicted.
3. False Positive (FP): Cases with the abnormality, that are incorrectly predicted.
4. False Negative (FN): Cases without the abnormality, that are incorrectly predicted.

Accuracy can be defined as the measurement of actual classification. It is the percentage of correctness of the measurement value. It can be said that, with changing methods and different data sets, different accuracy level is achieved. The accuracy is defined by Eq. (16.5), as follows:

$$Accuracy = \frac{TP + TN}{TP + TN + FP + FN} \tag{16.5}$$

Sensitivity of the test can be defined as the test's ability to designate an individual actually suffering from the abnormality, as positive. The value of sensitivity is inversely proportional to the number of false negative results. Sensitivity, also known as Recall, gives the measure of correct results [4]. The sensitivity is defined by Eq. (16.6), as follows:

$$Sensitivity(or\ Recall) = \frac{TP}{TP + FN} \tag{16.6}$$

Specificity of the test is its ability to designate an individual actually not suffering from the abnormality, as negative. The value of specificity is inversely proportional to the number of false positive results. The specificity is defined by Equ. (16.7), as follows:

$$Specificity = \frac{TN}{FP + TN} \tag{16.7}$$

Precision of the test is a measurement of correct classified instances among the ones classified as positive. By viewing and analysing the scan results, possible negative and positive cases can be predicted. Now, the success rate of this prediction is termed as Precision. It is defined by Eq. (16.8), as follows:

$$Precision = \frac{TP}{TP + FP} \tag{16.8}$$

F1 Score is a quantity which captures both precision and recall values, and combines them in a single property. From precision and recall values, average result for balancing is calculated from Eq. (16.9), as follows:

$$F1\ Score = 2 \times \frac{Precision \times Recall}{Precision + Recall} \tag{16.9}$$

These are some terms that plays vital role when the whole process becomes automated. These terms define performance quantification and the whole detection process relies on these.

16.4 Proposed Method

The methodology used in this study is designed keeping in mind the overall objective of the task at hand. Since we are interested in classifying two of the most common brain tumor types, i.e., Meningioma and Glioma, the imaging process must perform a comprehensive evaluation task by differentiating different abnormal tissue cells in the brain. Successful evaluation of the tissue types and the actual classification of the type of brain tumor are critical in making clinical decisions regarding successive treatment strategies and surgeries [55]. Since conventional imaging of a patient's brain using MRI scans is often not adequate to perform an absolutely accurate evaluation owing to a myriad of features that has to be taken into account for a successful assessment, automated DL tools are becoming more popular in medical diagnostic processes. Invasive procedures like biopsy, where the risks outweights the benefits are increasingly being replaced by DL medical diagnostic practices. Classification of brain tumors using DL practises will also be a much safer option instead of performing a histological examination on the brain tissues.

This work aims to automatically classify two types of brain tumors from MRI scans, namely Meningioma and Glioma. It uses supervised ML techniques to train the CNN model.

16.4.1 Proposed Model Architecture

A block diagram representing the functioning of the proposed model for classifying brain tumors, is demonstrated in Fig. 16.7. The CNN based classification model works in two phases, that is training and testing. At first, all the images are resized to 128×128 pixels as the images present in the dataset are of different sizes. In the training phase, a histogram equalization based pre-processing transformation function is performed on the images. The transformed images are fed to the CNN based proposed architecture, represented as a black-box. Features are automatically extracted from the images and are then used for training. After training was completed in each of the 10 folds, testing of the performance of the model is conducted. In the testing phase, the images to be tested are fed to the CNN based classification model. The model would calculate a prediction based on these test images. The prediction is now tallied with the ground truth (GT). If the prediction matches with the GT, the prediction is said to be true. Else, the prediction is said to be false. Performance metrics of a classification model such as accuracy, sensitivity, specificity and F1 scores are calculated from the correctness of the test predictions.

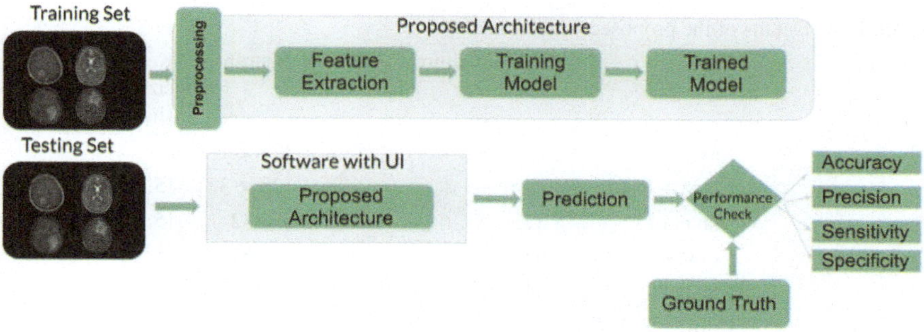

Fig. 16.7 Block Diagram of the proposed model

The proposed architecture which actually does the classification task, is a 13-layer CNN based DL algorithm. It is able to classify brain tumor MRI images as either Meningioma or Glioma. The proposed CNN architecture is constructed using convolutional, maxpool, and fully-connected layer. Five convolution layers with ReLU activation function and five max-pool layers are used alternatingly to each other. The convolution layers extract the special features from an image. The ReLU function discards the negative value of the images. The resultant feature maps are passed to the maxpool layers, which decrease the dimension size, and hence complexity of the images. The strides of the kernels in the convolution layers and the maxpool layers are taken as 1. The details about the kernel sizes, number of neurons and feature maps in each of the 13 layers, are given in Table 16.2. A detailed diagram of the architecture is given in Fig. 16.8.

16.4.2 Modelling the Classification Task

The brain tumor positive/negative binary classification task is generalized as a multi-class classification task, where every image could be classified into one of C classes. This is done so that the current binary classification task (to classify two types of brain tumor) could be extrapolated to a multi-class classification task (to classify more than two types of brain tumors) in the future with minimum amount of changes in the current algorithm. The CNN has C neurons in the final layer, each of them generating a score that can be represented as a vector, s. Meanwhile, the target vector or the ground truth vector, t is considered to be an one-hot vector. A softmax activation function is applied to the output scores, which squashes the vector s in the range $(0, 1)$. The softmax activation function of a given class can be computed as per Eq. (16.10), where s_j are the scores deduced for each class in C.

$$f(s_i) = \frac{e^{s_i}}{\sum_j^C e^{s_j}} \tag{16.10}$$

Table 16.2 Details of the proposed CNN model

Layers	Type	No. of feature maps	No. of Neurons	Kernel size/activation shape
0	Input	1	128 × 128 × 1	–
1	Conv. + ReLU	32	128 × 128 × 32	[5, 5, 32]
2	Maxpool	32	26 × 26 × 32	[5, 5, 32]
3	Conv. + ReLU	64	26 × 26 × 64	[5, 5]
4	Maxpool	64	6 × 6 × 64	[5, 5]
5	Conv. + ReLU	64	6 × 6 × 64	[5, 5]
6	Maxpool	64	2 × 2 × 64	[5, 5]
7	Conv. + ReLU	64	2 × 2 × 64	[5, 5]
8	Maxpool	64	1 × 1 × 64	[5, 5]
9	Conv. + ReLU	32	1 × 1 × 32	[5, 5, 32]
10	Maxpool	32	1 × 1 × 32	[5, 5, 32]
11	FC + ReLU	–	1024	–
12	FC + ReLU	–	128	–
13	FC + Softmax	–	2	–

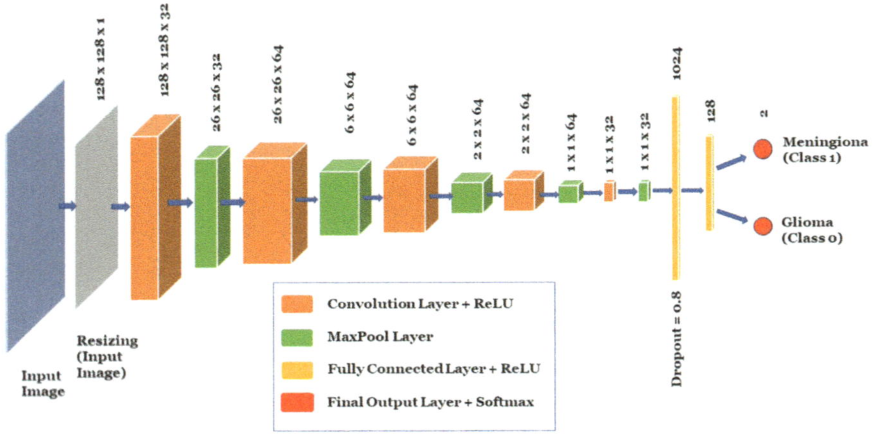

Fig. 16.8 Proposed CNN Architecture for the classification of Meningioma (Class-1) and Glioma (Class-0)

While training the CNN model, a cross-entropy loss is applied to the output of the softmax activation function as shown in Fig. 16.9. The combination of softmax activation plus a cross-entropy loss is known as categorical cross-entropy loss, and is used for multi class classification [14].

In this specific classification problem, the labels are considered to be one-hot encoded. This is done so that the expression for loss also takes into account the term

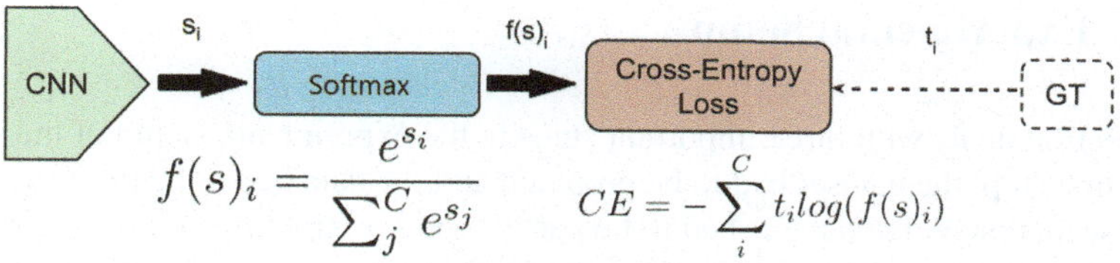

Fig. 16.9 Computation of categorical cross-entropy loss, for multi-class classification

due to the positive class C_p. Considering this, the final expression for cross-entropy loss can be written as per Eq. (16.11), where s_p is the positive class score.

$$CE = -\ log \frac{e^{s_p}}{\sum_j^C e^{s_j}} \tag{16.11}$$

After defining the loss, its gradient with respect to each CNN class score in s is calculated. This is used in the backpropagation algorithm. The defined loss function is optimized by tuning the network hyper-parameters. The derivative with respect to the positive class can be obtained as per Eq. (16.12), and the same with respect to the other (negative) classes can be obtained as per Eq. (16.13), where s_n is the negative class score.

$$\frac{\partial}{\partial s_p}[-\ log \frac{e^{s_p}}{\sum_j^C e^{s_j}}] = \frac{e^{s_p}}{\sum_j^C e^{s_j}} - 1 \tag{16.12}$$

$$\frac{\partial}{\partial s_n}[-\ log \frac{e^{s_p}}{\sum_j^C e^{s_j}}] = \frac{e^{s_n}}{\sum_j^C e^{s_j}} \tag{16.13}$$

The proposed CNN model is trained using back propagation with categorical cross-entropy loss calculated over mini-batch size of 32 for 50 epochs. In the forward pass, the error is calculated and in the backward pass, the weights are adjusted by finding the error contribution for each parameter. The learning parameters of the CNN architecture are optimized using the default setting of Adam optimizer, with learning rate, $\alpha = 0.001$, exponential decay rates for first moment estimate, $\beta_1 = 0.9$, exponential decay rates for second moment estimate, $\beta_2 = 0.999$, and epsilon, $\epsilon = 10^{-8}$. The optimizer, Adam, estimates the adaptive learning rate based on momentum. Implementation of this optimizer is widespread among the DL research groups. Based on the probability scores, the trained model classifies brain tumor images into either of the two classes, Class-1 (Meningioma) or Class-0 (Glioma). This model is developed and built in TensorFlow framework of Python using its TFLearn library.

16.5 Experimental Setup

This section deals with three important steps in the experimental setup of the study. In the first step, the dataset had to be prepared and the data had to be pre-processed. In the second step, the dataset had to be partitioned into training and testing sets. In the final step, the model had to be trained with the training sets and validation of the model was performed using testing sets.

16.5.1 Dataset Preparation and Pre-processing

For developing the model, T1-weighed MRI images were downloaded from "brain tumor dataset", available at Cheng's Figshare repository [8]. The dataset was presented at [9] and is used for the current research. These MRI images were collected between 2005 and 2010 from two well-known hospitals of China. It consists of a total number of 3064 T1-weighted axial, sagittal and coronal plane MRIs from 233 patients distributed in four folders. The MRI scans are of patients suffering from three different kinds of brain tumor; namely Meningioma (consisting of 708 images), Glioma (consisting of 1426 images) and Pituitary tumor (consisting of 930 images). The images are provided along with their labels, masks and patient IDs, in a data file (with *.mat* extension).

The T1-weighted MRI images of the dataset were saved in *.mat* format. The images were converted to *.jpg* format, so that they can be analysed. As shown in Fig. 16.10, these images are very hard to be distinguished by an ordinary person through naked eyes. Therefore, one of the primary objective as a pre-processing task should be to improve the graphic features of an image through contrast enhancement [28]. This pre-processing step has been used in many biomedical imaging applications [10, 26, 27, 29, 42]. In our present study, the dataset consists of low-contrast T1-weighted MRI images. Since the tumors are not visible, feature extraction would

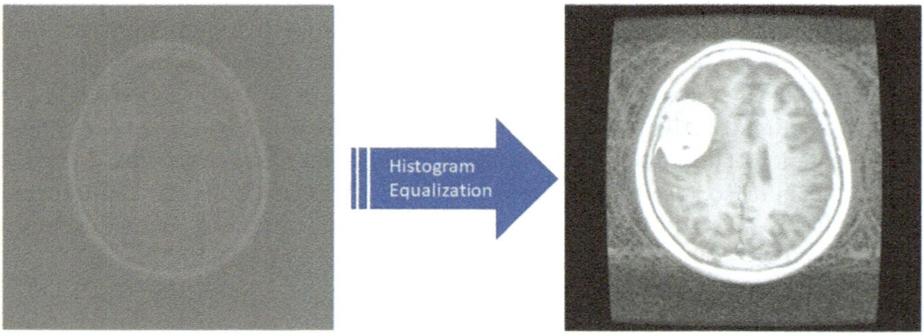

Fig. 16.10 Applying histogram equalization transformation function on the original T1-weighted MRI images to improve clarity

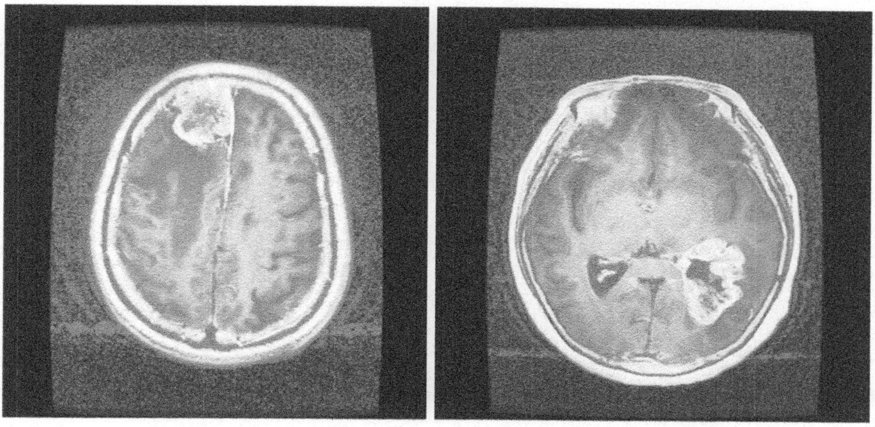

(a) (b)

Fig. 16.11 Two pre-processed T1 weighted MRI images showing **a** Meningioma, and **b** Glioma

be error prone. Therefore, discrete histogram equilization transformation function as given by Eqs. (16.15, 16.16) was performed as a necessary pre-processing tool to improve the contrast of these images, resulting in their enhanced clarity.

If the probability of occurence of a particular gray level in an image is approximated by Eq. (16.14), the discrete histogram transformation function is given by Eqs. (16.15, 16.16). It is accomplished by spreading out the intensity values which are more frequent, i.e. stretching out the intensity range of the image. Two pre-processed MRI images of the brain affected by Meningioma and Glioma, are shown in Fig. 16.11.

$$p_r(r_k) = \frac{n_k}{n} \quad where\ k = 0, 1, ..., L-1 \tag{16.14}$$

$$s_k = T(r_k) = (L-1)\sum_{j=0}^{k} p_r(r_j) \tag{16.15}$$

$$= (L-1)\sum_{j=0}^{k} \frac{n_j}{n} \quad where\ k = 0, 1, ..., L-1 \tag{16.16}$$

16.5.2 Data Partitioning

To develop and demonstrate the effectiveness of any deep learning algorithm, the given data (images) are partitioned into training and testing datasets. The partition is done randomly in a certain ratio, to negate any possible sampling bias. The training

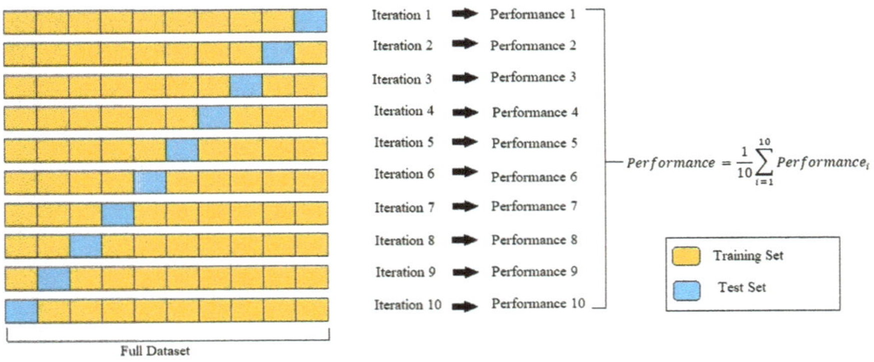

Fig. 16.12 Train/Test split in 10-fold Cross validation

dataset is used to train the model, while the testing dataset is used for testing the effectiveness of the trained model in the presence of unseen data of a similar kind.

A total of 257 (119 Melingioma and 138 Glioma) axial MRI slides from [8] were selected to train, test, and analyse the classification accuracy of the model. The proposed model was validated using a 10-fold cross-validation method, since it is the standard procedure in most of the medical image analysis researches. As demonstrated in Fig. 16.12, the training dataset was partitioned into 10 equal subsets, with 25 images in each of them. Among these 10 subsets, one of them was retained as a test set and rest of the nine subsets were used to train the model. This method was iterated for 10 times with the test subset being substituted for a new subset after each iteration and rest of the subsets being used for training the model. This ensures that the entire dataset is used for both training and testing, and each of the images is used once for testing. After 10 iterations, the results were averaged to get an exhaustive analysis of the model.

16.5.3 Training and Testing

The model was simulated in a laptop manufactured by Lenovo with a CPU of Intel Core i5-8250U @ 1.60 GHz, and having 8 GB RAM as primary memory. The prediction model took almost 12 min to be built in each of the folds.

The model was trained using many alterable hyperparameters which were already discussed. A list of all the trainable hyperparameters which produced the highest performance metrics, are summarised below:

- **Optimizer**: Adam
- **Epochs**: 50
- **Batch Size**: 32

16.6 Results, Analysis and Discussions

The system performance metrics were calculated for the model, considering the classification of Meningioma as the abnormality to be detected. In other words, Meningioma has been considered as Class-1 or positive. On the other hand, Glioma has been considered as Class-0 or negative. The proposed system gives the average validation accuracy of 1.0 (or 100%) after performing 10-fold cross validation. This optimal performance of the proposed CNN Architecture is obtained after the completion of 50 epochs. A table showing all the system parameters in each fold of a 10-fold cross-validation process as obtained from the confusion matrix for the architecture is shown in Table 16.3.

In any predictive model design based on neural network architecture, obtaining the highest training accuracy should not be the aim, rather obtaining higher validation accuracy (obtained from test data set) should be the conclusive objective. In the proposed architecture, the training accuracy increases more or less with every iteration as the weights get updated by the training data set, but when the network keeps getting more trained, it might causes overfitting, i.e., fails to predict generalized test cases. The model has been trained for 50 epochs, as it has been found that the model does not overfit in this range. The variation of validation accuracy and validation loss with epochs, for Fold 1, is illustrated in Fig. 16.13. It can be observed from the graph that the validation accuracy saturates to 100% after epoch 9, for Fold 1. Consequently, as given by Fig. 16.14, the confusion matrix obtained in Fold 1 shows that both the types of tumor, that is Meningioma (Class-1) and Glioma (Class-0) have been correctly detected for all the test images.

Table 16.3 System performance metrics calculated for the classification of Meningioma (Class-1) for the proposed architecture from the confusion matrix

Fold No.	TP	FP	TN	FN	Accuracy	Sensitivity/ Recall	Specificity	Precision	F1 Score
1	8	0	17	0	1.000	1.000	1.000	1.000	1.000
2	13	0	12	0	1.000	1.000	1.000	1.000	1.000
3	11	0	14	0	1.000	1.000	1.000	1.000	1.000
4	14	0	11	0	1.000	1.000	1.000	1.000	1.000
5	12	0	13	0	1.000	1.000	1.000	1.000	1.000
6	15	0	10	0	1.000	1.000	1.000	1.000	1.000
7	10	0	15	0	1.000	1.000	1.000	1.000	1.000
8	13	0	12	0	1.000	1.000	1.000	1.000	1.000
9	11	0	14	0	1.000	1.000	1.000	1.000	1.000
10	11	0	14	0	1.000	1.000	1.000	1.000	1.000
Average					1.000	1.000	1.000	1.000	1.000

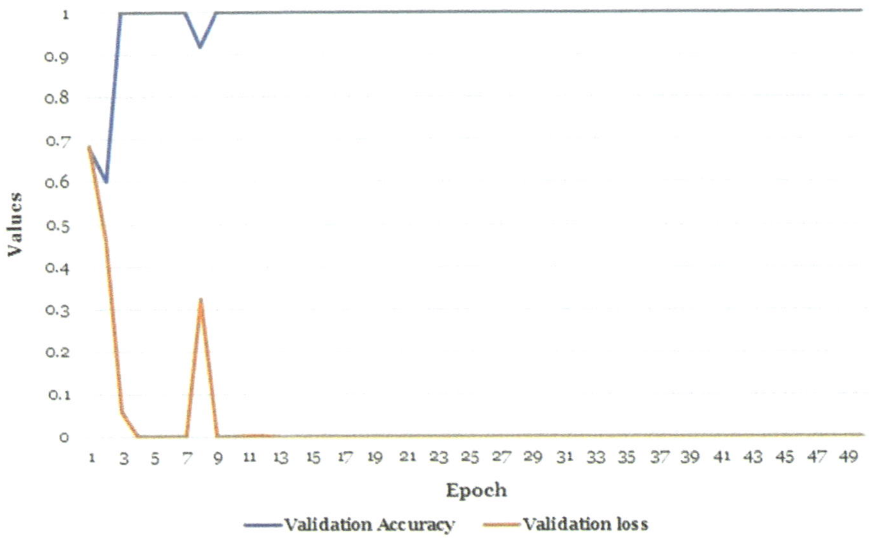

Fig. 16.13 Variation of validation accuracy and validation loss with epochs, in Fold 1

Fig. 16.14 Confusion Matrix obtained in Fold 1

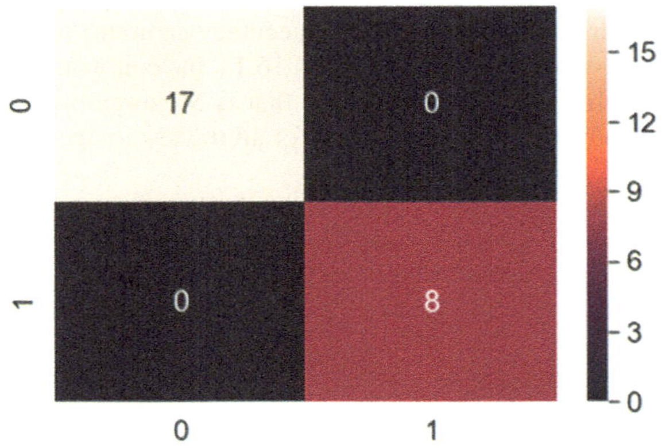

The proposed model gives the net accuracy of the classification task as 1.0. Also, the accuracies obtained for each of the folds are 1.0. This might seem unusually optimistic at first, but it only reinforces the fact that with the right selection of hyperparameters, and the right selection of the number of layers and filters in each layers for a dedicated DL based classification task, it is possible to obtain the highest possible performance metrics.

16.6.1 Comparison with Existing Works

In all of the literature surveyed in Sect. 16.2, different approaches have been tested on a diverse set of medical databases of brain tumors. To perform a comparative analysis of the proposed model with other similar representative studies, only those papers which used the same MRI image dataset (Cheng's "brain tumor dataset") that was used in the current study, were considered. The comparison is shown in Table 16.4. The accuracy obtained in the prposed model has been compared with these literatures, and has been represented graphically in Fig. 16.15. Most of the existing works on the same dataset were performed for a 3-class classification task (classifying Meningioma or Glioma or Pituitary Tumor). Meanwhile, the pituitary tumor cases are the most easy ones to classify since they occur only in the pituitary gland. On the other hand, the classification of Meningioma and Glioma is difficult. Kaldera et al. [24] developed a model to classify Meningioma and Glioma, taking into account a total of 257 axial MRIs (119 Meningioma and 138 Glioma), and had obtained a net accuracy of 94.6%. We have also trained the proposed model discussed in this study, with a similar number of axial MRIs for Meningioma and Glioma cases, to benchmark this classification model with that of [24]. This is by far and ever, the

Table 16.4 A comparative analysis of performance of the proposed model with other studies performed on Cheng's "brain tumor dataset"

Author	Year	No. of images used	Method	Task	Performance
Bhanothu et al. [5]	2020	Entire dataset (3064 images: 708 Meningioma, 1426 Glioma, 930 Pituitary tumor)	VGG16	Classification: Meningioma/ Glioma/ Pituitary Tumor	Precison : 77.60%
Kaplan et al. [25]	2020		KNN		Accuracy : 95.56%
Rehman et al. [43]	2020		VGG16		Accuracy : 98.69
Sarhan et al. [44]	2020		WCNN		Accuracy : 99.30%
Tahir et al. [50]	2019		SVM		Accuracy : 86.00%
Ismael et al. [22]	2019		ResNet50		Accuracy : 99.00% Precision : 99.00% Recall : 99.00% F1- Score : 99.00%
N. Abiwinanda et al. [1]	2018		CNN		Accuracy : 90.89%
Parian Afshar et al. [2]	2018		Capsnets		Accuracy : 90.89%
Abdel-Quader et al. [21]	2018		ANN		Accuracy : 91.90%
A. Pashaei et al. [36]	2018		KELM+CNN		Accuracy: 93.68%
J. Paul et al. [37]	2017		CNN		Accuracy : 91.43%
Cheng et al. [9]	2015		SVM (BoW)		Accuracy : 91.28%
Kaldera et al. [24]	**2019**	**257 axial images (119 Meningioma, 138 Glioma)**	**CNN**	**Classification: Meningioma/ Glioma**	**Accuracy (Glioma) : 87.50%** **Accuracy (Meningioma) : 94.00%** **Accuracy (Net) : 94.60%**
Proposed model	**2020**		**Proposed method**		**Accuracy : 100%** **Precison : 100%** **F1 Score : 100%** **Sensitivity : 100%**

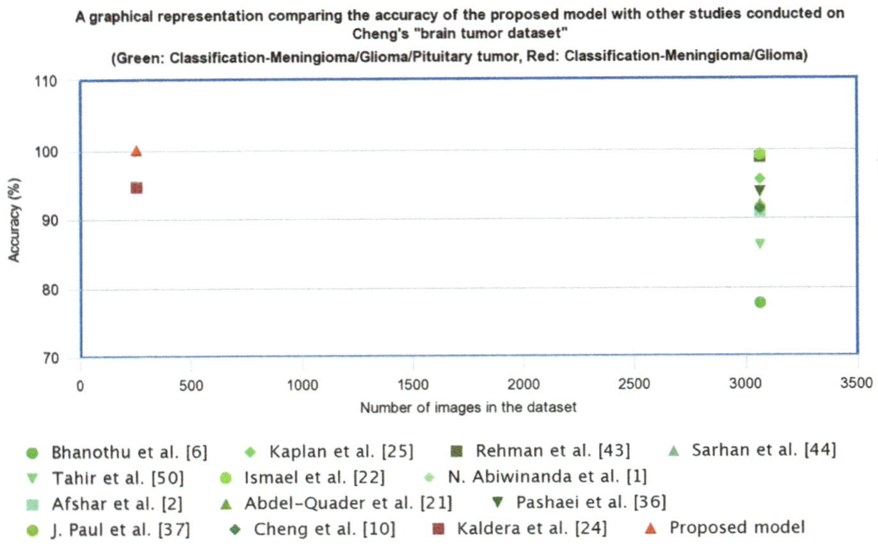

Fig. 16.15 A graphical representation comparing the accuracy of the proposed model with other studies conducted on Cheng's "brain tumor dataset"

best results that one can get for a classification model, that too by training a model with a fraction of images of the entire dataset.

The designed CNN model is simpler than existing architectures that employs pre-trained neural networks. Since, the proposed model requires much less resources for both training and testing, it can be easily deployed in an ordinary personal computer or mobile platform. This would significantly aid in diagnosis in most developing countries where optimal utilization of resources is the key for testing.

16.7 Conclusion

A novel DL model utilising a CNN was implemented in the proposed study to classify two types of brain tumor from MRI scans, namely Meningioma and Glioma. The problem was designed as a binary classification task. This custom-designed DL model gives the average validation accuracy of 100% after performing 10-fold cross validation. It also gives an average sensitivity of 100%, specificity of 100%, precision of 100% and F1 Score of 100%. This is by far, the best results that has been obtained on a binary classification task on two types of brain tumor namely, Meningioma and Glioma, benchmarked against Cheng's brain tumor dataset. The performance metrics obtained for the binary classification task is also significantly higher compared to other studies which performed a ternary classification task (classifying Meningioma or Glioma or Pituitary tumor) on the same dataset. Since the number of MRI images used to train the network is pretty low (119 axial Meningioma MRIs and 138 axial Glioma MRIs), it can be said that the impressive performance metrics obtained only shows the novelty involved in designing the CNN architecture to specifically classify two types of brain tumors.

The proposed method can be further improved by segmenting and analysing the lesions related to every type brain tumors, which could help the system to localize as well as classify the severity of the disease. Also, in the proposed study, only axial MRI images were used for the classification task. Focus will be on developing a model which can work on every type of MRI images, namely axial, sagittal and temporal images. The algorithm used in the proposed model can be extended in the next stage towards segmentation of brain tumor, i.e., if a brain tumor is detected, the model would be able to localize the affected area. It would assist the operators using MRI machines for deciding the orientation and coverage area of the scan. This could further aid physicians in detecting and analysing brain tumors.

References

1. Abiwinanda, N., Hanif, M., Hesaputra, S.T., Handayani, A., Mengko, T.R.: Brain tumor classification using convolutional neural network. In: World Congress on Medical Physics and Biomedical Engineering, pp. 183–189. Springer (2019)
2. Afshar, P., Plataniotis, K.N., Mohammadi, A.: Capsule networks for brain tumor classification based on mri images and coarse tumor boundaries. In: ICASSP 2019-2019 IEEE International Conference on Acoustics, Speech and Signal Processing (ICASSP), pp. 1368–1372. IEEE (2019)
3. Badža, M.M., Barjaktarović, M.Č.: Classification of brain tumors from mri images using a convolutional neural network. Appl. Sci. **10**(6), 1999 (2020)
4. Baratloo, A., Hosseini, M., Negida, A., El Ashal, G.: Part 1: Simple definition and calculation of accuracy, sensitivity and specificity. In: Archives Of Academic Emergency Medicine (Emergency). vol. 3, pp. 48–49. Shahid Beheshti University of Medical Sciences, Tehran (2015). https://www.sid.ir/en/journal/ViewPaper.aspx?id=438756. Accessed 11 July 2020
5. Bhanothu, Y., Kamalakannan, A., Rajamanickam, G.: Detection and classification of brain tumor in MRI images using deep convolutional network. In: 2020 6th International Conference on Advanced Computing and Communication Systems (ICACCS), pp. 248–252. IEEE (2020)
6. Bini, S.A.: Artificial intelligence, machine learning, deep learning, and cognitive computing: what do these terms mean and how will they impact health care? J. Arthroplasty **33**(8), 2358–2361 (2018)
7. Cha, S., Yang, L., Johnson, G., Lai, A., Chen, M.H., Tihan, T., Wendland, M., Dillon, W.: Comparison of microvascular permeability measurements, ktrans, determined with conventional steady-state t1-weighted and first-pass t2*-weighted MR imaging methods in gliomas and meningiomas. Amer. J. Neuroradiol. **27**(2), 409–417 (2006)
8. Cheng, J.: brain tumor dataset. https://figshare.com/articles/brain_tumor_dataset/1512427/5 (2017). Accessed 11 July 2020
9. Cheng, J., Huang, W., Cao, S., Yang, R., Yang, W., Yun, Z., Wang, Z., Feng, Q.: Enhanced performance of brain tumor classification via tumor region augmentation and partition. PloS One **10**(10) (2015)
10. Chouhan, V., Singh, S.K., Khamparia, A., Gupta, D., Tiwari, P., Moreira, C., Damaševičius, R., De Albuquerque, V.H.C.: A novel transfer learning based approach for pneumonia detection in chest x-ray images. Appl. Sci. **10**(2), 559 (2020)

11. Cicchetti, D.: Neural networks and diagnosis in the clinical laboratory: state of the art. Clin. Chem. **38**(1), 9–10 (1992)
12. Damodharan, S., Raghavan, D.: Combining tissue segmentation and neural network for brain tumor detection. Int. Arab J. Inform. Technol. (IAJIT) **12**(1) (2015)
13. DeAngelis, L.M.: Brain tumors. New England J. Med. **344**(2), 114–123 (2001)
14. Gomez, R.: Understanding categorical cross-entropy loss, binary cross-entropy loss, softmax loss, logistic loss, focal loss and all those confusing names. https://gombru.github.io/2018/05/23/cross_entropy_loss. Accessed 20 July 2020
15. Gomez, R.: BRATS-SICAS Medical Image Repository. https://www.smir.ch/BRATS/Start2015 (2015). Accessed 20 July 2020
16. Gonzalez, R.C., Woods, R.E.: Digital Image Processing. Prentice Hall, Upper Saddle River, N.J. (2008). http://www.amazon.com/Digital-Image-Processing-3rd-Edition/dp/013168728X
17. He, K., Zhang, X., Ren, S., Sun, J.: Deep residual learning for image recognition. In: Proceedings of the IEEE Conference on Computer Vision and Pattern Recognition, pp. 770–778 (2016)
18. Huettel, S.A., Song, A.W., McCarthy, G., et al.: Functional Magnetic Resonance Imaging, vol. 1. Sinauer Associates Sunderland, MA (2004)
19. Imgur.com: https://i.stack.imgur.com/6WbWu.png. Accessed 11 July 2020
20. IndoML.com: Convolutional Neural Networks (CNN) Introduction. https://indoml.com/2018/03/07/student-notes-convolutional-neural-networks-cnn-introduction/ (2018). Accessed 2 July 2020
21. Ismael, M.R., Abdel-Qader, I.: Brain tumor classification via statistical features and back-propagation neural network. In: 2018 IEEE international conference on electro/information technology (EIT), pp. 0252–0257. IEEE (2018)
22. Ismael, S.A.A., Mohammed, A., Hefny, H.: An enhanced deep learning approach for brain cancer MRI images classification using residual networks. Artif. Intell. Med. **102** (2020)
23. Ivezić, Ž., Connolly, A.J., VanderPlas, J.T., Gray, A.: Statistics, Data Mining, and Machine Learning in Astronomy: A Practical Python Guide for the Analysis of Survey Data. Updated Edition, Princeton University Press (2019). https://press.princeton.edu/books/hardcover/9780691198309/statistics-data-mining-and-machine-learning-in-astronomy. Accessed 11 July 2020
24. Kaldera, H., Gunasekara, S.R., Dissanayake, M.B.: Brain tumor classification and segmentation using faster r-cnn. In: 2019 Advances in Science and Engineering Technology International Conferences (ASET), pp. 1–6. IEEE (2019)
25. Kaplan, K., Kaya, Y., Kuncan, M., Ertunç, H.M.: Brain tumor classification using modified local binary patterns (lbp) feature extraction methods. Medical Hypotheses, p. 109696 (2020)
26. Ke, Q., Zhang, J., Wei, W., Połap, D., Woźniak, M., Kośmider, L., Damaševicius, R.: A neuro-heuristic approach for recognition of lung diseases from x-ray images. Expert Syst. Appli. **126**, 218–232 (2019)
27. Khan, M.A., Rubab, S., Kashif, A., Sharif, M.I., Muhammad, N., Shah, J.H., Zhang, Y.D., Satapathy, S.C.: Lungs cancer classification from CT images: An integrated design of contrast based classical features fusion and selection. Pattern Recogn. Lett. **129**, 77–85 (2020)
28. Khan, M.A., Ashraf, I., Alhaisoni, M., Damaševičius, R., Scherer, R., Rehman, A., Bukhari, S.A.C.: Multimodal brain tumor classification using deep learning and robust feature selection: a machine learning application for radiologists. Diagnostics **10**(8), 565 (2020)
29. Khan, M.A., Sharif, M., Akram, T., Bukhari, S.A.C., Nayak, R.S.: Developed newton-raphson based deep features selection framework for skin lesion recognition. Pattern Recogn. Lett. **129**, 293–303 (2020)
30. Khodamoradi, F., Ghoncheh, M., Pakzad, R., Gandomani, H., Salehiniya, H.: The incidence and mortality of brain and central nervous system cancer and their relationship with human development index in the world. World Cancer Res. J. **4**(4), 5 (2017)
31. Maclin, P.S., Dempsey, J., Brooks, J., Rand, J.: Using neural networks to diagnose cancer. J. Med. Syst. **15**(1), 11–19 (1991)

32. Mohsen, H., El-Dahshan, E.S.A., El-Horbaty, E.S.M., Salem, A.B.M.: Classification using deep learning neural networks for brain tumors. Future Comput. Inform. J. **3**(1), 68–71 (2018)
33. National Brain Tumor Society: Tumor types: Understanding brain tumors. https://braintumor.org/brain-tumor-information/understanding-brain-tumors/tumor-types. Accessed 20 July 2020
34. O'Shea, K., Nash, R.: An introduction to convolutional neural networks. arXiv preprint arXiv:1511.08458 (2015)
35. Özyurt, F., Sert, E., Avci, E., Dogantekin, E.: Brain tumor detection based on convolutional neural network with neutrosophic expert maximum fuzzy sure entropy. Measurement **147** (2019)
36. Pashaei, A., Sajedi, H., Jazayeri, N.: Brain tumor classification via convolutional neural network and extreme learning machines. In: 2018 8th International Conference On Computer and Knowledge Engineering (ICCKE), pp. 314–319. IEEE (2018)
37. Paul, J.S., Plassard, A.J., Landman, B.A., Fabbri, D.: Deep learning for brain tumor classification. In: Medical Imaging 2017: Biomedical Applications in Molecular, Structural, and Functional Imaging. vol. 10137, p. 1013710. International Society for Optics and Photonics (2017)
38. Pavan, M.S., Jagadeesh, P.: Brain tumor segmentation using covolutional neural network in MRI images. Int. J. Pure Appl. Math. **119**(17), 1585–1592 (2018)
39. Piper, R.J., Mikhael, S., Wardlaw, J.M., Laidlaw, D.H., Whittle, I.R., Bastin, M.E.: Imaging signatures of meningioma and low-grade Glioma: a diffusion tensor, magnetization transfer and quantitative longitudinal relaxation time MRI study. Magnetic Reson. Imaging **34**(4), 596–602 (2016)
40. Radiopaedia: https://radiopaedia.org. Accessed 20 July 2020
41. Rao, V., Sarabi, M.S., Jaiswal, A.: Brain tumor segmentation with deep learning. MICCAI Multimodal Brain Tumor Segmentation Challenge (BraTS), pp. 56–59 (2015)
42. Rehman, A., Khan, M.A., Mehmood, Z., Saba, T., Sardaraz, M., Rashid, M.: Microscopic melanoma detection and classification: a framework of pixel-based fusion and multilevel features reduction. Microscopy Res. Technique **83**(4), 410–423 (2020)
43. Rehman, A., Naz, S., Razzak, M.I., Akram, F., Imran, M.: A deep learning-based framework for automatic brain tumors classification using transfer learning. Circuits Syst. Signal Process. **39**(2), 757–775 (2020)
44. Sarhan, A.M., et al.: Brain tumor classification in magnetic resonance images using deep learning and wavelet transform. J. Biomed. Sci. Eng. **13**(06), 102 (2020)
45. Scarpace, L., Mikkelsen, L., Cha, T., Rao, S., Tekchandani, S., Gutman, S., Pierce, D.: Radiology data from the cancer genome atlas glioblastoma multiforme [tcga-gbm] collection. Cancer Imaging Arch. **11**(4), 1 (2016)
46. Seetha, J., Raja, S.S.: Brain tumor classification using convolutional neural networks. Biomed. Pharmacolo. J. **11**(3), 1457 (2018)
47. Simes, R.J.: Treatment selection for cancer patients: application of statistical decision theory to the treatment of advanced ovarian cancer. J. Chronic Diseases **38**(2), 171–186 (1985)
48. Singh, A., et al.: Detection of brain tumor in MRI images, using combination of fuzzy c-means and SVM. In: 2015 2nd International Conference on Signal Processing and Integrated Networks (SPIN), pp. 98–102. IEEE (2015)
49. Sirsat, M.: What is confusion matrix and advanced classification metrics? https://manisha-sirsat.blogspot.com/2019/04/confusion-matrix.html (2019). Accessed 11 July 2020
50. Tahir, B., Iqbal, S., Usman Ghani Khan, M., Saba, T., Mehmood, Z., Anjum, A., Mahmood, T.: Feature enhancement framework for brain tumor segmentation and classification. Microscopy Res. Technique **82**(6), 803–811 (2019)
51. Thai, L., Hai, T., Thuy, N.T.: Image classification using support vector machine and artificial neural network. Int. J. Inform. Technol. Comput. Sci. (IJITCS) **4**(5), 32–38 (2012)
52. Walker, A.E., Robins, M., Weinfeld, F.D.: Epidemiology of brain tumors: the national survey of intracranial neoplasms. Neurology **35**(2), 219–219 (1985)

53. Wen, P.Y., Kesari, S.: Malignant gliomas in adults. New England J. Med. **359**(5), 492–507 (2008)
54. Wu, M.N., Lin, C.C., Chang, C.C.: Brain tumor detection using color-based k-means clustering segmentation. In: Third International Conference on Intelligent Information Hiding and Multimedia Signal Processing (IIH-MSP 2007). vol. 2, pp. 245–250. IEEE (2007)
55. Zacharaki, E.I., Wang, S., Chawla, S., Soo Yoo, D., Wolf, R., Melhem, E.R., Davatzikos, C.: Classification of brain tumor type and grade using MRI texture and shape in a machine learning scheme. Magnetic Reson. Med.: Official J. Int. Soc. Magn. Reson. Med. **62**(6), 1609–1618 (2009)

The manufacturer's authorised representative in the EU is Springer Nature Customer Service Centre GmbH, Europaplatz 3, 69115 Heidelberg, Germany. If you have any concerns regarding our products, please contact ProductSafety@springernature.com

Printed and bound by CPI Group (UK) Ltd, Croydon, CR0 4YY
30/09/2026
02225294-0016